Biomarkers: Techniques, Methods and Applications

Biomarkers: Techniques, Methods and Applications

Edited by Gloria Rhodes

hayle
medical

New York

Hayle Medical,
750 Third Avenue, 9th Floor,
New York, NY 10017, USA

Visit us on the World Wide Web at:
www.haylemedical.com

ISBN: 978-1-63241-832-6

Cataloging-in-Publication Data

Biomarkers : techniques, methods and applications / edited by Gloria Rhodes.
p. cm.
Includes bibliographical references and index.
ISBN 978-1-63241-832-6
1. Biochemical markers. 2. Biochemistry. 3. Indicators (Biology). I. Rhodes, Gloria.
R853.B54 B56 2020
610.28--dc23

Table of Contents

Preface

The purpose of the book is to provide a glimpse into the dynamics and to present opinions and studies of some of the scientists engaged in the development of new ideas in the field from very different standpoints. This book will prove useful to students and researchers owing to its high content quality.

A biological marker or biomarker is an indicator of a biological condition. It is evaluated to examine pathogenic processes in the living system or observe normal biological processes or to understand the pharmacologic responses to a therapeutic intervention. Biomarkers are used in medicine to examine organ function or other aspects of human health or to determine a diagnosis of a disease state by testing for its presence or absence. A commonly used biomarker is prostate-specific antigen or PSA, which is used as an indicator of prostate cancer. Biomarkers are also used in personalized medicine for prognostic and predictive purposes. Prognostic biomarkers indicate patient outcome regardless of a specific treatment, while predictive biomarkers help to optimize treatments and increase the chances of benefitting from a therapy. This book unravels the recent studies in the field of biomarkers. It elucidates new techniques and applications of biological markers in a multidisciplinary manner. Coherent flow of topics, student-friendly language and extensive use of examples make this book an invaluable source of knowledge.

At the end, I would like to appreciate all the efforts made by the authors in completing their chapters professionally. I express my deepest gratitude to all of them for contributing to this book by sharing their valuable works. A special thanks to my family and friends for their constant support in this journey.

Editor

1

Higher plasma prorenin concentration plays a role in the development of coronary artery disease

Gakuro Yoshida[1], Masanori Kawasaki[2*], Ichijiro Murata[1], Yuka Hayakawa[2], Takuma Aoyama[2], Nagisa Miyazaki[1], Yoshihisa Yamada[2], Kazuhiko Nishigaki[2], Yoshie Arai[3], Fumiaki Suzuki[3] and Shinya Minatoguchi[2]

Abstract

Background: Prorenin and renin are both involved in atherosclerosis. However, the role of plasma prorenin and renin in the development and progression of coronary artery disease (CAD) is still not clear. Thus, we aimed to examine the relationships among plasma prorenin concentration, CAD and clinical parameters.

Methods: We measured plasma prorenin and renin concentrations and other parameters in 85 patients who underwent coronary angiography. Patients were divided into a CAD group (≥75 % stenosis in one or more coronary arteries) and a non-CAD group.

Results: There was a weak correlation between prorenin and plasma renin concentration (r =0.35, p =0.001), and plasma renin activity (r =0.34, p =0.001). There was no significant difference in the plasma prorenin concentration between the CAD group and non-CAD group. However, patients with a high plasma prorenin concentration frequently suffered CAD. Receiver-operating-characteristic curve analysis showed that the optimal cutoff value of plasma prorenin concentration to detect CAD was 1,100 pg/ml, with a positive predictive value of 94 % and a negative predictive value of 36 %.

Conclusion: The plasma prorenin concentration increases with increases in plasma renin concentration. Higher plasma prorenin concentration (>1,100 pg/ml) plays a role in the development of CAD.

Keywords: Prorenin, Renin, Coronary artery disease

Introduction

The renin-angiotensin system is a key regulator of the cardiovascular system. The principal effector hormone of the classic renin-angiotensin system is angiotensin II. The conversion of angiotensinogen to angiotensin I by renin is the rate limiting step in the synthesis of renin-angiotensin II. Chronic activation of renin-angiotensin system is a major contributing factor to the pathogenesis and progression of cardiovascular disease. In fact, higher plasma renin activity (PRA) was reported to be associated with an increased risk of myocardial infarction in the patients with hypertension [1]. Furthermore, another recent study demonstrated that high PRA was associated with an increased cardiac morbidity and mortality in patients with coronary artery disease (CAD) [2].

For many years, prorenin was considered to be an inactive precursor of renin. However, since the discovery of (pro)renin receptors, prorenin is now regarded as an important regulator of the renin-angiotensin system. Both prorenin and renin bind to (pro)renin receptors, and stimulation of (pro)renin receptors has been reported to be involved in the development of diabetic nephropathy [3] cardiac injury [4] and vascular damage [5]. Prorenin is released constitutively from the kidney, and its blood plasma levels are approximately 10-fold higher than those of renin. Chronic stimulation of the renin-angiotensin system usually increases renal prorenin-renin conversion, thereby decreasing the relative amount of prorenin in the circulation [6]. Furthermore, plasma prorenin concentration is markedly increased in diabetes mellitus patients

* Correspondence: masanori@ya2.so-net.ne.jp
[2]Department of Cardiology, Gifu University Graduate School of Medicine, Yanagido 1-1, Gifu 501-1194, Japan

with complications [7]. However, the plasma prorenin concentration and its pathophysiological role in patients with CAD are not clear. Therefore, in the present study, we aimed to examine the relationships among plasma prorenin concentration, CAD and clinical parameters.

Methods

Study patients

We initially enrolled 100 consecutive patients with chest pain and/or chest discomfort who underwent elective coronary angiography for suspicion of CAD. We excluded subjects with unstable angina or myocardial infarction within the previous three months and severe heart failure (NYHA class IV and/or a left ventricular ejection fraction ≤ 30 %). The final study population consisted of 85 patients who underwent coronary angiography. Patients were diagnosed with CAD when one or more of their coronary arteries had a stenosis ≥75 %. According to the angiographical diagnosis, patients were divided into two groups (CAD group or non-CAD group). Risk factors for CAD were evaluated in enrolled patients, including hypertension (HTN) (medication-dependent or systolic BP ≥140 and/or diastolic BP ≥90 mmHg), type 2 diabetes mellitus (DM) (medication-dependent or hemoglobin (Hb) A1c ≥ 6.5 %) and dyslipidemia (medication-dependent, LDL cholesterol ≥140 mg/dl and/or HDL cholesterol <40 mg/dl). The protocol was approved by the ethics committee of Gifu University Graduate School of Medicine. All of the patients gave informed consent before the start of study. The investigation conformed with the principles outlined in the Declaration of Helsinki (Br Med J 1964; ii:177).

Hemodynamic parameters

Blood pressure and pulse rate were measured. Left ventricular ejection fraction (LVEF) left ventricular end-diastolic dimension (LVEDd) and left ventricular end-systolic dimension (LVESd) were obtained by echocardiography. Echocardiographic measurements were used to calculate LVEF based on a disk summation method using the apical 2- and 4-chamber views.

Measurements of plasma prorenin and renin concentration

Blood samples were obtained from the antecubital vein in the morning while the patients were in a fasting state on the day of cardiac catheterization. The samples were collected into sterile tubes, immediately placed on ice, centrifuged at 3,000 x g for 10 min at 4 °C, and rapidly frozen and stored at −80 °C until analysis. Plasma prorenin concentrations were measured using an ELISA kit (LINCO Research Inc., St. Charles, MO, USA). Plasma renin concentrations were also measured using an ELISA kit (LINCO Research Inc., St. Charles, MO, USA). Plasma brain natriuretic peptide (BNP) levels were measured by immunoradiometric assay (Shionoria BNP RIA kit; Shionogi, Osaka, Japan). We also measured hemoglobin A1c (HbA1c), total cholesterol, LDL-cholesterol, HDL-cholesterol and estimated glomerular filtration rate (eGFR).

Statistical analysis

The data are shown as the mean ± one standard deviation. Categorical data were summarized as percentages and compared with a chi-square test or Fisher's exact test. The normality of data distributions was tested using the Kolmogorov-Smirnov test. The significance of the differences between groups for variables that were normally distributed and had similar variances was determined by an unpaired Student's t test. Otherwise, a Mann–Whitney U test was used to compare the differences between groups. Linear regression analysis was performed to examine the correlations between plasma prorenin concentration and other parameters. A p value <0.05 was considered significant. All statistical analyses were performed using Stat View version 5.0 (SAS Institution Inc, Cary, NC, USA).

Results

Patient's characteristics

Patient characteristics are shown in Table 1. The patients were taking oral angiotensin-converting enzyme inhibitors (ACEIs) or angiotensin II receptor blockers (ARBs) (n =24), calcium channel blockers (n =30), beta-blockers (n =12), or diuretics (n =9). There were no significant differences between the two groups in history of hypertension, current smoking or concomitant medication use. However, history of DM, history of dyslipidemia and age were significantly greater in the CAD group than in the non-CAD group.

Hemodynamic parameters

As shown in Table 2, there were no significant differences in heart rate, systolic blood pressure, diastolic blood pressure or LVEDd between the CAD group and the non-CAD group. The LVEF was significantly greater in the non-CAD group than in the CAD group.

Plasma prorenin concentration and plasma renin concentration

There was a weak correlation between the plasma prorenin concentration and plasma renin concentration (r =0.35, p =0.001), and plasma renin activity (r =0.34, p =0.001) (Fig. 1). However, there was no correlation between the plasma prorenin concentration and aldosterone (p =0.15), BNP (p =0.17) or eGFR (p =0.16) (Fig. 1). The LVEF was not correlated with the plasma prorenin concentration (p =0.83).

Table 1 Patient clinical characteristics and echocardiographic parameters

	Non-CAD group (n = 26)	CAD group (n = 59)	p-value
Clinical characteristics			
Men (%)	20 (76.9)	39 (66.1)	0.27
Age, years	62 ± 15	69 ± 9	0.007
Body mass index	22.7 ± 3.1	23.8 ± 3.0	0.12
Hypertension, n (%)	12 (46.1)	36 (61.0)	0.15
Diabetes mellitus, n (%)	5 (19.2)	28 (47.5)	0.010
Dyslipidemia, n (%)	5 (19.2)	32 (56.1)	0.002
Systolic blood pressure (mmHg)	125 ± 18	130 ± 18	0.21
Diastolic blood pressure (mmHg)	75 ± 11	75 ± 12	0.85
Echocardiographic parameters			
Left ventricular ejection fraction (%)	70 ± 6	62 ± 11	0.001
LVEDd (mm)	45 ± 7	47 ± 5	0.15
LVSWth (mm)	9.2 ± 1.7	9.5 ± 1.3	0.41
LVPWth (mm)	9.6 ± 1.5	9.7 ± 1.5	0.72
Medications			
ARBs or ACEIs, n (%)	8 (30.8)	16 (27.1)	0.81
Beta-blockers, n (%)	3 (11.5)	9 (15.2)	0.61
Calcium channel blockers, n (%)	7 (26.9)	23 (39.0)	0.23
Diuretics, n (%)	2 (7.7)	7 (11.9)	0.71

LVEDd: Left ventricular end-diastolic dimension, LVSWth: left ventricular septal wall thickness, LVPWth: left ventricular posterior wall thickness, ACEIs: angiotensin-converting enzyme inhibitors, ARBs: Angiotensin II receptor blockers

Table 2 Patient laboratory characteristics

	Non-CAD group (n = 26)	CAD group (n = 59)	p-value
Prorenin (pg/ml)	490 (321–786)	522 (297–1097)	0.70
Plasma renin concentration (pg/ml)	5.8 (3.3 - 9.8)	6.3 (4.4 - 12.0)	0.84
Plasma renin activity (ng/ml/hr)	1.0 (0.5 - 2.1)	1.1 (0.6 - 2.4)	0.83
Aldosterone (pg/ml)	85 (65–130)	74 (59–98)	0.40
Brain natriuretic peptide (ng/ml)	20 (14–55)	32 (14–62)	0.38
Cystatin C (mg/dl)	1.09 ± 0.87	1.09 ± 0.38	0.97
Creatinine (mg/ml)	1.01 ± 1.48	0.85 ± 0.27	0.42
Estimated GFR (ml/min/1.73 m^2)	77.1 ± 28.3	69.6 ± 19.2	0.16
Blood urea nitrogen (mg/dl)	18.0 ± 20.1	15.9 ± 4.1	0.45
Hemoglobin A1c (%)	5.7 ± 0.7	6.1 ± 1.1	0.16
Total cholesterol (mg/dl)	191 ± 43	187 ± 33	0.75
LDL cholesterol (mg/dl)	115 ± 39	112 ± 31	0.71
HDL cholesterol (mg/dl)	51 ± 13	48 ± 14	0.39
Triglycerides (mg/dl)	114 ± 56	139 ± 72	0.11
C-reactive protein (mg/dl)	0.24 ± 0.52	0.18 ± 0.21	0.52
Total protein (g/dl)	6.68 ± 0.52	6.72 ± 0.43	0.68
Albumin (g/dl)	3.99 ± 0.32	4.13 ± 0.30	0.054
Sodium (mEq/l)	141.1 ± 2.1	140.3 ± 2.3	0.57
Potassium (mEq/l)	4.10 ± 0.41	4.05 ± 0.35	0.53
Cl (mEq/l)	105.3 ± 3.2	105.4 ± 2.7	0.92

Numerical data are expressed as the mean ± one standard deviation. Non-parametric data are expressed as the median (interquartile range). GFR: glomerular filtration rate

Plasma prorenin concentration and coronary artery stenosis

There was also no significant difference in the plasma renin activity or plasma prorenin concentration between the CAD group and non-CAD group (Fig. 2). There was also no significant difference in the plasma prorenin concentration between patients with and without DM (635 ± 541 and 824 ± 533 pg/ml, respectively). There were also no significant differences in the plasma prorenin concentration in the patients with one-vessel disease, two-vessel disease and three-vessel disease (780 ± 681, 651 ± 507 and 884 ± 580 pg/ml, respectively). However, patients with a high plasma prorenin concentration frequently suffered from CAD (Fig. 2). Receiver-operating-characteristics curve analysis showed that the optimal cut-off value of the plasma prorenin concentration to detect CAD was 1,100 pg/ml with a positive predictive value for estimating CAD of 94 % and a negative predictive value of 36 % (Table 3) (Fig. 3). Only one of 26 patients with elevated plasma prorenin concentration (>1,100 pg/ml) did not have CAD (Fig. 2). The optimal cutoff value of the plasma renin activity to detect CAD was 0.8 ng/ml/hr with a positive predictive value of 72 %, and a negative predictive value of 32 %. A higher plasma prorenin concentration was more accurate than a higher PRA for the detection of CAD. Laboratory and clinical characteristics in the CAD group with patients stratified based on prorenin levels are shown in Table 4.

Discussion

The key findings in the present study were as follows: (1) the optimal cutoff value of plasma prorenin concentration to detect CAD was 1,100 pg/ml with a positive predictive value of 94 % and a negative predictive value of 36 %; (2) patients with high plasma prorenin concentration (>1,100 pg/ml) frequently suffered CAD; (3) the plasma prorenin concentration was positively correlated with the plasma renin concentration; (4) the plasma prorenin concentration was not correlated with LVEF, HbA1c, BNP or eGFR.

Plasma prorenin concentration and coronary artery disease

Prorenin is an inactive precursor of renin. Both prorenin and renin bind to (pro)renin receptors, and stimulation of these receptors activates intracellular cascades such as

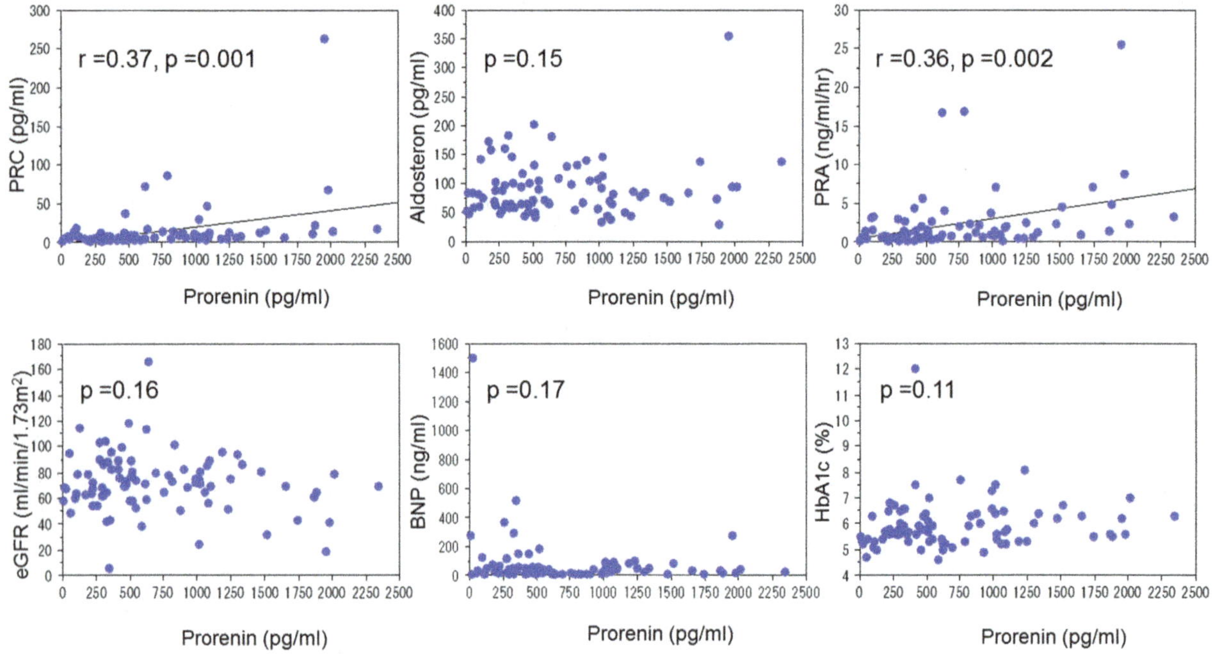

Fig. 1 Relationship between plasma prorenin concentration and laboratory parameters. PRC: plasma renin concentration, PRA: plasma renin activity, HbA1c: hemoglobin A1c, BNP: brain natriuretic peptide, eGFR: estimated glomerular filtration rate

MAP kinases ERK1/2 and p38 pathways, and heat shock protein 27. Activation of these pathways leads to enhanced synthesis of DNA, upregulation of TGF-β1, PAI-1, collagen-1, fibronectin and cyclooxygenase-2, independent of the classic renin-angiotensin-aldosterone system [8, 9]. This suggests that stimulation of (pro)renin receptors may exert important effects on the cardiovascular system. (Pro)renin receptors have been localized in various tissues such as the brain, kidneys, heart and vascular smooth muscle cells [10]. Stimulation of (pro)renin receptors has been reported to cause diabetic nephropathy, [3] cardiac injury [4] and vascular damage

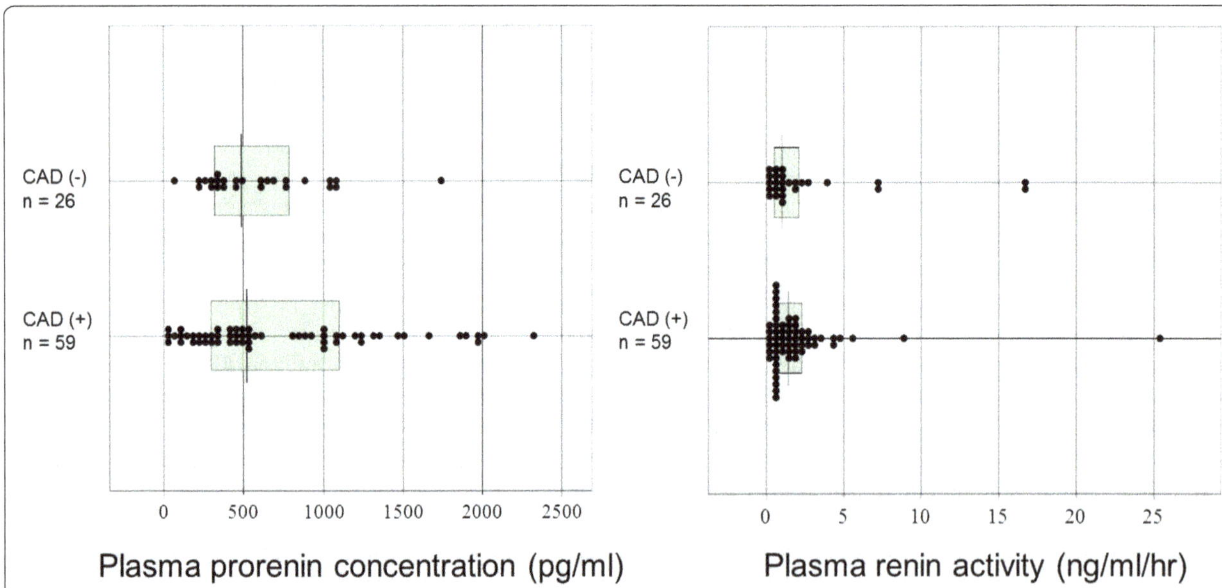

Fig. 2 Plasma prorenin concentrations and renin activity in coronary artery disease and non- coronary artery disease groups. Non-parametric data are shown in box plots. A line in each box indicates the median. The upper and lower limits of each box are the 1st and 3rd quartiles, respectively

Table 3 Accuracy of plasma prorenin and PRA for detecting coronary artery disease

	Cutoff	Sensitivity	Specificity	PPV	NPV
Prorenin (pg/ml)	1,100	25 (15–34)	96 (92–100)	94 (88–99)	36 (25–46)
PRA (ng/ml/hr)	0.8	36 (26–46)	69 (59–79)	72 (63–81)	32 (22–42)

The optimal cutoff values were determined by receiver-operating-characteristic curve analysis. Data are percentages. Numbers in parentheses are 95 % confidence intervals. PPV: positive predictive value, NPV: negative predictive value. PRA: plasma renin activity

[5]. Furthermore, the plasma prorenin level was markedly increased in patients with diabetes mellitus with end-organ damage [7, 11]. This suggests that increased plasma prorenin that stimulated (pro)renin receptors resulted in kidney damage.

We measured plasma prorenin concentration in patients with CAD and found that there were patients with CAD that had low plasma prorenin concentration, although patients with high plasma prorenin concentration frequently had CAD. This suggested that there may be two types of coronary stenosis: one type that is sensitive to prorenin and another type that is not. Increased plasma prorenin may have affected coronary artery stenosis through activation of (pro)renin receptors in vascular smooth muscle cells, since activation of (pro)renin receptors has been reported to cause vascular damage [5].

In the present study, patients with a high plasma prorenin concentration (>1,100 pg/ml) frequently suffered CAD (94 %), and accuracy of an elevated plasma prorenin concentration to detect CAD was greater than that of an elevated PRA (>0.8 ng/ml/hr). A previous study demonstrated that high PRA was an independent predictor of major vascular events and mortality in a stable population of high-risk patients with atherosclerosis and/or diabetes [12]. The results of the present study suggested that the plasma prorenin concentration may also be a marker of CAD and/or atherosclerosis. Although, there were patients with CAD that had a low plasma prorenin concentration, patients with a high plasma prorenin concentration frequently had CAD. This may be because a high plasma prorenin concentration induces coronary stenosis by a mechanism that does not involve endothelial injury or lipid accumulation in plaque. A previous study showed that prorenin induced the growth of extracellar matrix components rather than endothelial damage [13]. Another study reported that prorenin enhanced human vascular smooth muscle cell proliferation due to activation of extracellular-signal-related protein kinase in a dose- and time-dependent manner [14]. Therefore, prorenin may induce stenosis from a medial site due to vascular smooth muscle cell proliferation. The detailed mechanisms by which prorenin induces coronary artery stenosis are still

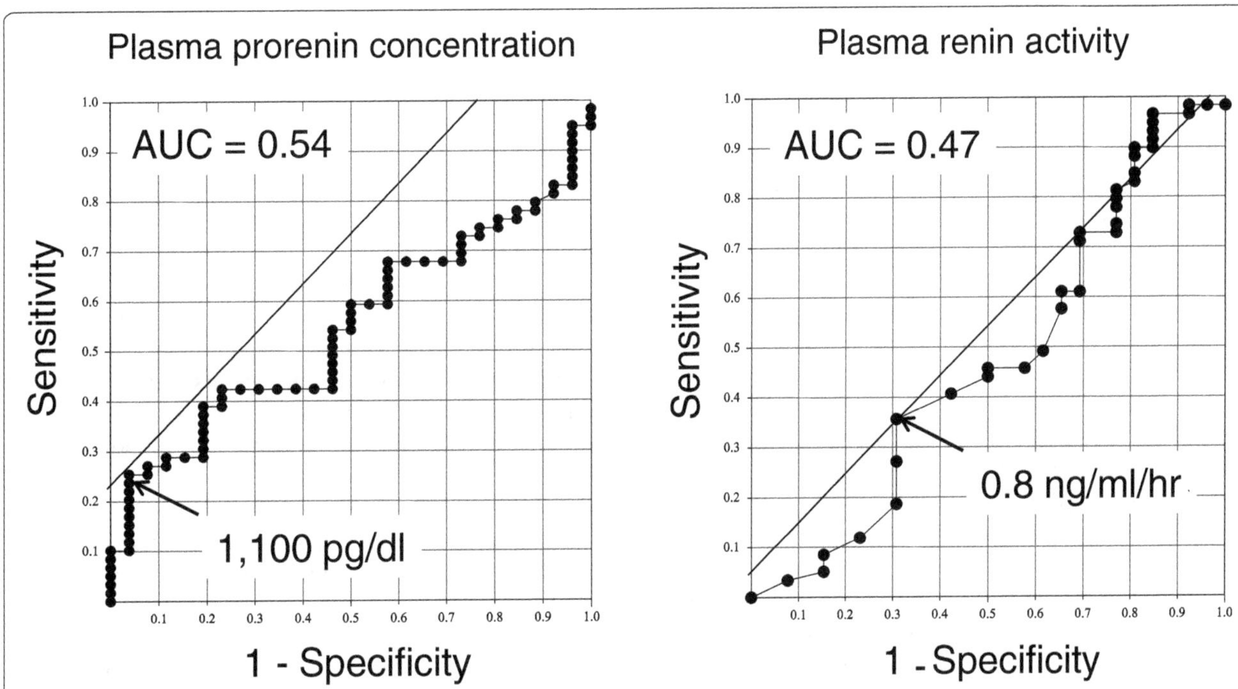

Fig. 3 Receiver operating characteristic curves (ROC) analysis. AUC: area under the curve

Table 4 Laboratory and clinical characteristics in the CAD group with patients stratified based on prorenin levels

	Prorenin ≥ 1,100 (n = 15)	Prorenin < 1,100 (n = 44)	p-value
Age, years	72 ± 6	67 ± 9	0.047
Body mass index	24.4 ± 3.3	23.7 ± 2.9	0.43
Prorenin (ng/ml)	1521 (1261–1937)	435 (227–601)	<0.001
Plasma renin concentration (pg/ml)	12.1 (6.9 - 17.5)	5.6 (4.1 - 8.5)	0.001
Plasma renin activity (ng/ml/hr)	2.3 (1.1 - 4.2)	0.8 (0.6 - 1.6)	0.017
Aldosterone (pg/ml)	82 (69–92)	69 (58–104)	0.63
Brain natriuretic peptide (ng/ml)	43 (24–76)	25 (12–60)	0.23
Cystatin C (mg/dl)	1.19 ± 0.54	1.05 ± 0.29	0.21
Creatinine (mg/ml)	0.91 ± 0.34	0.83 ± 0.24	0.32
Estimated GFR (ml/min/1.73 m^2)	65.8 ± 21.8	70.9 ± 18.3	0.38
Blood urea nitrogen (mg/dl)	17.2 ± 4.5	15.4 ± 3.9	0.16
Hemoglobin A1c (%)	6.2 ± 0.7	6.0 ± 1.2	0.67
Total cholesterol (mg/dl)	178 ± 33	191 ± 33	0.19
LDL cholesterol (mg/dl)	101 ± 29	115 ± 31	0.14
HDL cholesterol (mg/dl)	49 ± 12	48 ± 14	0.74
Triglycerides (mg/dl)	141 ± 60	138 ± 77	0.91
C-reactive protein (mg/dl)	0.13 ± 0.17	0.20 ± 0.22	0.32
Total protein (g/dl)	6.80 ± 0.24	6.70 ± 0.42	0.43
Albumin (g/dl)	4.15 ± 0.24	4.12 ± 0.32	0.74
Sodium (mEq/l)	139.6 ± 2.8	140.6 ± 2.1	0.13
Potassium (mEq/l)	4.27 ± 0.37	3.97 ± 0.32	0.005
Cl (mEq/l)	104.9 ± 3.8	105.5 ± 2.7	0.42

Numerical data are expressed as the mean ± one standard deviation. Non-parametric data are expressed as the median (interquartile range). GFR: glomerular filtration rate

unknown. However, the present study provides new insight into the relationship between plasma prorenin and CAD.

Plasma prorenin concentration and other diseases

Plasma prorenin concentration is determined by the balance between clearance of prorenin from the circulation and production of prorenin. We assessed the relationship between plasma prorenin concentration and eGFR, and there was no correlation between them. This suggests that clearance of prorenin from the kidney is not decreased and a higher plasma prorenin concentration is not due to decreased clearance of prorenin from the circulation. The plasma prorenin concentration was not correlated with LVEF or plasma BNP levels, suggesting that plasma prorenin concentration is not affected by cardiac function.

In the present study, there was also no significant difference in the plasma prorenin concentration between patients with and without DM. However, the plasma prorenin concentration has been reported to be increased in patients who have DM with complications [6]. This discrepancy may be because the present study included DM patients both with and without complications.

Study limitations

There are several limitations of the present study. First, the relationship between renin and cardiovascular disease may be obscured by the use of various drugs such as ACEIs, ARBs, beta-blockers and diuretics because these drugs modify PRA. In addition, the role of plasma prorenin in patients with CAD is still unclear. Second, a relatively small number of the patients were enrolled in the present study. Thus, the study may have been underpowered to definitively determine the relationship between the incidence of CAD and plasma prorenin concentration. A study in a larger population is needed to elucidate the relationship between the plasma prorenin concentration and the progression of CAD.

Conclusions

Although, there were patients with CAD that had a low plasma prorenin concentration (≤1,100 pg/ml), patients with a high plasma prorenin concentration

(>1,100 pg/ml) frequently had CAD. This may be because a high plasma prorenin concentration (>1,100 pg/ml) induces coronary stenosis by a mechanism that does not involve endothelial injury or lipid accumulation in plaque. The present study is a first report that demonstrated the relationship between plasma prorenin concentration and CAD.

Abbreviations

PRA: plasma renin activity; CAD: coronary artery disease; HTN: hypertension; DM: diabetes mellitus; LVEF: left ventricular ejection fraction; LVEDd: left ventricular end-diastolic dimension; LVESd: left ventricular end-systolic dimension; BNP: plasma brain natriuretic peptide; HbA1c: hemoglobin A1c; ACEI: angiotensin-converting enzyme inhibitors; ARB: angiotensin II receptor blockers.

Competing interests

The authors declare that they have no competing interests.

Authors' contributions

GY, MK and IM analysed data and wrote the manuscript. YH, TA and NM analysed data. YY, KN, YA measured data. FS and SM revised the manuscript. All authors read and approved the final manuscript.

Acknowledgements

The authors thank Ms. Akiko Tsujimoto for technical assistance. This work was supported by a grant from Gifu University Graduate School of Medicine (to S Minatoguchi).

Author details

[1]Department of Nephrology, Gifu University Graduate School of Medicine, Gifu, Japan. [2]Department of Cardiology, Gifu University Graduate School of Medicine, Yanagido 1-1, Gifu 501-1194, Japan. [3]Faculty of Applied Biological Sciences, Gifu University, Gifu, Japan.

Reference

1. Alderman MH, Madhavan S, Ooi WL, Cohen H, Sealey JE, Laragh JH. Association of the renin-sodium profile with the risk of myocardial infarction in patients with hypertension. N Eng J Med. 1991;324:1098–104.
2. Muhlestein JB, May HT, Bair TL, Prescott MF, Horne BD, White R, et al. Relationship of elevated plasma renin activity at baseline to cardiac events in patients with angiographically proven coronary artery disease. Am J Cardiol. 2010;106:764–9.
3. Ichihara A, Hayashi M, Kaneshiro Y, Suzuki F, Nakagawa T, Tada Y, et al. Inhibition of diabetic nephropathy by a decoy peptide corresponding to the 'handle' region for non-proteolytic activation of prorenin. J Clin Invest. 2004;114:1128–35.
4. Susic D, Zhou X, Frohlich ED, Lippton H, Knight M. Cardiovascular effects of prorenin blockade in genetivcally spontaneously hypertensive rats on normal and high-salt diet. Am J Physiol Heart Circ Physiol. 2008;295:H1117–21.
5. Veniant M, Menard J, Bruneval P, Morley S, Gonzales MF, Mullins J. Vascular damage without hypertension in transgenic rats expressing prorenin exclusively in the liver. J Clin Invest. 1996;98:1966–70.
6. Jan Danser AH, Batenburg WW, van Esch JH. Prorenin and the (pro)renin receptor–an update. Nephrol Dial Transplant. 2007;22:1288–92.
7. Luetscher JA, Kraemer FB, Wilson DM, Schwartz HC, Bryer-Ash M. Increased plasma iactive renin in diabetes mellitus. A marker of microvascular complications. N Eng J Med. 1985;312:1412–7.
8. Huang Y, Wongamornthan S, Kasting J, McQuillan D, Owens RT, Yu L, et al. Renin increases mesangial cell transforming growth factor-beta1 and matrix proteins through receptor-mediated, angiotensin II-independent mechanisms. Kidney Int. 2006;69:105–13.
9. Ichihara A, Suzuki F, Nakagawa T, Kaneshiro Y, Takemitsu T, Sakoda M, et al. Prorenin receptor blockade inhibits development of glomerulosclerosis in diabetic angiotensin II type 1a receptor-deficient mice. J Am Soc Nephrol. 2006;17:1950–61.
10. Nguyen G, Delarue F, Burcklé C, Bouzhir L, Giller T, Sraer JD. Pivotal role of the renin/prorenin receptor in angiotensin II production and cellular responses to renin. J Clin Invest. 2002;109:1417–27.
11. Nguyen G, Danser AH. Prorenin and (pro)renin receptor: a review of available data from in vitro studies and experimental models in rodents. Exp Physiol. 2008;93:557–63.
12. Verma S, Gupta M, Holmes DT, Xu L, Teoh H, Gupta S, et al. Plasma renin activity predicts cardiovascular mortality in the Heart Outcomes Prevention Evaluation (HOPE) study. Eur Heart J. 2011;32:2135–42.
13. Kim S, Iwao H. Molecular and cellular mechanisms of angiotensin II-mediated cardiovascular and renal diseases. J Pharmacol Sci. 2003;91:177–81.
14. Sakoda M, Ichihara A, Kaneshiro Y, Takemitsu T, Nakazato Y, Nabi AH, et al. (Pro)renin receptor-mediated activation of mitogen-activated protein kinases in human vascular smooth muscle cells. Hypertens Res. 2007;30:1139–46.

2

Elevation of brain-enriched miRNAs in cerebrospinal fluid of patients with acute ischemic stroke

Sofie Sølvsten Sørensen[1*], Ann-Britt Nygaard[2], Anting Liu Carlsen[3], Niels H. H. Heegaard[3], Mads Bak[4] and Thomas Christensen[1]

Abstract

Background: The purpose of this study was to investigate the potential of cerebrospinal fluid miRNAs as diagnostic biomarkers of acute ischemic stroke using three different profiling techniques in order to identify and bypass any influence from technical variation.

Methods: Cerebrospinal fluid (CSF) from patients with acute ischemic stroke (n = 21) and controls (n = 21) was collected by lumbar puncture. miRNA analysis was performed with three different methods: 1) Trizol RNA extraction followed by Illumina Next Generation Sequencing (NGS) on all small RNAs, 2) Exiqon RNA extraction protocol and miRNA qPCR assays, and 3) validation of 24 selected miRNAs with Norgen Biotek RNA extraction protocol and Applied Biosystems qPCR assays.

Results: NGS detected 71 frequently expressed miRNAs in CSF of which brain-enriched miR-9-5p and miR-128-3p were significantly higher in CSF of stroke patients compared to controls. When dividing stroke patients into groups according to infarct size several brain-enriched miRNAs (miR-9-5p, miR-9-3p, miR-124-3p, and miR-128-3p) were elevated in patients with infarcts >2 cm3. This trend appeared in data from both NGS, qPCR (Exiqon), and qPCR (Applied Biosystems) but was only statistically significant in some of the measurement platforms.

Conclusions: Several brain-enriched miRNAs are elevated in the CSF three days after stroke onset, suggesting that these miRNAs reflect the brain damage caused by ischemia. The expression differences seem, however, limited to patients with larger ischemic brain injury, which argues against the use of CSF miRNAs as diagnostic biomarkers of stroke based on current methods.

Keywords: Stroke, MicroRNA, Biomarkers, Brain ischemia, Cerebrospinal fluid

Background

Ischemic stroke is a frequent cause of death and disability all over the world. In patients with atypical or discrete symptoms the diagnosis of ischemic stroke can be difficult and determining the cause of stroke in each individual is even more complicated. Despite thorough clinical and paraclinical evaluation comprising brain computed tomography (CT) or magnetic resonance imaging (MRI), blood tests, cardiac workup, and ultrasound examination of the carotid arteries, the cause of acute ischemic stroke remains unknown in 25% of all patients [1]. A biomarker with the ability to distinguish between different stroke etiologies (large-artery atherosclerosis, small-artery occlusion, and cardio-embolism) could potentially aid the physicians in choosing the best secondary prevention for their patients since treatment of the different stroke subtypes is not the same. In patients with large-artery atherosclerosis or small artery occlusion, anti-platelet drugs are first choice treatment for reducing the risk of stroke recurrence [2]. In contrast, in patients with cardio-embolic stroke, anticoagulant therapy is the most effective prevention [3, 4]. Surgical intervention with carotid endarterectomy is considered in large-artery atherosclerosis as it reduces recurrent strokes in patients with a

* Correspondence: sofiess83@gmail.com
[1]Department of Neurology, Nordsjællands Hospital, University of Copenhagen, Dyrehavevej 29, 3400 Hillerød, Denmark

significant ipsilateral carotid artery stenosis [5]. The current and most widely used system for categorization of ischemic stroke subtypes, the TOAST classification, is based on clinical and paraclinical test results and has only moderate inter-rater reliability [6, 7]. Furthermore, many stroke patients have competing possible causes, such as concurrent atrial fibrillation and carotid artery stenosis, making it impossible to establish a specific etiology. Therefore, new diagnostic and prognostic biomarkers in relation to ischemic stroke are warranted and could potentially benefit stroke patients in various ways.

MicroRNAs (miRNAs) are small non-coding RNA molecules involved in numerous physiological processes in which they function as posttranscriptional inhibitors of gene expression. Their presence in different body fluids such as blood and CSF combined with their stability during long term storage make them interesting as biomarker candidates [8–10]. Recently, several clinical stroke studies have suggested a diagnostic value of miRNAs extracted from plasma/serum and circulating blood cells [11–15], although the results points in various directions. Since CSF is separated from the blood by the blood brain barrier (BBB) and because of its proximity to the brain tissue, it is obvious to assume that the CSF could contain unique signatures of miRNA expression specific for various central nervous system (CNS) pathologies, and therefore serve as a more valid biomarker source compared to other body fluids.

Within few minutes after stroke onset, various brain functions begin to break down as a direct consequence of ischemia including changes in gene expression [16, 17]. Microarray studies have identified several gene families, e.g. immediate early genes, heat shock protein genes, and genes related to apoptosis and inflammation that are regulated by focal brain ischemia [18–20]. Several experimental studies have shown changes in the expression of miRNAs in rat brain tissue following middle cerebral artery occlusion [21–26]. Based on this knowledge, we hypothesized that the changes in miRNA expression in the brain of acute ischemic stroke patients are reflected in the cerebrospinal fluid (CSF) surrounding the central nervous system.

Previously, we have explored the expression of miRNAs in CSF of acute stroke patients in a pilot study [27]. We found 21 frequently expressed miRNAs in the CSF of which two miRNAs (miR-221-3p and let-7c-5p) appeared to be up-regulated in stroke patients compared to controls, although not statistically significant after correction for multiple testing.

The purpose of this follow-up study was 1) to investigate the potential of CSF miRNAs as biomarkers of acute ischemic stroke using three different profiling techniques in order to identify and bypass any influence from technical variation and 2) to validate our previous findings in a larger group of patients.

Methods

Patient material and sample collection

Patients admitted with acute ischemic stroke at the Department of Neurology, Nordsjællands Hospital, University of Copenhagen, from June 2013 to December 2014 were asked to participate in accordance with the approval from the Danish Research Ethics Committee (project ID: H-I-2011-094).

As in our previous study, the stroke diagnoses were based on patient history, thorough neurologic examination and CT scan of the brain on admission. In addition, all patients were scanned on a 3 Tesla System Philips Achieva MRI scanner on the third day after symptom onset. The imaging protocol consisted of diffusion-weighted and T_2-weighted sequences. Infarct volumes were calculated from MR diffusion-weighted images by multiplying the summed areas of infarction with the distance between each section [28]. After additional Doppler Ultrasound of carotid arteries and cardiac telemetry for at least 48 h during admission patients were categorized according to stroke subtype using the TOAST classification [6]. Controls were recruited from our outpatient neurology clinic as they underwent planned lumbar punctures as part of their investigation program for neurologic diseases others than stroke. A total of 42 patients were included, n = 21 ischemic stroke patients, and n = 21 controls. Patient characteristics are given in Table 1. A more detailed description of the different diagnoses and stroke parameters in each individual patient is given in Additional file 1. The

Table 1 Patient characteristics

Characteristics	Stroke (n = 21) Mean (range) or n (%)	Control (n = 21) Mean (range) or n (%)
Age (years)	66.6 (47–78)	66.0 (31–86)
Male sex	12 (57.1)	13 (61.9)
NIHSS	2.5 (0–10)	-
Infarct (cm^3)	6.7 (0.3–32.4)	-
SAO	11 (52.4)	-
LAA	5 (23.8)	-
CE	2 (9.5)	-
U	3 (14.3)	-
Dementia	-	7 (33.3)
MCI	-	2 (9.5)
Multiple sclerosis	-	1 (4.8)
ALS	-	1 (4.8)
No CNS disease	-	10 (47.6)

NIHSS National Institute of Health Stroke Scale, *SAO* stroke caused by small-artery occlusion *LAA*, stroke caused by large-artery atherosclerosis, *CE* stroke caused by cardioembolism, *U* stroke of undetermined etiology,*MCI* mild cognitive impairment, *ALS* amyotrophic lateral sclerosis, *No CNS disease* patients with no evidence of disease in the central nervous system (benign headache, Bell's palsy, polyneuropathy, restless legs or lower back pain) composition of diagnoses and severity of stroke symptoms were comparable to our previous study, Additional file 2.

Lumbar punctures were done by sterile technique on the third day after stroke onset with the use of a 0.7 mm spinal needle in accordance with local guidelines. At least 5 ml CSF were collected from each patient. For miRNA detection 1 ml CSF from each patient was centrifuged at 2000 x g at 4 °C for 15 min immediately after collection and the cell-free fractions were stored at −80.0 °C. Analyses of miRNAs were performed by three different methods as described below. A detailed description of the methodology is available online, Additional file 3.

Trizol RNA extraction followed by Illumina next generation sequencing

RNA was isolated from 100 μl CSF using TriZol reagent (Invitrogen) according to the manufacturer's protocol. Small RNA libraries were prepared using the TruSeq small RNA library preparation kit (Illumina). The resulting cDNA was amplified by PCR and all small RNA sequences were purified on gels and sequenced on a NextSeq500 (Illumina). The libraries from two stroke patient samples were of low quality and were therefore excluded from further analysis. Reads were trimmed for adapters and reads shorter than 15 nucleotides in length were discarded. Small RNAs were aligned to the human genome (hg19) and miRbase (v20) using sRNAbench [29]. miRNA counts were normalized in R Bioconductor package edger [30] using Trimmed Mean of M-values (TMM). Fold changes were based on the average count in each patient group.

Exiqon RNA extraction protocol and miRNA qPCR assays

RNA extractions and sample preparations were done by Exiqon Services, Denmark. Total RNA was extracted from 200 μl CSF using spin column chromatography (miRCURY™ RNA isolation kit for bio fluids). RNA was reverse transcribed using the miRCURY LNA™ Universal RT miRNA kit (Exiqon). Each miRNA was assayed once by qPCR on the miRNA Ready-to-Use PCR, Human panel I containing 372 specific miRNA primers. Amplification was performed in a LightCycler® 480 Real-Time PCR System (Roche) in 384 well plates. Using NormFinder [31] the best normalizer was identified as the average Ct value of the 9 miRNAs detected in all samples (miR-15a-5p, miR-21-5p, miR-23a-3p, miR-23b-3p, miR-99a-5p, miR-125b-5p, miR-145-5p, miR-204-5p, and miR-320a) and relative expression levels (RELs) were calculated by the formula $REL = 2^{miR\ average - miR}/2^{Global\ mean\ average - Global\ mean}$ based on the principle of $2^{-\Delta\Delta Ct}$ [32]. Fold changes were based on the median value of REL in each patient group (missing values excluded).

Norgen Biotek RNA extraction protocol and applied biosystems qPCR assays

Total RNA was extracted from 200 μl CSF using spin column chromatography (Total RNA Purification Kit, Norgen Biotek). Reverse transcription was performed by TaqMan microRNA Reverse Transcription Kit performed on a 2720 Thermal Cycler (Applied Biosystems). miRNA specific pre-amplification was accomplished using TaqMan PreAmp master mix and TaqMan MicroRNA Assays (Applied Biosystems). Pre-amplified samples and TaqMan miRNA assays for 24 selected miRNAs were applied to a 48.48 Dynamic Array IFC chip and amplified on a BioMark real-time microfluidic PCR system (Fluidigm).

Normfinder [31] identified two equally good normalizers: miR-320a and the average Ct value of the 20 miRNAs detected in all samples. Based on the assumption that most of the 24 miRNAs in this validation experiment were differentially expressed between our patient groups we wanted to avoid a global mean normalization that could potentially undermine any differences by comparing raw data to the average of all miRNAs. Therefore, miR-320a was chosen as normalizer and RELs were calculated using the formula $REL = 2^{miR\ average - miR}/2^{miR\text{-}320a\ average - miR\text{-}320a}$ based on the principle of $2^{-\Delta\Delta Ct}$ [32]. Fold changes were based on the median value of REL in each patient group (missing values excluded).

Statistics

Two-sided nonparametric Mann-Whitney tests were performed for REL comparisons between groups (SPSS software). In the NGS experiment differentially expressed miRNAs were detected by an exact test based on conditional maximum likelihood (CML) included in the R Bioconductor package edgeR [30]. *P* values from NGS and qPCR were corrected for multiple testing with the Benjamini-Hochberg (BH) procedure and $p < 0.05$ were considered significant. In all group comparisons missing expression values were treated as zero. The NGS heat map was generated using Multiple Experiment Viewer [33]. Selection of the best miRNA predictors was based on logistic lasso regression [34] performed on the top 15 most deregulated miRNAs detected by NGS. AUC and classification accuracy was estimated by leave-one-out cross-validation based on the seven predictors selected by the lasso. Differences in total numbers of miRNAs between groups as well as differences in age were analyzed by two-sided parametric t tests. Fischer's exact test was used for analysis of sex differences.

Results

Overall detection by NGS and Exiqon qPCR (human panel I)

A total of 246 miRNAs were detected in the CSF by NGS of which 71 miRNAs were expressed in more than 90% of the patient samples. Slightly fewer, 210 miRNAs, were detected by the qPCR screening (Exiqon, human panel I) of which only 21 miRNAs were expressed in more than 90% of the samples. With the exception of miR-1246 all of the differentially expressed miRNAs between stroke patients and controls were detected by both NGS and qPCR (Additional file 4) although the detection rate was generally lower in the qPCR experiment.

Results from NGS

In the NGS experiment only two miRNAs (miR-1246 and miR-128-3p) were significantly up-regulated in the stroke group compared to controls after BH correction. The up-regulation of miRNAs was most evident in patients with large-artery atherosclerosis or cardioembolism whose infarcts were larger (mean volume (range) = 16.5 cm^3 (2.5–32.4)) compared to patients with small-artery occlusion (mean volume (range) = 0.7 cm^3 (0.3–1.6)) (Fig. 1). When dividing patients into groups according to infarct size 8 miRNAs (miR-9-5p, miR-99b-5p, miR-103a-3p, miR-107, miR-128-3p, miR-181a-5p, miR-181b-5p, and miR-1246) were significantly up-regulated in patients with infarcts >2.5 cm^3 (n = 7) compared to stroke patients with smaller infarcts (n = 12).

Results from qPCR screening (Exiqon, human panel I)

Consistent with our previous findings [27] qPCR (human panel I, Exiqon) detected only 21 frequently expressed miRNAs in CSF of which none were differentially regulated between stroke patients and controls after BH correction. The up-regulation of miR-221-3p and let-7c-5p found in our previous pilot study could not be validated. By considering the expression in subgroups with different infarct sizes two miRNAs (miR-9-3p and miR-124-3p) were significantly up-regulated in stroke patients with infarcts >2 cm^3 (n = 8) compared to stroke patients with smaller infarcts (n = 13).

Validation of selected miRNAs by qPCR (applied biosystems)

Following the completion of NGS and the first qPCR experiment we selected miRNAs that showed differential expression between stroke patients and controls (and/or between patients with small and large infarcts) for technical validation. The selection was based on significant unadjusted p values ($p < 0.05$) and/or a large fold change (0.3 > FC > 3) in at least one of the two experiments. A total of 21 selected miRNAs were included in the validation study (normalizers excluded). Table 2 summarizes results for the 21 selected miRNAs measured with NGS, qPCR (Exiqon), and qPCR (Applied Biosystems), respectively. Five miRNAs (miR-9-5p, miR-9-3p, miR-107, miR-124-3p, and miR-128-3p) were consistently up-regulated in the group of patients with infarcts >2 cm^3, although not statistically significant throughout all measurement platforms. At least four of them (miR-9-5p, miR-9-3p, miR-124-3p, and miR-128-3p) are known as brain-enriched miRNAs with a high tissue specificity index [35]. miRNA-1246 showed the highest up-regulation by NGS (FC = 13.6; p = 0.01) but did not appear to be up-regulated by qPCR (Applied Biosystems) and was unfortunately not included in the human panel I (Exiqon). Fig. 2 illustrates the expression levels of the four brain-enriched miRNAs in different patient subgroups.

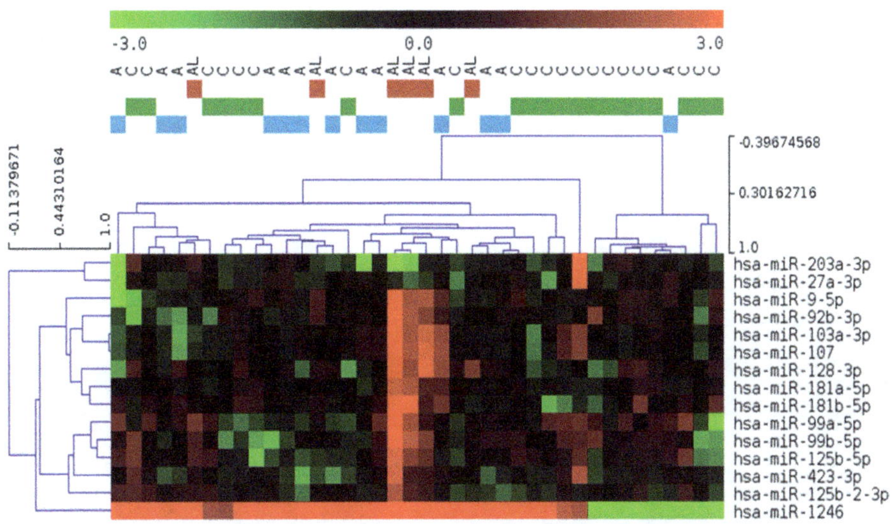

Fig. 1 Heatmap showing logFC expression of the top 15 most differentially expressed miRNAs between stroke patients and controls detected by Next Generation Sequencing. Fold changes were calculated as the expression in each sample (normalized count) relative to the average expression in the control group. *A*: stroke patients with infarcts <2 cm^3; *AL*: stroke patients with infarcts >2 cm^3; *C*: control patients

Table 2 Expression of 21 selected miRNAs detected by three different methods

miRNA	NGS			Exiqon qPCR			Applied Biosystems qPCR		
	Detection(%)	Stroke/Control FC (*P*)	Large/Small FC (*P*)	Detection(%)	Stroke/Control FC (*P*)	Large/Small FC (*P*)	Detection(%)	Stroke/Control FC (*P*)	Large/Small FC (*P*)
let-7b-5p	95	0.8 (0.99)	2.3 (0.73)	98	1.1 (0.99)	0.6 (0.29)	100	1.0 (0.89)	0.6 (0.57)
let-7c-5p	100	0.7 (0.99)	0.9 (0.99)	74	0.7 (0.99)	0.6 (0.11)	95	0.7 (0.71)	0.3 (0.88)
miR-9-5p	98	2.8 (0.06)	7.0 (0.00)	48	3.3 (0.90)	2.3 (0.07)	100	0.9 (0.95)	10.0 (0.01)
miR-9-3p	70	7.1 (0.08)	6.8 (0.28)	70	1.4 (0.85)	9.8 (0.01)	100	1.2 (0.73)	1.9 (0.66)
miR-15a-5p	63	1.0 (0.99)	2.0 (0.99)	100	1.0 (0.50)	2.2 (0.31)	100	1.0 (0.96)	2.4 (0.44)
miR-30d-5p	100	1.2 (0.99)	1.3 (0.79)	91	1.6 (0.45)	1.1 (0.48)	100	1.7 (0.01)	6.2 (0.09)
miR-99b-5p	100	1.9 (0.32)	4.2 (0.00)	38	0.7 (0.99)	0.9 (0.84)	72	0.4 (0.43)	0.5 (0.70)
miR-103a-3p	100	1.9 (0.17)	4.3 (0.00)	48	1.0 (0.84)	0.4 (0.80)	100	0.6 (0.49)	0.9 (0.85)
miR-107	100	2.0 (0.13)	4.5 (0.00)	31	0.6 (0.71)	n.d. small	100	3.6 (0.37)	3.5 (0.58)
miR-124-3p	58	2.7 (0.99)	11.0 (0.19)	83	0.9 (0.99)	3.6 (0.03)	100	1.1 (0.92)	1.7 (0.74)
miR-128-3p	100	2.5 (0.04)	5.5 (0.00)	41	1.0 (0.95)	2.7 (0.15)	100	0.6 (0.42)	1.5 (0.88)
miR-129-5p	60	2.6 (0.99)	2.3 (0.99)	26	1.1 (0.91)	3.1 (0.14)	100	1.5 (0.97)	1.0 (0.77)
miR-181a-5p	100	1.5 (0.40)	3.0 (0.00)	33	0.9 (0.78)	0.6 (0.49)	100	0.5 (0.33)	0.7 (0.76)
miR-181b-5p	100	1.8 (0.32)	3.1 (0.02)	5	n.d. control	n.d. small	100	0.9 (0.46)	0.7 (0.58)
miR-203a-3p	100	0.3 (0.02)	0.8 (0.99)	-	-	-	100	0.7 (0.85)	1.4 (0.78)
miR-204-5p	100	0.8 (0.99)	0.6 (0.73)	100	0.8 (0.90)	0.6 (0.13)	100	0.8 (0.46)	0.7 (0.06)
miR-210-3p	38	1.3 (0.99)	2.3 (0.99)	38	1.1 (0.99)	0.4 (0.06)	100	0.9 (0.52)	1.0 (0.81)
miR-221-3p	95	1.0 (0.99)	3.0 (0.63)	79	1.1 (0.97)	0.3 (0.33)	81	0.7 (0.32)	0.4 (0.52)
miR-485-5p	72	2.4 (0.99)	5.5 (0.46)	-	-	-	100	0.9 (0.54)	2.2 (0.73)
miR-497-5p	28	2.9 (0.99)	2.6 (0.99)	74	1.0 (0.94)	4.1 (0.32)	79	1.6 (0.44)	3.9 (0.65)
miR-1246	78	11.5 (0.02)	13.6 (0.01)	-	-	-	100	1.2 (0.40)	1.0 (0.80)

Detection (%): percentage out of 42 samples in which the miRNA was detected; *Stroke/Control FC*: fold change of median miRNA expression levels in the stroke group ($n = 21$) compared to the control group ($n = 21$); *Large/Small FC*: fold change of median miRNA expression levels in a stroke subgroup with infarcts >2 cm^3 ($n = 8$) compared to all other stroke patients ($n = 13$); *n.d.*: not detected. All *P* values were adjusted for multiple testing with the Benjamini-Hochberg procedure

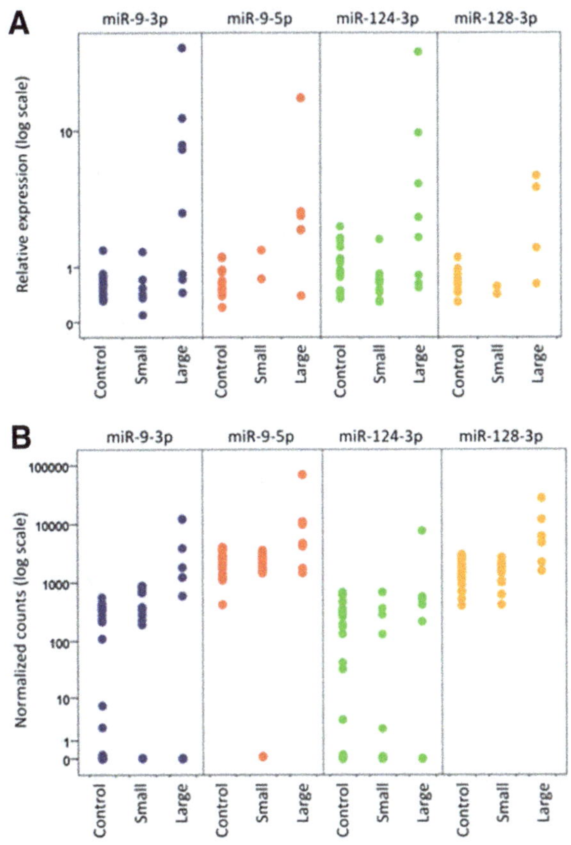

Fig. 2 Scatter plots of the expression levels of four brain-enriched miRNAs (miR-9-3p, miR-9-5p, miR-124-3p, and miR-128-3p) detected by Next Generation Sequencing (A) and Exiqon qPCR (B). *Large*: stroke patients with infarcts >2 cm^3 (n = 13); *Small*: stroke patients with infarcts <2 cm^3 (n = 8); *Control*: control patients with various neurological diseases other than stroke (n = 21)

Classification accuracy and ROC curve

Although the strongest miRNA changes were seen in patients with larger infarcts we attempted to analyze the predictive power of one or more miRNAs to separate stroke patients from controls. Logistic lasso regression performed on the top 15 most differentially expressed miRNAs detected by NGS identified a combination of 7 miRNAs that could discriminate stroke patients from controls with a classification accuracy of 0.75. Fig. 3 shows the receiver operating characteristic (ROC) curve estimated by leave-one-out cross validation (AUC = 0.80).

Discussion

Based on the hypothesis that acute stroke causes transcriptomic changes in the brain tissue which is reflected in the molecular profile of miRNAs in the CSF, we aimed to search for a miRNA expression profile that would uniquely identify stroke patients from other neurological patients. Such a marker could potentially be useful in situations where the diagnosis may be uncertain (e.g. transient ischemic attacks) or when the underlying cause of ischemic stroke remains unknown.

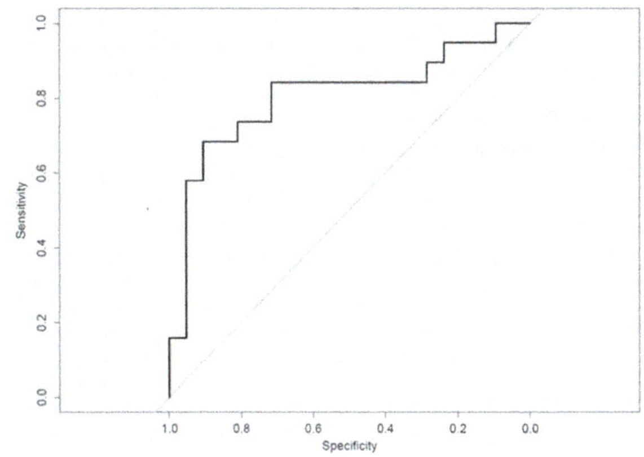

Fig. 3 Receiver operating characteristic (ROC) curve showing the diagnostic value of the combination of 7 miRNAs selected by logistic lasso regression to discriminate stroke patients from controls. AUC = 0.80, classification accuracy = 0.75. miRNAs included in the model: miR-9-3p, miR-92b-3p, miR-99a-5p, miR-128-3p, miR-181a-5p, miR-203a-3p, and miR-1246

Obtaining a blood sample for measurement of miRNA biomarkers is less invasive than a lumbar puncture. However, many organs are likely to contribute to the extracellular miRNA content in plasma. Blood cells, in particular, have been shown to be major sources of plasma miRNAs. Pritchard et al. [36] showed that 58% of plasma miRNAs, reported in the literature to be candidate biomarkers for various cancers, are highly expressed in blood cells. This raises the concern that many miRNAs reported as circulating biomarkers reflect a secondary effect of blood cells rather than a disease-specific effect. Since CSF is separated from the circulation by the BBB and because of the continuous interchange between CSF and interstitial fluid [37], it seems more likely that the composition of miRNAs in CSF reflects CNS pathology better than that of blood plasma. We therefore chose to examine miRNA expression in cell-free CSF samples.

In this comprehensive investigation of miRNAs in the CSF from 21 stroke patients and 21 controls, encompassing both NGS and two different qPCR protocols, we identified relatively few frequently expressed miRNAs in the CSF. In general, the expressional variations within groups and small fold changes between groups resulted in no statistically differences for most of the detected miRNAs. However, it is noteworthy that brain-enriched miR-9-5p, miR-9-3p, miR-124-3p, and miR-128-3p were consistently up-regulated in the group of patients with infarcts >2 cm^3 throughout all experiments.

Studies investigating the abundance of miRNAs in different human organs have identified miR-9-3p, miR-9-5p, miR-124-3p, and miR-128-3p as being enriched in various brain regions (midbrain, cortex, cerebellum and hippocampus) as well as being brain-specific with a high tissue specificity index [35, 38]. Cell studies suggest that miR-124 and miR-128 are predominantly expressed in neurons [39] and studies on embryonic stem cells imply that miR-9 and miR-124 play key roles in neural fate determination in mammalian brain development [40].

It is unknown whether disease-associated miRNAs in CSF are involved in the pathogenic mechanisms of ischemic cell death in the CNS or reflect a passive molecular response to cerebral damage. Stroke-associated miRNAs in the CSF may originate from cytoplasmic protein complexes released during neuronal and glial cell lysis caused by brain ischemia. In this study, the overall amount of miRNA in the CSF seemed slightly higher in patients with larger infarcts compared to other stroke patients, although not statistically significant. The total number of different miRNAs detected by both qPCR and NGS was significantly higher in the group of patients with infarcts >2 cm^3 (p = 0.03), which might indicate a general leak of miRNAs into the CSF following ischemic cell injury and ensuing cell lysis (Fig. 4).

Another possible origin of any miRNA in the CSF is active release of miRNAs enclosed in small membranous vesicles (exosomes) which may play a role in intercellular communication [41, 42]. Only one study has focused on exosome-derived miRNAs in stroke patients. Ji et al. [12] extracted exosomes from serum of 65 stroke patients and 66 non-stroke controls with matching age and cardiovascular risk factors. They found a generally higher concentration of exosomes and a significant increase of exosome derived miR-9 (FC = 16) and miR-124 (FC = 4) in the stroke group compared to controls, suggesting that exosomes from the brain can somehow cross the BBB and enter the peripheral circulation. Accordingly, Ogata et al. [43] have shown elevation of miR-9-3p in the hippocampus as well as in exosomes in peripheral blood of mice after administration of trimethyltin that selectively damages CNS neurons, indicating that miR-9-3p is a potential marker of brain damage.

If the elevation of specific miRNAs in the CSF of stroke patients is caused by expressional changes in the brain tissue, these changes could possibly both reflect the molecular chaos in the ischemic brain tissue as well as its counterregulatory mechanisms. To search for possible molecular functions we made a combined miRPath [44] (version 3.0) analysis of the up-regulated miR-9-3p, miR-9-5p, miR-107, miR-124-3p, and miR-128-3p (results merged by genes union, FDR correction, $P < 0.05$) which identified several KEGG pathways relevant to ischemic stroke, including pathways involved in p53 signaling, cell cycling, tumor necrosis factor (TNF) signaling, hypoxia inducible factor 1 (HIF-1) signaling and neurotrophin signaling.

In literature, the expression of miR-128 has been linked to alterations in the expression of genes implicated in

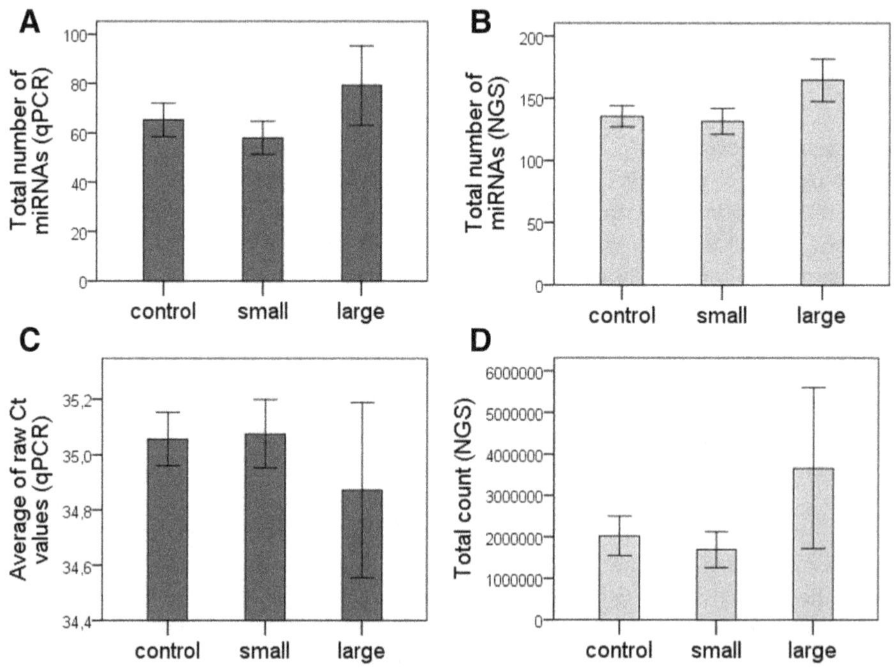

Fig. 4 Total number of different miRNAs detected by qPCR (A) and NGS (B). The general amount of miRNA is expressed as the average of raw Ct values (C), and NGS total counts (D). All variables are shown as mean values (with standard error bars) among controls, patients with infarcts <2 cm^3 (*small*), and patients with infarcts >2 cm^3 (*large*)

apoptosis (Bcl-2, Bax, p53, and Bak) as well as angiogenesis (VEGF) [45]. Yang et al. [46] found miR-128b significantly up-regulated in plasma from ischemic stroke patients compared to healthy controls. In addition, miR-124 has previously been associated with ischemic stroke. Liu et al. [47] as well as Sun et al. [48] found an increase of miR-124 in the ischemic penumbra after permanent middle cerebral artery occlusion in mice. In both studies cell culture experiments indicated that miR-124 is involved in apoptosis. Recently, Li et al. [13] reported up-regulation of three miRNAs in serum of stroke patients including miR-1246, which had the highest fold change (FC = 13.6; $p = 0.01$) in our NGS experiment. In summary, these results, although not fully comparable, support our findings. Only one study besides ours has focused on miRNAs in CSF of stroke patients. Peng et al. [49] analyzed the expression of let-7e and miR-338 in CSF from ischemic stroke patients and found up-regulation of let-7e in a group of patients included 1–7 days after symptom onset ($n = 11$) but they did not include any brain-specific miRNAs in their analysis.

Despite our consistent experimental setup, uniform sample handling, and data processing we were not able to validate the results from our previous pilot study [27]. This might be due to the small differences found in our pilot study, or the fact that none of our pilot study p values passed a BH correction for multiple testing. These results highlight the importance of performing follow-up studies, especially when patient numbers are small. Exiqon's protocol resulted in many missing values and had a lower detection rate for many miRNA sequences compared to NGS, which might explain why any potential differences in brain-enriched miRNAs were not detected in our previous pilot study. In addition, poorly elucidated factors like heterogeneity of genetic background, differences in BBB function, CSF turnover, and miRNA degradation might have influenced results differently in the two studies.

Limitations of our study include the relatively small study population and heterogeneous control group with regard to diagnoses. The various diagnoses represented in our control group may have influenced the fold changes calculated between stroke patients and controls. Nevertheless, if a stroke biomarker should be useful in the clinic, it should possess enough power to predict the diagnosis of ischemic stroke even when tested against non-healthy individuals. Therefore, and because of ethical issues in relation to doing lumbar punctures on healthy individuals, we decided to use neurological patients as controls.

We initially planned to include three equal groups of stroke patients with small-artery occlusion, large-artery atherosclerosis, and cardioembolism. However, we had to exclude patients from lumbar puncture if they were unable to give informed consent, received anticoagulant treatment, or had large infarctions with emerging vasogenic edema which contraindicated a lumbar puncture. Therefore, our study population mainly consisted of patients with lacunar infarctions and a smaller group of patients with larger infarcts having either cardioembolism or large-artery atherosclerosis, which prevented us from comparing miRNA expression profiles in subgroups based on stroke etiologies alone.

An advantage of our study is that it takes into consideration the technical uncertainties related to miRNA profiling by using three different profiling techniques on the same sample set. We observed quite significant discrepancies between results from NGS, qPCR (Exiqon), and qPCR (Applied Biosystems). The low quantities of miRNAs in the CSF combined with multiple factors such as RNA extraction quality, affinity of the primers, and PCR efficiency could influence the results in unpredictable ways. In addition, unknown biological factors such as BBB function and CSF clearance may have influenced our results.

Although the strongest miRNA expressional changes were seen in patients with larger infarcts, we attempted to analyze the predictive power of combining one or more miRNAs to separate stroke patients from controls with logistic lasso regression based on data from NGS. The best model combined 7 miRNAs but resulted in an overall unsatisfactory classification accuracy of 0.75.

Conclusion

In conclusion, several brain-enriched miRNAs are elevated in the CSF three days after stroke onset, suggesting that these miRNAs reflect the brain damage caused by ischemia. The expressional differences seem, however, limited to patients with larger ischemic injury, which argues against the use of CSF miRNAs as diagnostic biomarkers of stroke based on current methods.

Abbreviations

AUC: Area under the curve; BBB: Blood brain barrier; BH: Benjamini-Hochberg; CML: Conditional maximum likelihood; CNS: Central nervous system; CSF: Cerebrospinal fluid; Ct value: Cycle threshold value; CT: Computed tomography; FDR: False discovery rate; HIF-1: Hypoxia inducible factor 1; IFC chip: Integrated fluidic circuit chip; KEGG: Kyoto Encyclopaedia of Genes and Genomes; miRNAs: MicroRNAs; MRI: Magnetic resonance imaging; NGS: Next Generation Sequencing; qPCR: Quantitative Polymerase Chain Reaction; REL: Relative expression value; ROC: Receiver Operating Characteristics; TMM: Trimmed Mean of M-values; TNF: Tumor necrosis factor; TOAST: Trial of Org 10,172 in Acute Stroke Treatment; VEGF: Vascular endothelial growth factor

Acknowledgments

We sincerely thank all personnel at the Department of Neurology, University of Copenhagen, Nordsjællands Hospital, who helped us handling the study patients. Andreas Kryger Jensen, Department of Biostatistics, University of Copenhagen, is thanked for providing statistical assistance with the logistic regression analyses. We also thank the chief consultant at the Department of Neurology, Kai Jensen, who provided all facilities and helped to organize the study.

Funding

This project was supported by grants from the Research Foundation of Nordsjælland's Hospital, the Research Foundation for Health Research of the Capital Region of Denmark, and Helen Rude's Foundation.

Authors' contributions

SS participated in the design of the study, included the patients, collected the CSF samples, participated in the laboratory analyses and the data management, and drafted the manuscript. AN participated in the design of the study, helped to plan the laboratory analyses, contributed to the data management, and reviewed the manuscript. AC planned and carried out the qPCR (Applied Biosystems), contributed to the data management, and reviewed the manuscript. NH helped to organize the laboratory analyses, contributed to the data management, and reviewed the manuscript. MB participated in the design of the study, planned and carried out the NGS, contributed to the management and interpretation of data, and reviewed the manuscript. TC conceived the study, helped to plan and to organize the study, helped to include the patients, contributed to the interpretation of data, and reviewed the manuscript. All authors read and approved the final manuscript.

Competing interests

All the authors declare that they have no competing interests.

Author details

[1]Department of Neurology, Nordsjællands Hospital, University of Copenhagen, Dyrehavevej 29, 3400 Hillerød, Denmark. [2]Department of Clinical Biochemistry, Nordsjællands Hospital, Hillerød, Denmark. [3]Department of Autoimmunology and Biomarkers, Statens Serum Institut, Copenhagen, Denmark. [4]Department of Cellular and Molecular Medicine, Panum Institute, University of Copenhagen, Copenhagen, Denmark.

References

1. Hart RG, Diener HC, Coutts SB, Easton JD, Granger CB, O'Donnell MJ, et al. Embolic strokes of undetermined source: the case for a new clinical construct. Lancet Neurol. 2014;13:429–38.
2. Kernan WN, Ovbiagele B, Black HR, Bravata DM, Chimowitz MI, Ezekowitz MD, et al. AHA / ASA guideline guidelines for the prevention of stroke in patients with stroke and transient ischemic attack; 2014. doi:10.1161/STR.0000000000000024.
3. Diener H, Eikelboom J, Connolly SJ, Joyner CD, Hart RG, Lip GYH, et al. Apixaban versus aspirin in patients with atrial fi brillation and previous stroke or transient ischaemic attack: a predefi ned subgroup analysis from AVERROES , a randomised trial. Lancet Neurol. 2017;11:225–31.
4. Hart RG, Benavente O, McBride R, Pearce LA. Antithrombotic therapy to prevent stroke in patients with atrial fibrillation: a meta-analysis. Ann Intern Med. 1999;131:492–501.
5. Randomised trial of endarterectomy for recently symptomatic carotid stenosis: final results of the MRC European Carotid Surgery Trial (ECST). Lancet. 1998;351:1379–87.
6. Adams HP, Bendixen BH, Kappelle LJ, Biller J, Love BB, Gordon DL, et al. Classification of subtype of acute ischemic stroke. Definitions for use in a multicenter clinical trial. TOAST. Trial of org 10172 in acute stroke treatment. Stroke. 1993;24:35–41.
7. Goldstein LB, Jones MR, Matchar DB, Edwards LJ, Hoff J, Chilukuri V, et al. Improving the reliability of stroke subgroup classification using the trial of ORG 10172 in acute stroke treatment (TOAST) criteria. Stroke. 2001;32:1091 7.
8. Weber JA, Baxter DH, Zhang S, Huang DY, Huang KH, Lee MJ, et al. The microRNA spectrum in 12 body fluids. Clin Chem. 2010;56:1733–41.
9. Glinge C, Clauss S, Boddum K, Jabbari R, Jabbari J, Risgaard B, et al. Stability of circulating blood-based MicroRNAs – pre-analytic methodological considerations. PLoS One. 2017; doi:10.1371/journal.pone.0167969.
10. Balzano F, Deiana M, Giudici SD, Oggiano A, Baralla A, Pasella S, et al. MiRNA stability in frozen plasma samples. Molecules. 2015;20:19030–40.
11. Bam M, Yang X, Sen S, Zumbrun EE, Dennis L, Zhang J, et al. Characterization of Dysregulated miRNA in peripheral blood mononuclear cells from ischemic stroke patients. Mol Neurobiol. 2017; doi:10.1007/s12035-016-0347-8.
12. Ji Q, Ji Y, Peng J, Zhou X, Chen X, Zhao H, et al. Increased brain-specific MiR-9 and MiR-124 in the serum Exosomes of acute ischemic stroke patients. PLoS One. 2016;11:e0163645.
13. Li P, Teng F, Gao F, Zhang M, Wu J, Zhang C. Identification of circulating MicroRNAs as potential biomarkers for detecting acute ischemic stroke. Cell Mol Neurobiol. 2015;35:433–47.
14. Wang W, Sun G, Zhang L, Shi L, Zeng Y. Circulating MicroRNAs as novel potential biomarkers for early diagnosis of acute stroke in humans. J Stroke Cerebrovasc Dis. 2014;23:2607–13.
15. Tsai P-C, Liao Y-C, Wang Y-S, Lin H-F, Lin R-T, Juo S-HH. Serum microRNA-21 and microRNA-221 as potential biomarkers for cerebrovascular disease. J Vasc Res. 2013;50:346–54.
16. Hossmann K-A. Pathophysiology and therapy of experimental stroke. Cell Mol Neurobiol. 2006;26:1057–83.
17. Christensen T. Experimental Focal Cerebral Ischemia - pathophysiology, metabolism and pharmacology of the ischemic penumbra. Copenhagen: University of Copenhagen; 2007. p. 1–56. http://curis.ku.dk/ws/files/107825836/Disputats_TChristensen.pdf.
18. Schmidt-Kastner R, Zhang B, Belayev L, Khoutorova L, Amin R, Busto R, et al. DNA microarray analysis of cortical gene expression during early recirculation after focal brain ischemia in rat. Brain Res Mol Brain Res. 2002;108:81–93.
19. Lu XCM, Williams AJ, Yao C, Berti R, Hartings JA, Whipple R, et al. Microarray analysis of acute and delayed gene expression profile in rats after focal ischemic brain injury and reperfusion. J Neurosci Res. 2004;77:843–57.
20. Kinouchi H, Sharp FR, Hill MP, Koistinaho J, Sagar SM, Chan PH. Induction of 70-kDa heat shock protein and hsp70 mRNA following transient focal cerebral ischemia in the rat. J Cereb Blood Flow Metab. 1993;13:105–15.
21. Dharap A, Bowen K, Place R, Li L. Transient focal ischemia induces extensive temporal changes in rat cerebral MiroRNAome. J Cereb Blood Flow Metab. 2009;29:675–87.
22. Liu D-Z, Tian Y, Ander BP, Xu H, Stamova BS, Zhan X, et al. Brain and blood microRNA expression profiling of ischemic stroke, intracerebral hemorrhage, and kainate seizures. J Cereb Blood Flow Metab. 2010;30:92–101.
23. Wang W-X, Huang Q, Hu Y, Stromberg AJ, Nelson PT. Patterns of microRNA expression in normal and early Alzheimer's disease human temporal cortex: white matter versus gray matter. Acta Neuropathol. 2011;121:193–205.
24. Wang C, Pan Y, Cheng B, Chen J, Bai B. Identification of conserved and novel microRNAs in cerebral ischemia-reperfusion injury of rat using deep sequencing. J Mol Neurosci. 2014;54:671–83.
25. Jeyaseelan K, Lim KY, Armugam A. MicroRNA expression in the blood and brain of rats subjected to transient focal ischemia by middle cerebral artery occlusion. Stroke. 2008;39:959–66.
26. Gubern C, Camós S, Ballesteros I, Rodríguez R, Romera VG, Cañadas R, et al. miRNA expression is modulated over time after focal ischaemia: up-regulation of miR-347 promotes neuronal apoptosis. FEBS J. 2013;280:6233–46.
27. Sørensen SS, Nygaard A-B, Nielsen M-Y, Jensen K, Christensen T. miRNA expression profiles in cerebrospinal fluid and blood of patients with acute ischemic stroke. Transl Stroke Res. 2014;5:711–8.
28. Garcia-Finana M, Cruz-Orive LM, Mackay CE, Pakkenberg B, Roberts N. Comparison of MR imaging against physical sectioning to estimate the volume of human cerebral compartments. NeuroImage. 2003;18:505–16.
29. Rueda A, Barturen G, Lebron R, Gomez-Martin C, Alganza A, Oliver JL, et al. SRNAtoolbox: An integrated collection of small RNA research tools. Nucleic Acids Research. 2015. doi:10.1093/nar/gkv555.
30. Robinson MD, McCarthy DJ, Smyth GK. edgeR: a bioconductor package for differential expression analysis of digital gene expression data. Bioinformatics. 2009;26:139–40.
31. Andersen CL, Jensen JL, Ørntoft TF. Normalization of real-time quantitative reverse transcription-PCR Data : a model-based variance estimation

approach to identify genes suited for normalization, applied to bladder and colon cancer data sets. Cancer Res. 2004;64:5245–50.
32. Jolla L. Quantification strategies in real-time PCR. In: Bustin S, editor. A-Z of Quantitative PCR. La Jolla: International University Line (IUL); 2004. p. 87–112.
33. Saeed A, Sharov V, White J. TM4: a free, open-source system for microarray data management and analysis. BioTechniques. 2003;34:374–7.
34. Tibshirani R. Regression selection and shrinkage via the lasso. J R Stat Soc B. 1996;58:267–88.
35. Ludwig N, Leidinger P, Becker K, Backes C, Fehlmann T, Pallasch C, et al. Distribution of miRNA expression across human tissues. Nucleic Acids Res. 2016;44:3865–77.
36. Pritchard CC, Kroh E, Wood B, Arroyo JD, Dougherty KJ, Miyaji MM, et al. Blood cell origin of circulating microRNAs: a cautionary note for cancer biomarker studies. Cancer Prev Res (Phila). 2012;5:492–7.
37. Jessen NA, Munk ASF. Lundgaard1 I, Nedergaard M. The Glymphatic system – a Beginner's guide. Neurochem Res. 2016;8:583–92.
38. Landgraf P, Rusu M, Sheridan R, Sewer A, Iovino N, Aravin A, et al. A mammalian microRNA expression atlas based on small RNA library sequencing. Cell. 2007;129:1401–14.
39. Zeng Y. Regulation of the mammalian nervous system by MicroRNAs. Mol Pharmacol. 2009;75:259–64.
40. Krichevsky AM, Sonntag K-C, Isacson O, Kosik KS. Specific microRNAs modulate embryonic stem cell-derived neurogenesis. Stem Cells. 2006;24:857–64.
41. Lee Y, El Andaloussi S. Wood MJ a. Exosomes and microvesicles: extracellular vesicles for genetic information transfer and gene therapy. Hum Mol Genet. 2012;21:R125–34.
42. Valadi H, Ekström K, Bossios A, Sjöstrand M, Lee JJ, Lötvall JO. Exosome-mediated transfer of mRNAs and microRNAs is a novel mechanism of genetic exchange between cells. Nat Cell Biol. 2007;9:654–9.
43. Ogata K, Sumida K, Miyata K, Kushida M, Kuwamura M, Yamate J. Circulating miR-9* and miR-384-5p as potential indicators for trimethyltin-induced neurotoxicity. Toxicol Pathol. 2015;43:198–208.
44. Vlachos IS, Zagganas K, Paraskevopoulou MD, Georgakilas G, Karagkouni D, Vergoulis T, et al. DIANA-miRPath v3.0: deciphering microRNA function with experimental support. Nucleic Acids Res. 2015; doi:10.1093/nar/gkv403.
45. Adlakha YK, Saini N. Brain microRNAs and insights into biological functions and therapeutic potential of brain enriched miRNA-128. Mol Cancer. 2014;13:1–18.
46. Yang Z-B, Li T-B, Zhang Z, Ren K-D, Zheng Z-F, Peng J, et al. The diagnostic value of circulating brain-specific MicroRNAs for ischemic stroke. Intern Med. 2016;55:1279–86.
47. Liu X, Li F, Zhao S, Luo Y, Kang J, Zhao H, et al. MicroRNA-124-mediated regulation of inhibitory member of apoptosis-stimulating protein of p53 family in experimental stroke. Stroke. 2013;44:1973–80.
48. Sun Y, Gui H, Li Q, Luo Z-M, Zheng M-J, Duan J-L, et al. MicroRNA-124 protects neurons against apoptosis in cerebral ischemic stroke. CNS Neurosci Ther. 2013;19:813–9.
49. Peng G, Yuan Y, Wu S, He F, Hu Y, Luo B. MicroRNA let-7e is a potential circulating biomarker of acute stage ischemic stroke. Transl Stroke Res. 2015;6:437–45.

3

Gastric mucosa-associated lymphoid tissue lymphoma and *Helicobacter pylori* infection

Qinglong Hu[1*], Yizhuo Zhang[2], Xiaoyan Zhang[3] and Kai Fu[3]

Abstract

Helicobacter pylori (*H. pylori*)-associated gastritis is one of the most common infectious diseases in the United States, China and worldwide. Gastric mucosa-associated tissue lymphoma (MALT lymphoma) is a rare mature B-cell neoplasm associated with *H. pylori* infection that is curable by antibiotics therapy alone. The pathological diagnosis of gastric MALT lymphoma can be reached by histological examination, immunohistochemical staining and B-cell clonality analysis. *H. pylori* eradication is the choice of therapy for early-stage gastric MALT lymphoma. High response rates and long-term survival have been reported in refractory and localized diseases treated with low-dose radiation therapy. Systemic chemotherapy is recommended for advanced-stage gastric MALT lymphoma and cases with large B-cell lymphoma transformation. Recent advances in the pathological diagnosis and management of gastric MALT lymphoma are reviewed in this article.

Keywords: Gastric MALT, *Helicobacter pylori*

Background

Helicobacter pylori (*H. pylori*) infection of the stomach is one of the most common diseases worldwide. According to the World Health Organization, *H. pylori* infection contributes to approximately 75 % of stomach cancers and 5.5 % of all cancers worldwide [1]. The infection rate varies in different countries of the world and also in different regions of China, from 55 to 80 % in the mainland to 15 % in Hong Kong and 40 % in Taiwan [2–4]. The infection rate is higher in rural areas than in cities [4]. Gastric mucosa-associated lymphoid tissue (MALT) lymphoma is a clonal B-cell neoplasm arising from post-germinal center B-cells in the marginal zone of the lymphoid follicles. *H. pylori* was identified from the gastric mucosa of patients with active chronic gastritis more than 30 years ago by Marshall and Warren [5]. *H. pylori* infection of the stomach is considered a major cause of chronic active gastritis and a major risk factor for gastric MALT lymphoma. Since the discovery of the association of *H. pylori* gastritis with gastric MALT lymphoma [6], extensive basic studies and clinical trials have been performed worldwide, and treatment guidelines have been recommended for *H. pylori*-associated gastritis and gastric MALT lymphoma [7–11]. Gastric MALT lymphoma is a rare disease. The estimated incidence of gastric lymphoma was approximately 0.3–0.8 per 100,000 people in Europe [8]. The incidence of gastric MALT lymphoma was approximately 0.38 per 100,000 people in the United States, according to a recent study. The incidence rates increased with age [12]. No population-based studies have been reported in the Chinese literature, and the incidence of gastric MALT lymphoma is unknown in China. We searched literature of studies of *H. pylori* gastritis and gastric MALT lymphoma in English and Chinese and reviewed the recent advances in the diagnosis and management of these two closely related diseases. Current issues in the diagnosis and management of the disease are also discussed.

* Correspondence: qinglonghu@hotmail.com
[1]Tucson Pathology Associates, PC Carondelet Saint Joseph Hospital, 351 North Wilmot Road, Tucson, AZ 85711, USA

Diagnosis of gastric MALT lymphoma

The diagnosis of gastric MALT lymphoma relies on clinical symptoms, endoscopic features and pathohistological examination of gastric biopsy tissue, as well as noninvasive tests for *H. pylori* infection, such as the ^{13}C-urea breath test and the monoclonal stool antigen test. The clinical presentation of patients with gastric MALT lymphoma is nonspecific. The symptoms include dyspepsia, vague epigastric pain, bloating and heartburn; more severe and alarming symptoms are anemia, melena, hematemesis, vomiting and weight loss.

Endoscopic examination with biopsy and histopathologic examination is a standard practice in the diagnosis of gastric MALT lymphoma in the United States and the Western world. The macroscopic changes of the gastric mucosa in MALT lymphoma are nonspecific, including thickening of the mucosal folds, irregular nodules, polypoid lesions, petechiae, edema, erosion and ulcers. The distribution of the lesions is usually patchy, with multiple foci. Therefore, sampling at different anatomic sites is recommended during gastric endoscopic examination and biopsy. Biopsies should be taken from abnormal and normal areas, including the antrum, the greater and lesser curvatures, and the fundus. At least two biopsies should be taken from each site of the stomach, and the tissue from each biopsy site should be fixed in separate containers with 10 % buffered formalin [13]. Sampling from multiple sites may be difficult in practice as it increases risk of complications, such as acute gastric bleeding, especially in patients on anticoagulant therapy. *H. pylori*-associated chronic active gastritis is present in the majority of patients with gastric MALT lymphoma.

Histopathologic features of gastric MALT lymphoma

Under microscopic examination, the biopsy tissue usually shows dense lymphoid infiltration with monotonous features. Germinal centers may be observed with the expansion of the marginal zone. The lymphoma cells are typically small and monotonous with monocytoid features, with small, round nuclei and a scant to moderate amount of pink to clear cytoplasm. Some cases may show prominent plasmacytoid differentiation mixed with small lymphocytes. The lymphocytes may infiltrate the glandular epithelium, resulting in the destruction of the glands, forming so-called "lymphoepithelial lesions". The lymphocytes in the glands are B-cells, which may be identified by immunohistochemical staining for B-cell and epithelial markers such as CD20 and pancytokeratin. However, these stains are not used routinely. Common immunohistochemical stains may include the B-cell markers CD20 and CD79a and the T-cell markers CD3 and CD5. Staining for CD21 may be helpful to highlight residual lymphoid follicles and expanding marginal zones. Aberrant expression of CD43 by the B-cells may be identified, which is a supporting evidence for gastric MALT lymphoma. The diagnosis of gastric lymphoma can be established by morphologic examination and immunohistochemical evaluation. However, a majority of the cases may require clonality analysis of the B-cells by in situ hybridization for kappa and lambda light chains with formalin-fixed tissue sections. The expression of kappa/lambda light chain may be weak, and they often cannot be detected by in situ hybridization. Negative expression of the light chains cannot rule out the diagnosis of lymphoma. If the result of in situ hybridization is inconclusive, further molecular studies, such as polymerase chain reaction (PCR), for immunoglobulin heavy chain (IgH) gene rearrangement may be beneficial. A definitive diagnosis of gastric MALT lymphoma is supported if clonal IgH gene rearrangement is demonstrated by a PCR study. However, this result is not a prerequisite for the diagnosis of gastric MALT lymphoma [14]. A report of "atypical lymphoid proliferation, suspicious for MALT lymphoma" may be issued for ambiguous cases. Clinical follow-up and repeat biopsy may finally lead to a definitive diagnosis. Wotherspoon and colleagues [15] observed a spectrum of histological changes between normal gastric mucosa, chronic active gastritis and gastric MALT lymphoma, as shown in Table 1. This histological grading is helpful in differential diagnosis. Histopathologic changes of Types 3 and 4 requires immunohistologic staining and/or molecular investigation to reach a definitive diagnosis. The biopsy tissues taken by endoscopy are usually small, and the layer of muscularis propria may not be observed in most of the biopsies. The depth of invasion of the gastric wall by the lymphoma cells is important for disease staging, and it should be evaluated and documented if identified under a microscope. Monotonous and dense lymphoid infiltration in the gastric mucosa may raise the suspicion of gastric MALT lymphoma. This requires the pathologist's experience and may be affected by the adequacy of tissue processing, the thickness of the tissue sectioning, and the quality of histologic staining. Immunohistochemical staining may show expansion of the B-cell compartment with sheets of B-cells. The thickness of the tissue sections can significantly affect the interpretation of compartment expansion of B-cells or T-cells. The tissue sections of the gastric biopsy should not be more than 3 μm in thickness. A false impression of mixed B-cell and T-cell proliferation may be obtained due to inadequate thickness of the tissue sections during immunostaining.

Gastric MALT lymphoma is a type of low-grade B-cell lymphoma with tissue infiltration by small lymphocytes. High-grade transformation to large B-cell lymphoma is uncommon. If high-grade lymphoma is present, the infiltration of large lymphoma cells may be a predominant

Table 1 Wotherspoon scale of confidence of histological diagnosis of lymphoma [15]

Grade	Description	Histological features
0	Normal	Scattered plasma cells in the lamina propria. No lymphoid follicles.
1	Chronic active gastritis	Small clusters of lymphocytes in the lamina propria. No lymphoid follicles. No LELs.
2	Chronic active gastritis with florid lymphoid follicle formation	Prominent lymphoid follicles with surrounding mantle zone and plasma cells.
3	Suspicious lymphoid infiltrate, probably reactive	Lymphoid follicles surrounded by CCL cells that infiltrate diffusely into the lamina propria and occasionally into the epithelium.
4	Suspicious lymphoid infiltrate, probably lymphoma	Lymphoid follicles surrounded by CCL cells that infiltrate diffusely into the lamina propria and into the epithelium in small groups.
5	Low-grade B-cell lymphoma of MALT	Presence of dense diffuse infiltrate of CCL cells in the lamina propria with prominent lymphoepithelial lesions.

CCL cells centrocyte-like cells (or marginal zone cells), *LEL* lymphoepithelial lesion

component or a minor component depending on the stage of transformation. Identification of residual low-grade components of MALT lymphoma may be helpful for the differential diagnosis of large B-cell lymphoma transformed from gastric MALT lymphoma versus primary diffuse large B-cell lymphoma or secondary stomach involvement by diffuse large B-cell lymphoma arising from other primary organs. Focal large B-cell transformation of gastric MALT lymphoma is an unfavorable prognostic feature and should be documented in the pathology report when it presents [16–19].

The majority of gastric MALT lymphoma is associated with *H. pylori* infection. *H. pylori* were reported in 50–100 % of Chinese patients with gastric MALT lymphoma [20–22]. Similar observations were also reported in other areas of the world [23]. Searching for *H. pylori* is recommended in routine H&E slides of gastric biopsies, and the status of *H. pylori* should be documented in the pathology report. Immunostaining for *H. pylori* on tissue sections appears to be the most specific and sensitive and should be performed whenever available (Fig. 1). We found that immunostaining saved the pathologist's time while searching for the microorganisms under the microscope due to the unambiguous features of the staining (personal observation), although Giemsa and Alcian blue stains also serve well as alternative stains with high sensitivity and specificity [24]. Patients with gastric MALT lymphoma positive for *H. pylori* have better responses to antibiotics eradication therapy. The persistence of *H. pylori* in gastric biopsies after antibiotics eradication therapy usually indicates reinfection or the development of bacteria species resistant to the antibiotics. Therefore, a change in the therapeutic protocol is recommended [25].

Molecular cytogenetic findings of gastric MALT lymphoma

Many factors potentially affect the responsiveness of gastric MALT lymphoma to *H. pylori* eradication therapy. A balanced chromosomal translocation, t(11; 18)(q21;q21), results in a API2/MALT1 fusion gene, which is functional in activating the nuclear factor kappa B pathway and is associated with the pathogenesis of gastric MALT lymphoma. During translocation t(11;18)(q21;q21), the N-terminal region of API2 fuses to the C-terminal region of the MALT1 gene. Multiple breakpoints were identified in exons 7 and 8 of the API2 gene, and 3 major breakpoints were identified in the MALT1 gene. This cytogenetic abnormality could be demonstrated in approximately 20 % of gastric MALT lymphomas of Chinese patients, ranging from 14 to 22 % [26, 27]. The patients negative for translocation t(11; 18)(q21;q21) showed a higher response rate than those positive for the translocation (78 % versus 22 %); higher median survival time was also observed in the negative cases [18, 26]. Therefore, the status of t(11; 18)(q21;q21) with the lymphoma is a strong predictor for therapeutic response and patient prognosis. Interphase fluorescence in situ hybridization (FISH) may be performed using dual-color break-apart API2 and MALT1 probes or a dual-color dual-fusion probe. The test is highly sensitive and specific. Therefore, FISH for t(11; 18)(q21;q21) on formalin-fixed tissue sections should be performed routinely in newly diagnosed patients. Reverse transcriptase polymerase chain reaction (RT-PCR) was designed to detect the mRNA transcript of the API2/MALT1 fusion gene with high sensitivity and specificity. RT-PCR can be performed with tissue sections of paraffin-embedded, formalin-fixed tissue block. However, more tissue sections are required for the PCR reaction than for a FISH study. Other genetic abnormalities observed in gastric MALT lymphoma include translocations t(14;18)/IgH-MALT1, t(1;14)/BCL10-IgH and t(3;14)/FOXP1-IgH. However, these translocations are uncommon and their clinical significance has not been defined. Therefore, routine testing is not recommended [14].

The most common differential diagnosis of gastric MALT lymphoma is severe chronic gastritis. Careful morphologic examination of hematoxylin and eosin-stained biopsy tissue sections is essential for differential

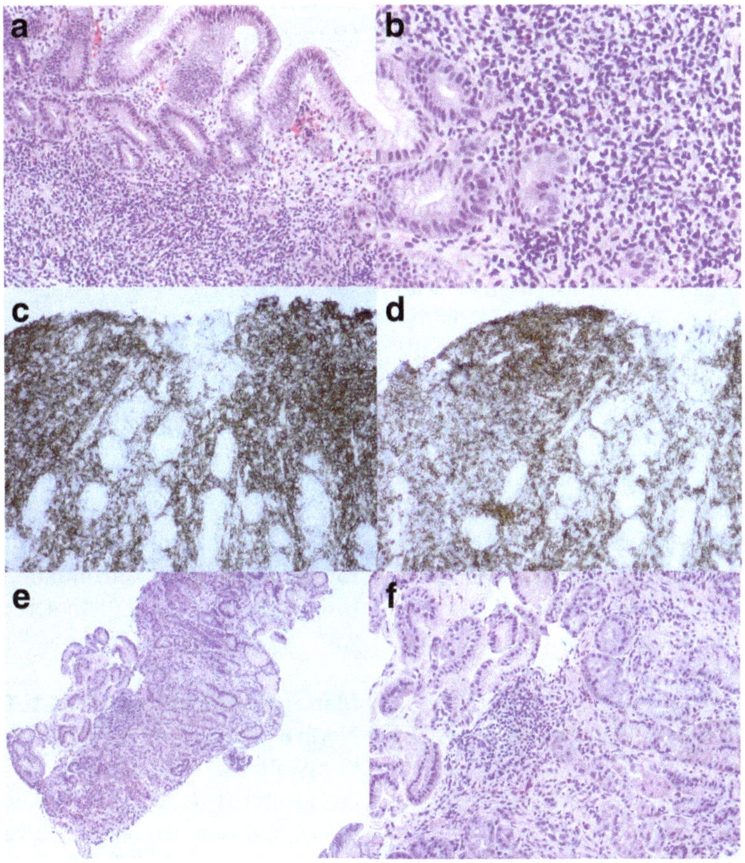

Fig. 1 Gastric biopsy showing intra-lamina small lymphocyte infiltrate with monotonous features (**a**, original magnification 100 X); foci of lymphoepithelial lesion (**b**, H&E, original magnification 200 X); CD20 immunostaining shows sheets of CD20+ small B-cells (**c**, original magnification 200 X); aberrant expression of CD43 is also detected (**d**, original magnification 200X). A repeat gastric biopsy 6 months after *H. pylori* eradication showed scattered intra-lamina infiltrates of small lymphocytes, plasma cells and a few small loose lymphoid aggregates, indicating complete remission (**e**, H&E, original magnification 100 X; **f**, 200 X)

diagnosis. Chronic gastritis usually shows less dense lymphoid infiltrates with mixed small lymphocytes and plasma cells and a lack of lymphoepithelial lesions, and it also appears more polymorphic. Immunostaining for B-cell and T-cell markers, such as CD20, CD3 and CD43, is helpful in difficult cases and may reveal well-preserved B-cell and T-cell compartments without evidence of lymphoepithelial lesions (Fig. 2).

Molecular diagnosis of gastric MALT lymphoma

In some cases, the histopathologic features are uncertain. Therefore, PCR for IgH gene rearrangement is helpful for

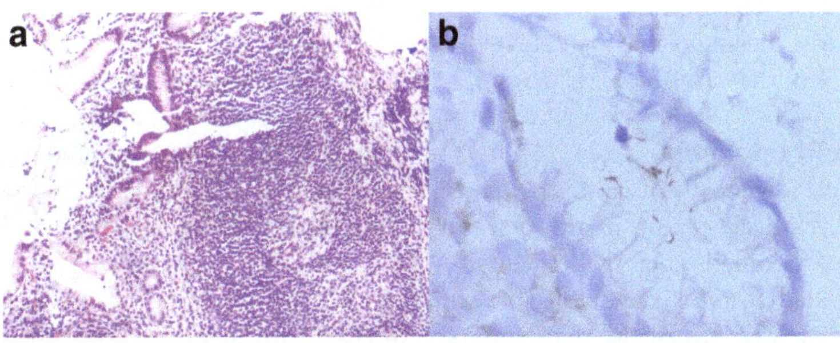

Fig. 2 Gastric biopsy shows *H. pylori*-associated chronic active gastritis with scattered small lymphocytes and plasma cells; a lymphoid follicle with a reactive germinal center and a slightly expanded marginal zone (**a**, H&E, original magnification 100 X). Immunostaining of *H. pylori* shows intra-foveolar bacteria with curving configuration, characteristic of *H. pylori* (**b**, immunohistochemical stain of *H. pylori*, original magnificantion 1000 X)

a definitive diagnosis. Some diagnostic laboratories in China have adapted PCR protocols for B-cell receptor gene clonality analysis, which were originally developed by European Biomed-2 Study Group [28]. The PCR for IgH gene rearrangement covers a majority of B-cell lymphomas with high clinical sensitivity and specificity. Routine testing for kappa light chain gene rearrangement is not recommended. Multiple sets of PCR primers are designed to detect more than 90 % cases of B-cell lymphomas. Adequate positive and negative controls together with patient specimens must be performed each time. The results of the controls should be included in the diagnostic report of the PCR analysis. A result cannot be reported if the control sample does not work or the DNA is disqualified or suboptimal for the test. Clinical false-positive and false-negative results have been reported in approximately 5–10 % of confirmed B-cell lymphoma cases. Therefore, it is important to interpret the PCR results in combination with histopathologic and immunophenotypic findings. A more conservative approach to the diagnosis may be taken for those atypical cases to avoid overdiagnosis and intervention with aggressive therapy.

Summary of pathologic diagnostic points of gastric MALT lymphoma

1. Infiltration of the gastric mucosa by dense, monomorphic small lymphocytes.
2. Lymphoepithelial lesions.
3. Dense B-cell infiltrates with sheet formation observed by immunohistochemical staining for CD20 and CD79a with aberrant expression of CD43.
4. *H. pylori* may be identified on hematoxylin and eosin-stained slides and confirmed by immunohistochemical staining.
5. In situ hybridization of the kappa and lambda light chains on tissue sections may show monoclonal light chain expression.
6. Monoclonal IgH gene rearrangement may be detected by PCR using formalin-fixed tissue and may be helpful in ambiguous cases.
7. API2/MALT1 gene rearrangement may be detected in approximately 20 % of the cases by FISH.

Staging of gastric MALT lymphoma

As soon as a pathological diagnosis of gastric MALT lymphoma is established, clinical staging of the disease should be performed. The modified Ann Arbor (Musshoff) system is recommended for the staging (Table 2) [25]. The majority of cases with gastric MALT lymphoma are in the early stage of disease, with lymphoma limited to the gastric mucosa, submucosa (stage I1E) and less commonly, in the superficial layer of the muscularis propria (stage I2E). Endoscopic ultrasound for the detection of lymphoma invasion of the stomach wall has been used in European countries. Routine abdominal CT scan is recommended for possible regional gastric lymph node involvement (stage II1E). Bone marrow involvement is uncommon, and routine bone marrow biopsy for staging is not recommended for patients with negative regional lymphadenopathy.

Table 2 Modified Ann Arbor (Musshoff) staging [25]

Modified Ann Arbor system	Extension of organ involvement by lymphoma
I1E	Mucosa, submucosa involvement
I2E	Muscularis propria, serosa, neighboring organs
II1E	Regional abdominal lymph nodes (compartment I + II)
II2E	Intra-abdominal distant lymph nodes
IIIE	Extra-abdominal lymph nodes
IV	Diffuse or disseminated infiltration of distant or extra-gastrointestinal organs, bone marrow

Management of gastric MALT lymphoma

Normal gastric mucosa lacks lymphoid aggregates; only rare scattered lymphocytes, plasma cells and eosinophils are identified in the gastric mucosa and submucosa. *H. pylori* infection triggers an inflammatory reaction with prominent neutrophil infiltration and lymphocytic proliferation. The lymphoid cells form lymphoid follicles with germinal center and minimal marginal zone expansion, which is characteristic for *H. pylori*-associated chronic active gastritis. The high prevalence of *H. pylori* infection and low incidence of gastric MALT lymphoma among the general population suggest that there is an interaction between *H. pylori* and host factors that determines the host susceptibility to MALT lymphoma. This observation has been supported by experimental studies. Certain genetic predispositions have been identified [29, 30]. An increased prevalence of both HLA-DQA1*0103 and HLA-DQB1*0601 alleles and DQA1*0103-DQB1*0601 haplotypes has been observed in patients with gastric MALT lymphoma [29]. Due to the close association of *H. pylori* with gastric MALT lymphoma, Wotherspoon, et al first used antibiotics to treat patients with gastric MALT lymphoma and induced dramatic regression of the lymphoma [6]. Since then, combined antibiotics for *H. pylori* eradiation has become a standard therapy for patients with gastric MALT lymphoma regardless of the status of *H. pylori* in the biopsy tissue. The majority of *H. pylori*-positive gastric MALT lymphomas are in early stage of disease, with involvement of the gastric mucosa and submucosa (stage I1E); invasion of the muscularis propria may be identified (stage I2E). Clinical studies have been performed for eradiation therapy of *H. pylori* gastritis and gastric MALT lymphoma over the last three decades. Guidelines for the diagnosis and management of *H. pylori* infection of the stomach were published and updated recently by the World Gastroenterology Organization, the American College of Gastroenterology, the Asian-Pacific Association of Gastroenterology and other professional organizations over the last decade (Table 3) [2, 7, 9, 11, 25, 31–36]. The guideline protocols are also adapted to *H. pylori* eradication therapy in gastric MALT lymphoma. A protocol combining a proton pump inhibitor (PPI) and two antibiotics, or "triple therapy," has been recommended as first-line therapy until recently. However, recent studies have shown an increase in drug resistance to "triple therapy" in China and other areas of the world [4, 33, 37]. Protocols with 14-day therapy appeared to have a higher response rate than 7-day therapy without an increase in side effects [9, 36]. Sequential therapy showed an advantage over conventional "triple therapy" and was recommended for the replacement of conventional "triple therapy" as the first-line *H. pylori* eradication therapy [38]. However, this result was not confirmed by recent studies in China and other countries of the world [11, 39, 40].

Although patients with gastric MALT lymphoma with no *H. pylori* are less responsive to *H. pylori* eradication, a portion of the *H. pylori*-negative cases are potentially curable by *H. pylori* eradication therapy alone [25]. The rationale for this finding has not been elucidated. It is suspected that some *H. pylori*-negative cases are false negatives due to patchy distribution of the microorganism in the gastric mucosa and limited tissue sampling during biopsy. PPI therapy before biopsy reduces the sensitivity of *H. pylori* detection. Therefore, PPI should be discontinued at least 2 weeks before *H. pylori* testing.

Follow-up examination was recommended in 3 months after finishing *H. pylori* eradication therapy. Tests such as the ^{13}C urea breath test or the monoclonal stool antigen test should be considered together with gastric endoscopic examination and biopsy. The patient's symptoms may disappear and *H. pylori* become undetectable with a negative breath test if the therapy is effective. The histological response usually lags behind the *H. pylori* eradication, and a lymphoma infiltrate may persist for 12 months or even longer. Scattered small lymphocytes and lymphoid aggregates may be identified with mild fibrosis (Fig. 2). The Groupe d'Etude des Lymphomes de l'Adult (GELA) grading system was recommended for the post-treatment evaluation of gastric MALT lymphoma (Table 4) [35, 38].

Immunohistochemical staining for B-cell and T-cell markers is helpful for the examination. The subsequent follow-up examinations may be arranged every 6 months in the first year, and then the frequency may be reduced to every 12 months. CT-scan or PCR study for IgH gene rearrangement is generally not recommended during follow-up.

If the above first-line therapy fails to eradicate *H. pylori*, a second-line protocol should be considered. Increased numbers of strains of *H. pylori* resistant to clarithromycin and metronidazole have been reported during the last decade, ranging from 30 to 100 % [4, 33, 37]. "Quadruple therapy" including PPI, bismuth, tetracycline and metronidazole has been recommended [7]. The patient's noncompliance may be one of the most common reasons for the failure of *H. pylori* eradication therapy. Discontinuation of medicine is common as soon as patients experience relief of symptoms or unexpected side effects. Therefore, patient education for therapy compliance is

Table 3 First-Line Regimens for *Helicobacter pylori* Eradication (ACG Guideline 2007) [7]

Regimen	Duration (days)	Eradication Rates	Comments
Triple therapy: *Standard dose PPI b.i.d. (esomeprazole is q.d.), clarithromycin 500 mg b.i.d., amoxicillin 1,000 mg b.i.d.	10–14	70–85 %	Consider in non-penicillin-allergic patients who have not previously received a macrolide
Triple therapy (penicillin allergic): Standard dose PPI b.i.d., clarithromycin 500 mg b.i.d., metronidazole 500 mg b.i.d.	10–14	70–85 %	Consider in penicillin-allergic patients who have not previously received a macrolide or are unable to tolerate bismuth quadruple therapy
Bismuth therapy: Bismuth subsalicylate 525 mg p.o. q.i.d. metronidazole 250 mg p.o. q.i.d., tetracycline 500 mg p.o. q.i.d., ranitidine 150 mg p.o. b.i.d. or standard dose PPI q.d. to b.i.d.	10–14	75–90 %	Consider in penicillin-allergic patients
Sequential therapy: PPI + amoxicillin 1 g b.i.d. ×5 followed by: PPI, clarithromycin 500 mg, tinidazole 500 mg b.i.d. ×5	10	>90 %	Requires validation in North America

Note: The above recommended treatments are not all FDA approved. The FDA-approved regimens are as follows:
Bismuth 525 mg q.i.d. + metronidazole 250 mg q.i.d. + tetracycline 500 mg q.i.d. × 2 weeks + H_2RA as directed × 4 weeks
Lansoprazole 30 mg b.i.d. + clarithromycin 500 mg b.i.d. + amoxicillin 1 g b.i.d. × 10 days
Omeprazole 20 mg b.i.d. + clarithromycin 500 mg b.i.d. + amoxicillin 1 g b.i.d. × 10 days
Esomeprazole 40 mg q.d. + clarithromycin 500 mg b.i.d. + amoxicillin 1 g b.i.d. × 10 days
Rabeprazole 20 mg b.i.d. + clarithromycin 500 mg b.i.d. + amoxicillin 1 g b.i.d. × 7 days
ACG American College of Gastroenterology, *PPI* proton pump inhibitor, *p.o.* orally, *q.d.* daily, *b.i.d.* twice daily, *t.i.d.* three times daily, *q.i.d.* four times daily
* Standard dosages for PPIs are as follows: lansoprazole 30 mg p.o., omeprazole 20 mg p.o., pantoprazole 40 mg p.o., rabeprazole 20 mg p.o., esomeprazole 40 mg p.o

Table 4 GELA grading system for post-treatment evaluation of gastric MALT lymphoma [35]

GELA category	Histological features	Clinical category
Complete histological response (CR)	Total disappearance of lymphoid infiltrate with only scattered small lymphocytes and plasma cells. Regressive stromal changes with fibrosis and separation of glands can be observed.	Complete remission
Probable minimal residual disease (pMRD)	Small lymphoid aggregates present, stromal regressive changes are usually present.	Complete remission
Responding residual disease (rRD)	Overt residual lymphoma with a nodular or diffuse infiltrate of neoplastic B-cells but with clear evidence of regressive stromal changes characterized by fine fibrosis and an "empty lamina propria."	Partial remission
No change (NC)	Persistence of overt lymphoma identical to that observed at diagnosis with no morphological features to suggest response to treatment (such as stromal fibrosis).	Stable or progressive disease

GELA Groupe d'Etude des Lymphomes de l'Adult, *MALT* mucosa-associated lymphoid tissue

important. The question should be raised about therapeutic compliance if the first-line therapy fails before starting the second-line therapy. Testing for drug sensitivity is recommended when drug resistance is suspected. However, in clinical practice, a culture-based approach is unfeasible, especially in the developing world and China. Recently, point mutation analysis of *H. pylori* genes by PCR, such as the 23S rRNA and gyrA genes, has been used for assessing *H. Pylori* susceptibility to clarithromycin and levofloxacin, respectively [41, 42]. Other factors may affect the result of *H. pylori* eradication therapy and gastric MALT lymphoma. Non-steroidal anti-inflammatory drugs potentially affect the result of *H. pylori* eradication therapy. *H. pylori* eradication therapy should be performed after the discontinuation of non-steroidal anti-inflammatory drugs, according to the Japanese Ministry of Health, Labor and Welfare [43]. Tinidazole is an analogue of metronidazole and has been used in the sequential therapy protocol for *H. pylori* eradication. The inhibitory effect of tinidazole on parasites, such as amoebae and bacteria is similar to metronidazole. However, the side effects are more tolerable and last a shorter time. The most common side effects include nausea, bitter taste and itchiness. Drinking alcohol while taking tinidazole may cause vomiting, headache, shortness of breath, flushing and an increase in blood pressure. Therefore, alcohol should be avoided during therapy with tinidazole. Lower rates of drug resistance of *H. pylori* were found with tinidazole than with metronidazole in a recent in vitro study [2].

Primary gastric large B-cell lymphoma may be a de novo large B-cell lymphoma or may be transformed from gastric MALT lymphoma. Large B-cell lymphoma transformation from gastric MALT lymphoma is uncommon, ranging from 0.5 % to 1 % in a 7-year observation period [44, 45]. It is a more aggressive lymphoma, and systematic chemotherapy is recommended for the first-line treatment. However, the current antibiotics protocols for *H. pylori* showed limited side effects, and complete remission has been observed in a portion of the patients with gastric large B-cell lymphoma. Therefore, antibiotics therapy may be beneficial for those cases with early-stage gastric large B-cell lymphoma [16–19].

Radiation therapy is effective for patients with localized gastric MALT lymphoma and is recommended for patients who have early-stage disease and are refractory to antibiotics therapy. The dosage of radiation has been reduced over the last two decades. Wirth et al. reported a study comprising 102 patients with gastric MALT lymphoma, 58 previously untreated cases and 44 with recurrent or residual disease after prior medical or surgical therapy. The overall 5-year recurrence-free survival rate was 97 % with low doses of less than or equal to 30 cGy based on a median follow-up time of 7.5 years [46]. Another recent study included 22 patients with stage IE and IIE gastric MALT lymphoma, including 8 cases with t(11;18)(q21;q21) translocation. All patients reached complete remission after radiation with 30 cGy without severe toxicity. The overall and 5-year relapse-free survival rates were 91 and 84 %, respectively at a median follow-up time of 74 months [47, 48]. The side effects of radiation are usually transient and tolerable, including nausea, anorexia and vomiting. Low-dosage radiation therapy preserves the function of the stomach and avoids nutritional disease induced by surgical resection. Surgical intervention is preserved only for those patients with ulcers, acute bleeding and/or perforation.

Systematic chemotherapy should be considered only for those patients with advanced-stage disease with involvement of distant lymph nodes and/or bone marrow and those patients with large B-cell transformation. It was reported recently that 95 % of MALT lymphoma patients who failed in *H. pylori* eradication antibiotics therapy showed 95 % complete remission after combined chlorambucil and rituximab therapy, which was superior to single-drug chemotherapy with chlorambucil or rituximab alone [44, 45, 49–51]. R-CHOP [Rituximab, Cyclophosphamide, Hydroxydaunorubicin (adriamycin), Oncovin (vincristine) and Prednisone] is recommended as a standard protocol for gastric large B-cell lymphoma [52].

Conclusions

H. pylori gastritis is one of the most common infectious diseases in China and worldwide. Gastric MALT lymphoma is a neoplasm associated with *H. pylori* infection and is the first malignant disease that can be cured by antibiotics therapy alone. The pathogenesis of gastric MALT lymphoma is not yet elucidated. The estimated incidence of gastric MALT lymphoma is low (0.3-0.4/100,000) in the United States and Europe, but the incidence is not known in China. The diagnosis of gastric MALT lymphoma can be challenging. Due to its rarity, most general pathologists may not be familiar with the diagnostic features of gastric MALT lymphoma. Therefore, underdiagnosis or overdiagnosis of this disease is not uncommon. Combined hematoxylin and eosin staining and immunohistochemical staining are routinely used for the pathologic diagnosis of the lymphoma. Special studies, such as molecular studies, are required to reach a definitive diagnosis in difficult cases. Expert consultation by hematopathologists may be beneficial for diagnosis. The *H. pylori* eradication regimen for early-stage gastric MALT lymphoma is similar to *H. pylori* gastritis. However, over-therapy, such as systemic chemotherapy for early-stage gastric MALT lymphoma, is not uncommon in the developing world, such as in China. *H. pylori* reinfection is common after eradication therapy due to cross-infection through person-to-person contact, especially among family members. Communication between gastroenterologists and oncologists is advised for the proper management of patients with gastric MALT lymphoma.

Abbreviations

H. pylori, Helicobacter pylori; IgH, immunoglobulin heavy chain; MALT, mucosa-associated lymphoid tissue; PCR, polymerase chain reaction; PPI, proton pump inhibitor

Acknowledgement

The authors appreciate Cheng Wang for preparing manuscript figures.

Funding

This study is partially supported by the Tucson Pathology Association, PC, Tucson, Arizona, United States.

Authors' contributions

QH selecting topic, collecting and reviewing literature, writing and editing the manuscript. KF selecting topic, editing and discussing the manuscript. YZ reviewing literature, discussing and editing the manuscript. XZ editing manuscript and preparing manuscript figures. All authors read and approved the final manuscript.

Competing interests

The authors declare that they have no competing interests.

Author details

[1]Tucson Pathology Associates, PC Carondelet Saint Joseph Hospital, 351 North Wilmot Road, Tucson, AZ 85711, USA. [2]Department of Hematology, Tianjin Medical University Cancer Institute and Hospital, National Clinical Research Center of Cancer, Tianjin Key Laboratory of Cancer Prevention and Therapy, Tianjin 300060, China. [3]Department of Pathology and Microbiology, University of Nebraska Medical Center, 983135 Nebraska Medical Center, Omaha, NE 68198, USA.

References

1. Arfaoui D, Elloumi H, Ben Abdelaziz A. Helicobacter pylori and gastric adenocarcinoma. Tunis Med. 2009;87(4):231–6.
2. Hunt RH, Xiao SD, Megraud F, Leon-Barua R, Bazzoli F, van der Merwe S, Vaz Coelho LG, Fock M, Fedail S, Cohen H, et al. Helicobacter pylori in developing countries. World Gastroenterology Organisation Global Guideline. J Gastrointestin Liver Dis. 2011;20(3):299–304.
3. Tu J, Chen Z, Cao W, Liu J, Zhao X, Wu X. Epidemiological survey of infection of Helicobacter pylori in health examing people in Lanzhou. Clinical Focus. 2012;27(20):1754–56. [in Chinese].
4. Gao L, Yang J, Guan J. Analysis on infection and drug resistance of Helicobacter pylori acquired in community and country. China Healthcare Front. 2009;18:104–5. [in Chinese].
5. Marshall BJ, Warren JR. Unidentified curved bacilli in the stomach of patients with gastritis and peptic ulceration. Lancet. 1984;1(8390):1311–5.
6. Wotherspoon AC, Ortiz-Hidalgo C, Falzon MR, Isaacson PG. Helicobacter pylori-associated gastritis and primary B-cell gastric lymphoma. Lancet. 1991; 338(8776):1175–6.
7. Chey WD, Wong BC, Practice Parameters Committee of the American College of G. American College of Gastroenterology guideline on the management of Helicobacter pylori infection. Am J Gastroenterol. 2007; 102(8):1808–25.
8. Ullrich A, Fischbach W, Blettner M. Incidence of gastric B-cell lymphomas: a population-based study in Germany. Ann Oncol. 2002;13(7):1120–7.
9. Zagari RM, Romano M, Ojetti V, Stockbrugger R, Gullini S, Annibale B, Farinati F, Ierardi E, Maconi G, Rugge M, et al. Guidelines for the management of Helicobacter pylori infection in Italy: The III Working Group Consensus Report 2015. Dig Liver Dis. 2015;47(11):903–12.
10. Lee SY. Current progress toward eradicating Helicobacter pylori in East Asian countries: differences in the 2013 revised guidelines between China, Japan, and South Korea. World J Gastroenterol. 2014;20(6):1493–502.
11. Chinese Society of Gastroenterology CSGoHp, Liu WZ, Xie Y, Cheng H, Lu NH, Hu FL, Zhang WD, Zhou LY, Chen Y, Zeng ZR, et al. Fourth Chinese National Consensus Report on the management of Helicobacter pylori infection. J Dig Dis. 2013;14(5):211–21.
12. Khalil MO, Morton LM, Devesa SS, Check DP, Curtis RE, Weisenburger DD, Dores GM. Incidence of marginal zone lymphoma in the United States, 2001-2009 with a focus on primary anatomic site. Br J Haematol. 2014; 165(1):67–77.
13. Sipponen P, Price AB. The Sydney System for classification of gastritis 20 years ago. J Gastroenterol Hepatol. 2011;26 Suppl 1:31–4.
14. Bacon CM, Du MQ, Dogan A. Mucosa-associated lymphoid tissue (MALT) lymphoma: a practical guide for pathologists. J Clin Pathol. 2007;60(4):361–72.
15. Wotherspoon AC, Doglioni C, Diss TC, Pan L, Moschini A, de Boni M, Isaacson PG. Regression of primary low-grade B-cell gastric lymphoma of mucosa-associated lymphoid tissue type after eradication of Helicobacter pylori. Lancet. 1993;342(8871):575–7.
16. Cavanna L, Pagani R, Seghini P, Zangrandi A, Paties C. High grade B-cell gastric lymphoma with complete pathologic remission after eradication of Helicobacter pylori infection: report of a case and review of the literature. World J Surg Oncol. 2008;6:35.
17. Mitsuhashi K, Yamashita K, Goto A, Adachi T, Kondo Y, Kasai K, Suzuki R, Saito M, Arimura Y, Shinomura Y. Gastric diffuse large B-cell lymphoma cured with Helicobacter pylori eradication regardless of whether it contains features of MALT lymphoma. Intern Med. 2014;53(7):695–8.
18. Zullo A, Hassan C, Andriani A, Cristofari F, Cardinale V, Spinelli GP, Tomao S,

Morini S. Primary low-grade and high-grade gastric MALT-lymphoma presentation. J Clin Gastroenterol. 2010;44(5):340–4.

19. Kuo SH, Yeh KH, Wu MS. Helicobacter pylori eradication therapy is effective in the treatment of early-stage H pylori-positive gastric diffuse large B-cell lymphomas. Blood. 2012;119:4838–44.
20. Liu G, Tang W, Yang J, Si Y. Analysis of association between gastric lymphoid lymphoma and helicobacter pylori. Clin Med China. 2005;21(4): 318–20. [in Chinese].
21. Wang J, Wang M. Analysis of 85 cases of gastric lymphoid lymphoma about helicobacter pylori. J Xinxiang Med Coll. 2005;22(4):358–59 [in Chinese].
22. Sun H. Analysis of 36 cases of gastric lymphoid lymphoma. Dalian Med Coll. 2010;5–40. [in Chinese].
23. Gong EJ, Ahn JY, Jung HY, Park H, Ko YB, Na HK, Jung KW, Kim DH, Lee JH, Choi KD, et al. Helicobacter pylori eradication therapy is Effective as the initial treatment for patients with H. pylori -negative and disseminated gastric mucosa-associated lymphoid tissue lymphoma. Gut Liver. 2016. [Epub ahead of print].
24. Hartman DJ, Owens SR. Are routine ancillary stains required to diagnose Helicobacter infection in gastric biopsy specimens? An institutional quality assurance review. Am J Clin Pathol. 2012;137(2):255–60.
25. Ruskone-Fourmestraux A, Fischbach W, Aleman BM, Boot H, Du MQ, Megraud F, Montalban C, Raderer M, Savio A, Wotherspoon A, et al. EGILS consensus report. Gastric extranodal marginal zone B-cell lymphoma of MALT. Gut. 2011;60(6):747–58.
26. Chen T, Cen L, Xiao R, Yang JH, Jiang NK, Lu XZ, Zhang Y, Lu JT. Prognostic value of t(11; 18) (q21; q21) for gastric mucosa-associated lymphoid tissue lymphoma. Zhonghua yi xue yi chuan xue za zhi = Zhonghua yixue yichuanxue zazhi = Chin J Med Genet. 2012;29(2):181–183.
27. Cui M. Pathology and gene fusion in gastric MALT lymphoma. Zhengzhou Coll. 2011;1–70. [in Chinese].
28. Evans PA, Pott C, Groenen PJ, Salles G, Davi F, Berger F, Garcia JF, van Krieken JH, Pals S, Kluin P, et al. Significantly improved PCR-based clonality testing in B-cell malignancies by use of multiple immunoglobulin gene targets. Report of the BIOMED-2 Concerted Action BHM4-CT98-3936. Leukemia. 2007;21(2):207–14.
29. Hussell T, Isaacson PG, Crabtree JE, Spencer J. The response of cells from low-grade B-cell gastric lymphomas of mucosa-associated lymphoid tissue to Helicobacter pylori. Lancet. 1993;342(8871):571–4.
30. Kawahara Y, Mizuno M, Yoshino T, Yokota K, Oguma K, Okada H, Fujiki S, Shiratori Y. HLA-DQA1*0103-DQB1*0601 haplotype and Helicobacter pylori-positive gastric mucosa-associated lymphoid tissue lymphoma. Clin Gastroenterol Hepatol. 2005;3(9):865–8.
31. Fischbach W, Goebeler ME, Ruskone-Fourmestraux A, Wundisch T, Neubauer A, Raderer M, et al. Most patients with minimal histological residuals of gastric MALT lymphoma after successful eradication of Helicobacter pylori can be managed safely by a watch and wait strategy: experience from a large international series. Gut. 2007;56(12): 1685–7.
32. Malfertheiner P, Megraud F, O'Morain CA, Atherton J, Axon AT, Bazzoli F, Gensini GF, Gisbert JP, Graham DY, Rokkas T, et al. Management of Helicobacter pylori infection–the Maastricht IV/Florence Consensus Report. Gut. 2012;61(5):646–64.
33. Fock KM, Katelaris P, Sugano K, Ang TL, Hunt R, Talley NJ, Lam SK, Xiao SD, Tan HJ, Wu CY, et al. Second Asia-Pacific Consensus Guidelines for Helicobacter pylori infection. J Gastroenterol Hepatol. 2009;24(10):1587–600.
34. Zucca E, Dreyling M, Group EGW. Gastric marginal zone lymphoma of MALT type: ESMO clinical recommendations for diagnosis, treatment and follow-up. Ann Oncol. 2009;20 Suppl 4:113–4.
35. Copie-Bergman C, Gaulard P, Lavergne-Slove A, Brousse N, Flejou JF, Dordonne K, de Mascarel A, Wotherspoon AC. Proposal for a new histological grading system for post-treatment evaluation of gastric MALT lymphoma. Gut. 2003;52(11):1656.
36. Rollan A, Arab JP, Camargo MC, Candia R, Harris P, Ferreccio C, Rabkin CS, Gana JC, Cortes P, Herrero R, et al. Management of Helicobacter pylori infection in Latin America: a Delphi technique-based consensus. World J Gastroenterol. 2014;20(31):10969–83.
37. Wang Y. Comparative studies of therapeutic protocols of Helicobacter pylori eradication and in vitro drug resistance. Hebei Univ Med Sci. 2009;1–52. [in Chinese].
38. Vaira D, Zullo A, Hassan C, Fiorini G, N. V. Sequential therapy for helicobacter pylori eradication: The time is now!. Therap Adv Gastroenterol. 2009;2(6):317–22.
39. Rakici H, Akdogan RA, Bedir R, Copur A, Yilmaz A. Comparison of standard triple therapy, sequential therapy and moxifloxacin-based triple therapy for Helicobacter pylori infection: Patients' compliance and bacterial eradication rates. J Dig Dis. 2014;15(9):508–13.
40. Zhou L, Zhang J, Chen M, Hou X, Li Z, Song Z, He L, Lin S. A comparative study of sequential therapy and standard triple therapy for Helicobacter pylori infection: a randomized multicenter trial. Am J Gastroenterol. 2014; 109(4):535–41.
41. Rimbara E, Noguchi N, Kawai T, Sasatsu M. Fluoroquinolone resistance in Helicobacter pylori: role of mutations at position 87 and 91 of GyrA on the level of resistance and identification of a resistance conferring mutation in GyrB. Helicobacter. 2012;17(1):36–42.
42. De Francesco V, Zullo A, Ierardi E, Giorgio F, Perna F, Hassan C, et al. Phenotypic and genotypic Helicobacter pylori clarithromycin resistance and therapeutic outcome: benefits and limits. J Antimicrob Chemother. 2010; 65(2):327–32.
43. Taniyama K, Shimbo T, Iwase H, Tanaka S, Watanabe N, Uemura N. Evidence-based therapy according to the guideline for gastric ulcers is cost-effective in Japan. J Physiol Pharmacol. 2011;62(6):627–35.
44. Martinelli G, Laszlo D, Ferreri AJ, Pruneri G, Ponzoni M, Conconi A, Crosta C, Pedrinis E, Bertoni F, Calabrese L, et al. Clinical activity of rituximab in gastric marginal zone non-Hodgkin's lymphoma resistant to or not eligible for anti-Helicobacter pylori therapy. J Clin Oncol. 2005;23(9):1979–83.
45. Olszewski AJ, Castillo JJ. Comparative outcomes of oncologic therapy in gastric extranodal marginal zone (MALT) lymphoma: analysis of the SEER-Medicare database. Ann Oncol. 2013;24(5):1352–9.
46. Wirth A, Gospodarowicz M, Aleman BM, Bressel M, Ng A, Chao M, Hoppe RT, Thieblemont C, Tsang R, Moser L, et al. Long-term outcome for gastric marginal zone lymphoma treated with radiotherapy: a retrospective, multi-centre, International Extranodal Lymphoma Study Group study. Ann Oncol. 2013;24(5):1344–51.
47. Abe S, Oda I, Inaba K, Suzuki H, Yoshinaga S, Nonaka S, Morota M, Murakami N, Itami J, Kobayashi Y, et al. A retrospective study of 5-year outcomes of radiotherapy for gastric mucosa-associated lymphoid tissue lymphoma refractory to Helicobacter pylori eradication therapy. Jpn J Clin Oncol. 2013; 43(9):917–22.
48. Okada H, Takemoto M, Kawahara Y, Nasu J, Takenaka R, Kawano S, Inoue M, Ichimura K, Tanaka T, Shinagawa K, et al. A prospective analysis of efficacy and long-term outcome of radiation therapy for gastric mucosa-associated lymphoid tissue lymphoma. Digestion. 2012;86(3):179–86.
49. Zucca E, Conconi A, Laszlo D, Lopez-Guillermo A, Bouabdallah R, Coiffier B, Sebban C, Jardin F, Vitolo U, Morschhauser F, et al. Addition of rituximab to chlorambucil produces superior event-free survival in the treatment of patients with extranodal marginal-zone B-cell lymphoma: 5-year analysis of the IELSG-19 Randomized Study. J Clin Oncol. 2013;31(5):565–72.
50. Zullo A, Hassan C, Andriani A, Cristofari F, De Francesco V, Ierardi E, Tomao S, Morini S, Vaira D. Eradication therapy for Helicobacter pylori in patients with gastric MALT lymphoma: a pooled data analysis. Am J Gastroenterol. 2009;104(8):1932–7. quiz 1938.
51. Hancock BW, Qian W, Linch D, Delchier JC, Smith P, Jakupovic I, Burton C, Souhami R, Wotherspoon A, Copie-Bergman C, et al. Chlorambucil versus observation after anti-Helicobacter therapy in gastric MALT lymphomas: results of the international randomised LY03 trial. Br J Haematol. 2009; 144(3):367–75.
52. Detterbeck F, Tanoue L, Reid A. National comprehensive cancer network. J Natl Compr Cancer Netw. 2013;11(4):365–6.

4

Burden of hepatocellular carcinoma among hispanics in South Texas

John Ha[1*], Aysha Chaudhri[1], Abhishek Avirineni[1] and Jen-Jung Pan[1,2]

Abstract

Background: Hepatocellular carcinoma (HCC) is one of the fastest rising causes of cancer-related mortality in the United States (U.S.). Despite improved HCC screening and surveillance guidelines, significant race/ethnicity-specific disparities in hepatocellular carcinoma remain, disproportionately affecting at risk racial minorities in the U.S. The current review aims to provide an updated analysis on race/ethnicity-specific disparities in HCC epidemiology with a focus on predisposing risk factors.

Conclusion: Among different race/ethnicities in the U.S., Hispanics experienced the greatest burden of HCC, particularly those residing in South Texas. It is important to understand that the underlying etiologies for these disparities are complex and multi-factorial. Some of these risk factors for developing chronic liver disease include non-alcoholic fatty liver disease/non-alcoholic steatohepatitis and alcohol use. In addition, population genetics, acculturation of ethnic minorities, and access to healthcare may be further contributing to the observed disparities in HCC. By increasing awareness, improved modalities for screening and surveillance for HCC are important in guiding future research for targeted preventive and therapeutic interventions.

Keywords: Hepatocellular carcinoma, Race disparities, Ethnic disparities, Non-alcoholic fatty liver disease, Metabolic syndrome, Healthcare access

Background

Hepatocellular Carcinoma (HCC) is the fifth leading cause of cancer-related death in the United States (U.S.) among men and ninth in women [1]. In the U.S., the incidence of HCC has more than doubled since the 1980's, becoming one of the fastest rising causes of cancer-related mortality, which may be attributed to the rising trend of chronic Hepatitis C Virus infection (HCV) and incidence of non-alcoholic fatty liver disease (NAFLD) [2]. Despite improvements in screening and surveillance efforts for HCC, the overall 5-year survival for HCC remains dismal. According to the Surveillance, Epidemiology, and End Results (SEER) registry, the overall 5-year survival for localized HCC is less than 31%, with more advanced HCC having significantly worse outcomes [3].

Among different race/ethnic populations in the U.S., significant disparities in HCC have been observed in recent years, where Hispanics experienced the greatest increase in HCC incidence by approximately 36% [4]. Hispanics accounted for nearly 50% of the U.S. population growth from 2000 to 2010 and are projected to reach 30% of the U.S. population within the next three decades [5]. It is conceivable for the incidence of HCC in the U.S. to increase proportionally with the rising Hispanic population. Although Texas accounts for the second greatest distribution of Hispanics by state, the incidence of HCC among Hispanics in Texas, particularly South Texas, was significantly higher than elsewhere in the U.S. [6]. This trend may be caused by the prevalence of unique regional risk factors, such as metabolic syndrome, NAFLD, population genetics, and different environmental exposures. The current review aims to provide an updated epidemiological analysis of the Hispanic cohort in South Texas and future implications of HCC in the region.

* Correspondence: Johnathan.s.ha@uth.tmc.edu
[1]Department of Internal Medicine, The University of Texas Health Science Center at Houston, 6431 Fanin St, MSB 1.150, Houston, TX 77030, USA

Epidemiology of HCC

HCC remains a leading cause of cancer-related morbidity and mortality in the U.S. There are over 20,000 new cases of HCC in the U.S. per year, where the incidence has tripled over the last three decades [7, 8]. Through analysis of the 2003–2011 SEER database, Ha et al. demonstrated the age-adjusted HCC incidence to be 9.4/100,000 (95% confidence interval (CI) 9.3–9.5). When evaluating HCC incidence between race/ethnicities, Asians has the highest overall incidence of HCC (18.6/100,000; 95% CI 18.2–19.0), followed by African Americans (15.7/100,000; 95% CI 15.4–16.1), Hispanics (11.8/100,000; 95% CI 11.6–12.2), and Non-Hispanic whites (7.0/100,000; 95% CI 6.9–7.1). During the same period, Hispanics were seen to have the greatest increase in HCC incidence (+35.8%) with an annual percent change of 4% [4]. When observing the overall trend in the incidence of HCC in the U.S., recent studies suggest HCC incidence to have stabilized; however, this trend may not be reflected among Hispanics residing in Texas, a region not included in the national SEER registry [4, 9, 10].

Compared to other 49 states in the U.S., Texas reported the highest age-adjusted incidence of HCC [11]. Hispanics residing in Texas make up approximately 20% of the overall U.S. Hispanic population, where 2,500 new cases of HCC are seen annually within this race/ethnic cohort [6, 12]. Approximately 70% of the population in South Texas is Hispanic, where the region accounts for more than half of the incident cases of HCC in Texas overall [6]. From 1995 to 2010, Hispanics of South Texas had the greatest incidence of HCC (12.1/100,000; 95% CI 11.7–12.5) compared to Hispanics in the rest of Texas (10.9/100,000; 95% 10.6–11.2) and the U.S. (8.4/100,000; 95% CI 8.2–8.7) [13]. The disproportionate incidence of HCC among Hispanics residing in South Texas may be attributed to the region's distribution of associated risk factors for HCC such diabetes mellitus and obesity, which contribute to NAFLD. Furthermore, there are likely cultural and socioeconomic factors in this population, which serve as barriers to care leading to higher rates of HCC in this region.

Unique Risk Factors for HCC among Hispanics

Among the general population, there are several well-known risk factors that play an important role in the development of HCC, such as chronic hepatitis B (HBV) and HCV, NAFLD, metabolic syndrome, environmental exposures, and population genetics. It is conceivable that Hispanics of South Texas are disproportionately affected by these risk factors, thus increasing their risk of developing HCC. Although difficult to evaluate precise prevalence of HCV in the U.S., Edlin et al. evaluated the possible under-representation of HCV prevalence by analyzing a 2003–2010 U.S. population-based database, National Health and Nutrition Examination Survey (NHANES), and determined at least 1 million persons were excluded and unaccounted for by the database [14]. Despite underreporting of HCV, the overall trend in the prevalence of HCV since 1992 seems to be downtrending from 2.4% to approximately 1.6%, and has remained stable since 2006 [15, 16]. There are limited studies when evaluating for race/ethnicity-specific disparities of HCV, particularly among the Hispanic population. Kuniholm et al. analyzed the NHANES database along with supplementing data from the Hispanic Community Health Study/Study of Latinos (HCHS/SOL) and reported a heterogeneous epidemiological make-up of HCV among Hispanics. Specifically, they found Mexican Americans to have an intermediate HCV prevalence (1.9%; 95% CI 1.1–3.4) compared to low HCV prevalence seen among South American Hispanics (0.4%; 95% CI 0.1–1.9) and high HCV prevalence seen among Puerto Rican Hispanics (11.6%; 95% CI 9.4–14.1) [17]. A randomized, population-based study cohort in a predominantly Mexican American community of south Texas (i.e. Cameron County Cohort) also reported similar findings with a weighted HCV prevalence of 2.3% ($n = 1,113$ 95% CI 2.1–3.4%) [18]. Race/ethnicity plays an important role among patients with HCV in the development of HCC. El-Serag et al. demonstrated among 149,407 U.S. Veterans with HCV viremia, only 6% were Hispanic; however, Hispanics had the highest annual incidence rate of cirrhosis (28.8%) and HCC (7.8%) compared to non-Hispanic whites (21.6 and 4.7%, respectively) [19]. Even after adjusting for co-morbid conditions, such as human immunodeficiency virus co-infection, obesity, and diabetes, Hispanics were still at higher risk of developing cirrhosis (hazard ratio (HR) 1.28; 95% CI 1.21–1.37) and HCC (HR 1.61; 95% CI 1.44–1.80) compared to non-Hispanic whites [19].

Due to the growing obesity epidemic, NAFLD has become the leading cause of elevated liver enzymes, where cirrhosis secondary to NAFLD is currently the most rapidly growing indication for liver transplantation within the U.S. [20–22]. Several studies in the past analyzed the NHANES database and determined Hispanics to have the greatest prevalence of NAFLD, ranging between 8.4 and 45%, compared to non-Hispanic whites and African Americans who experienced lower prevalence rates of NAFLD [23–28]. A recent study by Younossi et al. found similar findings when evaluating for race/ethnic disparities among patients with non-alcoholic steatohepatitis (NASH), where being Hispanic was significantly associated with developing NASH (odds ratio (OR) 1.75; 95% CI 1.28–2.33; $p = 0.0005$) [29]. In the setting of NAFLD, studies have shown that obesity and diabetes were independent risk factors for the development of HCC [30, 31]. A meta-analysis of 11 cohort-studies reported that compared to normal weight individuals, overweight patients (body mass index (BMI) 25.1 to 30 kg/m^2) had a 17% higher risk of developing HCC (relative risk (RR) 1.17; 95% CI 1.02–1.34), whereas obese patients (BMI greater than 30 kg/m^2) had an increased risk of 89% (RR 1.89; 95% CI 1.51–2.36) [32]. Similarly, Nair et al. evaluated 659 patients with HCC and determined obesity to be an independent predictor for HCC among those with cryptogenic cirrhosis (OR 11.1; 95% CI 1.5–87.4; $p = 0.02$) [33]. It may be difficult to associate obesity with HCC independent of diabetes mellitus, since both disease processes are strongly correlated with one another and are components of metabolic syndrome. Turati et al. conducted a multicenter case–control study to separately explore the association of obesity and diabetes mellitus among patients with 'hepatitis-free' HCC in Italy. Among 185 cases of HCC and 404 controls, obese patients were almost twice as likely of developing HCC (OR 1.92; 95% CI 1.03–3.79) and a 4-fold increased likelihood in patients with diabetes mellitus (OR 4.33; 95% CI 1.89–9.86). The risk of HCC further increased when combining more than one component of metabolic syndrome, such as being overweight and having diabetes mellitus (OR 4.75, 95% CI 1.75–12.89) [34]. Similar findings were noted in a U.S. study that calculated population attributable fractions (PAFs), which are utilized to better characterize the impact of specific HCC risk factors by evaluating both exposure and outcome associations along with the prevalence of each exposure in the population. Makarova-Rusher et al. reported metabolic disorders (i.e. obesity, diabetes, metabolic syndrome, and NAFLD) to carry the greatest HCC PAF risk, followed by HCV, alcohol use, smoking, HBV, and genetics disorders. Furthermore, they determined metabolic disorders carried the greatest HCC PAF risk among Hispanics (PAF 39.3%; 95% CI 31.9–46.7%), followed by non-Hispanic whites (PAF 34.8%; 95% CI 33.1–36.5%), Asians (PAF 21.8; 95% CI 16.5–27.1%), and African Americans (PAF 14.4%; 95% CI 6.4–22.3%) [35].

Between 2010 and 2011, approximately two-thirds of adults in the U.S. were at least overweight (68.5%; 95% CI 65.2–71.6%), 35% of those being obese. However, the prevalence of obesity disproportionately affected racial minorities, mainly African Americans (48.1%) and Hispanics (42.5%) [36]. When evaluating the Hispanic population in south Texas (i.e. Cameron County Hispanic Cohort – CCHC), Pan et al. reported 83.1% of their participants being either overweight (32.4%) or obese (50.7%) [37]. Similar trends were observed with diabetes mellitus where the overall prevalence of diabetes in the U.S. is estimated to be approximately 9.3%; however, the CCHC had a prevalence of 27.6% [37, 38]. The high prevalence of obesity and diabetes in Cameron County are likely contributing to the high rates of NAFLD [39, 40], which may explain why the annual incidence of HCC in this unique population is greater than Hispanics in other parts of the U.S.

Although obesity and insulin resistance are major contributing factors for the development of hepatic steatosis, the heterogeneous prevalence of hepatic steatosis between race/ethnicities may suggest other influencing factors, such as genetic variance [41]. From the Dallas Heart Study, Romeo et al. first demonstrated that the rs738409 [G] allele in the patatin-like phospholipase domain-containing 3 (*PNPLA3*) gene was significantly associated with increased hepatic fat levels ($p = 5.9 \times 10^{-10}$) and hepatic inflammation ($p = 3.7 \times 10^{-4}$), where the allele was more commonly seen among Hispanics (0.49) compared to non-Hispanic whites (0.23) and African Americans (0.17) [42]. Similarly, Wagenknecht et al. demonstrated *PNPLA3* rs738409 [G] to be two times more common in Hispanics compared African Americans (40% vs. 19%), which seems consistent with the greater prevalence of NAFLD among Hispanics compared to African Americans (24% vs. 9%) [43]. In addition to race/ethnic variance, G allele homozygotes have greater than a twofold increase of hepatic fat content compared to noncarriers [42]. *PNPLA3* genetic polymorphism may influence not only hepatic fat accumulation but also contribute to a more aggressive disease course. A meta-analysis of 16 studies performed by Sookoian et al. concluded GG homozygotes to have not only 73% higher hepatic fat content, but also a 3.24-fold greater risk for necroinflammatory scores and 3.2-fold greater risk of developing fibrosis compared to the CC homozygote control ($p < 1.0 \times 10^{-9}$). Furthermore, GG homozygotes were significantly more likely to develop NASH compared to the control group (OR 3.488; 95% CI 1.859–6.545; $p < 2.0 \times 10^{-4}$) [44].

Factors causing disparities in South Texas

As alluded to earlier, Asians have the highest incidence of overall HCC in the U.S. followed by African Americans, Hispanics, and Non-Hispanic whites; however, recent trends have noted the greatest percent increase in HCC incidence among Hispanics whereas Asians are experiencing a decline in the incidence of HCC [4, 45]. Furthermore, Hispanic individuals have a 5-fold greater risk of HCC mortality based on the Third NHANES, a nationwide survey from 1988 to 1994, with Hispanic ethnicity being an independent predictor of mortality (HR 5.14; 95% CI 1.75–15.06) [46]. Although the disease process of HCC and its associated risk factors, which include but are not limited to diabetes, NAFLD, HCV, HBV and metabolic syndrome, play an important role in race/ethnicity specific disparities of HCC, it is also important to understand complex psychosocial influences which may contribute to disparities seen in healthcare where it affects ethnic minorities to a greater degree.

Alcohol use, either as a primary factor or in combination with HBV, HCV or diabetes, is a key culprit for the development of HCC. The effect of alcohol on the liver is well studied where chronic alcohol use greater than 80 grams per day for more than 10 years leads to a 5-fold increase in the risk of HCC [47]. We want to focus on race/ethnic disparities in alcohol consumption, specifically affecting the Hispanic population since it is the largest and fastest growing minority group in the U.S. According to the 2012–2013 longitudinal study from the National Epidemiologic Survey on Alcohol and Related Conditions (NESARC), Hispanics had the greatest prevalence of heavy drinking (31.6%) compared to other race/ethnic minorities [48]. Additionally, cross-sectional and longitudinal data noted a declining trend of alcohol consumption in the U.S. when people reach their 30s; however, alcohol consumption in Blacks and Hispanics decreases less dramatically with age [48, 49]. One study analyzed the health of Hispanic men, including drinking habits, living on the Texas-Mexico border in an area with a 93.2% Hispanic population. This cross-sectional study included 945 Hispanic men in the CCHC from Brownsville, Texas between 2004 through 2015. In the study, "heavy drinking" was defined as more than 4 drinks on any day or 14 drinks per week and found that 7.3% reported heavy drinking and 60.3% reported occasional alcohol consumption [50].

Several theories have been proposed to explain the differences in drinking patterns among various racial/ethnic groups, including degree of acculturation and level of awareness of racial/ethnic stigma. Acculturation refers to how immigrants adapt to the behaviors, values and culture of the host society. One proposed theory is that more acculturated Hispanics have higher levels of alcohol use since acculturation has been associated with more liberal views towards drinking [51]. The Hispanic Americans Baseline Alcohol Survey (HABLAS) was used to study alcohol patterns in 5 major metropolitan areas in the United States. They concluded that Hispanic men of Puerto Rican and Mexican origin consume a higher number of drinks on average compared with Hispanics of Cuban or Dominican origin. This study also found that regardless of country of origin, the number of drinks per week for women, for instance, was positively correlated with level of acculturation [49]. In a prospective study of 36,864 Hispanics (18,485 US-born and 18,379 foreign-born) from Hawaii and California, the incidence of HCC was statistically greater in US-born Hispanics compared with foreign-born Hispanics even when controlling for age and gender (HR 1.61; 95% CI 1.20–2.17) [52]. It is conceivable that these observations are attributed to greater prevalence of HCC risk factors (e.g. HCV, alcohol consumption, and metabolic syndrome) among more acculturated US-born Hispanics [53]. Although there is no specific data on the population distribution of US-born versus foreign-born Hispanics in South Texas, U.S.-born Hispanics constitute 70% of the Hispanic population in Texas whereas foreign-born Hispanics account for 30% of Hispanics in Texas [54]. Another theory compared the level of awareness of racial/ethnic stigma on drinking patterns. A 2005 U.S. National Alcohol Survey, a nationally representative telephone-based survey of adults ages 18 and older, showed that Hispanics who self-reported experiences of racial/ethnic discrimination had a 2-fold greater risk of problem drinking [52]. Similarly, another study showed that Hispanics who self-reported major or lifetime discrimination attributed to race or ethnicity were 62% more likely of drinking heavily (OR 1.62; 95% CI 1.10–2.40) [55]. To our knowledge, there have not been studies specifically looking at the degree of racial/ethnic discrimination experienced by South Texas Hispanics. As mentioned previously, Hispanics of Mexican origin are the predominant Hispanic group in South Texas and studies have shown that Mexican Americans who are darker, more educated, and have more contact with Whites experience more discrimination [56].

Access to healthcare plays a vital role in treatment and survival in patients with HCC. A retrospective cohort study using SEER HCC registry evaluated early invasive therapy (i.e. tumor ablation, hepatic resection, liver transplant) and analyzed variations in survival across racial/ethnic groups. The study demonstrated median survival improvement from 4 to 6 months without treatment to 40 months with treatment among Hispanics. However, decreased utilization of invasive treatment strategies were noted among African American and Hispanic patients with HCC. In turn, there were higher rates of mortality among African Americans (HR 1.24; 95% CI 1.15–1.33) and Hispanic patients (HR 1.08; 95% CI 1.01–1.15) and lower rates of mortality in Asians (HR 0.87; 95% CI 0.82–0.93) compared with non-Hispanic whites [57]. Similarly, Altekruse et al. characterized trends of HCC mortality from 2000 to 2010 and noted significantly increased rates of HCC mortality among non-Hispanic whites, African Americans, and Hispanics, whereas decreased rates of HCC mortality was seen among Asians [9]. Although the exact etiology behind these disparate findings is unclear, these trends may be from greater awareness of HBV and greater awareness and implementation of HCC screening and surveillance programs among patients with chronic HBV, many of whom are Asian.

Conclusion

In summary, race/ethnicity-specific disparities persist in the epidemiology of HCC. Hispanics, particularly populations residing in south Texas, seem to experience more disparate trends in the incidence and prevalence of HCC. These may be attributed to increased exposures to well known risk factors, such as excessive alcohol consumption, obesity and diabetes mellitus, in turn resulting in the development of NAFLD/NASH. In addition, population genetics may predispose this unique race/ethnic cohort to a greater propensity of developing HCC compared to other race groups. Current literature suggests complex psychosocial factors that further complicate disparities seen in HCC including degree of acculturation, access to healthcare, and provider-specific variables of HCC screening and surveillance of at-risk patients. Improved awareness in screening and surveillance modalities of HCC among Hispanics are important in guiding future research for targeted preventive and therapeutic interventions.

Abbreviations

BMI: Body mass index; CCHC: Cameron county Hispanic cohort; HBV: Hepatitis B virus; HCC: Hepatocellular carcinoma; HCV: Hepatitis C virus; NAFLD: Non-alcoholic fatty liver disease; NASH: Non-alcohoic steatohepatitis; NESARC: National epidemiologic survey on alcohol and related conditions; NHANES: National health and nutritional examination survey; SEER: Surveillance, epidemiology, and end results; U.S.: United States

Acknowledgements

Not applicable.

Funding

No relevant funding or disclosures to be made.

Authors' contributions

JH – Conceptualization, design, investigation, drafting of manuscript, critical review and editing. AC – Investigation, contributor of manuscript, critical review and editing. AA – Investigation, contributor of manuscript. JP – Conceptualization, design, critical review and editing, supervision. All authors read and approved the final manuscript.

Competing interests

The authors declare that they have no competing interests.

Author details

[1]Department of Internal Medicine, The University of Texas Health Science Center at Houston, 6431 Fanin St, MSB 1.150, Houston, TX 77030, USA. [2]Division of Gastroenterology, Hepatology and Nutrition, Department of Internal Medicine, The University of Texas Health Science Center at Houston, 6431 Fanin St, MSB 4.234, Houston, TX 77030, USA.

References

1. Siegel RL, Miller KD, Jemal A. Cancer statistics, 2015. CA Cancer J Clin. 2015; 65(1):5–29.
2. Singal AG, El-Serag HB. Hepatocellular Carcinoma from Epidemiology to Prevention: Translating Knowledge into Practice. Clin Gastroenterol Hepatol. 2015;13(12):2140–51.
3. Surveillance E, and End Results (SEER) Program (http://www.seer.cancer.gov) SEER*Stat Database: Incidence - SEER 9 Regs Research Data, Nov 2012 Sub (1973–2010) < Katrina/Rita Population Adjustment > – Linked To County Attributes - Total U.S., 1969–2011 Counties, National Cancer Institute, DCCPS, Surveillance Research Program, Surveillance Systems Branch, released April 2013, based on the November 2012 submission. In
4. Ha J, Yan M, Aguilar M, Bhuket T, Tana MM, Liu B, et al. Race/ethnicity-specific disparities in cancer incidence, burden of disease, and overall survival among patients with hepatocellular carcinoma in the United States. Cancer. 2016;122(16):2512–23.
5. Ennis SR R-VM, Albert NG..The Hispanic population: 2010. 2010 Census brief. US Census Bureau 5/2011. Available from: URL: http://www.census.gov/prod/cen2010/briefs/c2010br-04.pdf.
6. Ramirez AG, Weiss NS, Holden AE, Suarez L, Cooper SP, Munoz E, et al. Incidence and risk factors for hepatocellular carcinoma in Texas Latinos: implications for prevention research. PLoS ONE. 2012;7(4), e35573.
7. El-Serag HB. Hepatocellular carcinoma. N Engl J Med. 2011;365(12):1118–27.
8. El-Serag HB, Kanwal F. Epidemiology of hepatocellular carcinoma in the United States: Where are we? Where do we go? Hepatology. 2014;60(5):1767–75.
9. Altekruse SF, Henley SJ, Cucinelli JE, McGlynn KA. Changing hepatocellular carcinoma incidence and liver cancer mortality rates in the United States. Am J Gastroenterol. 2014;109(4):542–53.
10. Njei B, Rotman Y, Ditah I, Lim JK. Emerging trends in hepatocellular carcinoma incidence and mortality. Hepatology. 2015;61(1):191–9.
11. White DL, Thrift AP, Kanwal F, Davila J, El-Serag HB. Incidence of Hepatocellular Carcinoma in All 50 United States, From 2000 Through 2012. Gastroenterology. 2016;48:538–543.e1.
12. Texas Department of State Health Services Texas Cancer Registry (http://www.dshs.state.tx.us/tcr) SEER*Stat Database, 1995–2010 Limited-Use Incidence, Texas statewide, Texas Department of State Health Services, created June 2013, based on NPCR-CSS Submission, cut-off 11/30/12.
13. Ramirez AG, Munoz E, Holden AE, Adeigbe RT, Suarez L. Incidence of hepatocellular carcinoma in Texas Latinos, 1995–2010: an update. PLoS ONE. 2014;9(6), e99365.
14. Edlin BR, Eckhardt BJ, Shu MA, Holmberg SD, Swan T. Toward a more accurate estimate of the prevalence of hepatitis C in the United States. Hepatology. 2015;62(5):1353–63.
15. Armstrong GL, Wasley A, Simard EP, McQuillan GM, Kuhnert WL, Alter MJ. The prevalence of hepatitis C virus infection in the United States, 1999 through 2002. Ann Intern Med. 2006;144(10):705–14.
16. Klevens RM, Hu DJ, Jiles R, Holmberg SD. Evolving epidemiology of hepatitis C virus in the United States. Clin Infect Dis. 2012;55 Suppl 1:S3–9.
17. Kuniholm MH, Jung M, Everhart JE, Cotler S, Heiss G, McQuillan G, et al. Prevalence of hepatitis C virus infection in US Hispanic/Latino adults: results from the NHANES 2007–2010 and HCHS/SOL studies. J Infect Dis. 2014; 209(10):1585–90.
18. Watt GP, Vatcheva KP, Beretta L, Pan JJ, Fallon MB, McCormick JB, et al. Hepatitis C virus in Mexican Americans: a population-based study reveals relatively high prevalence and negative association with diabetes. Epidemiol Infect. 2016;144(2):297–305.
19. El-Serag HB, Kramer J, Duan Z, Kanwal F. Racial differences in the progression to cirrhosis and hepatocellular carcinoma in HCV-infected veterans. Am J Gastroenterol. 2014;109(9):1427–35.
20. Flegal KM, Carroll MD, Kit BK, Ogden CL. Prevalence of obesity and trends in the distribution of body mass index among US adults, 1999–2010. JAMA. 2012;307(5):491–7.
21. Vernon G, Baranova A, Younossi ZM. Systematic review: the epidemiology and natural history of non-alcoholic fatty liver disease and non-alcoholic steatohepatitis in adults. Aliment Pharmacol Ther. 2011;34(3):274–85.
22. Wong RJ, Aguilar M, Cheung R, Perumpail RB, Harrison SA, Younossi ZM, et al. Nonalcoholic Steatohepatitis Is the Second Leading Etiology of Liver Disease Among Adults Awaiting Liver Transplantation in the United States. Gastroenterology. 2014;148:547–55.
23. Ruhl CE, Everhart JE. Determinants of the association of overweight with elevated serum alanine aminotransferase activity in the United States. Gastroenterology. 2003;124(1):71–9.
24. Clark JM, Brancati FL, Diehl AM. The prevalence and etiology of elevated aminotransferase levels in the United States. Am J Gastroenterol. 2003;98(5):960–7.
25. Browning JD, Szczepaniak LS, Dobbins R, Nuremberg P, Horton JD, Cohen JC, et al. Prevalence of hepatic steatosis in an urban population in the United States: impact of ethnicity. Hepatology. 2004;40(6):1387–95.
26. Lazo M, Hernaez R, Eberhardt MS, Bonekamp S, Kamel I, Guallar E, et al. Prevalence of nonalcoholic fatty liver disease in the United States: the Third National Health and Nutrition Examination Survey, 1988–1994. Am J Epidemiol. 2013;178(1):38–45.
27. Schneider AL, Lazo M, Selvin E, Clark JM. Racial differences in nonalcoholic fatty liver disease in the U.S. population. Obesity (Silver Spring). 2014;22(1):292–9.
28. Smits MM, Ioannou GN, Boyko EJ, Utzschneider KM. Non-alcoholic fatty liver disease as an independent manifestation of the metabolic syndrome: results of a US national survey in three ethnic groups. J Gastroenterol Hepatol. 2013;28(4):664–70.
29. Younossi ZM, Stepanova M, Negro F, Hallaji S, Younossi Y, Lam B, et al. Nonalcoholic fatty liver disease in lean individuals in the United States. Medicine. 2012;91(6):319–27.
30. Lee SS, Jeong SH, Byoun YS, Chung SM, Seong MH, Sohn HR, et al. Clinical features and outcome of cryptogenic hepatocellular carcinoma compared to those of viral and alcoholic hepatocellular carcinoma. BMC Cancer. 2013;13:335.

31. El-Serag HB, Tran T, Everhart JE. Diabetes increases the risk of chronic liver disease and hepatocellular carcinoma. Gastroenterology. 2004;126(2):460–8.
32. Larsson SC, Wolk A. Overweight, obesity and risk of liver cancer: a meta-analysis of cohort studies. Br J Cancer. 2007;97(7):1005–8.
33. Nair S, Mason A, Eason J, Loss G, Perrillo RP. Is obesity an independent risk factor for hepatocellular carcinoma in cirrhosis? Hepatology. 2002;36(1):150–5.
34. Turati F, Talamini R, Pelucchi C, Polesel J, Franceschi S, Crispo A, et al. Metabolic syndrome and hepatocellular carcinoma risk. Br J Cancer. 2013; 108(1):222–8.
35. Makarova-Rusher OV, Altekruse SF, McNeel TS, Ulahannan S, Duffy AG, Graubard BI, et al. Population attributable fractions of risk factors for hepatocellular carcinoma in the United States. Cancer. 2016;122(11):1757–65.
36. Ogden CL, Carroll MD, Kit BK, Flegal KM. Prevalence of childhood and adult obesity in the United States, 2011–2012. JAMA. 2014;311(8):806–14.
37. Pan JJ, Qu HQ, Rentfro A, McCormick JB, Fisher-Hoch SP, Fallon MB. Prevalence of metabolic syndrome and risks of abnormal serum alanine aminotransferase in Hispanics: a population-based study. PLoS ONE. 2011; 6(6), e21515.
38. Centers for Disease Control and Prevention. National Diabetes Statistics Report: Estimates of Diabetes and Its Burden in the United States, 2014. Atlanta: U.S. Department of Health and Human Services; 2014.
39. Pan JJ, Fisher-Hoch SP, Chen C, Feldstein AE, McCormick JB, Rahbar MH, et al. Burden of nonalcoholic fatty liver disease and advanced fibrosis in a Texas Hispanic community cohort. World J Hepatol. 2015;7(11):1586–94.
40. Jiao J, Watt GP, Lee M, Rahbar MH, Vatcheva KP, Pan JJ, et al. Cirrhosis and Advanced Fibrosis in Hispanics in Texas: The Dominant Contribution of Central Obesity. PLoS ONE. 2016;11(3), e0150978.
41. Caldwell SH, Ikura Y, Iezzoni JC, Liu Z. Has natural selection in human populations produced two types of metabolic syndrome (with and without fatty liver)? J Gastroenterol Hepatol. 2007;22 Suppl 1:S11–9.
42. Romeo S, Kozlitina J, Xing C, Pertsemlidis A, Cox D, Pennacchio LA, et al. Genetic variation in PNPLA3 confers susceptibility to nonalcoholic fatty liver disease. Nat Genet. 2008;40(12):1461–5.
43. Wagenknecht LE, Palmer ND, Bowden DW, Rotter JI, Norris JM, Ziegler J, et al. Association of PNPLA3 with non-alcoholic fatty liver disease in a minority cohort: the Insulin Resistance Atherosclerosis Family Study. Liver Int. 2011;31(3):412–6.
44. Sookoian S, Pirola CJ. Meta-analysis of the influence of I148M variant of patatin-like phospholipase domain containing 3 gene (PNPLA3) on the susceptibility and histological severity of nonalcoholic fatty liver disease. Hepatology. 2011;53(6):1883–94.
45. Centers for Disease C, Prevention. Hepatocellular carcinoma - United States, 2001–2006. MMWR Morb Mortal Wkly Rep. 2010;59(17):517–20.
46. Younossi ZM, Stepanova M. Hepatitis C virus infection, age, and Hispanic ethnicity increase mortality from liver cancer in the United States. Clin Gastroenterol Hepatol. 2010;8(8):718–23.
47. Morgan TR, Mandayam S, Jamal MM. Alcohol and hepatocellular carcinoma. Gastroenterology. 2004;127(5 Suppl 1):S87–96.
48. Dawson DA, Goldstein RB, Saha TD, Grant BF. Changes in alcohol consumption: United States, 2001–2002 to 2012–2013. Drug Alcohol Depend. 2015;148:56–61.
49. Ramisetty-Mikler S, Caetano R, Rodriguez LA. The Hispanic Americans Baseline Alcohol Survey (HABLAS): Alcohol consumption and sociodemographic predictors across Hispanic national groups. J Subst Use. 2010;15(6):402–16.
50. Watt GP, Vatcheva KP, Griffith DM, Reininger BM, Beretta L, Fallon MB, et al. The Precarious Health of Young Mexican American Men in South Texas, Cameron County Hispanic Cohort, 2004–2015. Prev Chronic Dis. 2016;13, E113.
51. Vaeth PA, Wang-Schweig M, Caetano R. Drinking, Alcohol Use Disorder, and Treatment Access and Utilization Among U.S. Racial/Ethnic Groups. Alcohol Clin Exp Res. 2017;41(1):6–19.
52. Mulia N, Ye Y, Zemore SE, Greenfield TK. Social disadvantage, stress, and alcohol use among black, Hispanic, and white Americans: findings from the 2005 U.S. National Alcohol Survey. J Stud Alcohol Drugs. 2008;69(6):824–33.
53. Setiawan VW, Wei PC, Hernandez BY, Lu SC, Monroe KR, Le Marchand L, et al. Disparity in liver cancer incidence and chronic liver disease mortality by nativity in Hispanics: The Multiethnic Cohort. Cancer. 2016;122(9):1444–52.
54. "Demographic Profile of Hispanics in Texas, 2014." Pew Research Center, Washington, D.C. Available from: http://www.pewhispanic.org/states/state/tx/.
55. Borrell LN, Diez Roux AV, Jacobs Jr DR, Shea S, Jackson SA, Shrager S, et al. Perceived racial/ethnic discrimination, smoking and alcohol consumption in the Multi-Ethnic Study of Atherosclerosis (MESA). Prev Med. 2010;51(3–4):307–12.
56. Ortiz V, Telles E. Racial Identity and Racial Treatment of Mexican Americans. Race Soc Probl. 2012;4:1.
57. Mathur AK, Osborne NH, Lynch RJ, Ghaferi AA, Dimick JB, Sonnenday CJ. Racial/ethnic disparities in access to care and survival for patients with early-stage hepatocellular carcinoma. Arch Surg. 2010;145(12):1158–63.

5

Engineering CAR-T cells

Cheng Zhang[1], Jun Liu[1], Jiang F. Zhong[2] and Xi Zhang[1*]

Abstract

Chimeric antigen receptor redirected T cells (CAR-T cells) have achieved inspiring outcomes in patients with B cell malignancies, and are now being investigated in other hematologic malignancies and solid tumors. CAR-T cells are generated by the T cells from patients' or donors' blood. After the T cells are expanded and genetically modified, they are reinfused into the patients. However, many challenges still need to be resolved in order for this technology to gain widespread adoption. In this review, we first discuss the structure and evolution of chimeric antigen receptors. We then report on the tools used for production of CAR-T cells. Finally, we address the challenges posed by CAR-T cells.

Keywords: Chimeric antigen receptor redirected T cells, CAR-T cells, Structure, Evolution, Production, Viral vector

Background

Chimeric antigen receptors (CARs) are engineered receptors that can graft an arbitrary specificity onto an immune effector cell (T cell). CARs include three parts: an extracellular antigen recognition domain of the single-chain Fragment variant (scFv) derived from an antibody), a transmembrane domain and an intracellular T cell activation domain of CD3ζ [1]. CAR-T cell therapy is designed to redirect a patient's or donor's T cells to specifically target and destroy tumor cells. This approach shows great promise for haematologic malignancies and solid tumors without major histocompatibility complex restriction [2]. In this review, we first discuss the structure and evolution of CARs. We then report on the tools used for production of CAR-T cells. Finally, we address the challenges posed by CAR-T cells.

Structure of CAR-T cells

CARs consist of an ectodomain, transmembrane domain and endodomain [3] (Fig. 1).

Ectodomain

The ectodomain is the domain of a membrane protein that is outside the cytoplasm and exposed to the extracellular space. The ectodomain in this case consists of signal peptide, antigen recognition region and spacer [1, 3].

The role of a signal peptide is to direct the nascent protein into the endoplasmic reticulum. The scFv, which serves as the signal peptide of the ectodomain in a CAR, is formed by the variable portions of heavy and light chains of an immunoglobulin fused through a flexible linker. An antigen recognition domain is usually a scFv with a simple ectodomain and more exotic recognition components, which can be used to recognize any antigen if it can bind targets with high affinity. The connection between the antigen binding domain and the transmembrane domain relied on the spacer. The simplest form of spacer is the hinge region of IgG1 and is sufficient for most scFv-based constructs.

Transmembrane domain

The transmembrane domain, from the most membrane-proximal component of the endodomain, consists of a hydrophobic alpha helix that spans the membrane [1, 3, 4]. The stability of the receptor is related to the transmembrane domain. The presence of the native CD3-zeta transmembrane can cause the incorporation of the artificial TCR into the native TCR. At present, the CD28 transmembrane domain is the most stable receptor.

Endodomain

The endodomain is the functional end of the receptor, and the most common component is CD3 ζ included three immunoreceptor tyrosine-based activation motifs (ITAMs) [3, 4]. After antigen recognition, the receptors

* Correspondence: zhangxxi@sina.com
[1]Department of Hematology, Xinqiao Hospital, Third Military Medical University, Chongqing 400037, People's Republic of China

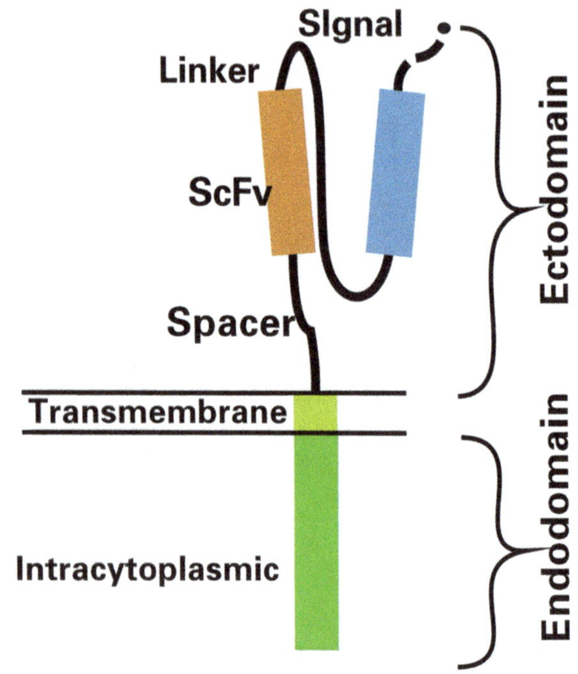

Fig. 1 Structure of chimeric antigen receptor (CAR). The CAR includes ectodomain, transmembrane domain and endodomain

cluster and signal was activated, then the sigal is transmitted to the T cell. Co-stimulatory signaling is needed during this profression.

Evolution of CAR-T cells

Since the initial development of CARs in 1989, CAR-T cells can be divided into four generations according to the structure of the endodomain (Fig. 2). The evolution of CAR therapy is an excellent example of the application of basic research to the clinic.

First generation

Single structure from the CD3 ζ- chain or FcεRIγ from the intracellular domain for the first generation of CARs is the typical characteristics, which is the primary transmitter of signals from endogenous T cell receptor (TCR) [5, 6]. However, these CAR-T cells could not produce enough interleukin-2 (IL-2), so in order to kill tumor cells it was necessary to administer exogenous IL-2. Therefore, the first generation of CAR-T cell therapy transfected with single-chain receptors benefitted substantially from the accompanying administration of cytokines [7].

Recent studies showed that the deletion of phosphorylation on ITAM A and C in the CD3ζ signaling moiety could decrease the apoptosis signal, which is beneficial for the continuous expression of the transgene [8, 9]. However, more studies were performed with CAR-T cells with the CD3ζ-chain than the FcεRIγ-chain in clinics. The reason may be that three ITAMs were included in CD3ζ-chain, but only one in the FcεRIγ-chain. On the other hand, the CAR-T cells with the CD3ζ-chain were more effective at activating T cells and killing tumor cells, although they had lower expression levels *in vitro*. The transmembrane domain of CAR-T cells consists of a dimer of homologous or heterologous in combinations of CD3, CD8 and CD28, which can mediate optimal cellular activation via the dimerization of CARs and the functional interaction of this receptor with the endogenous TCR. Carcinoembryonic Ag-specific CD3ζ (MFEζ) -CAR-T cells, alpha-folate receptor (FR) -CAR-T cells, CE7R-CAR-T cells, scFv(G250)-CAR-T cells, GD2-

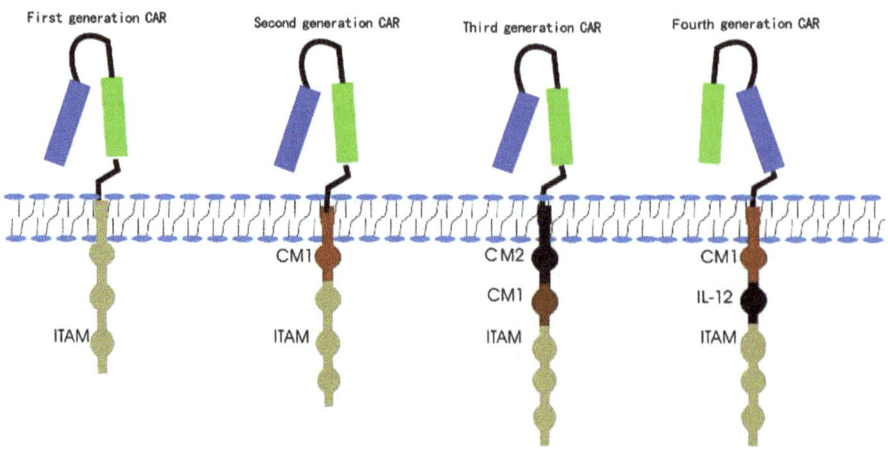

Fig. 2 Evolution of chimeric antigen receptor (CAR) from the first generation to the fourth generation. Single chain antibody (CD3ζ or FcεRIγ) links the ITAM at transmembrane region for the first generation. Costimulatory molecule (CM1), such as CD28, has been engineered to the signal transduction region for the second generation. Another costimulatory molecule (CM2) based on the second generation for the third generation has been engineered to the signal transduction region, such as combining CD134 or CD137. The interleukin-12 (IL-12) based on the second generation for the fourth generation has been engineered to the signal transduction region. ITAM: Immunoreceptor tyrosine-based activation motifs

CAR-Tcells and CD10- CAR-T cells were used to treat different tumors [10–15]. However, most of these studies with first-generation CAR-T cells did not achieve the desired outcomes because of inadequate proliferation, a short life span *in vivo* and insufficient secreted cytokines.

Second generation

Dual signal was the typical characteristics for T cell activation. Three different receptor types including the T-cell antigen receptors, cytokine receptors and co-stimulatory receptors are included in this progression. The first signal is the special signal that, triggered by the TCR, recognizes the antigenic peptide-MHC complex on the surface of antigen-presenting cells. The second signal is the co-stimulatory signal, produced by a co-stimulatory molecule such as CD28/B7, which promotes the IL-2 synthesis to complete the activation of T cells and avoid apoptosis. Naïve T cells cannot perform their normal role if the co-stimulatory signal is absent, and the same is true even if the T cells are stimulated by the antigen. Therefore, CARs that only include the CD3ζ sequence cannot activate CAR-T cells without a co-stimulatory signal. Accordingly, second generation CARs added intracellular signaling domains from various co-stimulatory protein receptors to the cytoplasmic tail of the CARs to provide additional signals to the T cell, such as CD28 or CD137(4-1BB and CD134(OX40)), which can improve the proliferation, cytotoxicity, and sustained response, and prolong the life of CAR-T cells *in vivo* [16–18]. CD28-mediated co-stimulation is very important in the regulation of proliferation and survival for lymphocytes, and plays a key role for the establishment of memory cells and effector cells. CD134 can sustain proliferation and strengthen IL-2 production. CD137 can maintain the response signal of T cells, which plays a key role in the survival of T cells and the memory of $CD8^+$ T cells [19–21]. The scFvCD19-CD137-CD3-CAR-T cells, MOv19-BBζ-CAR-T cells and scFvCD19-CD28-CD3ζ-CAR-T cells were used to treat B cell malignancies, and achieved better outcomes than the first generation [22, 23]. It seems that the 4-1BBζ-CAR-T cells have a longer persist time than CD28ζ-CAR-T cells, however, the direct comparisons is absent [24]. The CD28ζ-CAR-T cells can cause constitutively stimulation, proliferation and growth [25]. However, the 4-1BBζ-CAR-T cells can induce early exhaustion, which may limit antitumor efficacy [26, 27].

Third generation

The third-generation CARs were made by combining multiple signaling domains, such as CD3ζ-CD28-OX40 or CD3ζ-CD28-41BB, to augment potency with stronger cytokine production and killing ability [28]. These scFv CD20-CD28-CD137-CD3ζ-CAR-T cells and HER2-CAR-T cells were used to treat lymphoma and colon cancer; however, outcomes were not improved relative to the second generation [29, 30]. The reason may be that the number of cases studied was small. Therefore, further studies are needed to explore the safety and efficacy of these treatments, and the selection of co-stimulatory molecules is also important.

Fourth generation

The fourth-generation CARs were generated by adding IL-12 to the base of the second-generation constructs, and are known as T cell redirected for universal cytokine-mediated killing (TRUCKs). TRUCKs augment T-cell activation and activate and attract innate immune cells to eliminate antigen-negative cancer cells in the targeted lesion. It would be worthwhile to explore the role of TRUCKs in shaping the tumor environment by the inducible release of transgenic immune modifiers. Such TRUCK T cells can also treat viral infections, metabolic disorders and auto-immune diseases [31].

Altogether, these successive generations of CAR-T cell therapy have generated a great deal of enthusiasm in cancer treatment [32].

Tools of transduction for CAR-T cells

A tool is needed for the delivery of the foreign gene into human cells. At present, there are two ways to accomplish gene incorporation with vectors, i.e., viral systems and non-viral systems.

The major vectors for gene therapy in basic research and clinical study are viruses, because of the high transfer efficiency, the relatively short time needed to reach the clinically necessary numbers of cultured T cells and the availability of different viruses with different expression characteristics. Most viral systems can accommodate genes from helpful and interesting cells and can provide the viral structural enzymes and proteins to allow for the generation of vector-containing infectious viral particles. The virus vectors include retroviruses (including lentivirus), adenovirus and adeno-associated virus. Among them, the most popular tools for gene delivery are genetically engineered retroviruses [33]. Retroviridae is a family of retroviruses. In this family, amino acid and nucleotide sequence, genome structure, pathogenicity and host range is difference. However, the virus vectors pose a potential safety hazard. The insertion mutation used to induce the immune reaction can lead to tumorigenesis and toxicity, the carrier capacity is limited and the titer achieved is not high enough [33, 34].

Non-viral gene therapy has maintained its position as an approach for treating cancer because of its higher efficiency, target specificity, non-infectiousness, unlimited carrier capacity, controlled chemical constitution and generous production, [35, 36]. Non-viral vectors include nude DNA, liposomes, polymerizers and molecular conjugates. Minicircle DNA vectors free of plasmid bacterial DNA sequences are novel non-viral vectors which are generated in bacteria from a parental plasmid, and can persistently express transgene with high levels *in vivo*. It is practicable in clinics for this method [37, 38].

Production of CAR-T Cells

Several steps are required for the production of CAR-T cells. It is also very important to conduct quality control testing throughout the entire protocol [39].

First, leukocytes are taken from the patient's or donor's body using leukapheresis. Second, The T cells are enriched and washed to separate them from the leukocytes [40]. Third, the T cell subsets at the level of CD4/CD8 composition are separated using specific antibody bead conjugates or markers. Culture is then needed to activate the T cells. This process requires purifying autologous antigen-presenting cells (APCs) from the patients or donors, or beads coated with anti-CD3/anti-CD28 monoclonal antibodies, or anti-CD3 antibodies alone or in combination with feeder cells and growth factors, such as IL-2. IL-2 is the most commonly used agent because it induces rapid T cell growth. In order to polarize T cells to a specific phenotype, the culture conditions are further refined [41].

CARs are encoded with viral vectors, which guide the RNA to reverse-transcribe into DNA and permanently integrate into the genome of the patient cells. The viral vector is washed out of the culture via medium exchange and/or dilution during the activation process. Lentiviral vectors are more commonly used than gammaretroviral vectors in clinical trials because of their safer integration site profile [42]. The other methods includes Sleeping Beauty transposon system and mRNA transfection. However, many concerns remain, such as the requirement for several rounds of infusion using transient mRNA transfection and the unknown potential of insertional mutagenesis and remobilization of transposons when using the Sleeping Beauty transposon system [43].

Three bioreactor culture systems are used to culture CAR-T cells: WAVE Bioreactor, G-Rex and CliniMACS Prodigy [44]. The major drawback of the former two systems is that the flask must be opened during cell inoculation. However, the CliniMACS Prodicy system is a single device that can effectively enrich, activate, transducer and expand the cells [45]. After the cells reach the numbers required for clinical uses, they are collected and transfused into the patients.

Challenges for CAR-T cell therapy

Although CAR-T cells have been used in clinics, many questions still need to be addressed, such as the optimal vector and the long-term safety profile.

The key raw material for the CAR-T cell product is the viral vector that transduces the CARs into the T cells. The viral vector encoding the CARs can be made in large quantities and stored at −80 °C even for about 9 years [46]. Therefore, the sterility of the vector is crucial because these cells will be infused into the patients. The third-generation minimal lentiviral vector may be the safest one that has been developed thus far [47]. Quality control testing on the safety, sterility, titer, purity and potency is absolutely crucial. The comparison of vector purity, stability, and function is also important because vectors can be obtained from different suppliers. It would be most desirable to control these variables by using a single vector for the generation of CAR-T cells.

The potential for insertional mutagenesis caused by the integration of vector DNA into host cells is a concern. Lentiviral vectors may have a lower risk of mutagenesis than others [48]. However, both lentiviral and retroviral vectors are potentially oncogenic. The long-term safety of using viral vectors for CAR-T cell therapy remains unknown. Therefore, it is necessary to monitor carefully for any potential delayed adverse event related to these vectors for an extended period of time. The effects of persistent CAR-T cells on future pregnancies are also unknown.

Effective coordination among the collection, manufacturing, and treatment sites is crucial in order to ensure correct handling of the material and appropriate scheduling of patients during the therapeutic process. It is therefore very important to develop a standardized manufacturing process for CAR-T cells in order to establish the critical quality characteristics and target product profile. It is also important to gain more experience with these procedures because the CARs positivity, phenotype and viability vary among different products [49]. Comparing products is difficult because of the variability between the starting materials generated from leukapheresis.

The good results were observed in clinics with CAR-T cells therapy in hematological malignancies, however, it is still a change in the solid tumors because of antigen loss in tumor cells, the lack of unique antigens and the immune-suppressive tumor microenvironment of solid tumors [50, 51]. So in order to improve the effect of CAR-T cells therapy, many progresses have been made by incorporating CARs with another effector molecules such as PD1 switch receptors, anti-oxidant enzymes, matrix degradation enzymes and so on [52–56].

The major adverse effect observed after CAR-T cell therapy is severe cytokine release syndrome (CRS). Although most of the adverse events subsequent to

CAR-T cell therapy can be managed with currently available interventions, it is nevertheless important to reduce the adverse effects while maintaining the efficacy of the treatment [57]. Similarly, it is also important to increase the safety of CAR-T cell therapy when improving the specificity of the modified T cells.

Conclusion

CAR-T treatment for patients with tumors has shown promising outcomes; however, many remaining challenges need to be considered [58]. The high quality of CAR-T products needs to be ensured through optimization of protocols, and the long-term safety requires further study [59].

Abbreviations

CARs: Chimeric antigen receptors; CAR-T cells: Chimeric antigen receptor redirected T cells; scFv: Single-chain Fragment variant; ITAMs: immunoreceptor tyrosine-based activation motifs; IL-2: Interleukin-2; TCR: T cell receptor; TRUCKs: T cell redirected for universal cytokine-mediated killing; APCs: Antigen-presenting cells; CRS: Cytokine release syndrome

Acknowledgements

Not applicable.

Funding

This study was funded by the clinical key foundation of Xinqiao Hospital of Third Military Medical University (No. 2016YLC03).

Authors' contributions

LJ and ZC wrote the paper. ZX and ZJF revised the paper. All authors collected the data, read and approved the final manuscript.

Competing interests

The authors declare that they have no competing interests.

Author details

[1]Department of Hematology, Xinqiao Hospital, Third Military Medical University, Chongqing 400037, People's Republic of China. [2]Division of Periodontology, Diagnostic Sciences & Dental Hygiene, and Division of Biomedical Sciences, Herman Ostrow School of Dentistry, University of Southern California, Los Angeles, CA, USA.

References

1. Ramos CA, Dotti G. Chimeric antigen receptor (CAR)-engineered lymphocytes for cancer therapy. Expert Opin Biol Ther. 2011;11(7):855–73.
2. Lipowska-Bhalla G, Gilham DE, Hawkins RE, Rothwell DG. Targeted immunotherapy of cancer with CAR T cells: achievements and challenges. Cancer Immunol Immunother. 2012;61(7):953–62.
3. Liu J, Zhong JF, Zhang X, Zhang C. Allogeneic CD19-CAR-T cell infusion after allogeneic hematopoietic stem cell transplantation in B cell malignancies. J Hematol Oncol. 2017;10(1):35.
4. Tasian SK, Gardner RA. CD19-redirected chimeric antigen receptor-modified T cells: a promising immunotherapy for children and adults with B-cell acute lymphoblastic leukemia (ALL). Ther Adv Hematol. 2015;6(5):228–41.
5. Gross G, Waks T, Eshhar Z. Expression of immunoglobulin-T-cell receptor chimeric molecules as functional receptors with antibody-type specificity. Proc Natl Acad Sci U S A. 1989;86(24):10024–8.
6. Eshhar Z, Waks T, Gross G, Schindler DG. Specific activation and targeting of cytotoxic lymphocytes through chimeric single chains consisting of antibody-binding domains and the gamma or zeta subunits of the immunoglobulin and T-cell receptors. Proc Natl Acad Sci U S A. 1993;90(2):720–4.
7. Brocker T. Chimeric Fv-zeta or Fv-epsilon receptors are not sufficient to induce activation or cytokine production in peripheral T cells. Blood. 2000; 96(5):1999–2001.
8. Heuser C, Hombach A, Lösch C, Manista K, Abken H. T-cell activation by recombinant immunore-ceptors: impact of the intracellular signalling domain on the stability of receptor expression and antigen-speciic activation of grafted T cells. Gene Ther. 2003;10(17):1408–19.
9. Zhao Y, Wang QJ, Yang S, Kochenderfer JN, Zheng Z, Zhong X, et al. A herceptin-based chimeric antigen receptor with modified signaling domains leads to enhanced survival of transduced T lymphocytes and antitumor activity. J Immunol. 2009;183(9):5563–74.
10. Bridgeman JS, Hawkins RE, Bagley S, Blaylock M, Holland M, Gilham DE. The optimal antigen response of chimeric antigen receptors harboring the CD3zeta transmembrane domain is dependent upon incorporation of the receptor into the endogenous TCR/CD3 complex. J Immunol. 2010;184(12): 6938–49.
11. Kershaw MH, Westwood JA, Parker LL, Wang G, Eshhar Z, Mavroukakis SA, et al. A phase I study on adoptive immunotherapy using gene-modified T cells for ovarian cancer. Clin Cancer Res. 2006;12(20 Pt 1):6106–15.
12. Julie RP, David LD, Marilyn S, Wright C, Naranjo A, Wagner J, et al. Adoptive transfer of chimeric antigen receptor re-directed cytolytic T lymphocyte clones in patients with Neuroblastoma. Mol Ther. 2007;15(4):825–33.
13. Lamers CH, Langeveld SC, Groot-van Ruijven CM, Debets R, Sleijfer S, Gratama JW, et al. Gene-modified T cells for adoptive immunotherapy of renal cell cancer maintain transgene-specific immune functions in vivo. Cancer Immunol Immunother. 2007;56(12):1875–83.
14. Pule MA, Savoldo B, Myers GD, Rossig C, Russell HV, Dotti G, et al. Virus-specfic T cells engineered to coexpress tumor-speciic receptors: Persistence and antitumor activity in individuals with neuroblastoma. Nat Med. 2008; 14(11):1264–70.
15. Till BG, Jensen MC, Wang J, Chen EY, Wood BL, Greisman HA, et al. Adoptive immunotherapy for indolent non-Hodgkin lymphoma and mantle cell lymphoma using genetically modified autologous CD20-specific T cells. Blood. 2008;112(6):2261–71.
16. Finney HM, Lawson AD, Bebbington CR, Weir AN. Chimeric receptors providing both primary and costimulatory signaling in T cells from a single gene product. J Immunol. 1998;161(6):2791–7.
17. Dotti G, Savoldo B, Brenner M. Fifteen years of gene therapy based on chimeric antigen receptors: Are we nearly there yet? Hum Gene Ther. 2009; 20(11):1229–39.
18. Park TS, Rosenberg SA, Morgan RA. Treating cancer with genetically engineered T cells. Trends Biotechnol. 2011;29(11):550–7.
19. Acuto O, Michel F. CD28-mediated co-stimulation: a quantitative support for TCR signalling. Nat Rev Immunol. 2003;3(12):939–51.
20. Finney HM, Akbar AN, Lawson AD. Activation of resting human primary T cells with chimeric receptors: Costimulation from CD28, inducible costimulator, CD134, and CD137 in series with signals from the TCR zeta chain. J Immunol. 2004;172(1):104–13.
21. Croft M. The role of TNF superfamily members in T-cell function and diseases. Nat Rev Immunol. 2009;9(4):271–85.
22. Cai B, Guo M, Wang Y, Zhang Y, Yang J, Guo Y, et al. Co-infusion of haplo-identical CD19-chimeric antigen receptor T cells and stem cells achieved full donor engraftment in refractory acute lymphoblastic leukemia. J Hematol Oncol. 2016;9(1):131.
23. Hu Y, Sun J, Wu Z, Yu J, Cui Q, Pu C, et al. Predominant cerebral cytokine release syndrome in CD19-directed chimeric antigen receptor-modified T cell therapy. J Hematol Oncol. 2016;9(1):70.
24. Porter DL, Hwang WT, Frey NV, Lacey SF, Shaw PA, Loren AW, et al. Chimeric antigen receptor T cells persist and induce sustained remissions in relapsed refractory chronic lymphocytic leukemia. Sci Transl Med. 2015; 7(303):303ra139.
25. Frigault MJ, Lee J, Basil MC, Carpenito C, Motohashi S, Scholler J, et al. Identification of chimeric antigen receptors that mediate constitutive or inducible proliferation of T cells. Cancer Immunol Res. 2015;3(4):356–67.
26. Long AH, Haso WM, Shern JF, Wanhainen KM, Murgai M, Ingaramo M, et al. 4-1BB costimulation ameliorates T cell exhaustion induced by tonic signaling of chimeric antigen receptors. Nat Med. 2015;21(6):581–90.

27. Kawalekar OU, O'Connor RS, Fraietta JA, Guo L, McGettigan SE, Posey AD Jr, et al. Distinct signaling of coreceptors regulates specific metabolism pathways and impacts memory development in CAR T cells. Immunity. 2016;44(2):380–90.
28. Marin V, Pizzitola I, Agostoni V, Attianese GM, Finney H, Lawson A, et al. Cytokine-induced killer cells for cell therapy of acute myeloid leukemia: improvement of their immune activity by expression of CD33-specific chimeric receptors. Haematologica. 2010;95(12):2144–52.
29. Till BG, Jensen MC, Wang J, Qian X, Gopal AK, Maloney DG, et al. CD20-specific adoptive immunotherapy for lymphoma using a chimeric antigen receptor with both CD28 and 4-1BB domains: pilot clinical trial results. Blood. 2012;119(17):3940–50.
30. Morgan RA, Yang JC, Kitano M, Dudley ME, Laurencot CM, Rosenberg SA. Case report of a serious adverse event following the administration of T cells transduced with a chimeric antigen receptor recognizing ERBB2. Mol Ther. 2010;18(4):843–51.
31. Chmielewski M, Abken H. TRUCKs: the fourth generation of CARs. Expert Opin Biol Ther. 2015;15(8):1145–54.
32. Sha HH, Wang DD, Yan DL, Hu Y, Yang SJ, Liu SW, et al. Chimaeric antigen receptor T-cell therapy for tumour immunotherapy. Biosci Rep. 2017;37(1).
33. Hu WS, Pathak VK. Design of retroviral vectors and helper cells for gene therapy. Pharmacol Rev. 2000;52(4):493–511.
34. Wang GP, Garrigue A, Ciuffi A, Ronen K, Leipzig J, Berry C, et al. DNA bar coding and pyrosequencing to analyze adverse events in therapeutic gene transfer. Nucleic Acids Res. 2008;36(9):e49.
35. El-Aneed A. An overview of current delivery systems in cancer gene therapy. J Control Release. 2004;94(1):1–14.
36. Pahle J, Walther W. Vectors and strategies for nonviral cancer gene therapy. Expert Opin Biol Ther. 2016;16(4):443–61.
37. Chen ZY, He CY, Kay MA. Improved production and purification of minicircle DNA vector free of plasmid bacterial sequences and capable of persistent transgene expression in vivo. Hum Gene Ther. 2005;16(1):126–31.
38. Kay MA, He CY, Chen ZY. A robust system for production of minicircle DNA vectors. Nat Biotechnol. 2010;28(12):1287–9.
39. Levine BL. Performance-enhancing drugs: design and production of redirected chimeric antigen receptor (CAR) T cells. Cancer Gene Ther. 2015; 22(2):79–84.
40. Lee G, Arepally GM, et al. J Clin Apher. 2012;27:117–25.
41. Guedan S, Chen X, Madar A, Carpenito C, McGettigan SE, Frigault MJ, et al. (2014). ICOS-based chimeric antigen receptors program bipolar TH17/TH1 cells. Blood. 2014;124(7):1070–80.
42. McGarrity GJ, Hoyah G, Winemiller A, Andre K, Stein D, Blick G, et al. Patient monitoring and follow-up in lentiviral clinical trials. J Gene Med. 2013;15(2):78–82.
43. Beatty GL, Haas AR, Maus MV, Torigian DA, Soulen MC, Plesa G, et al. Mesothelin-specific chimeric antigen receptor mRNA-engineered T cells induce anti-tumor activity in solid malignancies. Cancer Immunol Res. 2014; 2(2):112–20.
44. Bajgain P, Mucharla R, Wilson J, Welch D, Anurathapan U, Liang B, et al. Optimizing the production of suspension cells using the G-Rex "M" series. Mol Ther Methods Clin Dev. 2014;1:14015.
45. Mock U, Nickolay L, Cheung G, Zhan H, Peggs K, Johnston I, et al. Automated lentiviral transduction of T cells with CARs using the CliniMACS Prodigy. Blood. 2015;11(2):A26–6.
46. Przybylowski M, Hakakha A, Stefanski J, Hodges J, Sadelain M, Rivière I. Production scale-up and validation of packaging cell clearance of clinical grade retroviral vector stocks produced in cell factories. Gene Ther. 2006; 13(1):95–100.
47. Dull T, Zufferey R, Kelly M, Mandel RJ, Nguyen M, Trono D, et al. A third-generation lentivirus vector with a conditional packaging system. J Virol. 1998;72(11):8463–71.
48. Vannucci L, Lai M, Chiuppesi F, Ceccherini-Nelli L, Pistello M. Viral vectors: a look back and ahead on gene transfer technology. New Microbiol. 2013; 36(1):1–22.
49. Porter DL, Levine BL, Kalos M, Bagg A, June CH. Chimeric antigen receptor-modified T cells in chronic lymphoid leukemia. N Engl J Med. 2011;365(8): 725–33.
50. Yu S, Li A, Liu Q, Li T, Yuan X, Han X, et al. Chimeric antigen receptor T cells: a novel therapy for solid tumors. J Hematol Oncol. 2017;10(1):78.
51. Kato D, Yaguchi T, Iwata T, Morii K, Nakagawa T, Nishimura R, et al. Prospects for personalized combination immunotherapy for solid tumors based on adoptive cell therapies and immune checkpoint blockade therapies. Nihon Rinsho Meneki Gakkai Kaishi. 2017;40(1):68–77.
52. Morsut L, Roybal KT, Xiong X, Gordley RM, Coyle SM, Thomson M, et al. Engineering customized cell sensing and response behaviors using synthetic notch receptors. Cell. 2016;164(4):780–91.
53. Roybal KT, Rupp LJ, Morsut L, Walker WJ, McNally KA, Park JS, et al. Precision tumor recognition by T cells with combinatorial antigen-sensing circuits. Cell. 2016;164(4):770–9.
54. Newick K, O'Brien S, Sun J, Kapoor V, Maceyko S, Lo A, et al. Augmentation of CAR T-cell trafficking and antitumor efficacy by blocking protein kinase A localization. Cancer Immunol Res. 2016;4(6):541–51.
55. Caruana I, Savoldo B, Hoyos V, Weber G, Liu H, Kim ES, et al. Heparanase promotes tumor infiltration and antitumor activity of CAR-redirected T lymphocytes. Nat Med. 2015;21(5):524–9.
56. Rodgers DT, Mazagova M, Hampton EN, Cao Y, Ramadoss NS, Hardy IR, et al. Switch-mediated activation and retargeting of CAR-T cells for B-cell malignancies. Proc Natl Acad Sci U S A. 2016;113(4):E459–68.
57. Lee DW, Gardner R, Porter DL, Louis CU, Ahmed N, Jensen M, et al. Current concepts in the diagnosis and management of cytokine release syndrome. Blood. 2014;124(2):188–95.
58. Levine BL, Miskin J, Wonnacott K, Keir C. Global Manufacturing of CAR T Cell Therapy. Mol Ther Methods Clin Dev. 2016;4:92–101.
59. Wang Z, Wu Z, Liu Y, Han W. New development in CAR-T cell therapy. J Hematol Oncol. 2017;10(1):53.

6

A robust prognostic gene expression signature for early stage lung adenocarcinoma

Marcin Krzystanek[1*], Judit Moldvay[2], David Szüts[3], Zoltan Szallasi[1,4,5] and Aron Charles Eklund[1]

Abstract

Background: Stage I lung adenocarcinoma is usually not treated with adjuvant chemotherapy; however, around half of these patients do not survive 5 years. Therefore, a reliable prognostic biomarker for early stage patients would be critical to identify those most likely to benefit from early additional treatments. Several studies have searched for gene expression prognostic biomarkers for lung adenocarcinoma, but these have not yielded a widely accepted prognosticator.

Results: We analyzed gene expression from seven published lung adenocarcinoma cohorts for which we included only stage I and II patients who were not given adjuvant therapy. Seven genes consistently obtained statistical significance in Cox regression for overall survival. The combined signature has a weighted mean hazard ratio of 3.2 in all cohorts and 3.0 (C.I. 1.3–7.4, $p < 0.01$) in an independent validation cohort and is strongly correlated with previously published signatures of chromosomal instability and cell cycle progression.

Conclusions: The new prognostic signature, if validated prospectively, may enable better stratification and treatment of early stage lung cancer patients.

Keywords: Lung adenocarcinoma, Prognostic biomarker, Gene expression, Early stage cancer

Background

Lung cancer has the third highest incidence rate and the highest mortality rate of all cancer types. For non-small cell lung cancer (NSCLC), the 5-year survival rate remains below 15 % [1, 2]. Given the difficulties with treatment of advanced NSCLC, the most promising possibility of improving outcomes may be efficient diagnosis and treatment of early stage cases. One of the most important clinical decisions in these patients is whether to give adjuvant chemotherapy in addition to surgical resection. At present postoperative chemotherapy is not recommended for patients with completely resected stage IA NSCLC with 1A level of evidence, and can be considered in stage IB disease and a primary tumor >4 cm with 2B level of evidence [2]. Nonetheless, only up to 73 % of stage IA and 58 % of stage IB patients survive 5 years [1]. Therefore, identification of patients who are likely to benefit from adjuvant treatment – even with NSCLC of stage I – would be of strong diagnostic and prognostic relevance.

A similar problem has been extensively studied and to a significant extent answered in node negative estrogen receptor positive breast cancer. A gene expression signature was obtained that identifies patients with high risk of recurrence who benefit from additional chemotherapy [3]. Identification of such a gene expression signature often initiates with the quantification of a large number of genes on a patient cohort where outcome is known and then the most informative genes are selected and further validated.

Similar strategies have been applied to lung adenocarcinoma as well. Several cohorts containing early to mid stage lung cancer patients have been subjected to transcriptomic analysis, mainly by microarray [4–10]. However, no reliable, consistent gene expression based prognosticator has emerged from these efforts. One possible reason for this failure could be that some of these studies followed a suboptimal strategy in one or more possible ways: 1)

* Correspondence: marcin@cbs.dtu.dk
[1]Department of Systems Biology, Center for Biological Sequence Analysis, Technical University of Denmark, Lyngby, Denmark

searching for a general NSCLC prognosticator, as opposed to lung adenocarcinoma (LUAD)- or lung squamous carcinoma (LUSC)-specific signatures [4, 5], 2) doing the analysis in a treated/untreated mixed population [4, 6, 9], 3) ignoring the possibility of technical bias in the microarray data [11, 12]. On the other hand, a PCR-based gene expression signature of cell cycle progression (CCP), which was *not* derived from lung cancer patients, was found to be prognostic in three early stage LUAD cohorts and validated in a PCR-based study [13, 14].

The increasing availability of lung cancer datasets makes it possible to look for a robust signature comprising of genes that would not otherwise be found if the study had been conducted on only a single dataset. Therefore, we set out to perform a meta-analysis of several lung cancer microarray datasets to see if we could identify a gene expression signature that is prognostic in early stage lung adenocarcinoma patients who were not given chemotherapy.

Methods

Microarray data were downloaded from the GEO database (GSE8894, GSE14814, GSE30219, GSE31210, GSE37745, GSE50081), except Shedden et al., which was downloaded from caarraydb.nci.nih.gov (Table 1). All calculations were performed using the R programming language. Each gene expression dataset was normalized with the RMA algorithm except GSE9984, for which we were unable to obtain the original raw data, and therefore we used the version downloaded directly from GEO which had been normalized with the GCRMA algorithm [4]. Each dataset, except GSE9984, was also corrected for two sources of potential bias: the RNA degradation captured as the average decrease in expression between 5' probes and 3' probes (degradation bias metric) and the diversity of starting mRNA (RMA IQR bias metric) that remained after RMA normalization. This step was performed using "bias" package version 0.0.5 [11]. Weighted average of hazard ratios was calculated as a mean weighted by size of each dataset.

Table 1 Number of patients in the cohorts included in this study

Cohort	Available	Included[a]		
		Stage I	Stage II	Total
Lee et al. 2008 [4]	138	39	12	51
Zhu et al. 2010 [5]	133	20	12	32
Shedden et al. 2008 [6]	505	164	43	207
Rousseaux et al. 2013 [7]	307	81	3	84
Okayama et al. 2012 [8]	246	162	42	204
Botling et al. 2013 [9]	196	31	4	35
Der et al. 2014 [10]	181	92	35	127

[a]passed inclusion criteria: adenocarcinoma, no chemotherapy

Gene expression and clinical covariates from the validation cohort were downloaded from the TCGA Data Portal using Data Matrix (https://tcga-data.nci.nih.gov/tcga/dataAccessMatrix.htm), selecting all available tumors on 15th Jan 2016, disease: LUAD and data type: RNASeqV2. Expression values were extracted from files containing RSEM gene-normalized results and we normalized them across samples using the average gene expression of each tumor [15, 16].

Results

We performed a literature and database search and identified seven publicly available gene expression data sets with overall or recurrence-free survival data and with at least 30 patients meeting the following criteria: 1) profiled on the Affymetrix HG-U133A or HG-U133 Plus 2.0 platform; 2) adenocarcinoma subtype by histological report; 3) pathological stage I or II; and 4) not given neoadjuvant, adjuvant, or targeted therapy (Table 1). Each data set (except Lee et al. [4]) was normalized individually and adjusted to reduce technical bias [11].

To identify genes whose expression level is prognostic, we applied the following procedure to each of the 22,277 common probe sets. We split each cohort into two groups according to the expression value of the probe set, and applied Cox proportional hazards regression and a log-rank test of statistical significance on these two groups. If the hazard ratio had the same directionality in all cohorts, and the P value was below 0.05 in any six of the seven cohorts, the probe set was considered prognostic. We expect this procedure to yield an individual type I error rate of 1.0×10^{-7}, and with Bonferroni correction for 22,277 probe sets, a family-wise error rate of 0.00036. This procedure resulted in seven probe sets, each representing a unique gene (Table 2).

The expression values of the seven probe sets were strongly positively correlated, so we defined a prognostic score of an individual tumor as the mean $\log_2$ expression value of the seven probe sets (termed "ESLA-7", for early stage lung adenocarcinoma). We found that the ESLA-7 score, when used to stratify each cohort into two groups of equal size, is prognostic in six of the seven individual cohorts (Table 2 and Fig. 1). Notably, the ESLA-7 score was more prognostic than any of the individual probe sets. Overall, the weighted average hazard ratio of ESLA-7 was 3.2, or 3.6 if the Botling cohort was omitted (Fig. 1).

We next performed a multivariate analysis, adjusting for stage, age and stratifying for gender. No other clinical data types were available in all cohorts. In this analysis, ESLA-7 showed a HR ranging between 1.1–4.9 in the individual cohorts, with a weighted mean of 2.7 and statistical significance in all cohorts except Botling et al. 2008 (Table 3).

Table 2 Hazard ratios for the individual ESLA-7 genes in each cohort

Gene	ADAM10		DLGAP5		RAD51AP1		FGFR1OP		NCGAP		KIF15		ASPM	
Probe set	202604_x_at		203764_at		204146_at		205588_s_at		218663_at		219306_at		219918_s_at	
Cohort	HR	p	HR	p	HR	p	HR	p	HR	p	HR	p	HR	p
Lee et al. 2008 [4]	3.0	**	2.3	*	4	***	2.9	**	2.3	*	2.5	*	2.5	*
Zhu et al. 2010 [5]	0.7		3.1	*	3.7	*	3.2	*	4.7	**	3.9	*	4.1	**
Shedden et al. 2008 [6]	1.7	*	1.7	*	1.7	*	1.6	*	1.8	*	1.6	*	1.7	*
Rousseaux et al. 2013 [7]	2.6	**	2.4	**	2.7	**	1.9	*	2.3	**	2.3	**	1.9	*
Okayama et al. 2012 [8]	4.3	***	2.9	**	2.9	**	3.4	**	2.4	*	2.8	*	4.2	***
Botling et al. 2013 [9]	2.5	*	1.7		1.0		1.3		1.3		1.7		1.1	
Der et al. 2014 [10]	2.2	**	2.5	**	2	*	2.1	**	2.5	**	2.4	**	2	*

$^*p \leq 0.05$, $^{**}p \leq 0.01$, $^{***}p \leq 0.001$

To assess the performance of ESLA-7 in an independent cohort that was not used to derive the signature, we analyzed RNA-seq gene expression data from the TCGA LUAD cohort. To reduce the effects of varying chemotherapy regimes in the TCGA cohort, we analyzed recurrence-free survival (RFS) in stage I and II patients from this cohort. The majority of early stage LUAD patients do not receive chemotherapy until recurrence; therefore this analysis could be considered as a more accurate assessment of true prognostic performance. Here, ESLA-7 was statistically significant (HR = 1.8, C.I. 1.3–2.6, p < 0.001, Additional file 1: Figure S1A). Subsequently, we used available treatment information to censor the survival times at the time of initiation of chemotherapy, thus creating a subcohort of patients who did not receive chemotherapy during the followup period. RFS analysis of stage I and II, untreated patients (N = 95) showed HR = 3.0 (C.I. 1.3–7.4, p < 0.01, Figure 1 and Additional file 1: Figure S1B).

Since most of the seven genes were annotated with functions related to chromosomal instability (CIN), we asked whether we could achieve similar prognostic performance with our previously described CIN25 chromosomal instability signature or with the previously published cell cycle progression (CCP) signature [13, 14, 17]. We applied the CIN25 and the CCP signatures in the same way as the ESLA-7 signature and found that ESLA-7 on average performed better than both CIN25 and CCP (weighted mean hazard ratio of 3.2, 2.9 and 2.8 respectively, Fig. 2). CIN25 and CCP scores also showed trends similar to ESLA-7 when using TCGA LUAD RNAseq data (Additional file 1:

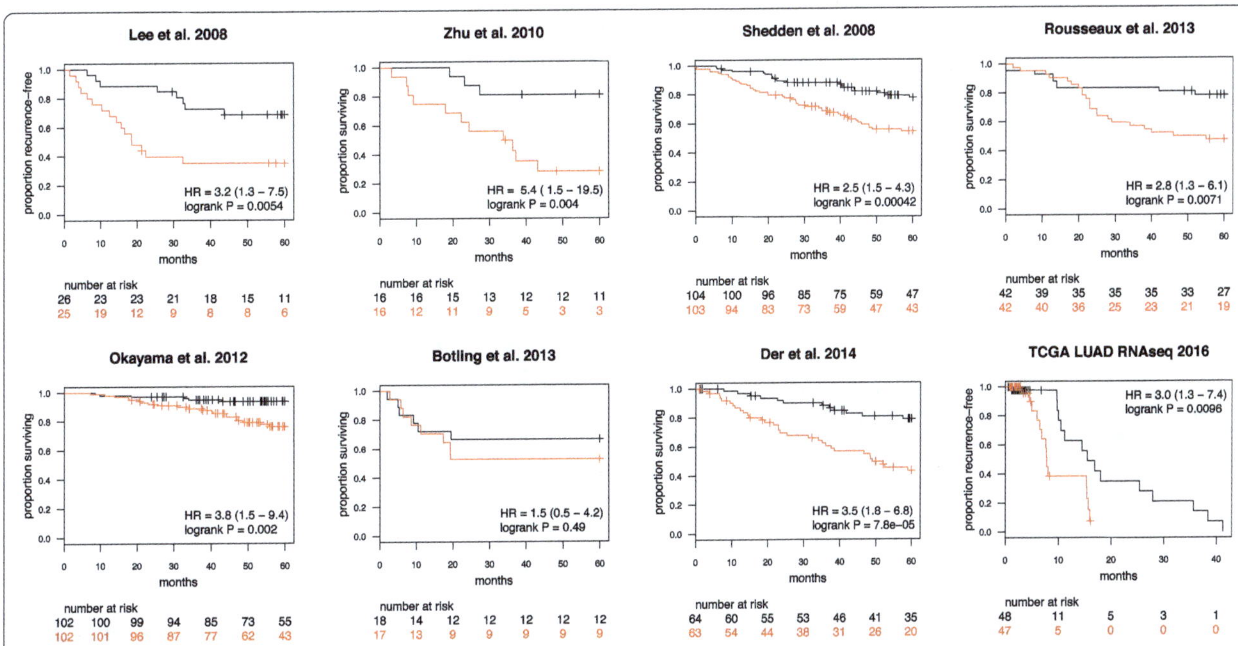

Fig. 1 Kaplan-Meier overall or recurrence-free survival estimates for seven early stage lung adenocarcinoma cohorts and the TCGA LUAD validation cohort [4–10, 16]. Each cohort was split according to ESLA-7 score (red: > median, black: ≤ median)

Table 3 Performance of ESLA-7 in multivariate setting when adjusted for age, stage and stratified for gender

Cohort	HR	CI	p	N	events
Lee et al. 2008 [4]	2.9	1.2–7.1	*	51	24
Zhu et al. 2010 [5]	4.9	1.3–18.1	*	32	14
Shedden et al. 2008 [6]	2.0	1.2–3.5	*	207	64
Rousseaux et al. 2013 [7]	2.6	1.2–5.8	*	84	31
Okayama et al. 2012 [8]	3.1	1.2–7.9	*	204	27
Botling et al. 2013 [9]	1.1	0.3–3.9		35	14
Der et al. 2014 [10]	3.2	1.6–6.2	***	127	44

$^{*}p \leq 0.05$, $^{**}p \leq 0.01$, $^{***}p \leq 0.001$

Figure S1C-F). Additionally, the correlation between ESLA-7 and CIN25 within each cohort was very high, ranging from 0.88 to 0.98, suggesting that ESLA-7 to a large extent quantifies CIN. Similarly correlation between ESLA-7 and CCP ranged from 0.89 to 0.99.

To assess the performance of ESLA-7 without arbitrary stratifying the cohorts into two equally sized groups, we performed Cox regression using ESLA-7 as a continuous variable. Association with overall survival (or recurrence-free survival in the Lee et al. 2008 cohort) was statistically significant in all cohorts except Botling et al. 2013 (weighted mean 2.1, Table 4). Additionally, we explored whether the ESLA-7 score might provide further prognostic stratification into more than two groups, using the ESLA-7 score to stratify each cohort into four groups of equal size. For cohorts with sufficient number of patients in each stratum a clear trend was apparent (Fig. 3). Patients in the first quartile had better survival than patients in the other three quartiles, and, especially, patients in the fourth quartile. No such trend was apparent in the Zhu et al. 2010 [5] and Botling et al. 2013 [9] cohorts, possibly due to the smaller numbers of patients in these two cohorts.

Finally, we applied ESLA-7 to five lung squamous cell carcinoma (LUSC) cohorts [4, 5, 7, 9]. Median split according to ESLA-7 value did not yield statistical significance in any of the LUSC cohorts (Additional file 2: Table S1 and Additional file 3). We attempted to create a separate signature for lung squamous cell carcinoma (LUSC). However, similar methodology applied to LUSC patients did not yield a robust expression signature (data not shown).

Discussion

We used simple methodology to derive a robust prognostic gene expression signature for early stage lung adenocarcinoma. The signature was validated in an independent cohort, however, with 95 patients in the regression, of which many left the study or were censored due to the methodology within the first semester of the follow-up, one should treat this result with caution. If successfully validated in an independent clinical trial, the ESLA-7 signature could potentially be used for guiding clinical onocologist decisions on whether an individual early stage lung adenocarcinoma patient, especially a patient with stage I disease, should receive chemotherapy after surgical resection of the tumor. The seven genes could be combined with an additional small panel of reference genes, as has been done in similar prognostic signatures for other cancer types [3, 14, 18].

High correlation among ESLA-7 and the two other signatures suggests that to a large degree they may be quantifying the same biological processes. CIN25 was developed as a signature of chromosomal instability from specific genes whose expression was consistently correlated with aneuploidy in several types of tumors. As with CIN25, net overexpression of ESLA-7 was predictive of poor clinical outcome. Both signatures contain genes with function connected directly with kinetochore assembly: KIF20A, KIF4A, TPX2, PRC1, and TTK in CIN25; and KIF15, DLGAP5, and ASPM in ESLA-7. Also, both contain genes that are part of condensin complexes: NCAPG in ESLA-7; and NCAPD2 in CIN25.

Study	Deaths	ESLA-7 HR	P	CIN25 HR	P	CCP HR	P
Lee et al. 2008	26/51	3.2(1.3-7.5)	0.0054	3.1(1.3-7.3)	0.0065	2.4(1.1-5.5)	0.032
Zhu et al. 2010	15/32	5.4(1.5-19.5)	0.004	2.1(0.7-6.3)	0.18	2.25(0.75-6.73)	0.14
Shedden et al. 2008	82/207	2.5(1.5-4.3)	0.00042	2.2(1.3-3.6)	0.0025	2.4(1.4-4)	9e-04
Rousseaux et al. 2013	45/84	2.8(1.3-6.1)	0.0071	2.8(1.3-6.1)	0.0071	2.8(1.3-6.1)	0.0071
Okayama et al. 2012	30/204	3.8(1.5-9.4)	0.002	3.8(1.5-9.3)	0.0021	3(1.3-7.2)	0.0081
Botling et al. 2013	22/35	1.5(0.5-4.2)	0.49	0.99(0.35-2.82)	0.98	1.5(0.5-4.2)	0.49
Der et al. 2014	51/127	3.5(1.8-6.8)	7.8e-05	3.5(1.8-6.8)	9e-05	3.6(1.8-6.9)	6.7e-05
Summary		**3.2**		**2.9**		**2.8**	
TCGA LUAD 2016	24/95	3.0(1.3-7.4)	0.0096	1.7(0.8-3.7)	0.15	2.6(1.1-6.2)	0.021

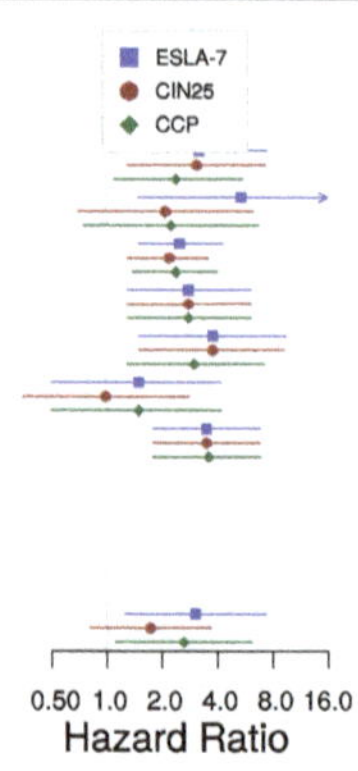

Fig. 2 Forest plot indicating the performance of the ESLA-7, CIN25 [17] and CPP [13] signatures in the seven early stage lung adenocarcinoma cohorts and in the TCGA LUAD validation cohort

Table 4 Hazard ratios of cox regression using ESLA-7 as continuous variable

Cohort	HR	CI	p	N	events
Lee et al. 2008 [4]	1.8	1.3–2.6	***	51	24
Zhu et al. 2010 [5]	3.8	1.1–12.1	*	32	14
Shedden et al. 2008 [6]	2.4	1.6–3.5	***	207	64
Rousseaux et al. 2013 [7]	2.2	1.5–3.3	***	84	31
Okayama et al. 2012 [8]	1.9	1.3–2.8	***	204	27
Botling et al. 2013 [9]	1.2	0.7–2.2		35	14
Der et al. 2014 [10]	1.6	1.1–2.2	*	127	44

*$p \leq 0.05$, **$p \leq 0.01$, ***$p \leq 0.001$

Both kinetochores and condensin complexes play central roles in chromosome assembly and segregation. Overall, both signatures point towards chromosomal instability as an important factor in early stage patient outcome.

Only a single gene, RAD51-associated protein 1 (RAD51AP1), is present in both signatures. This gene plays an important role in homologous recombination-mediated chromosome damage repair by enhancing the recombinase activity of RAD51.

The ESLA-7 signature includes genes ADAM10 and FGFR1OP, which have been reported to contribute to oncogenesis of various cancer types including lung cancer, and whose function indicates that they may take part in oncogenic transformation and/or increase cell proliferation by interaction with major signaling cascades (ERK1/2, p38 MAPK, and STAT, Notch1, RAS/MAPK, PLC-γ, and PI3K/AKT). The slightly better performance of ESLA-7 as compared to CCP might be due to additional information carried by ADAM10 and/or FGFR1OP, which are slightly less correlated with the remainder of the ESLA-7 genes (Additional file 4: Figure S2).

Interestingly, forkhead box MI (FOXM1), which takes part in the regulation of spindle assembly genes, nearly passed our criteria. This gene is also one of the top CIN25 and CCP genes and, more recently, was identified as predictor of adverse outcomes in various malignancies in a cross-platform, cross-cancer study [19].

While we found a monotonic correlation between the CIN signature and prognosis in LUAD, we previously found a non-monotonic relationship between CIN and prognosis in LUSC, in which very low and very high levels of CIN result in increased survival compared to the rest of the cohort [20].

Conclusions

If CIN is indeed highly prognostic in early stage lung cancer, as our results indicate, then this would suggest that LUAD and LUSC cohorts should be analyzed separately. The new prognostic signature, if further validated prospectively, will enable better stratification and reduce overtreatment of early stage lung cancer patients.

Statement on ethics approval

In this study we used publicly available data collected with patients consent approved by relevant institutional review board following declaration of Helsinki.

Data was approved by following institutional boards: Institutional review board of Samsung Medical Center, and written informed consent was obtained (IRB 2005-

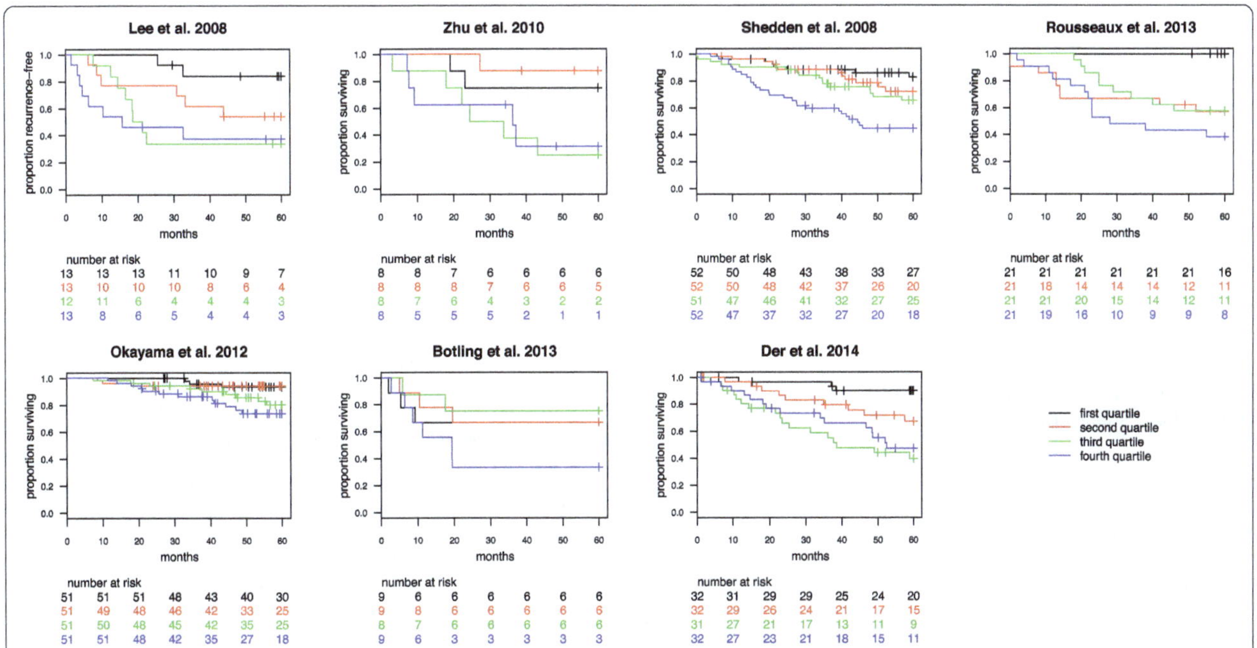

Fig. 3 Kaplan-Meier survival estimates for the seven early stage lung adenocarcinoma cohorts, split according to ESLA-7 score quartiles

12-034), The University Health Network Research Ethics Board, Institutional Review Board of each of the four institutions' (University of Michigan Cancer Center (UM), Moffitt Cancer Center (HLM), Memorial Sloan-Kettering Cancer Center (MSK) and the Dana-Farber Cancer Institute (CAN/DF)), Institutional Review Board of the National Cancer Center, Tokyo, Japan, Uppsala regional ethical review board, reference #2006/ 325 and Linkoeping regional ethical review board, reference #2010/44-31, Research Ethics Board of University Health Network (UHN181), for TCGA data used in this study declaration on ethics is as follows: All specimens were obtained from patients with appropriate consent from the relevant institutional review board.

Abbreviations

CCP: cell cycle progression (signature); CIN: chromosomal instability (signature); ESLA: early stage lung adenocarcinoma (signature); GEO: gene expression omnibus; LUAD: lung adenocarcinoma; LUSC: lung squamous carcinoma; NSCLC: non small lung cancer; OS: overall survival; PCR: polymerase chain reaction; RFS: recurrence-free survival.

Competing interests

ACE and ZS are named inventors on a patent related to the CIN25 chromosomal instability signature mentioned in this paper. For the remaining authors none were declared.

Authors' contributions

MK and ZS designed the study. MK, ACE and ZS performed the analysis. MK, ZS, JM, DS and ACE wrote the manuscript. DS, JM contributed to critical review of the manuscript. All authors read and approved the final manuscript.

Funding

This work was supported by the Danish Council for Independent Research [09-073053/FSS]; the Breast Cancer Research Foundation, the Széchenyi Progam, Hungary [KTIA_NAP_13-2014-0021], MTA Homing Program 2013, MTA-TKI643/ 2012 and the Novo Nordisk Foundation [to ZS]; the Danish Cancer Society grants R72- R90-A6213 [to MK] and A4618-13-S2 [to ACE] and the MTA Momentum Program 2011 [to DS].

Author details

[1]Department of Systems Biology, Center for Biological Sequence Analysis, Technical University of Denmark, Lyngby, Denmark. [2]Department of Tumor Biology, National Koranyi Institute – Semmelweis University, Budapest, Hungary. [3]Institute of Enzymology, Research Centre for Natural Sciences, Hungarian Academy of Sciences, Budapest, Hungary. [4]Computational Health Informatics Program (CHIP), Boston Children's Hospital, Boston, USA. [5]Harvard Medical School, Boston, USA.

References

1. Crinò L, Weder W, van Meerbeeck J, Felip E. Early stage and locally advanced (non-metastatic) non-small-cell lung cancer: ESMO Clinical Practice Guidelines for diagnosis, treatment and follow-up. Ann Oncol. 2010;21 Suppl 5:v103–15.
2. Vansteenkiste J, Crinò L, Dooms C, Douillard JY, Faivre-Finn C, Lim E, Rocco G, Senan S, van Schil P, Veronesi G, Stahel R, Peters S, Felip E, Kerr K, Besse B, Eberhardt W, Edelman M, Mok T, O'Byrne K, Novello S, Bubendorf L, Marchetti A, Baas P, Reck M, Syrigos K, Paz-Ares L, Smit EF, Meldgaard P, Adjei A, Nicolson M, et al. 2nd ESMO consensus conference on lung cancer: Early-stage non-small-cell lung cancer consensus on diagnosis, treatment and follow-up. Ann Oncol. 2014;25:1462 74.
3. Paik S, Shak S, Tang G, Kim C, Baker J, Cronin M, Baehner FL, Walker MG, Watson D, Park T, Hiller W, Fisher ER, Wickerham DL, Bryant J, Wolmark N. A multigene assay to predict recurrence of tamoxifen-treated, node-negative breast cancer. N Engl J Med. 2004;351:2817–26.
4. Lee E-S, Son D-S, Kim S-H, Lee J, Jo J, Han J, Kim H, Lee HJ, Choi HY, Jung Y, Park M, Lim YS, Kim K, Shim Y, Kim BC, Lee K, Huh N, Ko C, Park K, Lee JW, Choi YS, Kim J. Prediction of recurrence-free survival in postoperative non-small cell lung cancer patients by using an integrated model of clinical information and gene expression. Clin Cancer Res. 2008;14:7397–404.
5. Zhu C-Q, Ding K, Strumpf D, Weir BA, Meyerson M, Pennell N, Thomas RK, Naoki K, Ladd-Acosta C, Liu N, Pintilie M, Der S, Seymour L, Jurisica I, Shepherd FA, Tsao M-S. Prognostic and predictive gene signature for adjuvant chemotherapy in resected non-small-cell lung cancer. J Clin Oncol. 2010;28:4417–24.
6. Shedden K, Taylor JMG, Enkemann SA, Tsao M-S, Yeatman TJ, Gerald WL, Eschrich S, Jurisica I, Giordano TJ, Misek DE, Chang AC, Zhu CQ, Strumpf D, Hanash S, Shepherd FA, Ding K, Seymour L, Naoki K, Pennell N, Weir B, Verhaak R, Ladd-Acosta C, Golub T, Gruidl M, Sharma A, Szoke J, Zakowski M, Rusch V, Kris M, Viale A, et al. Gene expression-based survival prediction in lung adenocarcinoma: a multi-site, blinded validation study. Nat Med. 2008;14:822–7.
7. Rousseaux S, Debernardi A, Jacquiau B, Vitte A-L, Vesin A, Nagy-Mignotte H, Moro-Sibilot D, Brichon P-Y, Lantuejoul S, Hainaut P, Laffaire J, de Reyniès A, Beer DG, Timsit J-F, Brambilla C, Brambilla E, Khochbin S. Ectopic activation of germline and placental genes identifies aggressive metastasis-prone lung cancers. Sci Transl Med. 2013;5:186ra66.
8. Okayama H, Kohno T, Ishii Y, Shimada Y, Shiraishi K, Iwakawa R, Furuta K, Tsuta K, Shibata T, Yamamoto S, Watanabe S, Sakamoto H, Kumamoto K, Takenoshita S, Gotoh N, Mizuno H, Sarai A, Kawano S, Yamaguchi R, Miyano S, Yokota J. Identification of genes upregulated in ALK-positive and EGFR/ KRAS/ALK-negative lung adenocarcinomas. Cancer Res. 2012;72:100–11.
9. Botling J, Edlund K, Lohr M, Hellwig B, Holmberg L, Lambe M, Berglund A, Ekman S, Bergqvist M, Pontén F, König A, Fernandes O, Karlsson M, Helenius G, Karlsson C, Rahnenführer J, Hengstler JG, Micke P. Biomarker discovery in non-small cell lung cancer: integrating gene expression profiling, meta-analysis, and tissue microarray validation. Clin Cancer Res. 2013;19:194–204.
10. Der SD, Sykes J, Pintilie M, Zhu C-Q, Strumpf D, Liu N, Jurisica I, Shepherd FA, Tsao M-S. Validation of a histology-independent prognostic gene signature for early-stage, non-small-cell lung cancer including stage IA patients. J Thorac Oncol. 2014;9:59–64.
11. Eklund AC, Szallasi Z. Correction of technical bias in clinical microarray data improves concordance with known biological information. Genome Biol. 2008;9:R26.
12. Krzystanek M, Szallasi Z, Eklund AC. Biasogram: visualization of confounding technical bias in gene expression data. PLoS One. 2013;8:e61872.
13. Wistuba II, Behrens C, Lombardi F, Wagner S, Fujimoto J, Raso MG, Spaggiari L, Galetta D, Riley R, Hughes E, Reid J, Sangale Z, Swisher SG, Kalhor N, Moran CA, Gutin A, Lanchbury JS, Barberis M, Kim ES. Validation of a Proliferation-Based Expression Signature as Prognostic Marker in Early Stage Lung Adenocarcinoma. Clin Cancer Res. 2013;19:6261–71.
14. Bueno R, Hughes E, Lanchbury JS, Gustafson C, Jones JT, Barberis M, Wistuba I, Wallace WA, Harrison DJ. Validation of a Molecular and Pathological Model for Five-Year Mortality Risk in Patients with Early Stage Lung Adenocarcinoma. J Thorac Oncol. 2015;10:67–73.
15. Li B, Dewey CN. RSEM: accurate transcript quantification from RNA-Seq data with or without a reference genome. BMC Bioinformatics. 2011;12:323.
16. Network TCGAR. Comprehensive molecular profiling of lung adenocarcinoma. Nature. 2014;511:543–50.
17. Carter SL, Eklund AC, Kohane IS, Harris LN, Szallasi Z. A signature of chromosomal instability inferred from gene expression profiles predicts

clinical outcome in multiple human cancers. Nat Genet. 2006;38:1043–8.
18. Paik S. Development and clinical utility of a 21-gene recurrence score prognostic assay in patients with early breast cancer treated with tamoxifen. Oncologist. 2007;12:631–5.
19. Gentles AJ, Newman AM, Liu CL, Bratman SV, Feng W, Kim D, Nair VS, Xu Y, Khuong A, Hoang CD, Diehn M, West RB, Plevritis SK, Alizadeh AA. The prognostic landscape of genes and infiltrating immune cells across human cancers. Nat Med. 2015;21:938–45.
20. Birkbak NJ, Eklund AC, Li Q, McClelland SE, Endesfelder D, Tan P, Tan IB, Richardson AL, Szallasi Z, Swanton C. Paradoxical relationship between chromosomal instability and survival outcome in cancer. Cancer Res. 2011;71:3447–52.

7

Tumor-associated macrophages, potential targets for cancer treatment

Li Yang[1] and Yi Zhang[1,2*]

Abstract

The fact that various immune cells, including macrophages, can be found in tumor tissues has long been known. With the introduction of concept that macrophages differentiate into a classically or alternatively activated phenotype, the role of tumor-associated macrophages (TAMs) is now beginning to be elucidated. TAMs act as "protumoral macrophages", contributing to disease progression. As the relationship between TAMs and malignant tumors becomes clearer, TAMs are beginning to be seen as potential therapeutic targets in these cases. In this review, we will discuss how TAMs can be used as therapeutic targets of cancer in clinics.

Keywords: Tumor-associated macrophages (TAMs), Tumor microenvironment, Therapeutic target, Cancer treatment, Protumoral activities

Background

Non-resolving inflammation in a tumor microenvironment is a hallmark of cancer. Leukocytes, fibroblasts, and vascular endothelial cells together form a tumor microenvironment, with immune cells representing its major component. These immune cells interact with tumor cells to influence the initiation, growth, and metastasis of tumors. Tumor-associated macrophages (TAMs), specifically, are often prominent immune cells that orchestrate various factors in the tumor microenvironment [1, 2].

In general, TAMs are thought to more closely resemble M2-polarized macrophages [3], also known as alternatively activated macrophages, which are activated by helper T cell 2 cytokines (e.g., interleukin (IL) -4, IL-10, and IL-13). TAMs play an important role in connecting inflammation with cancer. TAMs can promote proliferation, invasion, and metastasis of tumor cells, stimulate tumor angiogenesis, and inhibit antitumor immune response mediated by T cells, followed by the promotion of tumor progression [3]. There are strong evidences of tumor promotion by TAMs in different cancer models, and an increased TAM prevalence correlates with low survival rates in many human cancers.

With the unraveling of the relationship between TAMs and malignant tumors, TAMs are now being recognized as potential therapeutic targets for cancer. Targeting TAMs is a novel strategy for treatment of cancers. In this review, we summarize how TAMs are used as therapeutic targets in cancers.

Limiting monocyte recruitment

One strategy for targeting TAMs is to block monocyte recruitment into tumor tissues. Targeting the chemokine (C-C motif) ligand 2 (CCL2) - chemokine (C-C motif) receptor (CCR2) axis is promising due to its important role in monocyte recruitment in tumors. A CCL2-blocking agent (carlumab, CNTO88) has been shown to inhibit the growth of several cancers in animal models. A phase II study of carlumab in metastatic castration-resistant prostate cancer patients showed that this antibody was well-tolerated, but that neither blocked the CCL2/CCR2 axis nor showed antitumor activity as a single agent in these metastatic cancer patients [4] (NCT00992186, Table 1). Similar results from Brana et al. showed that carlumab in combination with four chemotherapy regimens for the treatment of patients with solid tumors was well-tolerated, although no long-term suppression of serum CCL2 or significant tumor responses were observed [5] (NCT01204996, Table 1).

* Correspondence: yizhang@zzu.edu.cn
[1]Biotherapy Center and Cancer Center, The First Affiliated Hospital of Zhengzhou University, No.1 Jianshe East Road, Zhengzhou, Henan Province 450052, China
[2]School of Life Sciences, Zhengzhou University, No.100 Kexue Road, Zhengzhou, Henan Province 450001, China

Table 1 Clinical trials of agents that target TAMs for cancer treatment

Action	Agent name	Target	Status	Phase	Tumor type	Effect	Trial number
Limiting monocyte recruitment	Carlumab	CCL2	Completed	II	Metastatic castration-resistant prostate cancer	Well-tolerated, no antitumor activity as a single agent	NCT00992186
			Completed	Ib	Solid tumors	Well-tolerated, no long-term suppression of serum CCL2 or significant tumor responses	NCT01204996
			Completed	I	Solid tumors	Transient CCL2 suppression, preliminary antitumor activity	NCT00537368
	PF-04136309	CCR2	Completed	Ib	Locally advanced pancreatic cancer	Safe and tolerable, objective tumor response	NCT01413022
	MLN1202	CCR2	Completed	II	Bone metastases	uNTX response rate: 14/43	NCT01015560
Targeting TAM activation	MCS110	CSF1	Recruiting	II	Advanced triple negative breast cancer	NA	NCT02435680
			Recruiting	Ib/II	Advanced malignancies	NA	NCT01643850
			Terminated	I/II	Prostate cancer, bone metastases	NA	NCT00757757
	IMC-CS4	CSF1R	Recruiting	I	Advanced solid tumors	NA	NCT01346358
			Recruiting	I	Advanced, refractory breast or prostate cancer	NA	NCT02265536
	AMG 820	CSF1R	Completed	I	Advanced solid tumors	NA	NCT01444404
			Recruiting	I/II	Pancreatic cancer, colorectal cancer, non-small cell lung cancer	NA	NCT02713529
	PLX7486	CSF1R	Recruiting	I	Advanced solid tumors	NA	NCT01804530
	PLX3397	CSF1R	Completed	II	Recurrent glioblastoma	Well tolerated, no efficacy	NCT01349036
			Completed	II	Relapsed or refractory Hodgkin's lymphoma	Safe, response rate: 1/20	NCT01217229
			Completed	II	Advanced castration-resistant prostate cancer	NA	NCT01499043
			Recruiting	I/II	Sarcoma, malignant peripheral nerve sheath tumors	NA	NCT02584647
			Recruiting	II	Advanced melanoma, other solid tumors	NA	NCT02452424
			Recruiting	Ib/II	Metastatic breast cancer	NA	NCT01596751
			Recruiting	I/II	Refractory leukemias, solid tumors	NA	NCT02390752
			Recruiting	I	Advanced solid tumors	NA	NCT01525602
	Alemtuzumab	CD52	Terminated	I	Ovarian, fallopian, or primary peritoneal cancers	NA	NCT00637390
			Completed	II	Kidney cancer	NA	NCT00073879
Reprogramming TAMs to antitumor macrophages	ChiLob 7/4	CD40	Completed	I	Advanced malignancies refractory to conventional anti-cancer treatment	Safe, activate B and NK cells	NCT01561911
	(GM.CD40L) vaccine with CCL21	CD40	Active, not recruiting	I/II	Lung cancer	NA	NCT01433172
	Tremelimumab and CP-870, 893	CD40	Active, not recruiting	I	Metastatic melanoma	NA	NCT01103635
	WP1066	STAT3	Not yet recruiting	I	Recurrent malignant glioma and brain metastases	NA	NCT01904123
	AZD9150 (ISIS-STAT3Rx)	STAT3	Completed	I/Ib	Advanced/metastatic hepatocellular	NA	NCT01839604

Table 1 Clinical trials of agents that target TAMs for cancer treatment *(Continued)*

					carcinoma		
	β-glucan	MAPK	Completed	II	Stage IV KRAS-mutant colorectal cancer	Compelling, albeit modest, clinical activity	NCT00912327
			Recruiting	I	Neuroblastoma	NA	NCT00911560
			Active, not recruiting	I	Metastatic neuroblastoma	NA	NCT00492167
	Hu5F9-G4	CD47	Recruiting	I	Solid tumor	NA	NCT02216409
	CC-90002 and Rituximab	CD47	Recruiting	I	Hematologic neoplasms	NA	NCT02367196

However, according to the results of other study, carlumab was well-tolerated with evidence of transient CCL2 suppression and preliminary antitumor activity [6] (NCT00537368, Table 1).

Sanford et al. demonstrates that a CCR2 antagonist (PF-04136309) can block the mobilization of CCR2$^+$ monocytes from bone marrow to tumors in a mouse model of pancreatic cancer and can lead to TAM depletion, causing the inhibition of tumor growth and distant metastasis [7]. PF-04136309, in combination with FOLFIRINOX chemotherapy, was used in a phase Ib trial (NCT01413022, Table 1). This therapy was found safe and tolerable with an objective tumor response [8]. Moreover, the efficiency of the humanized antibody specific for CCR2 (MLN1202) was determined in a clinical investigation (NCT01015560, Table 1).

Treatment with systemic CD11b-neutralizing monoclonal antibodies has been shown to prevent the recruitment of myeloid cells to tumors. It has been shown that the use of Mac-1 (CD11b/CD18) antibodies leads to an improved response to radiation therapy in squamous cell carcinoma xenografts of mice, which is accompanied by reduced infiltration of myeloid cells expressing matrix metallopeptidase-9 and S100A8 inside tumors [9].

Because targeting monocytes, prior to being recruited to tumors, has been effective in various cancer models and partial clinical trials, TAMs can be directly targeted as well by other approaches once they invade tumors.

Targeting the activation of TAMs

TAMs can be targeted at the level of activation using various strategies. Colony-stimulating factor 1 (CSF1)/CSF1 receptor (CSF1R) signaling is critical for the generation of monocyte progenitors in bone marrow and TAM polarization in tumor tissues. For these reasons, CSF1/CSF1R signaling is an attractive target for cancer treatment. Genetic loss of CSF1 results in significantly reduced metastasis and delayed tumor progression in breast and neuroendocrine tumor models [10]. Based on these results, several clinical trials of CSF1/CSF1R inhibitors have been completed or are ongoing (Table 1).

Macrophage surface markers can act as useful therapeutic targets. Mannose receptor CD206 can be exploited as a macrophage-specific target. A single-chain peptide bound to the CD206 receptor was attached to nanobodies that can selectively target CD206$^+$ TAMs [11]. Legumain, a stress protein and a member of the asparagine endopeptidase family, can serve as an efficient therapeutic target when overexpressed in TAMs [12]. Targeting surface markers such as scavenger receptor A and CD52 by using immunotoxin-conjugated monoclonal antibodies (mAbs) has been investigated in ovarian cancer [13]. Moreover, the efficiency of alemtuzumab (anti-CD52 antibody) as a tumor treatment in ongoing clinical trials is under investigation (NCT00637390, NCT00073879, Table 1).

Trabectedin (ET743, Yondelis®) was shown to decrease the number of TAMs in tumor tissues by inducing apoptosis of monocytes and macrophages [14]. Based on the favorable results of several phase I, II, and III clinical trials, trabectedin has gained full marketing approval from the European Commission for use in the treatment of ovarian cancer and soft tissue sarcomas and FDA approval in 2015 for use in unresectable or metastatic liposarcoma or leiomyosarcoma [15].

Reprogramming TAMs to antitumor macrophages

As discussed above, one of the key features of macrophages is their plasticity, which enables them to change their phenotype in the tumor microenvironment. Thus, reprogramming TAMs to an antitumor phenotype is an attractive therapeutic strategy. The results of our previous study showed that pseudomonas aeruginosa mannose-sensitive hemagglutinin, which is used in MPE treatment, re-educated CD163$^+$ TAMs to M1 macrophages in MPE, suggesting that reprogramming CD163$^+$ TAMs can be served as a potential therapeutic strategy of MPE [16].

Nanoparticles are gradually used in polarization of TAMs into antitumor macrophages. Recently, Zanganeh et al. found that ferumoxytol significantly inhibited growth of subcutaneous adenocarcinomas in mice, and this tumor growth inhibition was accompanied by an increase in pro-inflammatory M1 macrophages in tumor tissues [17].

Recent data suggest that bioconjugated manganese dioxide nanoparticles enhance the responses of chemotherapy by inducing TAM toward M1-like phenotype [18]. Synthesized nanoparticles with IL-12 payload can reverse macrophages to antitumor function [19].

CD40 is a surface marker of macrophages that can be used to inhibit cytotoxic functions. The combination of a CD40 agonist with gemcitabine in unresectable pancreatic cancer resulted in regression of tumors by promoting antitumor macrophages [20]. ChiLob 7/4 is an intermediate CD40 agonist and chimeric IgG1, which was also shown to induce pro-inflammatory cytokines, with promising results in CD40-expressing solid tumors and diffuse large B-cell lymphoma resistant to conventional therapy in a phase I clinical trial [21] (NCT01561911, Table 1). Other clinical trials of molecules targeting CD40 for cancer treatment are ongoing (NCT01433172, NCT01103635, Table 1).

Activation of the nuclear factor κB pathway also plays an important role in polarization of TAMs to an antitumor phenotype using Toll-like receptor agonists, anti-CD40 mAbs and IL-10 mAbs [22]. In addition, regulation of STAT1 activity is an attractive strategy to induce an antitumor phenotype in macrophages because of the increase production of IL-12 in a murine carcinoma model. A small molecule inhibitor of STAT3 (WP1066) was found to reverse immune tolerance in patients with malignant gliomas and to selectively induce the expression of costimulatory molecules CD80, CD86, and IL-12 on peripheral and tumor-infiltrating macrophages [23]. An investigation of this agent to treat recurrent malignant gliomas and brain metastasis are ongoing (NCT01904123, Table 1).

Thymosin-α is an immunomodulating hormone that can reeducate TAMs into dendritic cells, which participate in antitumor host responses and produce high level of pro-inflammatory cytokines. Nanodelivery of thymosin-α is a feasible approach to increase immune activity in cancer patients. Moreover, several clinical trials have confirmed that thymosin-α prolongs survival in patients with metastatic melanomas and advanced non-small cell lung cancers [24].

β-glucan, a yeast-derived polysaccharide, has been shown to differentiate TAMs into an M1 phenotype, and is a potent immunomodulator with anti-cancer properties. The use of β-glucan is currently under investigation in a phase I clinical trial of patients with neuroblastoma [25] (NCT00911560, Table 1). In another clinical trial, a β-glucan polymer (PGG) showed compelling but modest activity in a phase II multicancer study [26] (NCT00912327, Table 1). Furthermore, the efficiency of β-glucan is currently under phase I clinical investigation (NCT00492167, Table 1).

In addition, CD47 has been identified as an important "don't eat me" signal expressed on malignant cells [27]. Blockade of the CD47:SIRP-α axis between tumor cells and macrophages increases tumor cell phagocytosis in both solid tumors and hematological malignancies. Two phase I dose escalation trials are currently underway with anti-CD47 antibodies as a monotherapy for the treatment of advanced solid tumors and hematological cancers [27] (NCT02216409, NCT02367196, Table 1). CD47 blocking agents are expected to be well tolerated, efficacious and broadly applicable for cancer therapies.

TAMs as a carry of anti-cancer drugs

TAMs can also be used as a carry of anti-cancer drugs, which is one of the most promising strategies of cancer treatment. It has been reported that macrophages can actively internalize gold nanoshells and deliver them into hypoxic regions of tumors [28], inducing cancer cell death around these macrophages. Wang et al. found that macrophages loaded by a magnetic shell combined with topoisomerase I inhibitor SN38 could deliver into the tumor site and exert an anti-cancer effect [29]. In addition, similar combination therapy was showed by Ikehara et al. [30]. Nanoparticles coated with mannose and loaded with 5-fluorouracil were internalized by macrophages. The tumor growth inhibition was observed when an electromagnetic field was applied in a mouse intraperitoneal metastatic model.

Targeting TAMs in combination with standard therapies

Radiotherapy and chemotherapy are useful treatments in many cancers, and studies have shown that infiltrated-myeloid increases after irradiation. However, the interaction between tumor cells and stroma after these therapies remains poorly defined. DNA damage, cell death, and increased hypoxia have been observed in tumors after radiotherapy, which has been shown to lead to macrophage recruitment and promote tumor progression in animal models [31]. Therefore, it is essential to combine TAM targeting with standard therapies for effective tumor treatment.

The hypoxia-inducible factor-1 (HIF-1) pathway is stimulated by radiation-induced tumor hypoxia and the HIF-1 inhibitor can result in decreased infiltration of myeloid cells into tumors [32]. Even more strikingly, blocking CSF1R signaling appears to enhance the efficacy of several other standard therapies. As such, CSF1R blockade has been shown to increase the efficacy of chemotherapy for pancreatic tumors [33].

Conclusions

Targeting TAMs is a promising strategy for cancer treatment. Recent ongoing experimental, pre-clinical, and clinical studies of TAMs have shown encouraging progress. We believe that TAM-targeted therapies would be applied in cancer patients in the future.

Abbreviations

CCL2: Chemokine (C-C motif) ligand 2; CCR2: Chemokine (C-C motif) receptor 2; CSF1: Colony-stimulating factor; CSF1R: CSF1 receptor; HIF-1: Hypoxia-inducible factor 1; IL: Interleukin; TAMs: Tumor-associated macrophages

Acknowledgements

Not applicable.

Authors' contributors

LY wrote and edited the manuscript, YZ revised the manuscript. All authors read and approved the final manuscript.

Funding

This study was supported by grants from the National Natural Science Foundation of China (No.81171986, No.81602024), Funding from State's Key Project of Research and Development Plan (No. 2016YFC1303500), International Research Cooperation Grant from Science and Technology Department of Henan Province (No.162102410059), Research Grant from the Ministry of Public Health (No.201501004).

Competing interests

The authors declare that they have no competing interests.

References

1. Quail DF, Joyce JA. Microenvironmental regulation of tumor progression and metastasis. Nat Med. 2013;19:1423–37.
2. Li L, Yang L, Wang L, Wang F, Zhang Z, Li J, Yue D, Chen X, Ping Y, Huang L, et al. Impaired T cell function in malignant pleural effusion is caused by TGF-β derived predominantly from macrophages. Int J Cancer. 2016;139: 2261–9.
3. Grivennikov SI, Greten FR, Karin M. Immunity, inflammation, and cancer. Cell. 2010;140:883–99.
4. Pienta KJ, Machiels JP, Schrijvers D, Alekseev B, Shkolnik M, Crabb SJ, Li S, Seetharam S, Puchalski TA, Takimoto C, et al. Phase 2 study of carlumab (CNTO 888), a human monoclonal antibody against CC-chemokine ligand 2 (CCL2), in metastatic castration-resistant prostate cancer. Investig New Drugs. 2013;31:760–8.
5. Brana I, Calles A, LoRusso PM, Yee LK, Puchalski TA, Seetharam S, Zhong B, de Boer CJ, Tabernero J, Calvo E. Carlumab, an anti-C-C chemokine ligand 2 monoclonal antibody, in combination with four chemotherapy regimens for the treatment of patients with solid tumors: an open-label, multicenter phase 1b study. Target Oncol. 2015;10:111–23.
6. Sandhu SK, Papadopoulos K, Fong PC, Patnaik A, Messiou C, Olmos D, Wang G, Tromp BJ, Puchalski TA, Balkwill F, et al. A first-in-human, first-in-class, phase I study of carlumab (CNTO 888), a human monoclonal antibody against CC-chemokine ligand 2 in patients with solid tumors. Cancer Chemother Pharmacol. 2013;71:1041–50.
7. Sanford DE, Belt BA, Panni RZ, Mayer A, Deshpande AD, Carpenter D, Mitchem JB, Plambeck-Suess SM, Worley LA, Goetz BD, et al. Inflammatory monocyte mobilization decreases patient survival in pancreatic cancer: a role for targeting the CCL2/CCR2 axis. Clin Cancer Res. 2013;19:3404–15.
8. Nywening TM, Wang-Gillam A, Sanford DE, Belt BA, Panni RZ, Cusworth BM, Toriola AT, Nieman RK, Worley LA, Yano M, et al. Targeting tumour-associated macrophages with CCR2 inhibition in combination with FOLFIRINOX in patients with borderline resectable and locally advanced pancreatic cancer: a single-centre, open-label, dose-finding, non-randomised, phase 1b trial. Lancet Oncol. 2016;17:651–62.
9. Ahn GO, Tseng D, Liao CH, Dorie MJ, Czechowicz A, Brown JM. Inhibition of Mac-1 (CD11b/CD18) enhances tumor response to radiation by reducing myeloid cell recruitment. Proc Natl Acad Sci U S A. 2010;107:8363–8.
10. Pyonteck SM, Gadea BB, Wang HW, Gocheva V, Hunter KE, Tang LH, Joyce JA. Deficiency of the macrophage growth factor CSF-1 disrupts pancreatic neuroendocrine tumor development. Oncogene. 2012;31:1459–67.
11. Movahedi K, Schoonooghe S, Laoui D, Houbracken I, Waelput W, Breckpot K, Bouwens L, Lahoutte T, De Baetselier P, Raes G, et al. Nanobody-based targeting of the macrophage mannose receptor for effective in vivo imaging of tumor-associated macrophages. Cancer Res. 2012;72:4165–77.
12. Smahel M, Duskova M, Polakova I, Musil J. Enhancement of DNA vaccine potency against legumain. J Immunother. 2014;37:293–303.
13. Pulaski HL, Spahlinger G, Silva IA, McLean K, Kueck AS, Reynolds RK, Coukos G, Conejo-Garcia JR, Buckanovich RJ. Identifying alemtuzumab as an anti-myeloid cell antiangiogenic therapy for the treatment of ovarian cancer. J Transl Med. 2009;7:49.
14. Allavena P, Signorelli M, Chieppa M, Erba E, Bianchi G, Marchesi F, Olimpio CO, Bonardi C, Garbi A, Lissoni A, et al. Anti-inflammatory properties of the novel antitumor agent yondelis (trabectedin): inhibition of macrophage differentiation and cytokine production. Cancer Res. 2005;65:2964–71.
15. Gordon EM, Sankhala KK, Chawla N, Chawla SP. Trabectedin for soft tissue sarcoma: current status and future perspectives. Adv Ther. 2016;33:1055–71.
16. Yang L, Wang F, Wang L, Huang L, Wang J, Zhang B, Zhang Y. CD163+ tumor-associated macrophage is a prognostic biomarker and is associated with therapeutic effect on malignant pleural effusion of lung cancer patients. Oncotarget. 2015;6:10592–603.
17. Zanganeh S, Hutter G, Spitler R, Lenkov O, Mahmoudi M, Shaw A, Pajarinen JS, Nejadnik H, Goodman S, Moseley M, et al. Iron oxide nanoparticles inhibit tumour growth by inducing pro-inflammatory macrophage polarization in tumour tissues. Nat Nanotechnol. 2016;11:986–94.
18. Song M, Liu T, Shi C, Zhang X, Chen X. Bioconjugated manganese dioxide nanoparticles enhance chemotherapy response by priming tumor-associated macrophages toward M1-like phenotype and attenuating tumor hypoxia. ACS Nano. 2016;10:633–47.
19. Wang Y, Lin YX, Qiao SL, An HW, Ma Y, Qiao ZY, Rajapaksha RP, Wang H. Polymeric nanoparticles promote macrophage reversal from M2 to M1 phenotypes in the tumor microenvironment. Biomaterials. 2017;112:153–63.
20. Beatty GL, Chiorean EG, Fishman MP, Saboury B, Teitelbaum UR, Sun W, Huhn RD, Song W, Li D, Sharp LL, et al. CD40 agonists alter tumor stroma and show efficacy against pancreatic carcinoma in mice and humans. Science. 2011;331:1612–6.
21. Johnson P, Challis R, Chowdhury F, Gao Y, Harvey M, Geldart T, Kerr P, Chan C, Smith A, Steven N, et al. Clinical and biological effects of an agonist anti-CD40 antibody: a Cancer Research UK phase I study. Clin Cancer Res. 2015;21:1321–8.
22. Seya T, Shime H, Matsumoto M. TAMable tumor-associated macrophages in response to innate RNA sensing. Oncoimmunology. 2012;1:1000–1.
23. Hussain SF, Kong LY, Jordan J, Conrad C, Madden T, Fokt I, Priebe W, Heimberger AB. A novel small molecule inhibitor of signal transducers and activators of transcription 3 reverses immune tolerance in malignant glioma patients. Cancer Res. 2007;67:9630–6.
24. Garaci E, Pica F, Serafino A, Balestrieri E, Matteucci C, Moroni G, Sorrentino R, Zonfrillo M, Pierimarchi P, Sinibaldi-Vallebona P. Thymosin alpha1 and cancer: action on immune effector and tumor target cells. Ann N Y Acad Sci. 2012;1269:26–33.
25. Kushner BH, Cheung IY, Modak S, Kramer K, Ragupathi G, Cheung NK. Phase I trial of a bivalent gangliosides vaccine in combination with beta-glucan for high-risk neuroblastoma in second or later remission. Clin Cancer Res. 2014;20:1375–82.
26. Segal NH, Gada P, Senzer N, Gargano MA, Patchen ML, Saltz LB. A phase II efficacy and safety, open-label, multicenter study of Imprime PGG injection in combination with Cetuximab in patients with stage IV KRAS-mutant colorectal cancer. Clin Colorectal Canc. 2016;15:222–7.
27. McCracken MN, Cha AC, Weissman IL. Molecular pathways: activating T cells after cancer cell Phagocytosis from blockade of CD47 "Don't eat me" signals. Clin Cancer Res. 2015;21:3597–601.
28. Choi M-R, Stanton-Maxey KJ, Stanley JK, Levin CS, Bardhan R, Akin D, Badve S, Sturgis J, Robinson JP, Bashir R, et al. A cellular Trojan horse for delivery of therapeutic nanoparticles into tumors. Nano Lett. 2007;7:3759–65.

29. Wang H, Shrestha TB, Basel MT, Dani RK, Seo GM, Balivada S, Pyle MM, Prock H, Koper OB, Thapa PS, et al. Magnetic-Fe/Fe(3)O(4)-nanoparticle-bound SN38 as carboxylesterase-cleavable prodrug for the delivery to tumors within monocytes/macrophages. Beilstein J Nanotechnol. 2012;3:444–55.
30. Ikehara Y, Niwa T, Biao L, Ikehara SK, Ohashi N, Kobayashi T, Shimizu Y, Kojima N, Nakanishi H. A carbohydrate recognition-based drug delivery and controlled release system using intraperitoneal macrophages as a cellular vehicle. Cancer Res. 2006;66:8740–8.
31. De Palma M, Lewis CE. Macrophage regulation of tumor responses to anticancer therapies. Cancer Cell. 2013;23:277–86.
32. Kioi M, Vogel H, Schultz G, Hoffman RM, Harsh GR, Brown JM. Inhibition of vasculogenesis, but not angiogenesis, prevents the recurrence of glioblastoma after irradiation in mice. J Clin Invest. 2010;120:694–705.
33. Mitchem JB, Brennan DJ, Knolhoff BL, Belt BA, Zhu Y, Sanford DE, Belaygorod L, Carpenter D, Collins L, Piwnica-Worms D, et al. Targeting tumor-infiltrating macrophages decreases tumor-initiating cells, relieves immunosuppression, and improves chemotherapeutic responses. Cancer Res. 2013;73:1128–41.

8

Bone biomarker for the clinical assessment of osteoporosis

Tsung-Rong Kuo[1,2] and Chih-Hwa Chen[3,4*]

Abstract

Bone biomarkers included formation, resorption and regulator are released during the bone remodeling processes. These bone biomarkers have attracted much attention in the clinical assessment of osteoporosis treatment in the past decade. Combination with the measurement of bone mineral density, the clinical applications of bone biomarkers have provided comprehensive information for diagnosis of osteoporosis. However, the analytical approaches of the bone biomarkers are still the challenge for further clinical trials. In this mini-review, we have introduced the functions of bone biomarkers and then recently developed techniques for bone biomarker measurements have been systematically integrated to discuss the possibility for osteoporosis assessment in the early stage.

Keywords: Bone biomarker, Bone formation, Bone resorption, Regulators, Bone turnover, Osteoporosis

Background

Osteoporosis is a worldwide disease with reduction of bone mass and decrease of bone strength to result in bone fragility and fracture. Based on the report of World Health Organization (WHO), the disease of osteoporosis has been diagnosed by bone mineral density (BMD) at the hip and/or the spine at least 2.5 standard deviations below in comparison with the bone mass of young healthy adults as determined by dual-energy X-ray absorptiometry (DXA) [1]. The people with osteoporosis are steadily increased because of aging society occurring worldwide. There are about 200 million people are suffered from osteoporosis in the word and approximately 8.9 million fractures are caused by osteoporotic fracture [2]. In the osteoporotic fractures, hip fractures have led to mortality rates up to 20–24% within the first year and then the death rate has steadily increased for at least 5 years [3]. After hip fractures, the survivors may lose the capability of action and independence with 40% unable to walk independently and 60% requiring assistance at least 1 year. Due to the loss of capability, around 33% patients are totally dependent or in a nursing home in the year following a hip fracture. Nowadays, osteoporosis is a major concern of public health because of its healthcare cost. Moreover, the fracture caused by osteoporosis is the most important factor for the decreases of quality of life and survival rate in aging people.

Osteoporosis is a silent disease without obvious symptom and evidence until occurrence of fracture. Early diagnosis of osteoporosis is the key issue for efficient treatment and for identification of osteoporotic patient with high risk of fracture. At present, diagnosis of osteoporosis and assessment of fracture risk are based on the quantitative analysis of BMD by DXA. However, the gold standard method of BMD assessment of bone mass by DXA only partially provides the information about bone strength. The osteoporosis is characterized by bone fragility. Bone fragility is evaluated by its microarchitectural quality which is identified by all bone features such as microarchitecture, microdamage and remodeling rates with the influence of bone's ability for resistant fracture. The two-dimensional technique of DXA reveals the intrinsic limitations to discriminate cortical from cancellous bone and characterize changes because of bone geometry. Recently, several approaches have been developed to provide supplementary information for the assessment of fracture risks except BMD. For example,

* Correspondence: chihhwache@tmu.edu.tw
[3]Bone and Joint Research Center, Department of Orthopedics and Traumatology, Taipei Medical University Hospital, Taipei 11031, Taiwan
[4]School of Medicine, College of Medicine, Taipei Medical University, Taipei 11031, Taiwan

quantitative computed tomography (QCT) has been developed to evaluate bone loss [4, 5]. In QCT, the true value of mineral density for trabecular bone has been obtained from cortical portion of bone [6]. Moreover, the instrument of ultrasound has been applied to examine bone condition and fracture risk [7, 8]. The novel ultrasonic instrument is the first tool to characterize bone and assess microarchitecture with the detection of central axial reference sites (lumbar vertebrae and proximal femur) without the uses of ionizing radiations. However, these imaging techniques still have some limitations such as bulky device, high cost and limited accessibility to impede their applications for widespread uses and primary care inspection. Besides imaging techniques, the alternative method is still essential to be developed for the early and correct diagnosis of osteoporosis because the accurate diagnosis of osteoporosis in the early stage leads to a better management for the prevention and treatment.

The biomarkers of bone turnover have been investigated in the past decade. As shown in Fig. 1, the mechanism of bone remodeling is composed by bone resorption and bone formation [9]. Bone biomarkers are produced from the bone remodeling process included bone formation biomarkers, bone resorption biomarkers and regulators of bone turnover. Detections of bone metabolism have been studied with the biomarkers of enzymes, proteins and by-products during the bone remodeling process [10–13]. Various biomarkers are now available for specific and sensitive assessment of the rate for bone formation and bone resorption as shown in Table 1 [14]. For example, the bone formation biomarkers are total alkaline phosphatase (ALP), bone-specific alkaline phosphatase (BALP), osteocalcin (OC), procollagen type 1 N-terminal propeptide (P1NP) and procollagen type 1 C-terminal propeptide (P1CP). The bone resorption biomarkers are hydroxyproline (HYP), hydroxylysine (HYL), deoxypyridinoline (DPD), pyridinoline (PYD), bone sialoprotein (BSP), osteopontin (OP), tartrate-resistant acid phosphatase 5b (TRAP 5b), carboxy-terminal crosslinked telopeptide of type 1 collagen (CTX-1), amino-terminal crosslinked telopeptide of type 1 collagen (NTX-1) and cathepsin K (CTSK). The regulators of bone turnover are receptor activator of NF-kB ligand (RANKL), osteoprotegerin (OPG), dickkopf-1 (DDK-1) and sclerostin. These biomarkers are useful to provide the early assessment of osteoporosis when the BMD measurement of DXA does not offer enough information to make the diagnosis. Therefore, the combination of BMD measurement by DXA and bone biomarker detections shows the great potential to improve the early assessment of people with the high risk of osteoporosis. Herein, we present the recent studies and breakthroughs in the detections of bone related biomarkers for the assessment of osteoporosis. We hope to provide a comprehensive mini-review starting from

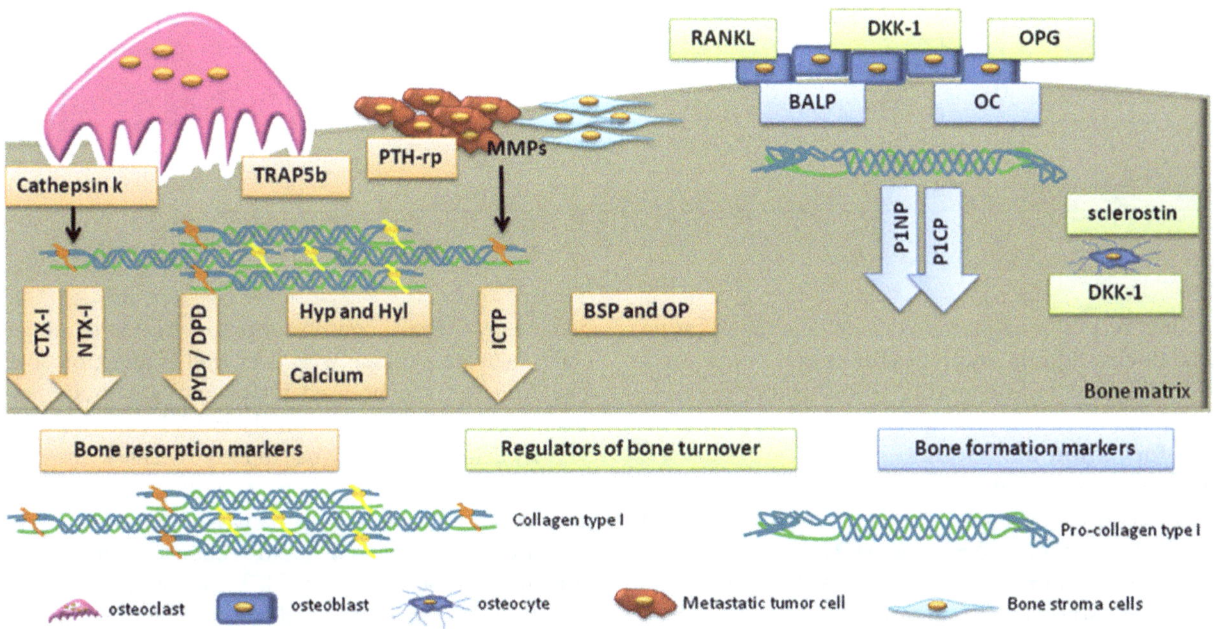

Fig. 1 Biochemical biomarkers of bone turnover. *Blue* boxes/arrows represent bone formation markers: bone-specific alkaline phosphatase (BALP); osteocalcin (OC); propeptides of type I procollagen (P1NP and P1CP). Orange boxes/arrows represent bone resorption markers: pyridinoline (PYD); deoxypyridoline (DPD); carboxy-terminal crosslinked telopeptide of type 1 collagen (CTX-1); amino-terminal crosslinked telopeptide of type 1 collagen (NTX-1); hydroxyproline (HYP); hydroxylysine (HYL); bone sialoprotein (BSP); osteopontin (OP); tartrate-resistant acid phosphatase 5b (TRAP 5b); cathepsin K (CTSK). *Green* boxes represent regulators of bone turnover: receptor activator of NF-κB ligand (RANKL), osteoprotegerin (OPG), dickkopf-1 (DDK-1) and sclerostin.

Table 1 Summary of detection techniques for bone biomarkers

Biomarker	Method	Concentration	Reference
Total ALP	standard Technicon Auto-analyzer	113 U/L	[12]
Total ALP	Roche COBAS Integra 800	>129 U/L	[13]
Total ALP	Olympus AU 5200 analyzer	64.8–79.7 U/L	[14]
BALP	enzyme immunoassay	24.9–19.7 U/L	[24]
BALP	enzyme immunoassay	66.4 ± 8.7 U/L	[25]
OC	antibody immunoassay	4.1 ± 0.5 ng/mL	[27]
OC	ELISA	16.16 ± 4.5 ng/mL	[28]
P1NP	Elecsys 2010 automated analyzer	54.1 μg/L	[29]
P1CP	radioimmunoassay	97–116 ng/mL	[32]
HYP	Bergman and Loxley method	34.7 mg/g creatinine	[35]
GHYL	HPLC	1.35 ± 0.82 mmol/mol	[39]
GHYL	HPLC	1.93–6.07 μmol/L	[40]
DPD	HPLC	11.3–22.3 nmol/L	[40]
DPD	chemiluminescence immunoassay	4.7 nmol/L	[42]
DPD	enzyme immunoassay	4.4 nmol/L	[42]
PYD	HPLC	28.8 μmol/mol creatinine	[45]
BSP	radioimmunoassay	12.1 ± 5.0 μg/L	[48]
BSP	radioimmunoassay	8.0 μg/L	[49]
OP	ELISA	20.75 ± 5.36 ng/mL	[51]
TRAP 5b	enzyme immunoassay	4.0 U/L	[54]
TRAP 5b	enzyme immunoassay	3.40 ± 0.87 U/L	[55]
CTX-1	ELISA	0.17–0.30 ng/ml	[56]
NTX-1	ELISA	37 ± 15 nmol BCE/mmol Cr	[57]
CTSK	ELISA	10.17 pmol/L	[59]
RANKL	ELISA	0.08 pmol/L	[61]
OPG	ELISA	1.8 pmol/L	[61]
DDK-1	ELISA	34.3 pmol/L	[65]
Sclerostin	ELISA	29.5 pmol/L	[65]

the functions of bone biomarkers included bone formation, bone resorption and regulator of bone turnover to the applications in osteoporotic assessment at the end.

Bone formation biomarkers

Total alkaline Phosphatase (ALP)

Alkaline phosphatase is an enzyme found in the bloodstream. The different forms of ALPs can break down proteins in the human body. Most of ALPs are produced in liver and some of ALPs are generated in the bones, intestines and kidneys. The total ALP is examined by the measurement of the amount of alkaline phosphatase enzyme in the bloodstream. The measurement of total ALP only needs a simple blood draw and is often a routine part of blood tests. The normal levels of ALP with people are various by age, blood type, gender and pregnancy. Unusual concentrations of ALP in blood generally indicate an issue with liver, gall bladder, or bones. The ALP test can be used for diagnosis of bone problems such as rickets, osteomalacia and Paget's disease. The ALP level also can be applied to check the treatment efficiency for the above conditions. For example, the standard Technicon Autoanalyzer has been used to measure the serum ALP for osteoporotic patients with inflammatory bowel disease [15]. The spinal bone mineral content has revealed significant correlations with serum total ALP. Recent study has also shown that the activity of serum total ALP >129 U/L is used as an indicator for osteoporosis in men [16]. Moreover, the decrease of total ALP has been demonstrated with the treatment with alendronate from 79.7 U/L to 64.8 U/L [17]. The results indicate that total ALP can be used as an indicator to reflect the efficiency of drug treatment for osteoporosis. However, small change and wide extensive range of total ALP may be led to wrong diagnosis of osteoporosis for postmenopausal women.

Bone-specific alkaline Phosphatase (BALP)

With normal liver function in adults, about 50% of total ALP is produced from bone in serum. The ALP isoenzymes produced from bone are difficult to distinguish with the isoenzymes from liver because they are only different by posttranslational glycosylation. Several approaches have been applied to specific measurements of BALP such as agarose electrophoresis, heat and chemical inactivation, wheat germ agglutinin precipitation, wheat germ agglutinin-high performance liquid chromatography, immunoradiometric assay and enzyme immunoassay [18–26].

For the enzyme immunoassay of BALP, the detection limit is 0.7 U/L and the mean values are 24.9 ± 7.0 U/L and 19.7 ± 5.6 U/L for men and premenopausal women, respectively. [27] With osteoporosis, the BALP activity of 66.4 ± 8.7 U/L has been detected with women aged over 59 years [28]. As an indicator of osteoblastic activity, the measurement of BALP is applied as the assistance for the management of osteoporosis in premenopausal and postmenopausal women.

Osteocalcin (OC)

Osteocalcin, also known as bone gamma-carboxyglutamic acid-containing protein, is a small protein composed by 49 amino acids. OC is synthesized by mature osteoblasts, odontoblasts and hypertrophic chondrocytes. Moreover, OC is the most abundant non-collagenous protein in bone comprised about 2% of total protein in the human body. OC produced by osteoblasts plays an important role for metabolic regulation, bone mineralization and calcium ion homeostasis [29]. OC has been demonstrated that the level of serum OC is highly correlated with the increase of BMD during treatment with bone formation drugs for osteoporosis. Serum OC has been considered a specific biomarker of osteoblast function for evaluation of bone formation rate in osteoporosis. In many studies, osteocalcin has been demonstrated as an important biomarker to investigate the efficiency for the drug on bone formation. For instance, with the RNAse-enriched-LF supplementation, the change of OC from baseline (7.2 ± 2.8%) has shown a promising and favorable effect in postmenopausal women [30]. Furthermore, the mean levels of osteocalcin have revealed a significant difference between the postmenopausal osteoporotic (16.16 ± 4.5 ng/ml) and non-osteoporotic (11.26 ± 3.07 ng/ml) women [31]. The uses of osteocalcin as a bone formation biomarker could provide the advantages such as tissue specificity, wide availability and low variation. The bone remodeling biomarker of serum OC may be useful for the assessment of osteoporosis and for the prediction of the fracture risk in elderly persons, especially in women.

Procollagen type 1 N-terminal Propeptide (P1NP)

Type 1 collagen can be found in the organic bone matrix (> 90%), which is developed in bone from procollagen type 1. Procollagen type 1 is synthesized by fibroblasts and osteoblasts. Procollagen type 1 has N-terminal and C-terminal extensions, which are removed by specific proteases during conversion of procollagen to collagen. The procollagen type 1 included P1CP and P1NP are subsequently conjugated onto the bone matrix. The bone formation biomarker of P1NP is a specific indicator of type 1 collagen deposition. P1NP is released during the formation of type 1 collagen into the intracellular space and P1NP eventually exists in the blood stream. P1NP is usually released in the trimeric structure (derived from the trimeric collagen structure) and then is rapidly broken down to a monomeric form by thermal degradation effects. Antibodies of P1NP are used to detect the trimeric structure of P1NP by enzyme-linked immunosorbent assay (ELISA) or radioimmunoassay. Recently, for the postmenopausal women with osteoporosis participating in the Parathyroid Hormone and Alendronate for Osteoporosis study, the mean value (54.1 μg/L) of total P1NP before initiating therapy is 74% higher than that in healthy premenopausal women with the age above 35 [32]. P1NP has been demonstrated to be a more sensitive bone biomarker to measure the bone formation rate in osteoporosis. The measurement of P1NP is being developed for clinical application.

Procollagen type 1 C-terminal Propeptide (P1CP).

P1CP is a single protein with molecular weight of 115 kDa containing mannose-rich carbohydrate side chains inserted post-translationally. PICP is cleared by liver endothelial cells via the mannose receptor and therefore has a short serum half-life of 6–8 min [33, 34]. Recent study shows that the P1CP in serum is used as a biomarker of bone formation to evaluate the effect of nandrolone decanoate and female sex hormones. The mean initial PICP concentration in the women with a vertebral fracture (97 ± 23 ng/mL) is significantly lower than that in the women with a forearm fracture (116 ± 27 ng/mL) [35]. Currently, both of P1NP and P1CP are analyzed by specific immunoassays. However, for the analyses of procollagen type 1, the biomarker of P1NP is more extensively investigated in the literature than that of P1CP. Several studies have also demonstrated good correlations between serum P1CP levels and the rate of bone formation [36].

Bone Resorption biomarkers

Hydroxyproline (HYP)

HYP is an amino acid derived from the post-translational hydroxylation of proline. HYP provides about 12–14% of the total amino acid content of mature collagen. During the degradation of bone collagen, about 90% of the HYP is released and then the HYP is primarily metabolized in the liver [37]. The level of HYP has significantly increased in urine with postmenopausal osteoporosis women in comparison with the postmenopausal nonosteoporosis women [38]. The increase of urinary HYP indicates that the degradation of collagen type I from the bone matrix is raised in osteoporotic women. Although the HYP is principally used as a resorption biomarker, about 10% of the HYP is derived from newly synthesized procollagen peptides during bone formation. Moreover, HYP can be found in other tissues such as skin and cartilage and also can be liberated from the metabolism of elastin and C1Q [39]. HYP is consequently considered as a non-specific bone resorption biomarker of collagen turnover. The use of HYP has been replaced by more sensitive and specific biomarkers for the assessment of osteoporosis [40].

Hydroxylysine (HYL)

HYL is an amino acid derived from a post-translational hydroxy modification of lysine. HYL has two forms included galactosyl hydroxylysine (GHYL) and glucosyl-galactosyl-hydroxylysine (GGHYL) [41]. GHYL and GGHYL are both released into the circulation during collagen degradation. GHYL is a more specific for bone biomarker because it is only derived from bone resorption. On the other hand, GGHYL can be found in skin and complement molecule of C1Q. Therefore, GHYL is considered as a better bone resorption biomarker than GGHYL and HYP. In previous work, the concentration of GHYL in urinary excretion has been applied to evaluate the occurrence of fracture in postmenopausal osteoporotic women without fragility fractures and postmenopausal osteoporotic women with fragility fractures [42]. The high levels of GHYL in fracture patients suggest a possible defect in bone collagen and the urinary GHYL may indeed identify such an abnormality. Furthermore, GHYL can be easily measured without preanalytical hydrolysis and extraction by high performance liquid chromatography (HPLC) [43]. Although the GHYL has revealed the potential as a biomarker of bone resorption, the use of GHYL has not been extensively studied for the assessment of osteoporosis and the evaluation of osteoporotic treatment. The clinical application of GHYL is still limited because of the absence of facile routine methods for its measurement.

Deoxypyridinoline (DPD)

DPD is a molecule to mechanically stabilize collagen by crosslinking between individual collagen peptides [44]. During the process of bone resorption, the crosslinked collagens are proteolytically broken down and then the DPD is released into the circulation and excreted by urine. Most of DPD are found in the bone and dentin. Therefore, DPD is used as a specific biomarker for bone resorption. In previous work, the DPD has been pre-treated with preanalytical hydrolysis and extraction before HPLC analysis because DPD is excreted in the urine in free (40%) and peptide-bound (60%) forms. To improve the accuracy, the peptide-bound form is transferred into free form for the HPLC measurement. The drawbacks for HPLC measurement of DPD are complicated procedure and variable recovery [43]. Recently, the automated chemiluminescence immunoassay and enzyme immunoassay have been developed for the direct detection of urinary free DPD. The experimental results of chemiluminescence immunoassay and enzyme immunoassay methods have shown the correlation with HPLC measurement of urinary free DPD [45–47]. The measurements of free DPD in urine by the immunoassay approaches have provided the possibility for the clinical application in the monitoring of patients with bone pathology and metabolic bone disease.

Pyridinoline (PYD)

Collagen crosslink of PYD is produced during the extracellular maturation of fibrillar collagens and released into the circulation from degradation of mature collagens. Previous study shows that the PYD exhibits long-term chemical stability in both the free and conjugated forms by HPLC analyses [48]. However, PYD is found in cartilage, bone, ligaments and blood vessels. Therefore, PYD is a non-specific bone resorption biomarker in comparison with DPD.

Bone Sialoprotein (BSP)

BSP is a phosphorylated glycoprotein with an apparent molecular weight of 60–80 kDa [49]. BSP is an element of mineralized tissues such as bone, dentin, cementum and calcified cartilage. BSP is an important component of the bone extracellular matrix and has been demonstrated to for the formation of approximately 8% of all non-collagenous proteins found in bone and cementum [50]. BSP is generated by osteoblasts, odontoblasts and osteoclasts. Therefore, BSP is considered as an important factor for cell-matrix adhesion processes and stimulation of osteoclast-mediated bone resorption. Many studies have developed immunoassays for the measurement of BSP in serum. For example, radioimmunoassay measurements have obtained mean serum BSP concentrations of 12.1 ± 5.0 μg/L from 90 healthy controls and 32.3 ± 17.3 μg/L from patients with Paget disease [51]. Serum levels of BSP have been also demonstrated the significant correlation with BALP and OC in osteoporosis patients [52]. BSP has shown great potential as a bone resorption biomarker for osteoporotic assessment.

Osteopontin (OP)

OP is a phosphorylated glycoprotein expressed by transformed cells, macrophages, activated T-lymphocytes, specialized epithelial cells and bone cells [53]. Recent study shows that women with OP over-expression reveal less resistance to postmenopausal osteoporosis than women with normal OP levels [54]. The levels of plasma OP could be used as a biomarker to evaluate the treatment of intermittent parathyroid hormone in menopausal osteoporosis.

Tartrate-resistant acid Phosphatase 5b (TRAP 5b)

TRAP 5b is normally secreted by osteoclasts during bone resorption [55, 56]. Thus, TRAP 5b is used as a reference for osteoclast activity and numbers. In the circulation, the hydrolyzed TRAP 5b is metabolized in the liver and then excreted in the urine. TRAP 5b can be specifically detected in serum by immunoassays. Previous report shows that serum TRAP 5b has been used to identify limited or extensive bone metastasis in breast cancer patients [57]. Furthermore, serum TRAP 5b has been applied to monitor the efficiency of alendronate treatment [58]. The bone resorption biomarker of TRAP 5b is extensively studied and revealed good specificity and high sensitivity in comparison with other bone biomarkers.

Carboxy-terminal Crosslinked Telopeptide of type 1 collagen (CTX-1),

Telopeptides of type 1 collagen are extensively investigated and used bone resorption biomarkers included carboxy-terminal crosslinked (CTX-1) and amino-terminal crosslinked (NTX-1). CTX-1 and NTX-1 are both are released during collagen degradation. ELISA is used to measured CTX-1 with a monoclonal antibody against an octapeptide sequence (EKAHD-β-GGR) in the α-1 (I) chain of the β-isoform. Recent study has shown that CTX-1 is a specific and sensitive biomarker of bone resorption that can rapidly indicate the response to bisphosphonate therapy for postmenopausal osteoporosis [59]. However, serum CTX-1 is influenced by food intake and blood withdrawal must take place in the fasting state because food intake substantially decreases the levels of CTX-1 [60].

Amino-terminal Crosslinked Telopeptide of type 1 collagen (NTX-1)

NTX-1 is stable in urine at room temperature for up to 24 h and is usually quantified by ELISA with urine sample. The urinary NTX-1 has been used as a bone resorption biomarker to assess the risk of fracture in postmenopausal women [60]. The urinary NTX-1 is selected as the preferred biomarker compared with serum CTX-1 for practical application because it is not affected by food intake and it prevents blood withdrawal.

Cathepsin K (CTSK)

Cathepsins are members of the cysteine protease family with 11 isoforms. CTSK is defined by its high specificity for kinins. CTSK is mainly expressed at the ruffled border of actively resorbing osteoclasts [61]. Osteoclasts secrete CTSK into bone resorption defect for degradation of bone matrix proteins included type 1 collagen, osteopontin and osteonectin. Therefore, CTSK is an important factor in process of bone resorption. The level of CTSK has revealed significantly different between controls and patients with osteoporosis [62]. The result indicates that serum level of CTSK could serve as a potential biomarker for fracture prediction and bone-mineral density.

Regulators of bone turnover

Receptor activator of NF-κB ligand (RANKL)

During the process of bone remodeling, osteoblasts produce RANKL and OPG to regulate the differentiation and maturation of osteoclasts. Recently, dextromethorphan has been demonstrated the inhibition of RANKL-induced osteoclastogenesis and bone resorption by abrogating the activation of NF-κB signaling in vitro. The oral administration of dextromethorphan improves ovariectomy-induced osteoporosis in vivo [63]. Serum levels of RANKL from humans have been observed for assessments of the states in metabolic bone diseases [64]. Although the serum RANKL has been studied for fracture risk prediction and evaluation of the response from osteoporosis treatment, many works still need to be investigated for the clinical application of RANKL.

Osteoprotegerin (OPG)

OPG is generally considered to be a secreted soluble receptor and is produced by many different tissues and cell types including osteoblasts. The role of OPG is used as a decoy receptor for RANKL and inhibitor of osteoclastogenesis [65]. Studies in mice have revealed that the OPG knockout mouse develops severe osteoporosis, whereas the overexpression of OPG in transgenic mouse models and OPG treatment of normal mice leads to osteopetrosis [66]. OPG can be measured in serum, plasma EDTA, citrate and heparin samples. There are commercially available sandwich ELISA assays for analyzing OPG by using a monoclonal capture and polyclonal detection antibodies [64]. However, the clinical use of serum OPG as a biomarker for evaluation of bone disease activity still needs additional demonstration.

Dickkopf-1 (DDK-1)

DKK-1 and sclerostin are the inhibitors of Wnt signaling and are applied as bone remodeling biomarkers. DKK-1 is produced by osteoblasts and is secreted into circulation. The serum levels of DDK-1 reflect the inhibition of bone formation [67]. DKK-1 levels have decreased from 34.3 pmol/L at baseline to 29.7 pmol/L at the 24-month of the breast cancer patients with anastrozole treatment [68]. DKK-1 has shown the correlation with the BMD of the femoral neck and of the total hip. Further long-term studies are necessary to identify the clinical application of the regulator DKK-1 as a biomarker for assessment of osteoporosis.

Sclerostin

In the presence of sclerostin, the Wnt pathway is downregulated and consequently osteoblastic differentiation is inhibited. Sclerostin is produced by osteocytes. Sclerostin is secreted into circulation, and serum levels reflect inhibition of bone formation [67]. In previous work, the concentrations of serum sclerostin have significantly increased from 29.5 pmol/L at baseline to 43.2 pmol/L after 24 months of treatment with anastrozole in breast cancer patients [68]. However, the clinical trial is further needed for the use of sclerostin as a biomarker of bone turnover.

Conclusions

In this mini-review, we reviewed several investigations and developments for the applications of bone biomarkers in the assessments of bone related diseases. From laboratory tests to clinical trials, the possibility of bone biomarkers to evaluate bone remodeling processes has been extensively demonstrated in physiological and pathological states. Bone biomarkers have shown great potential to serve as powerful indicators to evaluate the osteoporosis therapy and even to assist the clinical diagnosis of osteoporosis in the early stage. **Among these bone biomarkers, P1NP has shown the great potential as a sensitive and stable bone biomarker for the early detection of osteoporosis.**

Abbreviations

ALP: Total alkaline phosphatase; BALP: Bone-specific alkaline phosphatase; BMD: Bone mineral density; BSP: Bone sialoprotein; CTSK: Cathepsin K; CTX-1: Carboxy-terminal crosslinked telopeptide of type 1 collagen; DDK-1: dickkopf-1; DPD: Deoxypyridinoline; DXA: Dual-energy X-ray absorptiometry; HYL: Hydroxylysine; HYP: Hydroxyproline; NTX-1: Amino-terminal crosslinked telopeptide of type 1 collagen; OC: Osteocalcin; OP: Osteopontin; OPG: Osteoprotegerin; P1CP: Procollagen type 1 C-terminal propeptide; P1NP: Procollagen type 1 N-terminal propeptide; PYD: Pyridinoline; QCT: Quantitative computed tomography; RANKL: Receptor activator of NF-kB ligand; TRAP 5b: Tartrate-resistant acid phosphatase 5b (TRAP 5b); WHO: World Health Organization

Acknowledgements

We would like to thank the support from Taipei Medical University.

Funding

This work was supported by 105TMU-TMUH-09, TMU104-AE1-B28, MOST 105-2119-M-038-002 -MY2, MOST 103-2113-M-003-003-MY3, Taipei Medical University and Taipei Medical University Hospital.

Author's contributions

The present manuscript was drafted by TRK and revised by TRK and CHC. Both authors read and approved the final manuscript.

Competing interest

The authors declare that they have no competing interests.

Author details

[1]Graduate Institute of Nanomedicine and Medical Engineering, College of Biomedical Engineering, Taipei Medical University, Taipei 11031, Taiwan. [2]International Ph.D. Program in Biomedical Engineering, College of Biomedical Engineering, Taipei Medical University, Taipei 11031, Taiwan. [3]Bone and Joint Research Center, Department of Orthopedics and Traumatology, Taipei Medical University Hospital, Taipei 11031, Taiwan. [4]School of Medicine, College of Medicine, Taipei Medical University, Taipei 11031, Taiwan.

References

1. Genant HK, Cooper C, Poor G, Reid I, Ehrlich G, Kanis J, et al. Interim report and recommendations of the World Health Organization task-force for osteoporosis. Osteoporos Int. 1999;10:259–64.
2. Pisani P, Renna MD, Conversano F, Casciaro E, Di Paola M, Quarta E, et al. Major osteoporotic fragility fractures: risk factor updates and societal impact. World J Orthop. 2016;7:171.
3. Leibson CL, Tosteson ANA, Gabriel SE, Ransom JE, Melton LJ. Mortality, disability, and nursing home use for persons with and without hip fracture: a population-based study. J Am Geriatr Soc. 2002;50:1644–50.
4. Lang TF, Guglielmi G, Van Kuijk C, De Serio A, Cammisa M, Genant HK. Measurement of bone mineral density at the spine and proximal femur by volumetric quantitative computed tomography and dual-energy X-ray Absorptiometry in elderly women with and without vertebral fractures. Bone. 2002;30:247–50.
5. Adams JE. Radiogrammetry and radiographic Absorptiometry. Radiol Clin N Am. 2010;48:531–40.
6. Alexeeva L, Burkhardt P, Christiansen C, Cooper C, Delmas P, Johnell O, et al. Assessment of fracture risk and its application to screening for postmenopausal osteoporosis; 1994. p. 1–129.
7. Pisani P, Greco A, Renna M, Conversano F, Casciaro E, Quarta L, et al. An innovative ultrasound-based method for the identification of patients at high fracture risk; 2014. p. e50–e3.
8. Conversano F, Franchini R, Greco A, Soloperto G, Chiriaco F, Casciaro E, et al. A novel untrasound methodology for estimating spine mineral density. Ultrasound Med Biol. 2015;41:281–300.
9. Ferreira A, Alho I, Casimiro S, Costa L. Bone remodeling markers and bone metastases: from cancer research to clinical implications. BoneKEy reports. 2015;4
10. Eastell R, Hannon RA. Biomarkers of bone health and osteoporosis risk. Proc Nutr Soc. 2008;67:157–62.
11. Shi X, Li C, Liang B, He K, Li X. Weak cation magnetic separation technology and MALDI-TOF-MS in screening serum protein markers in primary type I osteoporosis. Genet Mol Res. 2014;14:15285–94.
12. He W-T, Wang B, Li M, Liang B-C, Shi Y-Z, Li X-Y, et al. Weak cation exchange magnetic beads coupled with MALDI-TOF-MS in screening serum

markers in perimenopausal women with osteopenia. Int J Clin Exp Med. 2016;9:8136–44.

13. Liu L, Webster TJ. In situ sensor advancements for osteoporosis prevention, diagnosis, and treatment. Curr Osteoporos Rep. 2016;14:386–95.
14. Delmas PD, Eastell R, Garnero P, Seibel MJ, Stepan J, Comm Sci Advisors Int O. The use of biochemical markers of bone turnover in osteoporosis. Osteoporos Int. 2000;11:2–17.
15. Compston J, Judd D, Crawley E, Evans W, Evans C, Church H, et al. Osteoporosis in patients with inflammatory bowel disease. Gut. 1987;28:410–5.
16. Fink HA, Litwack-Harrison S, Taylor BC, Bauer DC, Orwoll ES, Lee CG, et al. Clinical utility of routine laboratory testing to identify possible secondary causes in older men with osteoporosis: the osteoporotic fractures in men (MrOS) study. Osteoporos Int. 2016;27:331–8.
17. Kyd P, De Vooght K, Kerkhoff F, Thomas E, Fairney A. Clinical usefulness of bone alkaline phosphatase in osteoporosis. Ann Clin Biochem. 1998;35:717–25.
18. PetitClerc C. Quantitative fractionation of alkaline phosphatase isoenzymes according to their thermostability. Clin Chem. 1976;22:42–8.
19. Štěpán J, Volek V, Kolář J. A modified inactivation-inhibition method for determining the serum activity of alkaline phosphatase isoenzymes. Clin Chim Acta. 1976;69:1–9.
20. Whitaker KB, Whitby L, Moss D. Activities of bone and liver alkaline phosphatases in serum in health and disease. Clin Chim Acta. 1977; 80:209–19.
21. Behr W, Barnert J. Quantification of bone alkaline phosphatase in serum by precipitation with wheat-germ lectin: a simplified method and its clinical plausibility. Clin Chem. 1986;32:1960–6.
22. Schreiber WE, Whitta L. Alkaline phosphatase isoenzymes resolved by electrophoresis on lectin-containing agarose gel. Clin Chem. 1986;32:1570–3.
23. Van Hoof V, Lepoutre L, Hoylaerts M, Chevigne R, De Broe M. Improved agarose electrophoretic method for separating alkaline phosphatase isoenzymes in serum. Clin Chem. 1988;34:1857–62.
24. Gonchoroff DG, Branum EL, Cedel SL, Riggs BL, O'Brien JF. Clinical evaluation of high-performance affinity chromatography for the separation of bone and liver alkaline phosphatase isoenzymes. Clin Chim Acta. 1991; 199:43–50.
25. Crofton P. Wheat-germ lectin affinity electrophoresis for alkaline phosphatase isoforms in children: age-dependent reference ranges and changes in liver and bone disease. Clin Chem. 1992;38:663–70.
26. Day A, Saward S, Royle C, Mayne P. Evaluation of two new methods for routine measurement of alkaline phosphatase isoenzymes. J Clin Pathol. 1992;45:68–71.
27. Gomez B, Ardakani S, Ju J, Jenkins D, Cerelli MJ, Daniloff GY, et al. Monoclonal antibody assay for measuring bone-specific alkaline phosphatase activity in serum. Clin Chem. 1995;41:1560–6.
28. Lumachi F, Ermani M, Camozzi V, Tombolan V, Luisetto G. Changes of bone formation markers osteocalcin and bone-specific alkaline phosphatase in postmenopausal women with osteoporosis. Ann N Y Acad Sci. 2009;1173:E60–E3.
29. Lee NK, Sowa H, Hinoi E, Ferron M, Ahn JD, Confavreux C, et al. Endocrine regulation of energy metabolism by the skeleton. Cell. 2007;130:456–69.
30. Bharadwaj S, Naidu A, Betageri G, Prasadarao N, Naidu A. Milk ribonuclease-enriched lactoferrin induces positive effects on bone turnover markers in postmenopausal women. Osteoporos Int. 2009;20:1603–11.
31. Singh S, Kumar D, Lal AK. Serum osteocalcin as a diagnostic biomarker for primary osteoporosis in women. J Clin Diagn Res. 2015;9:RC04–7.
32. Garnero P, Vergnaud P, Hoyle N. Evaluation of a fully automated serum assay for total N-terminal propeptide of type I collagen in postmenopausal osteoporosis. Clin Chem. 2008;54:188–96.
33. Olsen BR, Guzman NA, Engel J, Condit C, Aase S. Purification and characterization of a peptide from the carboxy-terminal region of chick tendon procollagen type I. Biochemistry (Mosc). 1977;16:3030–6.
34. Smedsrød B, Melkko J, Risteli L, Risteli J. Circulating C-terminal propeptide of type I procollagen is cleared mainly via the mannose receptor in liver endothelial cells. Biochem J. 1990;271:345–50.
35. Hassager C, Jensen L, Johansen J, Riis B, Melkko J, Pødenphant J, et al. The carboxy-terminal propeptide of type I procollagen in serum as a marker of bone formation: the effect of nandrolone decanoate and female sex hormones. Metabolism. 1991;40:205–8.
36. Eriksen EF, Charles P, Melsen F, Mosekilde L, Risteli L, Risteli J. Serum markers of type I collagen formation and degradation in metabolic bone disease: correlation with bone histomorphometry. J Bone Miner Res. 1993;8:127–32.
37. Lowry M, Hall DE, Brosnan JT. Hydroxyproline metabolism by the rat kidney: distribution of renal enzymes of hydroxyproline catabolism and renal conversion of hydroxyproline to glycine and serine. Metabolism. 1985;34:955–61.
38. Jagtap VR, Ganu JV. Effect of antiresorptive therapy on urinary hydroxyproline in postmenopausal osteoporosis. Indian J Clin Biochem. 2012;27:90–3.
39. Prockop DJ, Kivirikko KI, Tuderman L, Guzman NA. The biosynthesis of collagen and its disorders. N Engl J Med. 1979;301:77–85.
40. Delmas P, Eastell R, Garnero P, Seibel M, Stepan J, Foundation CoSAotIO. The use of biochemical markers of bone turnover in osteoporosis. Osteoporos Int. 2000;11:S2–S17.
41. Cunningham LW, Ford JD, Segrest JP. The isolation of identical hydroxylysyl glycosides from hydrolysates of soluble collagen and from human urine. J Biol Chem. 1967;242:2570–1.
42. Cascio VL, Bertoldo F, Gambaro G, Gasperi E, Furlan F, Colapietro F, et al. Urinary galactosyl-hydroxylysine in postmenopausal osteoporotic women: a potential marker of bone fragility. J Bone Miner Res. 1999;14:1420–4.
43. Bettica P, Baylink D, Moro L. Galactosyl hydroxylysine and deoxypyridinoline: a methodological comparison. Clin Chem Lab Med. 1993;31:459–66.
44. Seibel MJ. Biochemical markers of bone turnover part I: biochemistry and variability. Clin Biochem Rev/Australian Association of Clinical Biochemists. 2005;26:97.
45. Seyedin SM, Kung VT, Daniloff YN, Hesley RP, Gomez B, Nielsen LA, et al. Immunoassay for urinary pyridinoline: the new marker of bone resorption. J Bone Miner Res. 1993;8:635–41.
46. Robins SP, Woitge H, Hesley R, Ju J, Seyedin S, Seibel MJ. Direct, enzyme-linked immunoassay for urinary deoxypyridinoline as a specific marker for measuring bone resorption. J Bone Miner Res. 1994;9:1643–9.
47. Rosano TG, Peaston RT, Bone HG, Woitge HW, Francis RM, Seibel MJ. Urinary free deoxypyridinoline by chemiluminescence immunoassay: analytical and clinical evaluation. Clin Chem. 1998;44:2126–32.
48. Gerrits MI, Thijssen J, Van Rijn H. Determination of pyridinoline and deoxypyridinoline in urine, with special attention to retaining their stability. Clin Chem. 1995;41:571–4.
49. Fisher LW, Whitson SW, Avioli LV, Termine JD. Matrix sialoprotein of developing bone. J Biol Chem. 1983;258:12723–7.
50. Fisher L, McBride O, Termine J, Young M. Human bone sialoprotein. Deduced protein sequence and chromosomal localization. J Biol Chem. 1990;265:2347–51.
51. Karmatschek M, Maier I, Seibel MJ, Woitge HW, Ziegler R, Armbruster FP. Improved purification of human bone sialoprotein and development of a homologous radioimmunoassay. Clin Chem. 1997;43:2076–82.
52. Fassbender W, Ruf T, Kaiser H, Stracke H. Serum levels of immunoreactive bone sialoprotein in osteoporosis: positive relations to established biochemical parameters of bone turnover, vol. 14. Athens: In vivo; 1999. p. 619–24.
53. Zhang Q, Wana JL, Sodek J. Characterization of the promoter region of the porcine opn (osteopontin, secreted phosphoprotein 1) gene. Eur J Biochem. 1992;207:649–59.
54. Chiang T-I, Chang I-C, Lee H-S, Lee H, Huang C-H, Cheng Y-W. Osteopontin regulates anabolic effect in human menopausal osteoporosis with intermittent parathyroid hormone treatment. Osteoporos Int. 2011;22:577–85.
55. Halleen JM, Alatalo SL, Suominen H, Cheng S, Janckila AJ, Väänänen HK. Tartrate-resistant acid phosphatase 5b: a novel serum marker of bone resorption. J Bone Miner Res. 2000;15:1337–45.
56. Väänänen HK, Zhao H, Mulari M, Halleen JM. The cell biology of osteoclast function. J Cell Sci. 2000;113:377–81.
57. Chao T-Y, Yu J-C, Ku C-H, Chen MM, Lee S-H, Janckila AJ, et al. Tartrate-resistant acid phosphatase 5b is a useful serum marker for extensive bone metastasis in breast cancer patients. Clin Cancer Res. 2005;11:544–50.
58. Nenonen A, Cheng S, Ivaska KK, Alatalo SL, Lehtimäki T, Schmidt-Gayk H, et al. Serum TRACP 5b is a useful marker for monitoring alendronate treatment: comparison with other markers of bone turnover. J Bone Miner Res. 2005;20:1804–12.
59. Baim S, Miller PD. Perspective: assessing the clinical utility of serum CTX in postmenopausal osteoporosis and its use in predicting risk of osteonecrosis of the jaw. J Bone Miner Res. 2009;24:561–74.
60. Christgau S. Circadian variation in serum CrossLaps concentration is reduced in fasting individuals. Clin Chem. 2000;46:431.
61. Pérez-Castrillón JL, Pinacho F, De Luis D, Lopez-Menendez M, Dueñas LA. Odanacatib, a new drug for the treatment of osteoporosis: review of the results in postmenopausal women. J Osteoporos. 2010;2010:401581.

62. Holzer G, Noske H, Lang T, Holzer L, Willinger U. Soluble cathepsin K: a novel marker for the prediction of nontraumatic fractures? J Lab Clin Med. 2005;146:13–7.
63. Wu K, Lin T-H, Liou H-C, Lu D-H, Chen Y-R, Fu W-M, et al. Dextromethorphan inhibits osteoclast differentiation by suppressing RANKL-induced nuclear factor-κB activation. Osteoporos Int. 2013;24:2201–14.
64. Rogers A, Eastell R. Circulating osteoprotegerin and receptor activator for nuclear factor κB ligand: clinical utility in metabolic bone disease assessment. J Clin Endocrinol Metab. 2005;90:6323–31.
65. Yasuda H, Shima N, Nakagawa N, Yamaguchi K, Kinosaki M, S-i M, et al. Osteoclast differentiation factor is a ligand for osteoprotegerin/osteoclastogenesis-inhibitory factor and is identical to TRANCE/RANKL. Proc Natl Acad Sci U S A. 1998;95:3597–602.
66. Yasuda H, Shima N, Nakagawa N, Mochizuki S-I, Yano K, Fujise N, et al. Identity of osteoclastogenesis inhibitory factor (OCIF) and osteoprotegerin (OPG): a mechanism by which OPG/OCIF inhibits osteoclastogenesis in vitro 1. Endocrinology. 1998;139:1329–37.
67. Anastasilakis AD, Polyzos SA, Gkiomisi A, Bisbinas I, Gerou S, Makras P. Comparative effect of zoledronic acid versus denosumab on serum sclerostin and dickkopf-1 levels of naive postmenopausal women with low bone mass: a randomized, head-to-head clinical trial. J Clin Endocrinol Metab. 2013;98:3206–12.
68. Kyvernitakis I, Rachner TD, Urbschat A, Hars O, Hofbauer LC, Hadji P. Effect of aromatase inhibition on serum levels of sclerostin and dickkopf-1, bone turnover markers and bone mineral density in women with breast cancer. J Cancer Res Clin Oncol. 2014;140:1671–80.

9

Assessing biological and technological variability in protein levels measured in pre-diagnostic plasma samples of women with breast cancer

Christine Y. Yeh[1,2,3†], Ravali Adusumilli[2†], Majlinda Kullolli[2], Parag Mallick[2,4], Esther M. John[4,5] and Sharon J. Pitteri[2,4*]

Abstract

Background: Quantitative proteomics allows for the discovery and functional investigation of blood-based pre-diagnostic biomarkers for early cancer detection. However, a major limitation of proteomic investigations in biomarker studies remains the biological and technical variability in the analysis of complex clinical samples. Moreover, unlike 'omics analogues such as genomics and transcriptomics, proteomics has yet to achieve reproducibility and long-term stability on a unified technological platform. Few studies have thoroughly investigated protein variability in pre-diagnostic samples of cancer patients across multiple platforms.

Methods: We obtained ten blood plasma "case" samples collected up to 2 years prior to breast cancer diagnosis. Each case sample was paired with a matched control plasma from a full biological sister without breast cancer. We measured protein levels using both mass-spectrometry and antibody-based technologies to: (1) assess the technical considerations in different protein assays when analyzing limited clinical samples, and (2) evaluate the statistical power of potential diagnostic analytes.

Results: Although we found inherent technical variation in the three assays used, we detected protein dependent biological signal from the limited samples. The three assay types yielded 32 proteins with statistically significantly (p < 1E-01) altered expression levels between cases and controls, with no proteins retaining statistical significance after false discovery correction.

Conclusions: Technical, practical, and study design considerations are essential to maximize information obtained in limited pre-diagnostic samples of cancer patients. This study provides a framework that estimates biological effect sizes critical for consideration in designing studies for pre-diagnostic blood-based biomarker detection.

Keywords: Breast cancer, Protein, Mass spectrometry, Immunoassay, Blood plasma

Background

Early detection of breast cancer greatly increases prognosis with a 5-year survival rate of >98% for localized disease versus 29.6% survival for disease diagnosed at a metastatic stage [1]. Systematic blood-based studies using a variety of protein assay technologies have profiled hundreds of proteins and identified candidate targets that differentiate between cancer patients and matched controls [2, 3]. Only a small subset of these targets has been validated in additional samples [4]. One major limitation is that most of these discovery studies have relied on samples that were collected at the time of cancer diagnosis. Using such samples makes the key assumption that proteins indicative of disease pathology in cancer patients can be extrapolated to pre-diagnostic samples. Due to the relative scarcity of pre-diagnostic blood samples, few biomarker studies have

* Correspondence: spitteri@stanford.edu
†Equal contributors
[2]Department of Radiology, Canary Center at Stanford for Cancer Early Detection, Stanford University School of Medicine, Palo Alto, CA 94304, USA
[4]Stanford Cancer Institute, Stanford University School of Medicine, Stanford, CA 94305, USA

used such samples, and they were primarily used in validation studies, often with negative results even with initially high-confidence protein targets [5]. Molecular profiles of blood in cancer progression have been shown to change in longitudinal studies [6], indicating that particular protein analytes are only predictive of disease outcomes within a limited lead time [4]. This henceforth reinforces the need to conduct exploratory studies in pre-diagnostic samples to identify early cancer diagnostic protein targets.

Despite valuable progress in the limited efforts to detect biomarkers in pre-diagnostic breast cancer samples [7–9], challenges of small samples sizes and technical/biological noise persist. Meta-analyses of the proteomic revolution and its application to cancer biomarker discovery highlights the amount of inter-individual variability that interferes with true analytical variability in clinical samples [9]. Some of the variation may be due to lifestyle factors [10], and twin studies measuring plasma proteins have emphasized the need to account for genetic, environmental, and temporal variability [11]. Moreover, variability in clinical samples may also arise from therapies received by cancer patients. Studies based on samples from patients using menopausal hormone therapy [12–14] have highlighted the need for cancer biomarker studies to consider the confounding effect of hormone therapy on protein levels.

Given the known variability in protein expression in the blood, the implications of technical and practical choices for biomarker discovery on often limited numbers of samples need to be considered. Immuno-based methods once dominated the field, and are still commonly used in biomarker studies [15]. However, technical advancements in mass spectrometry now allow for shotgun proteomics that provide unbiased relative protein measurements with higher coverage. Emerging reaction monitoring [16], and sequential window acquisition of all theoretical mass spectra [17] mass spectrometry-based technologies have also started to build quantitative assays for larger numbers of proteins. Each type of platform comes with advantages, disadvantages, and varying ability to detect true analytical signals beyond the biological noise. We thus present, to our knowledge, the most extensive characterization of pre-diagnostic samples of ten breast cancer cases with side-by-side comparison of select proteomics platforms with the goals of characterizing technical and biological variation.

Methods

Human plasma samples

The blood plasma samples used in this study were obtained from the Northern California site of the Breast Cancer Family Registry (BCFR) [18]. Women with newly diagnosed breast cancer (probands) were enrolled in the family registry from 1996 to 2011, as well as their sisters and other relatives, and followed prospectively to 2017. At enrollment, probands completed a cancer family history questionnaire and all participants completed a questionnaire on epidemiologic risk factors for breast cancer, including personal history of cancer, and provided a blood sample that was stored in -70C freezers for future research. Other health conditions were not assessed at enrollment. Probands were interviewed annually and asked about new cancer diagnoses among family members. More extensive follow-up questionnaires were administered to probands and relatives in 2012–2014 and 2015–2017. For this pilot study, we selected stored plasma samples from 10 sister pairs from women who did not have a personal history of breast cancer when they enrolled in the family registry. They included 10 women who were diagnosed with breast cancer within 24 months of providing the blood sample and 10 of their biological full sisters who did not develop breast cancer within 24 months of providing the blood sample.

Case samples. The ten women with breast cancer were diagnosed between 1997 and 2007 and nine diagnoses were confirmed by pathology reports, medical records, or the cancer registry. One diagnosis was based on a proband report only, as the affected individual did not participate in follow-up. None of these 10 women had a cancer diagnosis before enrollment in the family registry.

Control samples. Nine of the 10 control women completed follow-up questionnaires between 2012 and 2017 and did not report any cancer diagnosis. Three of the control women were California residents and linkage with the California Cancer Registry in 2013 did not reveal any cancer diagnoses. One control woman had a cervical cancer diagnosis 10 years before enrollment and a breast cancer diagnosis 18 years after enrollment in the family registry; both diagnoses were confirmed by the cancer registry. (Additional file 1: Table S1).

Sample preparation for shotgun proteomic analysis

The plasma mass spectrometry-based proteomics workflow used in this study was adapted from a previously described workflow [13] (Fig. 1a). Briefly 250 μL aliquots of each plasma sample were subjected to immunodepletion. The fourteen most abundant proteins (including albumin, immunoglobulins G (IgG) and A (IgA), transferrin, haptoglobin, α-1-antitrypsin, fibrinogen, α-2-macroglobulin, apolipoprotein A1, and acid-1-glycoprotein) were removed from the plasma samples using CaptureSelect™ HumanPlasma14 depletion material [19]. The proteins in the depleted plasma samples were then isotopically labeled with the control samples receiving "light" ^{12}C3-acrylamide and the case samples receiving "heavy" ^{13}C3-acrylamide [20]. The case and control samples were mixed and fractionated by reversed phase chromatography using a C8 column (POROS R2). Fractions were then lyophilized and digested with trypsin in solution.

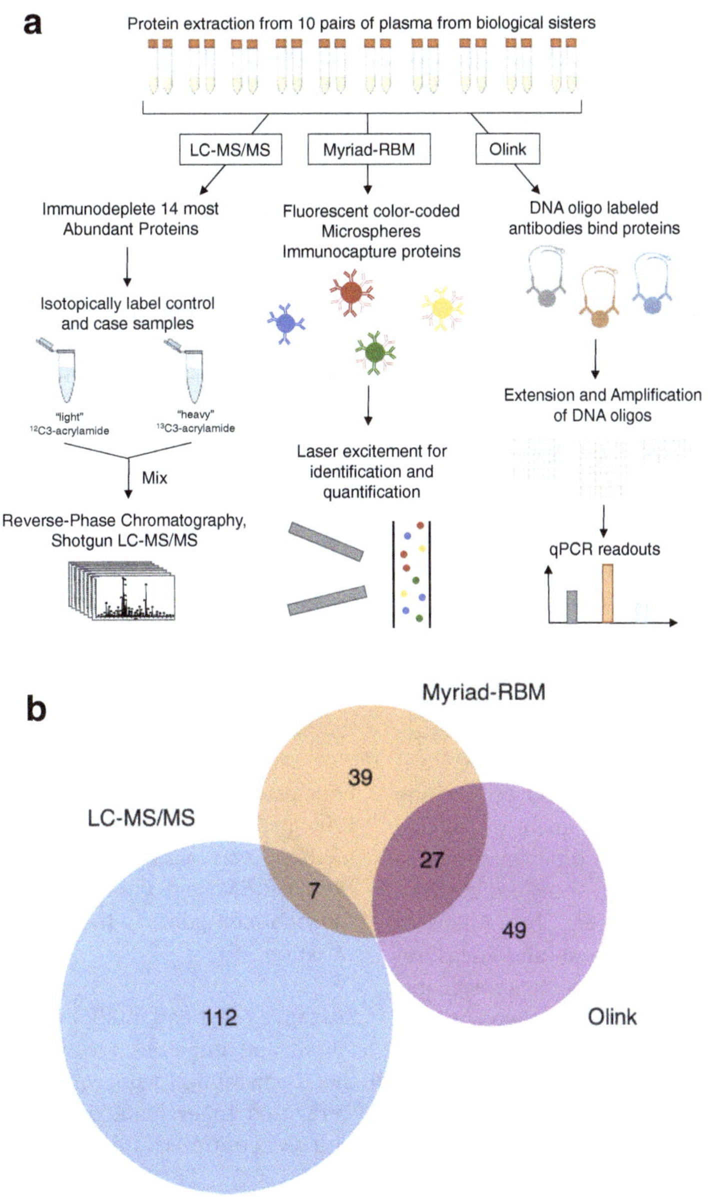

Fig. 1 Overview and Summary of Study. **a** Study design and workflow. **b** Number of distinct proteins measured across the three platforms; LC-MS/MS, Myriad-RBM, and Olink

LC-MS/MS protein quantification

The tryptic peptide samples were analyzed by liquid chromatography-tandem mass spectrometry (LC-MS/MS) on a LTQ-Orbitrap Velos mass spectrometer coupled with an Eksigent nanoLC. The resulting LC-MS/MS data were searched against the human UniProtKB database using the Computational Protein Analysis System from X!Tandem. Search results were analyzed by PeptideProphet [21] and peptides with a score > 0.75 were retained for protein identification and quantitation. Quantitative information from peptide signal intensities was then extracted using Q3ProteinParser, and ratios of heavy-to-light acrylamide-labeled peptides were computed for each protein in each of the ten sample pairs (Additional file 2) [20]. The estimated absolute protein abundance levels for the LC-MS/MS method were based on a reference database of 1200 canonical proteins [22].

Myriad-RBM analysis

We used the Human OncologyMAP® v.1.0 assay (Luminex xMap technology, Myriad-RBM Inc., Austin TX) from Myriad-RBM Inc. to measure a targeted panel of 101 potential protein biomarkers such as cancer antigens, interleukins, and proteases (Additional file 1: Table S2) in the 20 samples. Two hundred microliters of each plasma sample was submitted for analysis. This assay uses color-coded microspheres with antibodies specific to each of the target protein to capture and detect specific analytes in each sample. Lasers then simultaneously excite the reporter dye that quantifies the analyte specific to each microsphere, and the internal fluorescent dye that identifies the microsphere (Fig. 1a). The Myriad-RBM analysis provides the measured concentration of each target analyte in a sample, the least detectable concentration (LDD), as well as the low to high normal range for all analytes (Additional file 2).

Olink analysis

Protein levels of an additional 96 potential biomarkers (Additional file 1: Table S2) were analyzed in the 20 samples using the Olink Proseek Multiplex Oncology I 96 × 96 kit (Additional file 2) [23]. Twenty microliters of each plasma sample was submitted for analysis. For each target analyte in this assay, a pair of oligonucleotide-labelled antibodies probes bind to the protein in each sample. When the two probes are near each other after binding to the target protein, a PCR target sequence is formed by a proximity-dependent DNA polymerization event. The resulting sequence is subsequently detected and quantified using standard real-time quantitative polymerase chain reaction (qPCR) on the Fluidigm BioMark HD real-time PCR platform (Fig. 1a). All assay characteristics including detection limits and measurements of assay performance and validations are available from the manufacturer's webpage (http://www.olink.com/products/oncology/).

Data filtering

In the LC-MS/MS analysis, only proteins quantified in all ten case-control mixed samples were used in downstream quantitative analysis. For Myriad-RBM and Olink analyses, only analytes with at least 80% of valid measurements (defined as measurements above LDD for Myriad-RBM platform) across all samples were kept for downstream quantitative analyses. These cutoffs were made to retain statistical power in downstream quantitative analyses.

Inter-assay comparisons

Inter-assay comparisons were visualized by standard boxplots and linear regression scatter plots. The adjusted R^2 metric defined the strength of correlation between measurements of the same proteins across different platforms.

Intra-assay technical variation

Protein assays have inherent variability known as technical variation across technical replicates. The statistical metric used to evaluate technical variation in the LC-MS/MS and Olink platforms was relative error (defined as the standard deviation divided by the mean across multiple replicates). The intra-assay technical variation of the LC-MS/MS method was evaluated by the density of relative error for case-to-control ratios; the relative error was calculated for all proteins using multiple peptides for the same protein as replicates. Meanwhile, for the Olink analysis we evaluated relative error for triplicate measurements for each protein analyte.

Biological versus technical variance

For the Olink assay, technical variation was calculated as the mean of standard deviation across each protein analyte and biological variation was calculated as the standard deviation of mean measurements across each protein analyte. The variance was first analyzed by comparing biological variance with technical variance. Furthermore, to assess variance decomposition, we then averaged the type-II ANOVA sum of squares to evaluate the proportions of variance.

Principal component analysis (PCA)

Principal Component Analysis, an unsupervised learning method, was used to reduce the multi-dimensional Myriad-RBM and Olink datasets into the first two orthogonal components that capture the major sources of variation.

Student's *t*-test and multiple hypothesis correction

Paired and unpaired *t*-tests with *p*-values corrected by the Benjamini-Hochberg multiple hypothesis testing were used to evaluate quantitative differences between case and control samples.

Results

As shown in Fig. 1b, the LC-MS/MS method measured relative levels of 119 proteins, while the Myriad-RBM and Olink methods measured absolute levels of 73 and 76 proteins, respectively, for all samples. No proteins were measured by all three methods. Seven proteins were measured by both LC-MS/MS and Myriad-RBM, and 27 proteins were measured by both the Olink Biosciences and Rules Based Medicine assays. The three methods provided ample information to evaluate the variability of current protein assays in detecting protein biomarkers for early breast cancer diagnosis.

Depth and frequency of protein measurements

The LC-MS/MS method provided relative quantitation values for proteins over six orders of magnitude (Fig. 2a).

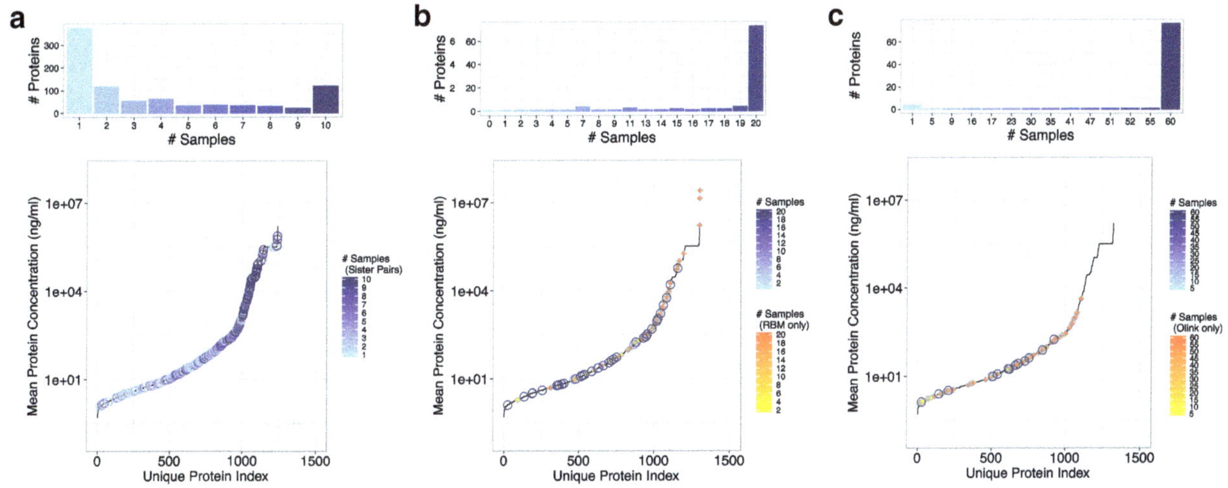

Fig. 2 Depth of analyses and measurement frequency across platforms. Histogram (top) of frequency that a protein is quantified in *n* number of samples, and dynamic range plot (bottom) of mean concentrations measured for each unique protein quantified in platforms (**a**) LC-MS/MS, (**b**) Myriad-RBM, (**c**) Olink

Similarly, Fig. 2b shows that the Myriad-RBM method also quantified proteins over six orders of magnitude, whereas the Olink method quantified proteins over a relatively smaller range of four orders of magnitude (Fig. 2c). Overall, the Olink platform captured lower abundance and smaller range of protein levels compared to the other two methods.

The frequency of unique protein measurements across plasma samples is plotted in the histograms of Fig. 2a-c for the three methods. Most proteins were measured in all 20 samples by the Myriad-RBM and Olink methods. Conversely, the LC-MS/MS method quantified the largest total number of proteins (1200), but also yielded missing data: only 13.5% of the total number of quantified proteins was measured in all ten pairs of "heavy" and "light" mixed samples. We chose to focus on only the 119 proteins identified across all samples in the LC-MS/MS method for downstream analysis.

Assay-to-assay comparison in antibody-based technologies

The Myriad-RBM and Olink assays are both antibody-based technologies that aim to capture absolute concentrations of protein analytes in biological samples. We therefore compared the results from each of the two panels. Fig. 3a shows boxplots of protein measurements across all genes sorted by mean abundance for both methods. In general, the Myriad-RBM assay provided higher absolute level measurements than the Olink assay, even for analytes that were measured by both assays. This is particularly noteworthy as each method used absolute standards to determine values for protein concentrations.

Despite the discrepancy of absolute measurements between these two antibody-based assays, we saw that at least the measurements were mostly concordant for the 30 proteins measured by both methods (Fig. 3b), although the strength of correlation varied from protein analyte to analyte.

Technical variation in LC-MS/MS and Olink analysis

Each assay has inherent technical variation. We were able to measure variation across technical replicates for the LC-MS/MS and Olink Analyses. We concluded that the LC-MS/MS method had a mean relative error for each measured peptide at approximately 10% for this dataset (Fig. 4a). The relative error across the triplicates for each analyte in the Olink analysis was plotted as boxplots in Fig. 4c. This figure highlights that the average relative error was found to be approximately 20% across all analytes, but the relative error was not consistent across analytes. Moreover, as shown in Fig. 4b, there was no evidence that relative error is correlated with measured protein abundance. Together, Fig. 4b-c suggest that inherent technical variation is specific to analyte and not necessarily specific to measurement platform or measured protein abundance.

Biological versus technical variation

Figure 5a shows a scatterplot of technical variation versus biological variation in the Olink assay. Each point represents a protein and points above the line indicate that the biological variation in the measurements was higher than the technical variation of the measured protein levels. A variance decomposition ternary plot, shown in Fig. 5b, exhibits that variance is mostly captured by variability between individuals rather than

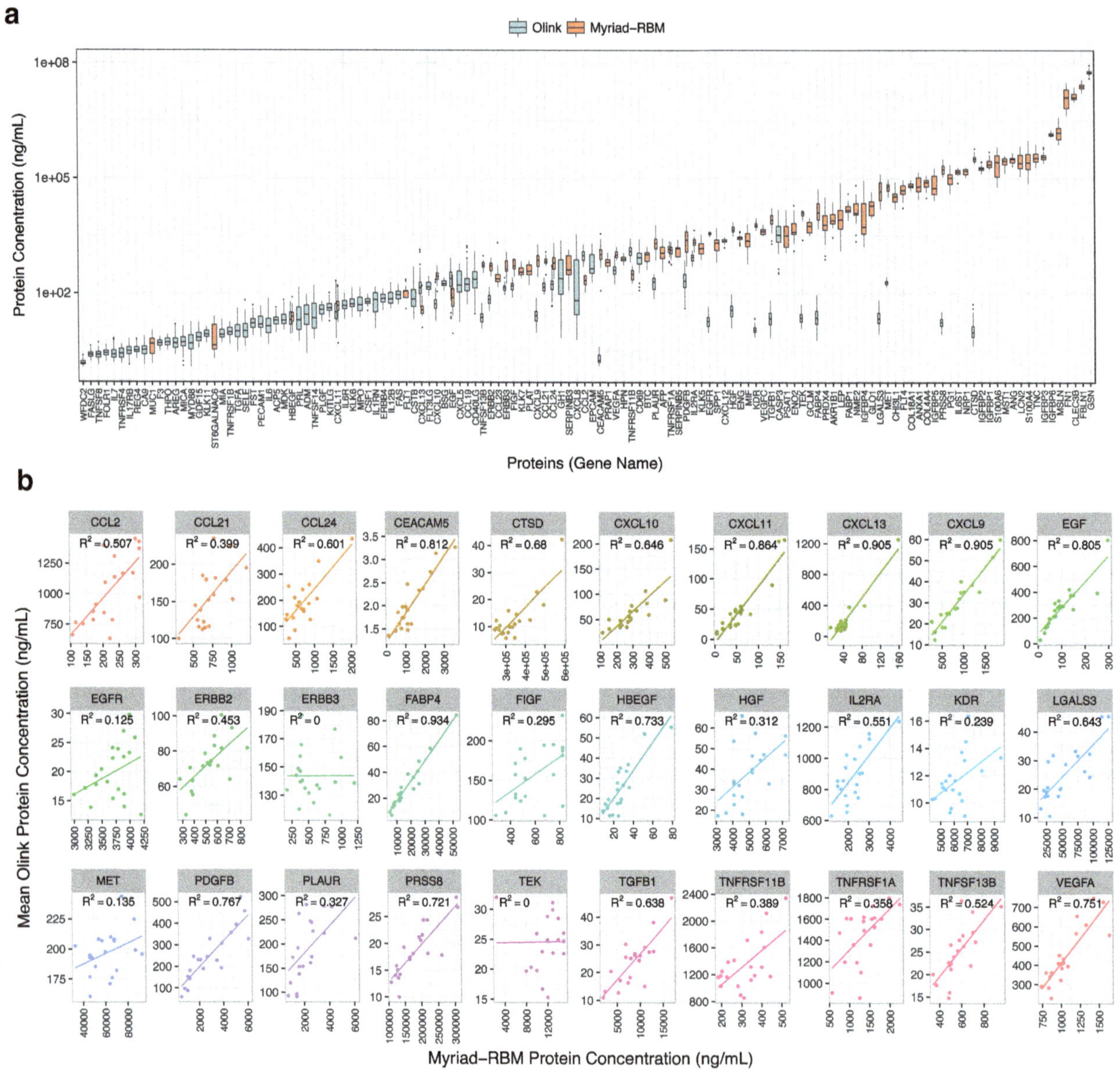

Fig. 3 Assay-to-Assay Comparison for Antibody-Based Technologies. **a** Myriad-RBM estimates higher absolute protein concentration in comparison to Olink platform. **b** Protein levels are concordant for most proteins measured in both antibody-based platforms

technical variance or random error. Though there was inherent technical variance in the Olink measurements as shown in Fig. 3, we were still able to detect biological signals across the individuals in the study.

Furthermore, it is noteworthy that both the biological and technical variations were specific to the protein analyte measured in the Olink Assay. The ratio of biological to technical variation for each protein was plotted in Fig. 5c. Some proteins show more biological variability than other proteins; it is expected that in plasma from breast cancer cases some proteins will behave similarly, whilst others would vary depending on personal variability. We observed that in the Olink analysis, variability was mostly bounded by biological variance, although a deeper look revealed that some individual protein analytes had inherently more individual personalized biological variability.

Case to control comparison

An unsupervised principal component analysis of the Myriad-RBM and Olink datasets showed that the two principal components captured more than 90% of the variation in both the antibody-based assay datasets. However, there was no observable discrimination between the case and control samples in this reduced dimensional space (Additional file 3: Figure S1A).

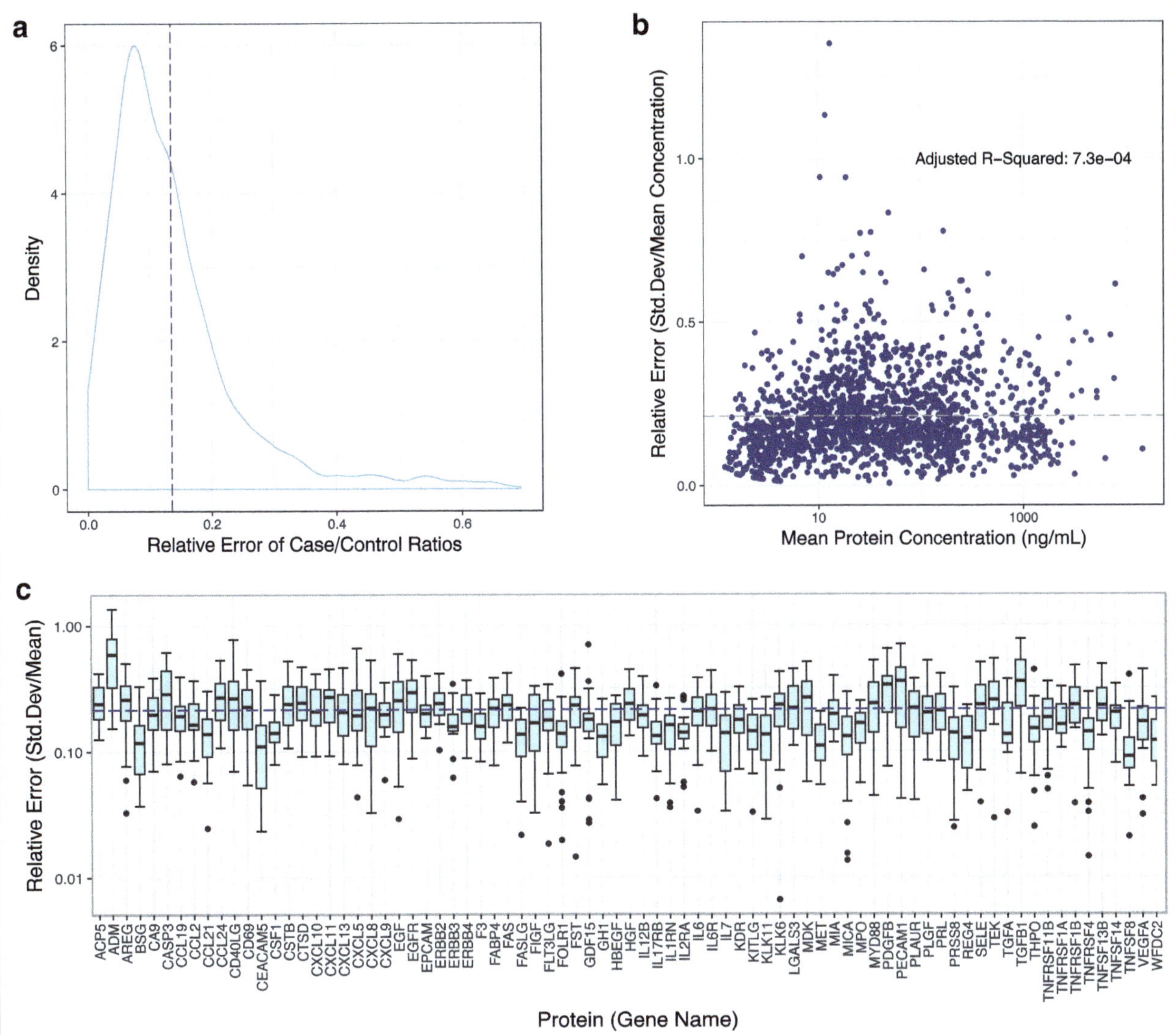

Fig. 4 Technical Variation. **a** Relative error of case/control ratios across all peptides per proteins average at 10% (dashed line) in LC-MS/MS platform. **b** Relative error independent to protein abundance in Olink analysis determined by adjusted R^2 value from linear regression. **c** Relative error across all proteins measured in the Olink analysis averages at 20% (dashed line)

Violin plots in Fig. 6a summarize the most significant proteins from unpaired and paired *t*-tests on measurements from the antibody-based assays. Only a few proteins showed differences with *p*-value less than 1E-01 in the Myriad-RBM analysis; and within the group of five significant analytes measured, we observed only minimal differences between the means of the cases and controls. We observed that the Olink platform identified more significant proteins (*p*-value <1E-01), with better separation of the case and control distributions. Fatty Acid Binding Protein 4 (FABP4), a protein highly expressed in the liver, was found to be significantly different between cases and controls from both Olink and Myriad-RBM measurements. Some significant analytes were mutually exclusive to the paired and unpaired analyses in the Myriad-RBM platform, but not in the Olink analysis.

Figure 6b shows ten proteins with both the largest absolute fold differences and most significant Benjamini-Hochberg corrected *p*-values from a parallel paired *t*-test analysis of the LC-MS/MS data. Amongst these top ten proteins, most are commonly observed in the blood but not previously explicitly linked to cancer-related molecular mechanisms.

Discussion

We evaluated three different types of assays (Fig. 1a) currently used for protein biomarker studies for their respective figures of merit and practical considerations. We found that each platform delivered varying degrees of depth and range

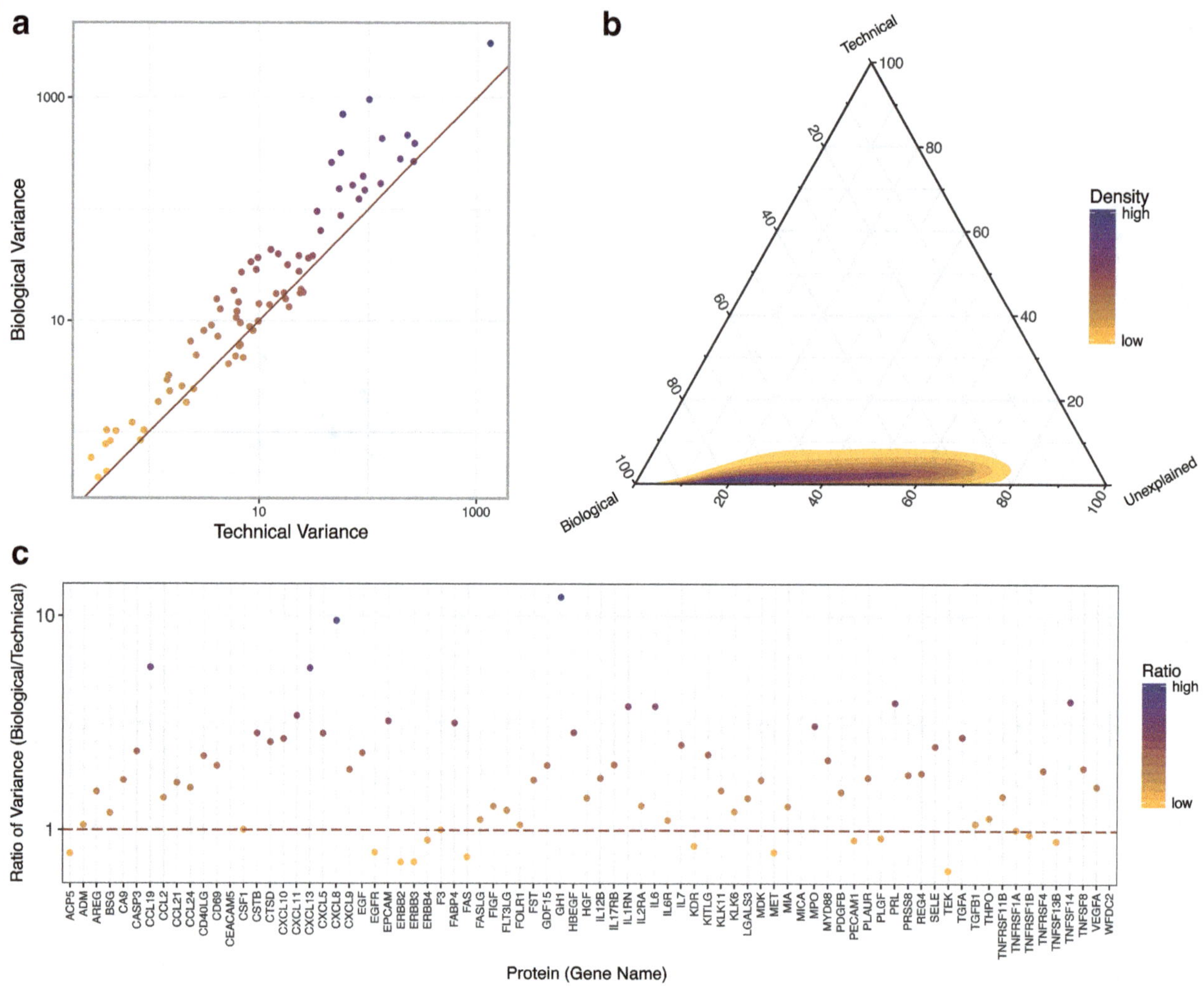

Fig. 5 Biological versus Technical Variation. **a** Biological variance is generally higher than Technical Variance in the Olink Assay. **b** Variance decomposition shows that most variance can be explained by biological variability across the samples. **c** Each protein measured has its own ratio of biological variance vs. technical variance

for each individual analyte measured (Fig. 2), even in the cases where the two immuno-based assays claim to measure the absolute values of the same protein (Fig. 3). We found that platforms had inherent technical variation evaluated with technical replicates (Fig. 4); however, we were still able to detect biological signal that generally surpassed technical variation (Fig. 5a, c). Despite that most variability was captured by biological effects (Fig. 5c), paired and unpaired comparisons of pre-diagnostic case and control samples yielded 32 significant proteins (Fig. 6) with altered expression levels, with a limited subset previously reported to be associated with cancer. No proteins, however, retained statistical significance after false discovery correction. We conclude that technical, practical, and study design considerations are essential to maximize information obtained in limited pre-diagnostic samples of cancer patients.

The motivation for this study was to perform an exploratory investigation of technical and study design implications for identifying potential protein biomarkers in a small sample (n = 10) of pre-diagnostic breast cancer biospecimens. The pre-diagnostic plasma samples from the BCFR in this study – and human clinical cancer biospecimens in general – are often relatively limited in number and amount and difficult to come by. Thus one often arrives, as we did in this study, at a situation wherein there are multiple available technologies to analyze precious samples. It is therefore critical to understand the implications of technical choices, and to carefully design experiments to maximize information obtained.

In this study, we selected three different types of assays (Fig. 1a) currently used for protein biomarker studies. We evaluated each type assay for their respective merit and practical considerations. We leveraged specimens from matched sisters who remained cancer-free as controls and compared them to pre-diagnostic specimens of sisters

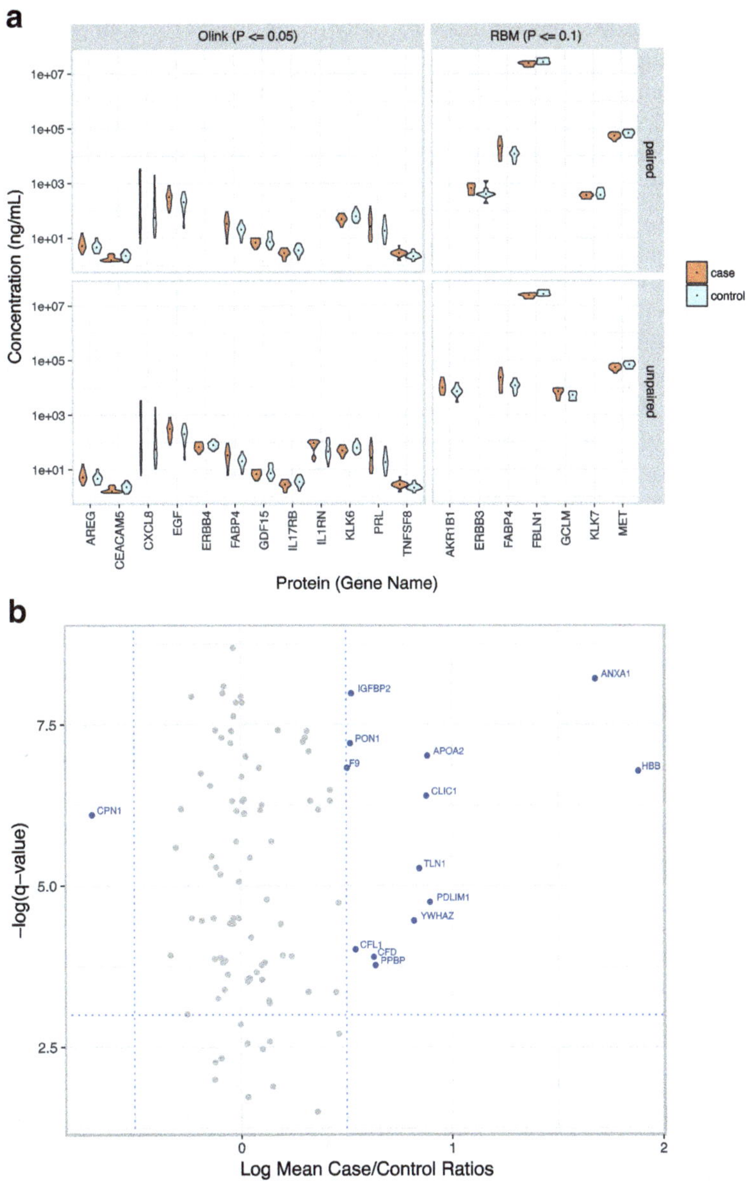

Fig. 6 Case and Control Differences. **a** Unpaired and paired *t*-tests reveal few case/control ratios that are significant in the targeted proteomics assays. **b** Volcano plots reveal protein analytes that characterize difference between case and controls (blue points) from shotgun LC-MS/MS measurements

who developed breast cancer within 2 years of providing the blood sample. Therefore, in addition to comparatively assessing the technical platforms, we also evaluated whether a paired design would bring more statistical power to account for confounding biological variability. Though modest in sample size, this study serves as a model pilot study and practical strategy to evaluate important factors before designing a larger study.

Each of the three methods evaluated in this study comes with their own advantages and disadvantages. The unbiased shotgun LC-MS/MS method not only avoids a constrained pre-selection of analytes of interest, but at the same time can also quantify many more proteins than targeted panels such as the Myriad-RBM and Olink platforms (Fig. 2a). However, LC-MS/MS and most other quantitative mass spectrometry-based methods provide relative rather than absolute quantitation. Absolute measurements require the use of internal standards, which is not feasible in an untargeted study of hundreds of proteins. In recent years, emerging mass spectrometry-based technologies [16] have started to build quantitative assays for larger numbers of proteins; however, these technologies require either a priori knowledge of analytes of interest, or peptide spectral libraries that still rely on data dependent acquisition methods as exhibited in this study. The LC-MS/MS approach is also more sensitive towards higher abundance proteins, thus impacted by a relatively large amount of missing data compared to the antibody-based approaches due to the inherent under-sampling of the mass spectrometer.

In contrast to the LC-MS/MS method, the Myriad-RBM and Olink approaches provide absolute measurements of specific protein levels (Additional file 1: Table S2) which are useful for targeted rather than exploratory studies. These platforms provide respective datasets with protein measurements for nearly every analyte in every sample, with little missing data (Fig. 2b-c). However, though the subset of proteins that were measured by both platforms provided mostly concordant values (Fig. 3b), there remained a clear discrepancy in absolute measurements between the platforms (Fig. 3a) which raises concerns about the reliability of these reported absolute values. This discrepancy is possibly due to differential calibrations used by the different technologies. Moreover, for protein measurements that were not concordant between the two antibody-based methods, it is possible that corresponding antibodies may not be measuring the same epitope of a protein and are henceforth capturing different protein forms. Another disadvantage of these antibody-based technologies is that antibodies can either be inherently biased due to their affinity to substrates, or unavailable for potential novel protein biomarkers.

In addition to the technical features of these assays, there are several practical considerations for each approach. The LC-MS/MS approach was the most time-consuming approach due to time needed to perform fractionation to overcome the large dynamic range of proteins in the blood and the time required for LC-MS/MS data acquisition. The Olink assays required the smallest volume of plasma samples of all the platforms, which is an important practical consideration when working with the precious and limited pre-diagnostic samples. Lastly, each assay comes at a different cost which may determine the feasibility of performing assays in duplicate, or even triplicate.

The three assay platforms provide both complementary and mutually exclusive information. Therefore, practical considerations and priorities may determine the choice of assay for evaluating clinical samples for biomarker discovery. All assays used in this this study had some inherent technical variation. We also chose to evaluate technical variation of the antibody-based Olink platform rather than the Myriad-RBM platform largely because the Olink assay requires significantly smaller volume of our limited biospecimens. We found some technical variation in the Olink assay, but it was not correlated with the type of analyte or measured protein abundance (Fig. 4b-c), thus establishing reliable scalability of the assay across all protein targets.

Despite technical variation detected with our triplicate analysis, we observed that the signal from biological variation of protein levels between samples was larger than the technical variation (Fig. 5a-b). Interestingly, each protein analyte in the same antibody-based platform has its own technical and biological variation (Fig. 5c), which cannot necessarily be predicted a priori, probably owing to inherent biases in the antibodies, or to confounding biological noise. For each analyte in a protein measurement study, it is thus important to evaluate the technical and biological variation to account for confounding in the analytical signal. Our findings therefore support the utility of replicates in studies to assess analyte variation.

Lastly, in addition to assessing the inherent variability within and between the different protein assays, we also evaluated whether a matched case and control sisters study design would yield more statistical power in uncovering significant early diagnostic biomarkers. We initially hypothesized that sisters of the breast cancer cases would serve as well-matched controls as they are naturally controlled for race/ethnicity and a large proportion of genetic background. Moreover, our choice to evaluate pre-diagnostic samples eliminates bias associated with sample collection as both case and control samples were collected under the same conditions without knowledge of cancer diagnosis at the time of collection.

However, the unbiased principal component analysis exhibited that even with our careful study design choices to minimize bias, samples showed relatively large individual variance along their two principal component axes in the antibody-based datasets. Samples from biological sisters did not generally appear to be more similar to each other than to other individual samples (Additional file 3: Figure S1B). Hence it was not surprising to discover that the case and control samples were not well separated in the two-dimensional space of components that captured a substantive amount of the overall variance (>90%) (Additional file 3: Figure S1A).

Henceforth, we focused our analysis efforts on identifying individual protein analytes with potential diagnostic power. While a small number of proteins showed statistically significant differences between cases and controls; the changes were small (less than two-fold) and the number of proteins showing differences was small (Fig. 6). This finding is not necessarily unexpected. Given that the samples were collected from women up to 2 years before they were diagnosed with breast cancer, it is highly likely that the analytical signal in the blood plasma associated with breast cancer cannot be detected above the biological noise that arises from inter-individual variation.

We observed in Fig. 6a that the paired statistical analysis in the Olink platform provided more significant analytes than the unpaired analysis, suggesting that for the Olink platform, the paired design had greater statistical power when evaluating each protein analyte independently. However, also shown in Fig. 6a, we observed that there were some significant analytes that were mutually exclusive to the paired and unpaired analysis in the Myriad-RBM platform. If evaluating this platform in isolation, these results echo our initial PCA (Additional file 3: Figure S1); it appears that on the Myriad-RBM platform, the sisters are not more similar to each other than across all the samples both when protein levels are analyzed independently, and in covariance. This result may be explained by factors including, but not limited to, noise introduced by technical variation that was not evaluated for this platform, coupled with person-to-person variation from the samples. The Myriad-RBM oncology panel was chosen specifically for this study, and our results suggest that these protein measurements show little utility in pre-diagnostic breast cancer samples. This suggests that there is still a need for the unbiased exploratory LC-MS/MS methods that yield novel significant biomarker candidates as seen in Fig. 6b. Although the protein analytes in Fig. 6b have not been validated, they serve as a proof of concept that an untargeted approach can yield candidates that would otherwise be missed by targeted panels applied to noisy clinical samples.

Conclusions

This study has comprehensively evaluated technical, practical and study design considerations for potential protein biomarker detection using the currently available technologies. Our findings provide a framework for larger studies and estimates of biological effect sizes for a more informed early protein cancer biomarker detection approach.

Abbreviations

BCFR: Breast Cancer Family Registry; FABP4: Fatty Acid Binding Protein 4; IgA: Immunoglobulin A; IgG: Immunoglobulin G; LC-MS/MS: Liquid chromatography-tandem mass spectrometry; LDD: Least detectable concentration; PCA: Principal component analysis; qPCR: quantitative polymerase chain reaction

Acknowledgements

We thank scientists from Olink Bioscience for helpful discussions. Inquiries about bioinformatics analyses should be directed to P.M.

Funding

The authors are grateful for support from a Developmental Cancer Research Award from the Stanford Cancer Institute (S.J.P and E.M.J.) and support from Canary Foundation (P.M. and S.J.P.). The Breast Cancer Family Registry (BCFR) is supported by grant UM1 CA164920 from the National Cancer Institute. The content of this manuscript does not necessarily reflect the views or policies of the U.S. National Cancer Institute or any of the collaborating centers in the BCFR, nor does mention of trade names, commercial products, or organizations imply endorsement by the U.S. Government or the BCFR. The work of P.M. and R.A. is partially supported by DARPA Deep Purple Program (program manager Dr. James Gimlett) through a DOI contract #D17AC00006, DARPA SIMPLEX W911NF-15-1-0555 by NIH 1R01GM11709701. Funding bodies played no role in the design of the study and collection, analysis, or interpretation of data.

Authors' contributions

CYY analyzed and interpreted the data and was a major contributor in writing the manuscript. RA contributed to data analysis strategies, and analyzed and interpreted the data. MK contributed to study design and generated and analyzed the data. PM contributed to data analysis and interpretation. EMJ contributed to study design, data interpretation, and was a major contributor in writing the manuscript. SJP contributed to study design, data generation, analysis, and interpretation and was a major contributor in writing the manuscript. All authors read and approved the final manuscript.

Competing interests

The authors declare that they have no competing interests.

Author details

[1]Department of Biomedical Informatics, Stanford University School of Medicine, Stanford, CA 93405, USA. [2]Department of Radiology, Canary Center at Stanford for Cancer Early Detection, Stanford University School of Medicine, Palo Alto, CA 94304, USA. [3]Department of Genetics, Stanford University School of Medicine, Stanford, CA 93405, USA. [4]Stanford Cancer Institute, Stanford University School of Medicine, Stanford, CA 94305, USA. [5]Cancer Prevention Institute of California, Fremont, CA 94538, USA.

References

1. SEER Cancer Statistics Review. [https://seer.cancer.gov/csr/1975_2014/].
2. Berghuis AM, Koffijberg H, Prakash J, Terstappen LW, IJzerman MJ. Detecting blood-based biomarkers in metastatic breast cancer: a systematic review of their current status and clinical utility. Int J Mol Sci. 2017;18(2):doi:10.3390/ijms18020363.
3. Pitteri SJ, Amon LM, Busald Buson T, Zhang Y, Johnson MM, Chin A, Kennedy J, Wong CH, Zhang Q, Wang H, et al. Detection of elevated plasma levels of epidermal growth factor receptor before breast cancer diagnosis among hormone therapy users. Cancer Res. 2010;70: 8598–606.
4. Anderson GL, McIntosh M, Wu L, Barnett M, Goodman G, Thorpe JD, Bergan L, Thornquist MD, Scholler N, Kim N, et al. Assessing lead time of selected ovarian cancer biomarkers: a nested case-control study. J Natl Cancer Inst. 2010;102:26–38.
5. Opstal-van Winden AW, Rodenburg W, Pennings JL, van Oostrom CT, Beijnen JH, Peeters PH, van Gils CH, de Vries A. A bead-based multiplexed immunoassay to evaluate breast cancer biomarkers for early detection in pre-diagnostic serum. Int J Mol Sci. 2012;13:13587–604.
6. Blyuss O, Gentry-Maharaj A, Fourkala EO, Ryan A, Zaikin A, Menon U, Jacobs I, Timms JF. Serial patterns of ovarian cancer biomarkers in a Prediagnosis longitudinal dataset. Biomed Res Int. 2015;2015:681416.
7. Amon LM, Pitteri SJ, Li CI, McIntosh M, Ladd JJ, Disis M, Porter P, Wong CH, Zhang Q, Lampe P, et al. Concordant release of glycolysis proteins into the plasma preceding a diagnosis of ER+ breast cancer. Cancer Res. 2012;72: 1935–42.
8. Opstal-van Winden AW, Krop EJ, Karedal MH, Gast MC, Lindh CH, Jeppsson MC, Jonsson BA, Grobbee DE, Peeters PH, Beijnen JH, et al. Searching for early breast cancer biomarkers by serum protein profiling of pre-diagnostic serum; a nested case-control study. BMC Cancer. 2011;11:381.

9. Hawkridge AM, Muddiman DC. Mass spectrometry-based biomarker discovery: toward a global proteome index of individuality. Annu Rev Anal Chem (Palo Alto, Calif). 2009;2:265–77.
10. Enroth S, Johansson A, Enroth SB, Gyllensten U. Strong effects of genetic and lifestyle factors on biomarker variation and use of personalized cutoffs. Nat Commun. 2014;5:4684.
11. Liu Y, Buil A, Collins BC, Gillet LC, Blum LC, Cheng LY, Vitek O, Mouritsen J, Lachance G, Spector TD, et al. Quantitative variability of 342 plasma proteins in a human twin population. Mol Syst Biol. 2015;11:786.
12. Pitteri SJ, Hanash SM, Aragaki A, Amon LM, Chen L, Busald Buson T, Paczesny S, Katayama H, Wang H, Johnson MM, et al. Postmenopausal estrogen and progestin effects on the serum proteome. Genome Med. 2009;1:121.
13. Katayama H, Paczesny S, Prentice R, Aragaki A, Faca VM, Pitteri SJ, Zhang Q, Wang H, Silva M, Kennedy J, et al. Application of serum proteomics to the Women's Health Initiative conjugated equine estrogens trial reveals a multitude of effects relevant to clinical findings. Genome Med. 2009;1:47.
14. Pitteri SJ, Hanash SM. Confounding effects of hormone replacement therapy in protein biomarker studies. Cancer Epidemiol Biomark Prev. 2011;20:134–9.
15. Solier C, Langen H. Antibody-based proteomics and biomarker research - current status and limitations. Proteomics. 2014;14:774–83.
16. Faria SS, Morris CF, Silva AR, Fonseca MP, Forget P, Castro MS, Fontes W. A timely shift from shotgun to targeted proteomics and how it can be groundbreaking for cancer research. Front Oncol. 2017;7:13.
17. Anjo SI, Santa C, Manadas B. SWATH-MS as a tool for biomarker discovery: from basic research to clinical applications. Proteomics. 2017;17(3-4). doi:10.1002/pmic.201600278.
18. John EM, Hopper JL, Beck JC, Knight JA, Neuhausen SL, Senie RT, Ziogas A, Andrulis IL, Anton-Culver H, Boyd N, et al. The breast cancer family registry: an infrastructure for cooperative multinational, interdisciplinary and translational studies of the genetic epidemiology of breast cancer. Breast Cancer Res. 2004;6:R375–89.
19. Kullolli M, Warren J, Arampatzidou M, Pitteri SJ. Performance evaluation of affinity ligands for depletion of abundant plasma proteins. J Chromatogr B Analyt Technol Biomed Life Sci. 2013;939:10–6.
20. Faca V, Coram M, Phanstiel D, Glukhova V, Zhang Q, Fitzgibbon M, McIntosh M, Hanash S. Quantitative analysis of acrylamide labeled serum proteins by LC-MS/MS. J Proteome Res. 2006;5:2009–18.
21. Ma K, Vitek O, Nesvizhskii AI. A statistical model-building perspective to identification of MS/MS spectra with PeptideProphet. BMC Bioinformatics. 2012;13(Suppl 16):S1.
22. Farrah T, Deutsch EW, Omenn GS, Campbell DS, Sun Z, Bletz JA, Mallick P, Katz JE, Malmstrom J, Ossola R, et al. A high-confidence human plasma proteome reference set with estimated concentrations in PeptideAtlas. Mol Cell Proteomics. 2011;10:M110.006353.
23. Assarsson E, Lundberg M, Holmquist G, Bjorkesten J, Thorsen SB, Ekman D, Eriksson A, Rennel Dickens E, Ohlsson S, Edfeldt G, et al. Homogenous 96-plex PEA immunoassay exhibiting high sensitivity, specificity, and excellent scalability. PLoS One. 2014;9:e95192.

antioxidant, anti-inflammatory, antipyretic and antinociceptive activities. Acquired ultraviolet (UV) and MS data will be used for dereplication and tentative identification of known compounds, as well as to pinpoint potentially new compounds. The chromatogram and the activity profile will then be matched to identify active peaks. Characterization will be done by analyzing the NMR data for eluted fractions or peaks recorded off-line using microprobe technology. Metabolomics-based phytochemical profiling and in vitro bioassays may establish the correlation between specific phytochemicals and different bioactivities leading to the identification of biomarkers. Synergistic multi-target biomarkers are expected to be identified and used for in vivo validation. This data could also be used in targeted metabolomics analysis, for lead identification and eventual downstream chemical production analyses and clinical development (Fig. 1).

Although there are some standardized anti-malarial phytomedicines in current use in some endemic countries [18], the continuous and unsafe use of non-standardized plant-derived products in many malaria endemic countries obliges new approaches.

Herewith an overview of the emerging methodological landscape in the application of the multi-target phytotherapeutic concept in malaria drug discovery. This interdisciplinary approach employs tailored technology platforms coupled to miniaturized biological assays to track and characterize the anti-malarial components of herbal medicines.

By combining the modified reverse pharmacology to the systems biology approaches, the bioactivities of different phytochemicals can be assessed, in view of the identification of potential biomarkers. This will facilitate unravelling of the multi-target phytotherapeutic mechanisms and the standardization of herbal medicines as well as facilitate lead discovery for prioritization and downstream clinical analyses. Therefore, its application in malaria drug discovery could be of immense importance.

Generation of a plant extract/compound library

A library can be defined as a collection of plant extracts/compounds stored in a standardized format and readily deliverable for screening assays. The information associated with each sample is usually stored in a database. Prior to establishing an extract library, key issues that have to be considered include the choice of plants and suitable extraction procedures to be applied to the samples.

Choice of plants

The choice of plants as test material remains the most challenging and a determinant factor in plant-based malaria drug discovery process. There are various approaches to select plant material for this process and these include the

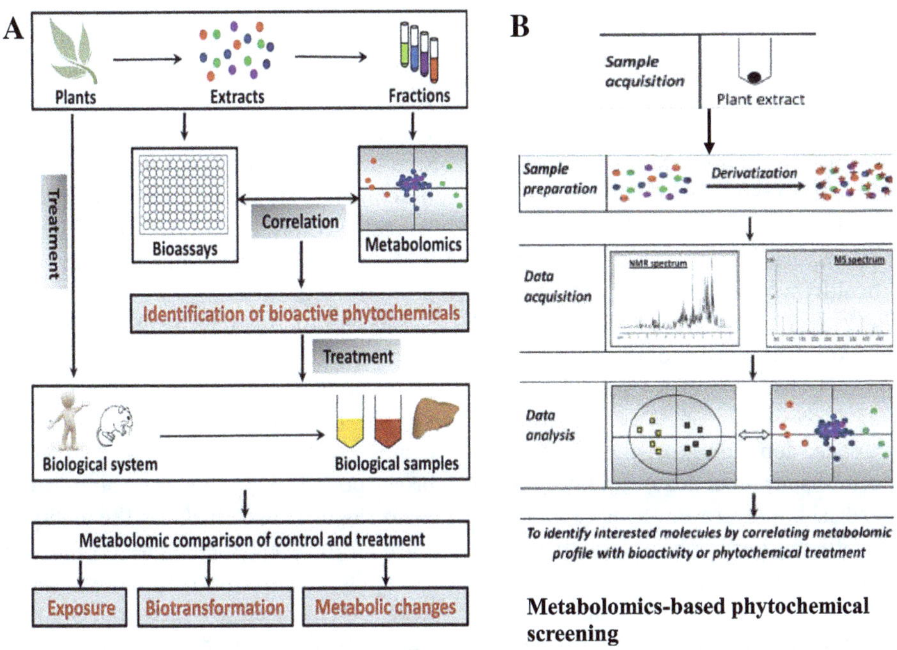

Fig. 1 Work flow for the application of metabolomics in analysis of HMs. **a** HPLC-based activity profiling. **b** Phytochemical profiling (untargeted metabolomics) Metabolomics-based phytochemical profiling and in vitro bioassays of bioactivities may establish the correlation between specific phytochemicals and different bioactivities leading to the identification of biomarkers

random selection, ethnopharmacological, chemosystematic (phylogenetic), ecological and computational approaches.

The random selection of extracts and/or fractions from different plant species on the basis of their availability can be highly advantageous when samples are derived from areas of high biodiversity and malaria endemism [19]. This is because the chemical diversity of natural products can reflect the biodiversity of their source organism. Random selection of plant material can potentially result in the unexpected identification of bioactivities that would not be predicted based on indigenous or existing knowledge [20].

Ethnopharmacology is the classical approach for the choice of plants for bioassays and involves the gathering of data on the indigenous use of the plants as a basis for their selection. This usually involves the observation, description, and experimental assessment of traditionally used medicines and their effects on humans. It represents a transdisciplinary concept between the natural (botany, chemistry, biochemistry, pharmacology and pharmacognosy) and the social sciences (anthropology, archeology, history and linguistics) [12, 21]. This approach has led to the prominent discovery of some vital anti-malarials. Examples include the isolation of quinine from Cinchona species 1820 and its derivatives, chloroquine and mefloquine which replaced it in the 20th century [22]. Artemisinin was isolated from *Artemisa annua* in 1971 and constitutes the core of artemisinin-based combination therapies (ACT) and its derivatives, artesunate and artemether which are widely in use currently [23]. A recently introduced plant-derived antimalarial drug is atovaquone, a synthetic naphthoquinone based on lapachol, a prenylnaphtoquinone, first isolated from *Tabebuia impetiginosa*, a South American member of the Bignoniaceae family [4]. Ethnopharmacological data is easily accessible in well-established traditional health systems such as the Traditional Chinese Medicine (TCM) and Ayurveda, which possess current documented evidence of centuries. However, this is not the case with other health systems such as the African Traditional health system, where knowledge is passed on from one generation to the other orally, and formulations in use are usually kept secret by the aging practitioners, rendering access to relevant information difficult [21, 24]. Hence, depending on the plant to be studied, there are various sources of acquiring information such as books on medical botany, review articles on medicinal plants used in different geographical regions or cultures [25] as well as computer databases [26].

The chemosystematic or phylogenetic approach is based on the chemotaxonomy and phylogeny taking into account that plant species from some genera or families are known to produce compounds and compound classes associated with a certain bioactivity or therapeutic potential [20]. The combination of phylogenetic information and ethnobotanical knowledge can be a very powerful tool in natural product drug discovery. The exploration of cross-cultural ethnomedical patterns within a phylogenetic framework can lead to high success rates [27, 28].

The ecological approach is based on the observation of interactions between organisms and their environment, considering that plant secondary metabolites possess ecological functions from which a potential therapeutic use for humans can be derived [20]. For example, compounds with antimalarial activity could be isolated from plant species eaten by chimpanzees and baboons in the wild [29].

The computational approach relies on *in silico* bioactivity predictions for constituents of certain plant species. These studies can focus on the main constituents of herbal remedies as well as on other natural compounds with anti-malarial effects directly retrieved from literature [30].

Having appropriately identified and sourced the plant(s) of choice, the next step in the value addition of medicinal plants bio-resources is the production of herbal preparations (extracts) using a variety of technologies from simple traditional technologies to advance extraction techniques, subject to the choice of assay.

Extraction procedure

Extraction is the separation of medicinally active components (secondary metabolites) of plant tissues, using relevant solvents and standard conditions. A key aspect to the characterization of plant-derived active components is the selection of an adapted extraction protocol that would be suitable for the detection of the biomarkers of interest. This is a fundamental and critical step with important consequences for the accuracy of outcomes [31]. To increase extraction yields, plants are typically ground to a fine powder. However, when fresh material is used, it is imperative for the grinding process to be done on ice.

The aim of characterizing the bioactive components in plants is to comprehensively profile the largest possible array of low molecular weight metabolites in a given sample. In order for this to be achieved, extraction procedures with solvents that can extract compounds over a broad polarity range need to be utilized. And since there is no single solvent that has the ability to extract and dissolve all the plant metabolites at once, several solvents of increasing polarity need to be used in succession, such as hexane > ethylacetate > methanol > ethanol > water. This is the classical approach used for phytochemical screening and bio-activity guided fractionation, and it is difficult to implement in modern characterization studies known as metabolomics, because it generates many different extracts per sample that have to be analyzed separately, which usually is not compatible with the large number of samples that need to be analyzed. A dependable alternative is a combination of various solvents, such as a multi-phase solvent system composed of a mixture of solvents, such as chloroform-methanol—water, which has been proposed for such studies which are performed with pure methanol or a mixture containing it [31]. In this regard, there are various parameters to be considered in the solvent systems to be utilized, which should make it compatible with the applicable analytical technique. These include the nature of the organic and aqueous solvents, the volumes, ratios and aqueous solvent pH. For example, an aspect that needs to be considered is that lipophilic compounds do not elute from C18 reversed phase columns and certain methanol—water mixtures do not extract chlorophyll from plant aerial parts, which might be an advantage for incorporating LC analysis in MS—based metabolomics [13].

To accelerate the extraction process, additional energy needs to be applied to reduce the extraction time. This can be achieved by directly heating the system and increasing the pressure by using techniques such as the microwave-assisted extraction, supercritical fluid extraction and the mostly used pressurized (or accelerated) solvent extraction [32, 33]. These enable an efficient extraction under standardized conditions and make use of very little quantities of the plant material to be extracted, which are compatible with miniaturization of assays and the generalization of the microplate format. Moreover, extraction temperatures are usually maintained below the solvent boiling points for yield optimization and preservation of metabolite chemistry.

A review of potential anti-malarial components that have been identified from plants cover a very wide range of phytochemicals classes, which include alkaloids, terpenoids, flavonoids, coumarins, phenolics, polyacetylenes, xanthones, quinones, steroids and lignans [3, 34, 35]. Extracting each necessitates specific extraction technique, making it cumbersome and time-consuming for the investigator, especially given the fact that there might be little or no activity after extraction and isolation, as has been the case with many small molecules that have been tested for their activity. Since this reverse pharmacology – systems biology approach entails a farm - to-clinic process, whereby the ethnopharmacological knowledge and pharmacological validation is vital before HPLC-based anti-malarial profiling, solvent extracts will be dried are stored in a standardized (usually microplate) format, readily available for screening assays, biomarker and target identification, while the information associated with each sample are stored in a database.

Choice of bioassays in in vitro efficacy and safety

In malaria drug discovery, efficacy and safety screening is a long and costly process confronted with low productivity, thereby limiting the number of new drugs. In order to improve on this, recent efforts have been dedicated to developing high throughput screening (HTS) platforms that mimic in vivo systems and provide more relevant information than biochemical assays, for the pipeline [36]. For the purposes of screening natural products, cell-based HTS methods are more relevant and typically make use of 96, 384 and 1536-well (in automated systems) microtitre plates and can be performed in a more biological relevant microenvironment. The main components are cells or parasites, culture device and detection system for quantification of cells or bioactivities. When used in screening plant extracts and other drugs, they provide representative tissue specific responses, which can be useful in efficacy and safety screening, biomarker and target identification, thereby facilitating standardization.

In vitro antiplasmodial efficacy

In vitro screening of malaria parasite laboratory strains and field isolates for susceptibility against test compounds provides an early indication of drug efficacy, failure or possible clinical resistance. These screens are usually whole-cell based and require screening both the erythrocyte and exo-erythrocytic stages [37]. They serve first and foremost to identify active extracts before subjecting them to metabolomics analysis and secondly for the identification of potential biomarkers after metabolomics characterization of their phytochemical constituents.

In the erythrocyte stage screening, inhibition is monitored by measures of growth and proliferation of *P. falciparum* strains, usually without knowledge of the molecular targets of the compounds that are being screened [38]. HTS methods currently being used to measure *P. falciparum* in vitro drug susceptibility include the ^{3}H-hypoxanthine incorporation assay [39], histidine-rich protein-2 enzyme linked immunosorbent assay (HRP-2 ELISA) [40, 41], parasite lactate dehydrogenase colorimetric assay (pLDH) [42] and the most recent SYBR Green-1 fluorescence assay [43, 44]. The titriated hypoxanthine uptake assay involves measuring parasite growth by recording levels of titriated hypoxanthine incorporation into the parasite DNA. Though accurate and reliable, its major shortcoming is the use of radioactivity, the safe disposal of which demands substantial resources. The HRP-2 method assesses parasite growth by using ELISA to measure *P. falciparum* HRP-2 and offers better result upon examining drug susceptibilities of field isolates using non-radioactive procedure. It is also more cost effective compared to the ^{3}H-hypoxathine method. The pLDH assay is an indirect method that measures *P. falciparum* LDH activity as an assessment of parasitaemia by colorimetry. Although this method is more cost effective when compared to the ^{3}H-hypoxanthine method, it is an ELISA method just like the HRP-2 method, which depends on the availability of specific antibodies. The recently developed SYBR Green-1 fluorescence assay is based on measuring the incorporation of the fluorescent SYBR Green-1 dye into parasite DNA. This requires a single step of DNA staining, it is less labour intensive and cost effective compared to the other methods and it is more amenable for HTS, which has become the gold standard in drug screening. This assay demonstrates the reliability of a simple, rapid, inexpensive and easy to use fluorescence-based method for drug susceptibility testing of *P. falciparum* laboratory strains and clinical isolates [45].

The exo-erythrocyte or liver stage is a very important life cycle stage with respect to the eradication programme. Recent progress has been made in the development of HTS for identification of active compounds against this stage of the parasite. There are billions of parasites present in the human blood stage infection, only a limited number of ookinetes, hypnozoites or early liver forms exists during transmission and re-infection, hence the unlikely emergence of resistance in the event of an intervention at these stages [46]. Parasites injected with the mosquito's saliva find their way into the host liver, where they multiply asexually as exo-erythrocytic forms (EEFs) during an asymptomatic incubation period of about a week prior to emerging into the blood stream. This initiates the asexual erythrocytic cycle that is responsible for the manifestation of malaria. Contrary to the limited life span of some *Plasmodium* species, *P. ovale* and *vivax* can persist within the liver as dormant hypnozoites for several months. Their reactivation, which is usually triggered by an unknown mechanism, could see rapidly growing parasites re-populate the blood, thereby causing a pathology. Hence, the persistence of the hypnozoites represents formidable barrier to the eradication process [47].

Amongst the blood stage forms of the parasite, a subset, in response to cues that are not well understood, can differentiate into male and female gametocytes in a process that takes about 8–12 days in *P. falciparum*. These parasites metabolize the host red cell hemoglobin while progressing through five morphological distinct stages that can be identified by light microscope [48]. These immature gametocytes can last in the host for up to 55 days and mature gametocytes are the only form that can survive in the mosquito midgut, mate, undergo meiosis and give rise to next generation of parasites to be transmitted to a new host [49]. The majority of compounds active against the erythrocyte stage are inactive against the liver stage and current first line artemisin-based treatment regimens do not block transmission [50]. A current focus of anti-malarial drug discovery is to screen for small molecules and HMs that are active against both liver and gametocytes in order to block malaria transmission. The complex chemical diversity of HMs is a sure source of such scaffolds in one system.

One of the major shortcomings of developing HTS assays to evaluate liver stage activity is that parasites cannot be maintained in culture. A recently developed assay that can be used to determine the efficacy of HMs with known blood stage activity is the high content screening (HCS) on *P. yoelli* infected hepatocytes. To detect likely prophylactic activity, *P. berghei* or *P. yoelli* sporozoites are seeded unto human hepatoma cells and the infection is imaged [51] or detected enzymatically [52]. Alternatively, using a medium throughput assay, the radical potential of a test compound could be tested using the hypnozoite-forming monkey model, *P. cynolmolgi*. *P. cynolmolgi* sporozoites are seeded unto primary monkey hepatocytes and HCS used to determine the ratio between large, rapidly developing schizonts and dormant "small forms" (supposed hypnozoites). All parasites including hypnozoites will be eliminated by radical cure agents whereas prophylactic compounds will act on growing schizonts [53].

Though assays are available for screening compounds with transmission-blocking potential, these assays are particularly difficult because the process of gametocytogenesis is not well understood. The first gametocyte screen was conducted using alamar blue, an oxido-reduction indicator that fluoresces and changes colour in response to chemical reduction of growth medium during metabolic activity of gametocytes [54]. Based on this principle, other screens have been implemented using lactate dehydrogenase [55]. During the 12 days it takes for gametocytes to mature from the early to the late (transmission) stage, they do not divide. Consequently, methods based on the detection of inhibited parasite proliferation are limited [37]. Alternative HTS assay techniques to detect gametocyte death have been developed, most of which use overall ATP hydrolysis to measure viability. Hence the loss of this activity would signify gametocyte death [54]. It is also possible to selectively count parasites expressing a gametocyte-stage specific GFP tag by flow cytometry [56]. However, most of the assays only attempt to predict transmission-blocking activity by measuring gametocyte death. Efforts have been focused on more predictive assays aimed at measuring viability at different stages, especially the later stage [57]. Recently, Plouffe et al. [58] developed a HTS and cost effective assay technique, the Saponin-Lysis

Sexual Stage Assay (SaLSSA) for identifying small molecules with transmission-blocking capacity, which clearly emphasizes substantial physiological difference between asexual and sexual parasite and provides a tool and starting point for the discovery and development of transmission-blocking drugs.

One of the limitations of the relevance of HTS antiplasmodial efficacy assays is their inability to provide information on some factors that influence the activity of substances in vivo such as absorption, distribution, metabolism, excretion and toxicity (ADME/T), which describes the disposition of bioactive compounds in in vivo systems. However, they still represent very important tools to identify and characterize active test substances [59] and this should be proceeded by toxicological screening. This is very important for the development of new drugs and for the extension of the therapeutic potential of existing molecules and herbal drugs, the first step of which is the screening on cell lines or cytotoxicity.

Cell viability and cytotoxicity screening

Despite the growing market demand for herbal medicines, there are still concerns associated with not only their use, but their safety. Less than 10% of herbal products in the world market are truly standardized to known active components and strict quality control measures are not always diligently adhered to [60]. Therefore, cell viability and cytotoxicity assays are essential for drug screening and in vitro safety of anti-malarial drug molecules and herbal products [61]. The importance of including these assays anti-malarial plant profiling, was emphasized by van Dyk et al. [62], when they eliminated nine out of fifty-nine organic solvent extracts of South African plants that exhibited anti-malarial activity. A simple, rapid, sensitive, reliable, safe and cost-effective measurement of cells viability is the ideal test for in vitro cell proliferation and cytotoxicity and it should not interfere with the compound to be tested. These cell-based tests are performed to predict potential toxicities, using cultured cells which may be normal or transformed cells. The procedure normally involves short term exposure of cultured cells to test compounds, to detect the effects on basal or specialized cell function, prior to performing safety studies on whole organisms. It can also provide insight towards the carcinogenic or genotoxic dispositions of the test substances. The ability of a plant extract or test compound to inhibit cellular growth and viability can be ascertained as an indication of its toxicity, parameters of which include inhibition of cell proliferation, cell viability markers (metabolic and membrane), morphologic and intracellular differentiation markers [63]. Some of the factors to be considered when conducting these assays include cell culture systems, cell type compatibility with solvent system used for extraction and final concentration of dimethyl sulphoxide (DMSO) to avoid toxicity [64]. DMSO is an important aprotic solvent that can solubilize a wide variety of otherwise poorly soluble polar and nonpolar molecules, due to its amphipathic nature. This, coupled with its apparent low toxicity at concentrations <10%, has led to its ubiquitous use and widespread application [65].

Another important factor to be considered is the selection of a wide range of high quality cell types for testing including normal cells of primary origin and permanent cell lines, due to the selective toxicity displayed by some plant extracts. The advantage of using these cell lines include unlimited supply, no genetic variation, which aids reproducibility and predictive power of an outcome, as well as access to the collective knowledge gained from global research conducted on the geno- and phenotype of the cell line in question [66]. However, primary cell cultures have an advantage over most perpetual cell lines in that they are the closest in vitro representation of the in vivo cell type under scrutiny. Hence, primary hepatocytes are considered the "gold standard" used for predictive toxicology because they are often employed with the expectation that chemicals will affect or be affected by an isolated cell in the same manner that would occur in the whole organ [67].

Cell-based assays can be used to predict the mechanism of toxicity depending on the endpoint that is assessed; these include cell death/survival, adaptive/prelethal mechanistic reactions, including mitochondrial homeostasis, generation of reactive oxygen species (ROS), lipid peroxidation, Ca^{2+} signaling, enzyme inhibition and transporters endpoints [66].

Toxicokinetics

Toxicokinetics deals with the prediction of toxicity due to pharmacokinetic disposition of an herb or pure compound derived from it, as a result of genetics or potential herb-drug interactions, especially given the increasing use of anti-malarial plants for therapy in endemic countries. Therefore, toxicokinetics of antimalarial components is of utmost important in evaluating the toxicity and drug interaction of anti-malarial components. Chung et al. [68] recently reported the toxicokinetics of anti-malarial artesunate in rats. This assay involves the use of human liver microsomal Cytochrome P450 isoforms and is aimed at the early identification of metabolites which are known to cause toxicological modulation in the cellular organization [69]. Cytochrome P450s are heme-containing monooxygenases located in the small intestine, liver and other tissues that play pivotal roles in the detoxification and bioactivation of diverse xenobiotics [70]. Approximately 75% of all known drugs are metabolized hepatically by mixed function oxidation reactions catalyzed by Cytochrome P450 isoforms (CYP3A4, CYP2C9, CYP2C19, CYP1A2 and CYP2D6) and they are highly subject to inhibition owing to their broad specificity for structurally diverse substrates. Modulation of Cytochrome P450 is of great significance in drug biotransformation to active or inactive forms. For drugs that are dependent on these enzymes for inactivation via conjugation to chemical polar groups prior to elimination, any herb that induces these enzymes would lead to rapid inactivation and clearance of such drugs. Herbs that inhibit enzyme activity will result to high concentrations of the drug whose inactivation relies on the enzyme activity. This could have serious implications for toxicity especially if the drug accumulated has a narrow therapeutic window. Hence, clinically significant drug-herb interactions can be observed when an herb interacts with the metabolism of a co-administered drug and either reduces its efficacy due to increased formation of an active metabolite or increases its toxicity due to reduced metabolite elimination [71]. This clinically significant effects can be predicted by analyzing in vitro metabolic data and correlating it with metabolic disposition of a test substance in vivo [72].

In vitro therapeutic index

The in vitro therapeutic index (TI), otherwise known as the selectivity index (SI) of test compounds in malaria drug discovery research is a measure of the amount of the therapeutic agent that causes toxicity relative to that which causes the therapeutic effect (antiplasmodial activity). That is, cytotoxicity (CC_{50})/antiplasmodial activity (EC_{50} or IC_{50}) [73, 74] and represents the therapeutic safety, which is the basis for selectivity of anti-malarial components for in vivo validation. In a recent study, Lima et al. [75] used SI values as a basis to select three among sixty-nine Amazonian plant extracts, for further in vivo studies. The higher the TI values for the herbal extracts or compounds derived from them, the more therapeutically safe they are considered, indicating that smaller quantities of such products will be needed to achieve high clinical efficacy with increased tolerability and safety [76]. It should be noted that although the minimum TI "cut-off" value for prioritizing samples is usually considered at $SI > 4$ [77], it is somewhat subjective because of the difference in susceptibilities of various cell lines and parasite strains to test compounds [78].

The effectiveness of any plant extract is dependent upon a favourable therapeutic ratio; that is the drug must kill or inhibit the parasite but have little or no toxicity to the host. The selectivity of a plant to inhibit the growth of a parasite and yet be less toxic to the host depends on differences in biochemistry between the parasite and the host. Such a plant could operate on a biochemical target in the parasite that is either absent or significantly different in the host [79].

Characterization of the interactions between herbal extracts

Despite the use of herb-herb combinations for therapy over the past millennia, scientific evidence of their therapeutic benefits is still lacking. With the increasing interest shifting from the "one-drug-one-target" to "multi-target" or combination therapy for optimum benefits, there is momentum to explore new knowledge by tapping the past empirical experiences of herb-herb combinations. Systematic screening of combinations of some approved drugs with natural products in certain disease models has started only recently [80] but the potential of combining anti-malarial drugs and/or herbs is not yet systematically explored. There is therefore the need to characterize the interactions between anti-malarial herbal extracts and/or bioactive compounds derived from them to understand the multi-target concept in phytotherapy. These combinations may exhibit synergy at some doses, while resulting in additivity or antagonism at others. Combination dose response in in vitro antiplasmodial assays over combined dose ranges provide critical information on how different compounds act together to affect different *Plasmodium* infection outcomes [81]. The method used in combining these plant extracts is known as the fixed ratio method [59] and a modified method of combining them at equipotencies and variable potencies in antiplasmodial assays have been reported to give reproducible results [82, 83].

Briefly, active solvent extracts (say A and B) are combined in pairs at equipotency ($5EC_{50}A:5EC_{50}B$) or in variable potency ($5EC_{50}A:0EC_{50}B$ to $0EC_{50}A:5EC_{50}B$) ratios and each combination screened on resistant strains of *Plasmodium falciparum*, (such as Dd2) in an appropriate HTS assay set-up, using anti-malarial drug combinations of chloroquine/chloroquine and chloroquine/artemisinin as drug-drug interaction controls [84].

Measurements to quantify these interactions include mathematical and graphical models [85–87]. The mathematical model requires plotting the logarithm of the extract combination concentrations against activity (for example represented by the fluorescence reading) to obtain a nonlinear regression curve-fitting and a variable slope sigmoidal dose–response curve, from which inhibitory coefficients (IC_{50}) of each extract in combination are determined. These are in turn used to calculate fractional inhibitory concentrations ($FIC_{50}A = IC_{50}A$ in combination/$IC_{50}A$ alone) and eventually combination indices ($CI = FIC_{50}A + FIC_{50}B$), recognized as the standard measure of combination effect that indicates a greater (synergistic, CI < 1), lesser (antagonistic, CI > 1) or similar (CI = 1) effect than the expected additive effect.

Graphical models require the use of the previously calculated FIC_{50}s of each extract in combination for each of the variable potency combination ratios to plot isoboles. These are plots with the line of additivity running from point (0,1) of the vertical axis to point (1,0) of the horizontal axis. Analysis of these isoboles, known as isobologram analysis, will enable the prediction of the type of interaction that exists between the plant extracts. Plant extracts in combination may produce effects that are greater than or less than their individual effects. The basis for predicting their effects in combination is based on relative potencies or dose equivalence. Therefore, a plot of the FIC_{50}s of plant extracts with a constant relative potency, will produce linear additive isoboles (curves of constant effect), whereas varying potency ratios produce nonlinear additive isoboles.

Synergy or antagonism will be revealed when the plotted FIC_{50} values is situated below or above the line of additivity, respectively. An illustration of these is shown in Fig. 2, in a study carried out by Tarkang et al. [84].

Based on Chinese herbal medicine, phyto-preparations are formulated deliberately according to the following basic modes of herb-herb interactions; reinforcement, potentiation, restrain, detoxification, counteraction and toxicity. The rational of this principle suggests four mechanisms: (i) synergistic multi-target effects on enzymes, substrates, metabolites, receptors, ion channels, transport proteins and antibodies (ii) pharmacokinetic or physicochemical effects based on improved solubility, resorption rate and enhanced bioavailability (iii) antagonistic interactions with resistance mechanisms of pathogens such as *P. falciparum* (iv) elimination or neutralization of adverse effects caused by other substances present in the mixture [80, 88]. Overall, the aim remains always an effective therapy with less adverse effects.

Besides quality assurance, the proof of efficacy of phyto-preparations and the determination of their mode of action remain permanent issues for an evidence-based approach. The "omics" technologies (genomics, proteomics and metabolomics) are high throughput platforms that can provide us with these possibilities, especially for the identification of the multiple targets of identified plant constituents [88].

These in vitro analyses of the effects of polyherbals gives us an idea of effects to expect in in vivo and clinical studies. Before translating this data further in the drug discovery process, the following considerations must be made during these combination analysis: (i) an appropriate use of concepts and methods (ii) a standard reference analysis framework for characterization (iii) adaptation of the analysis to each step of the research and development process (iv) optimization of dose ratio (v) interpretation of combinations effects guided by

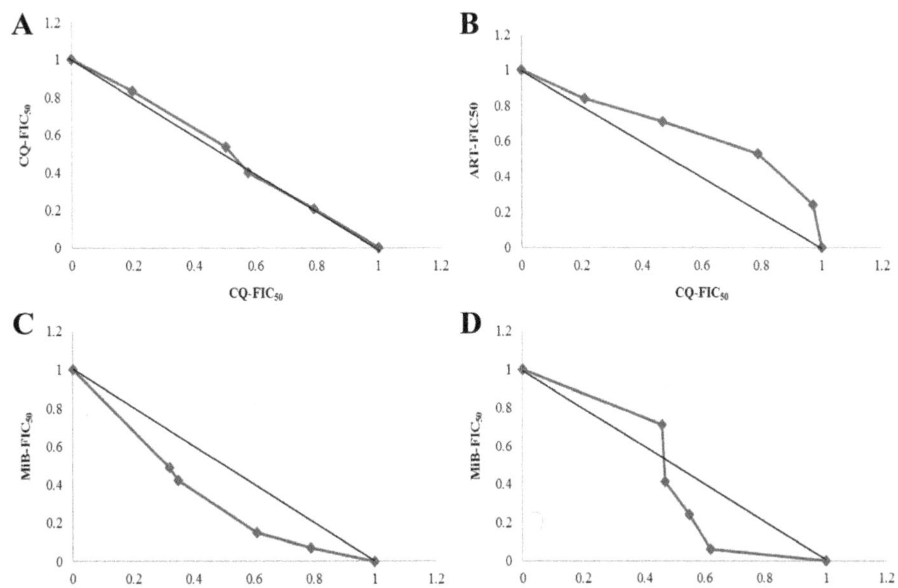

Fig. 2 Isobolograms of the in vitro interactions between differential solvent extracts of a polyherbal product at variable potency ratios (**a**)-Additive interaction: Chloroquine/chloroquine combination (**b**)-Antagonistic interaction: Chloroquine/Artemisinin combination (**c**)-Synergistic interaction: MiB/Pg aqueous extracts combination (**d**)-Synergistic and antagonistic interactions: MiB/Cs aqueous extracts at different potency combinations [79]

rigorous methodology (vi) combining more than two herbs as is usually the case with polyherbals [89].

Plant metabolomics

Metabolomics is increasingly playing a vital role in natural products drug discovery process. It aims at the comprehensive qualitative and quantitative analysis of the plant metabolome which consists of both primary and secondary metabolites, the end products of the cellular regulatory processes. This approach is based on the unbiased acquisition of MS and NMR data from specially prepared samples [13]. Application of state-of-the-art mining on this data leads to sample classification and identification of relevant biomarkers, which is very vital in lead discovery and understanding the multi-target mode of action in malaria phytotherapy. However, this method requires specific extraction (as discussed earlier) and sample preparation techniques. Since the aim is to comprehensively profile the largest possible array of low molecular weight metabolites in a given biological sample, techniques such as multiple-phase solvent systems [31] coupled to accelerated extraction processes such as microwave [90], ultrasonic [91], pressurized or accelerated liquid [92] can be applied to drastically reduce extraction times. Sample preparation usually involves the use of quality buffer and deuterated solvents that will minimize the chemical shift due to pH of the sample solution and result in good quality spectra [93].

There are various hyphenated chromatographic techniques for data acquisition such as the LC-MS, gas chromatography (GC)-MS and capillary electrophoresis (CE)-MS, as well as direct spectroscopic methods such as NMR and direct injection mass spectroscopy (DIMS). However, LC-MS is the most widely used technology in phytotherapeutic drug discovery due to its ability to detect and separate a diverse range of molecules with high sensitivity. When coupled to the NMR, it is even more versatile. The successful combination and application of these analytical tools, data mining and processing, in combination with bioassay profiling methods serve an important role in metabolomics for the purpose of dereplication in natural products-based drug discovery [17, 94].

HPLC-based anti-malarial profiling

HPLC-based anti-malarial profiling is a highly versatile strategy to accelerate deconvolution of active herbal extracts. The principle of this approach consists of separating bioactive components of herbal extracts by analytical and semi-preparative HPLC. The first step which is a microfractionation can be performed with the bioactive sample from the generated plant library, since very little quantities of extract can be used, thereby avoiding the time-consuming recollection and extraction of samples, which at times is non-reproducible. The generated ultraviolet and MS data are recorded on-line and in combination with data searches, can be used for early dereplication and tentative identification of bioactive compounds. In parallel, fractions can be collected into microplates via a T-split of the column effluent, dried and re-dissolved in suitable solvent [95]. These will then then be assayed in vitro for their activities blood and exo-erythrocytic stage malaria parasites, using appropriate HTS assay set-ups as discussed earlier. In order to assess the full bioactivities of each extract, they will also be assayed for other activities relevant in the pathogenesis of malaria, such as antioxidant [96, 97], anti-inflammatory, antinociceptive and antipyretic [98, 99]. By matching the chromatogram and the activity profile, active peaks can be identified.

NMR data for eluted fractions and peaks are recorded off-line using microprobe NMR technology. The collected HPLC peaks can be processed in parallel and an NMR autosampler allows unattended measurement of ^{1}H NMR spectra which serves as a basis for more advanced 1D and 2D analysis. If the need arises, subsequent HPLC preparative sample purification can be performed using a peak-guided strategy, since the chromatographic conditions can be easily transposed.

For a successful application of this methodology, the aspects that need to be considered include the choice of column diameter depending on the miniaturization (analytical or semi-preparative) and sensitivity of the bioassay, sample injection and column flow rates, choice of solvents for bioassays [94].

In the past decade, the application of HPLC-based anti-malarial profiling in targeted and untargeted metabolomics, for the analysis of plant extracts and HMs has been well established. Studies highlighting this potential include the quality control of various *Artemisia* species [100], correlation of antiplasmodial activities with the plants' metabolome and efficient tracking of metabolites [101, 102]. In addition to the efficient tracking of bioactive metabolites, activity profiles can be defined, which are vital for prioritization and chemical analyses. With this information, isolation capacities can be dedicated to bioactive portions in view of facilitating the formulation of standardized and effective phytomedicines for downstream clinical development. In a recent study, Suberu et al. [103] reported the use of multivariate analysis of generated metabolomics data, to identify the association and correlation of the metabolites of artemisinin and related compounds in extracts of varieties of *Artemisia annua*. This study was aimed at determining the effects of different growth conditions, species' origin and identification of adulterants. In another study, Allman et al. [104] reported that the metabolomics profiling of the malaria box revealed several major classes of metabolic disruption, which allows for the prediction of the mode-of-action for many of the Malaria Box compounds [104]. These results can influence the selection of appropriate drug combinations that simultaneously target multiple metabolic pathways, in future combination therapies, aimed of eliminating malaria and forestalling the expansion of drug-resistant parasites in the field.

Metabolomics has also been applied for the analysis of other biological systems such as the serum and urine of *Plasmodium*-infected hosts, in order to unveil host-pathogen interactions [105, 106]. Though still in its infancy, it enables the unveiling of novel aspects of parasite and vector biology. Furthermore, it provides insights into the biochemistry of the host, the nature of host-parasite interactions during infection, and makes it feasible for us to discover species-specific biomarkers that might correlate with various clinical manifestations of malaria.

Therefore, the metabolomics workflow and anti-malarial metabolomics profiling approach provide the malaria community with data that can be used to help prioritize the next generation of potent anti-malarial drugs for future testing in clinical trials.

Armed with the activity profile of the HMs, the next vital step is to validate these activities in animal pharmacology, as well as confirm the safety profile.

Animal pharmacology and safety studies

In accordance with the reverse pharmacology or target-directed approach, test substances identified with good in vitro antiplasmodial activity need to be tested in vivo in suitable animal models that can provide basic pharmacological and toxicological data prior to subsequent human clinical trials [59]. Despite the fact that these in vivo assays do not necessarily predict the outcomes of clinical trials in humans because the pathogen models in animals are different from the human pathogens, animal models remain very vital in malaria phytotherapy. However, due to the reasonably high homology and similarity between mammalian genomes and physiology, and to the relatively short reproductive cycle, mouse and rat models are the most used for assessment of antiplasmodial activity of plant extracts and products derived from them [107]. Therefore, these animal models remain crucial for malaria drug evaluation and validation because they provide an integrated response encompassing efficacy, bioavailability, side effects and toxicity (ADME/T) of test substances in a whole organism and can be used for pharmacokinetic and safety studies that are pre-requisite for human clinical trials [108–110].

Toxicity testing

While cell-based assays may be predictive of potential toxicity, use of the whole animal measures the critical toxicity of the test substance, to determine signs of toxicity as a result of gradual increase in the dose of the test substance. Many research groups are resorting to plants as a major source of new anti-malarial chemotherapeutic agents because of the extensive use of these plants for malaria therapy in African Traditional Medicine. Their use, however, does not take into consideration their safety [111]. It is therefore imperative to establish the pre-clinical safety profile of plants and their components that exhibit good anti-malarial activity in animal models. Standard guidelines have been established internationally for the care and use of animals in toxicity studies [112]. These guidelines take care of the preparation and administration of test substances, animal welfare considerations, choice of animals and regulatory requirements. The toxicity tests that are usually carried out include acute, sub-acute/sub-chronic and chronic toxicities. Exposure routes may be by oral gavage, inhalation, dermal, intraperitoneal or intramuscular, depending on the intended use and/or route of administration.

Acute toxicity testing measures relative toxicological response of an experimental organism to a single or brief exposure to a test substance [112]. This test is used to calculate lethal dose (LD_{50}) [113] and observation usually lasts for fourteen days. Sub-acute (28–30 days) and sub-chronic (60–90 days) are repeated-dose daily exposure to test substances with a view of evaluating the effects on the physiological, biochemical and histopathological parameters of the organ systems of test animals. Chronic toxicity testing which is similar to sub-chronic involves the exposure of test animals over a period of six to twenty-four months or more, to reveal the effects on organ systems [114]. In addition, specialized tests may follow to reveal specific toxicities, such as reproductive, developmental, eye, skin irritancy, neuro- and geno- toxicities [115].

In vivo antiplasmodial assays

In vivo tests are the oldest approach in the assessment of therapeutic responses and have enabled determination of the thresholds of treatment failure that are crucial for adjusting anti-malarial drug policies [116]. Test substances effective in in vitro tests are taken up for in vivo evaluation. Since *Plasmodium* species that cause human malaria are essentially unable to infect non primate animal models, in vivo evaluation of anti-malarial compounds begins with the use of rodent malaria parasites. These include *Plasmodium berghei*, *P. yoelii*, *P. chabaudi*, *P. vinckei* (blood and gametocyte stages screening) and *P. cynomolgi* (liver stage screening). In vivo models are usually employed in anti-malarial studies because they take into account the possible prodrug effect and probable involvement of the immune system in eradication of the pathogen [117]. These in vivo methods have been validated through the identification of standard drugs like mefloquine and artemisinin [118, 119] and thus remain a standard in herbal medicines drug discovery. They can be classified into primary, secondary and tertiary biological assessments [120]. In all methods, determination of percent inhibition of parasitemia is the most reliable parameter. A mean parasitemia level ≤ 90% to that of the vehicle treated animals (mock-treated control) usually indicates that the test compound is active [121].

The most widely used primary biological test is the *P. berghei* 4-Day suppressive test [122], which requires the infection of test mice with *P. berghei*, ANKA strain on day 0. 3 h post-infection and on day 1–3, the mice are treated with the test substance while using chloroquine and artemisinin as standards. On day four, blood smears from all groups of animals are prepared and stained with giemsa stain. Parasitaemia is determined from day 4 to 6 and substances identified as active are further subjected through several secondary biological assessments such as dose ranging, curative and prophylactic tests.

The dose ranging test requires a minimum of four different doses of the test substance (the "dose ranging, full 4-day test"). ED_{50} and ED_{90} values are calculated by plotting the log dose against probit activity and reflect the concentrations at which 50% and 90% of suppression of parasitaemia is achieved. This test also leads to information about the relative potency compared to an appropriate standard drug [121].

The Curative test, otherwise known as the Rane's test, involves the daily administration of the test substance to mice or rats, 72h (D3) post established infection, for a period of five days. Parameters followed up are measurement of the reduction in blood stage parasitemia and improved survival of test animals [123]. However, in the liver stage screening, the radical cure potential of a test compound is tested using the hypnozoite-forming monkey model. Monkeys are infected with *P. cynomolgi* sporozoites followed by treatment with a compound that eliminates all blood stage parasites, followed by the test compound. The monkeys are then monitored over several months to measure reductions in the frequency of hypnozoite-caused relapses as an evaluation the potential of the test compound for radical cure [124]. The transmission-blocking activity of the test compound could also be assayed by taking advantage of the ability of gametocytes to infect mosquitoes; this can be measured by using standard membrane feeding assay, using *P. falciparum* [125], or by direct feeding of an infected mouse [126]. After feeding, the number of oocysts per mosquito midgut are counted to determine the efficacy of the test compound.

For the prophylactic test, substances with a therapeutic lead are tested for prophylactic activity by administering them for three days prior to infection and smears continually examined daily for three days, to assess suppression of blood stage parasitaemia and improved survival [127].

Tertiary biological assessments are used to monitor cross resistance and in vivo generation of drug resistance. Cross resistance monitoring employs the 4-day suppressive test in order to determine whether the same ED_{50} and ED_{90} values are observed in drug-resistant strains of rodent malaria when compared to *P. berghei* ANKA infection [121]. To determine the potential of parasites to develop resistance to a new compound in vivo, the 2% relapse method is the most widely used for most classes of compounds [128]. This entails administering a dose of the test substance that when given 1 h before infection, delays the development of 2% parasitaemia until about 7–10 days post-infection. When this parasitaemia is attained, the procedure is repeated and the time to reach 2% parasitaemia is monitored on a daily basis. The degree of resistance is expressed as a reduction in "delay time to 2%". This method can be extended to demonstrate the stability of resistance following the removal of drug pressure and to select a partner compound that can slow the rate of development of resistance.

Pharmacokinetics

There is evidence that the crude extracts of whole plants or mixtures thereof, which are widely used for malaria therapy, exhibit greater in vitro and/or in vivo antiplasmodial activities than isolated compounds from them, at equivalent doses. This might be as a result of synergistic interactions between their components which result in an overall positive anti-malarial effect [129]. Pharmacokinetics (PK) of these anti-malarial plants remains a major problem due to the number of plant-derived molecules that are typically present in them. This presents a substantial challenge to chemical and pharmacological evaluation, in addition to the wide concentration range of these molecules. Furthermore, the dynamic nature of the type of chemical interactions between their bioactive components and endogenous molecules have a great influence on their PK, and consequently on treatment outcomes in humans [130]. Moreover, monitoring of chemical profiles have been made more complicated due to their complex biological matrices and the lack of authenticated standards. The evolutionary considerations in interdisciplinary expertise involving 'omics' technologies, pharmacology, biochemistry, bioinformatics and systems modeling, offers new opportunities [94]. However, understanding their metabolic fate is a critical step toward the development of next generation of combinatorial drugs, which will maximize the synergistic and/or antagonistic effects of bioactive components and minimize their undesirable metabolic side effects [131].

The advent of comprehensive profiling technologies offers tremendous new opportunities for understanding multicomponent PK. Phytochemical profiling and metabolomics, coupled to multivariate statistical tools to generate multiparametric assessments, enable us to create a concentration-time profile of these anti-malarial plants, in a process known as a "Poly-PK" approach. This approach uses the integrated diversity of chemical composition and metabolomics profiling strategy coupled to multivariate statistical to simultaneously monitor the complex effects on the metabolic pathways of the mammalian system [131, 132]. When anti-malaria plant extracts enter mammalian bodies, the following metabolite profile changes occur over time: (i) Plant-derived compounds are absorbed into the circulation (ii) new metabolites are generated by the chemical transformation of these compounds by hepatic enzymes and gut microbes (iii) endogenous metabolites are altered in response to their intervention.

Certain PK variables such as plasma and urine concentration can be collected over time of treatment, and characterized using UHPLC-MS, while parameters such as area under the curve and the elimination half-life ($t_{1/2}$) can be generated using PK modeling software [133]. Analysis of the various metabolomes of treated and non-treated mammals, can generate a correlation between the dynamic concentration profiles of bioactive components and the human metabolic response profile. Therefore, this approach of simultaneously monitoring the PK behaviours of multiple phytochemicals in vivo can lead to the direct elucidation of the pharmacological and molecular mechanisms underlying anti-malarial plants. This approach therefore reveals the interrelationship between xenobiotics and endobiotics, as well as the metabolic impact of these plants, using pharmacodynamics (PD) endpoints, to provide insight into the mechanisms of action and advance novel therapeutic development.

Conclusion

Drawing from the prolonged history of phytotherapy for the clinical management of malaria, there is evidence that plant extracts exert superior effects compared to isolated phytochemicals. This is as a result of the multi-target effects of their secondary metabolites. Therefore, the success rate of developing a new drug from herbal medicinal preparations should, in theory, be higher than that from chemical synthesis. By setting quality standards to this reductionist interdisciplinary approach, potential biomarkers as well as the cellular and molecular modes of action would be unraveled. This endeavor will not only facilitate a fast and convenient discovery of efficient and standardized improved traditional medicines, but eventually lead discovery for downstream chemical analyses and prioritization. Therefore, this approach should be an asset in natural products-based drug discovery, which might shift the paradigm from the capital intensive "one-drug-to-fit-all" to the new "less investment, more drugs" model. It is believed that the former will be unsustainable in the short run, hence the need for new approaches towards the latter. Another major asset of this approach is the ethnopharmacological information providing hints for therapeutically effective plants and miniaturization, thereby reducing random and indiscriminate harvest of plants and promoting the preservation of biodiversity.

Therefore, by unifying a complete state-of-the-art reductionist and holistic techniques, the application of the multi-target phytotherapeutic concept holds great promise in widening the therapeutic arsenal against malaria.

Acknowledgements
Not applicable.

Funding
The authors are grateful to Bill and Melinda Gates Foundation (BMGF) for financial support to PAT, for a Postdoctoral Fellowship in infectious diseases, under the Global Health Grant No. OPP52155 at Noguchi Memorial Institute for Medical Research (NMIMR), Accra, Ghana. However, the funders do not have any role to play in the design, execution, interpretation and drafting of this manuscript.

Authors' contributions
PAT wrote the manuscript; PAT, RA, MFO, LSA, AKN read, edited and approved of the manuscript.

Competing interests
The authors declare that they have no competing interests.

Author details
[1]Centre for Research on Medicinal Plants and Traditional Medicine, Institute of Medical Research and Medicinal Plants Studies (IMPM), P. O. Box 8013, Yaoundé, Cameroon. [2]Department of Clinical Pathology, Noguchi Memorial Institute for Medical Research, University of Ghana, P. O. Box LG 581, Legon, Accra, Ghana. [3]Department of Immunology, Noguchi Memorial Institute for Medical Research, University of Ghana, P. O. Box LG581, Legon, Accra, Ghana. [4]Malaria Research Laboratory, Centre Pasteur Cameroon, BP 1274 Yaoundé, Cameroon. [5]School of Pharmacy, University of Ghana, P.O. Box LG43, Legon, Accra, Ghana.

References

1. Snow RW, Marsh K. Malaria in africa: progress and prospects in the decade since the Abuja declaration. Lancet. 2010;376(9735):137–9.
2. World Health Organization. Traditional medicine. Fact sheet No. 134. Geneva: WHO; 2003. http://www.who.int/mediacentre/factsheet/fs134/en/.

3. Oliveira AB, Dolabela MF, Braga FC, Jacome RL, Varotti FP, Povoa MM. Plant-derived antimalarial agents: new leads and efficient phythomedicines. Part I. Alkaloids. An Acad Brasil Ciênc. 2009;81(4):715–40.
4. Castellanos JRG, Prieto JM, Heinrich M. Red lapacho (*tabebuia impetiginosa*) - a global ethnopharmacological commodity? J Ethnopharmacol. 2009; 121(1):1–13.
5. Ginsburg H, Deharo E. A call for using natural compounds in the development of new antimalarial treatments - an introduction. Malar J. 2011;10 Suppl 1:1–7.
6. Ariey F, Witkowski B, Amaratunga C, Beghain J, Langlois AC, Khim N, Kim S, et al. A molecular marker of artemisinin-resistant plasmodium falciparum malaria. Nature. 2014;505(7481):50–5.
7. Efferth T, Koch E. Complex interactions between phytochemicals. The multi-target therapeutic concept of phytotherapy. Curr Drug Targets. 2011;12(1): 122–32.
8. Long F, Yang H, Xu Y, Hao H, Li P. A strategy for the identification of combinatorial bioactive compounds contributing to the holistic effect of herbal medicines. Sci Rep. 2015;5(12361):1–11.
9. Wells TNC, Gutteridge WE. Malaria: new medicines for its control and eradication. In: Palmer MJ, Wells TNC, editors. Neglected diseases and drug discovery. Cambridge: Royal Society of Chemistry Publishing; 2012. p. 1–32. Ch. 1.
10. Rather AM, Bhat BA, Qurishi MA. Multicomponent phytotherapeutic approach gaining momentum: is the "one drug fit all" model breaking down? Phytomedicine. 2013;21(1):1–14.
11. Larson J, Gottfries J, Bohlin L, Backlund A. Expanding the Chem GPS chemical space with natural products. J Nat Prod. 2005;68(7):985–91.
12. Heinrich M. Ethnopharmacology in the 21st century – grand challenges. Front Pharmacol. 2010;1(8):1–3.
13. Wolfender J, Rudaz S, Choi YH, Kim HK. Plant metabolomics: from holistic data to relevant biomarkers. Curr Med Chem. 2013;20(8):1056–90.
14. Hamburger M, Hostettmann K. Bioactivity in plants: the link between phytochemistry and medicine. Phytochemistry. 1991;30(12):3864–74.
15. van de Greef J, McBurney RN. Innovation: rescuing drug discovery: in vivo systems pathology and systems pharmacology. Nat Rev Drug Discov. 2005;4:961–7.
16. Wang M, Lamers R-JAN, Korthout HAAJ, et al. Metabolomics in the context of systems biology: bridging traditional Chinese medicine and molecular pharmacology. Phytother Res. 2005;19:173–82.
17. Wolfender J, Marti G, Thomas A, Bertrand S. Current approaches and challenges for the metabolite profiling of complex natural products. J Chromatogr. 2015;1382:136–64.
18. Wilcox M. Improved traditional phytomedicines in current use for the clinical treatment of malaria. Planta Med. 2011;77(6):662–71.
19. Henrich CJ, Beutler JA. Matching the power of high throughput screening to the chemical diversity of natural products. Nat Prod Rep. 2013;30(10): 1284–98.
20. Barbosa WLR, do Nascimento MS, do Nascimento Pinto L, Maia FLC, Sousa AJA, Júnior JOCS, et al. Selecting Medicinal Plants for Development of Phytomedicine and Use in Primary Health Care, Bioactive Compounds in Phytomedicine, Prof. Iraj Rasooli (Ed.). InTech; 2012. doi:10.5772/26078. Available from: http://www.intechopen.com/books/bioactive-compounds-in-phytomedicine/selecting-medicinal-plants-for-development-of-phytomedicine-and-use-in-primary-health-care.
21. Fabricant DS, Farnsworth NR. The value of plants used in traditional medicine for drug discovery. Environ Health Perspect. 2001;109 Suppl 1:69–75.
22. Cragg GM, Newman DJ. Natural products: a continuing source of novel drug leads. Biochim Biophys Acta. 2013;1830(6):3670–95.
23. White NJ. Qinghaosu (artemisinin): the price of success. Science. 2008; 320(5874):330–4.
24. Brusotti G, Cesari I, Dentamaro A, Caccialanza G, Massolini G. Isolation and characterization of bioactive compounds from plant resources: the role of analysis in the ethnopharmacological approach. J Pharm Biomed Anal. 2014; 87:218–28.
25. Gairola S, Sharma J, Bedi YS. A cross-cultural analysis of Jammu, Kashmir and ladakh (India) medicinal plant use. J Ethnopharmacol. 2014;155(2):925–86.
26. Ningthoujam SS, Talukdar AD, Potsangbam KS, Choudhury MD. Challenges in developing medicinal plant databases for sharing ethnopharmacological knowledge. J Ethnopharmacol. 2012;141(1):9–32.
27. Saslis-Lagoudakis CH, Klitgaard BB, Forest F, Francis L, Savolainen V, Williamson EM, et al. The use of phylogeny to interpret cross-cultural patterns in plant use and guide medicinal plant discovery: an example from *Pterocarpus* (leguminosae). PLoS One. 2011;6(7):e22275.
28. Saslis-Lagoudakis CH, Savolainen V, Williamson EM, Forest F, Wagstaff SJ, Baral SR, et al. Phylogenies reveal predictive power of traditional medicine in bioprospecting. Proc Natl Acad Sci U S A. 2012;109(39):15835–40.
29. Krief S, Martin MT, Grellier P, Kasenene J, Sevenet T. Novel antimalarial compounds isolated in a survey of self-medicative behavior of wild chimpanzees in Uganda. Antimicrob Agents Chemother. 2004;48(8):3196–9.
30. Rollinger JM, Schuster D, Danzl B, Schwalger S, Markt P, Schmidtke M, et al. *In silico* target fishing for rationalized ligand discovery exemplified on constituents of *Ruta graveolens*. Planta Med. 2009;75(3):195–204.
31. Kim HK, Verpoorte R. Sample preparation for plant metabolomics. Phytochem Anal. 2010;21(1):4–13.
32. Kaufmann B, Christen P. Recent extraction techniques for natural products: microwave-assisted extraction and pressurized solvent extraction. Phytochem Anal. 2002;13(2):105–13.
33. Handa SS, Khanuja SPS, Longo G, Rakesh DD. Extraction technologies for medicinal and aromatic plants. Trieste: ICS-UNIDO International Centre for Science and High Technology; 2008.
34. Onguene PA, Ntie-Kang F, Lifongo LL, Ndom JC, Sippl W, Mbaze LM. The potential of anti-malarial compounds derived from African medicinal plants. Part I: a pharmacological evaluation of alkaloids and terpenoids. Malar J. 2013;12:449.
35. Ntie-Kang F, Onguene PA, Lifongo LL, Ndom JC, Sippl W, Mbaze LM. The potential of anti-malarial compounds derived from African medicinal plants. Part II: a pharmacological evaluation of non-alkaloids and non-terpenoids. Malar J. 2014;13:81.
36. Zang R, Li D, Tang I, Wang J, Yang S. Cell-based assays in high-throughput screening for drug discovery. Int J Biotechnol Wellness Ind. 2012;1:31–51.
37. Flannery EL, Chatterjee AK, Winzeler EA. Anti-malarial drug discovery: approaches and progress towards new medicines. Nat Rev Microbiol. 2013; 11(12):849–62.
38. Miller LH, Ackerman HC, Su X, Wellems TE. Discovery of anti-malarial drugs: new methods of screening chemical compounds for anti-malarial drugs available to the malaria community. In: Malaria biology and disease pathogenesis: insights for new treatments. 2013. p. 156–67.
39. Rieckmann KH. Visual in-vitro test for determining the drug sensitivity of plasmodium falciparum. Lancet. 1982;1(8285):1333–5.
40. Desjardins RE, Canfield CJ, Haynes JD, Chulay JD. Quantitative assessment of antimalarial activity in vitro by a semiautomated microdilution technique. Antimicrob Agents Chemother. 1979;16(6):710–8.
41. Noedl H, Attlmayr B, Wernsdorfer WH, Kollaritsch H, Miller RS. A histidine-rich protein 2-based malaria drug sensitivity assay for field use. Am J Trop Med Hyg. 2004;71(6):711–4.
42. Noedl H, Wernsdorfer WH, Miller RS, Wongsrichanalai C. Histidine-rich protein II: a novel approach to malaria drug sensitivity testing. Antimicrob Agents Chemother. 2002;46(6):1658–64.
43. Makler MT, Ries JM, Williams JA, Bancroft JE, Piper RC, Gibbins BL, Hinrichs DJ. Parasite lactate dehydrogenase as an assay for *Plasmodium falciparum* drug sensitivity. Am J Trop Med Hyg. 1993;48(6):739–41.
44. Johnson JD, Dennull RA, Gerena L, Lopez-Sanchez M, Roncal NE, Waters NC. Assessment and continued validation of the malaria SYBR green 1-based fluorescence assay for use in malaria drug screening. Antimicrob Agents Chemother. 2007;51(6):1926–33.
45. Akala HM, Eyase FL, Cheruiyot AC, Omondi AA, Ogutu BR, Waters NC, et al. Antimalarial drug sensitivity profile of western Kenya *Plasmodium falciparum* field isolates determined by a SYBR green-1 in vitro assay and molecular analysis. Am J Trop Med Hyg. 2011;85(1):34–41.
46. Derbyshire ER, Mota MM, Clardy J. The next generation in anti-malaria drug discovery: the liver stage. PLoS Pathog. 2011;7:e1002178.
47. Trampuz A, Jereb M, Muzlovic I, Prahbu RM. Clinical review: severe malaria. Crit Care. 2003;7:315.
48. Hanssen E, Knoechel C, Dearnley M, et al. Soft X-ray microscopy analysis of cell volume and hemoglobin content in erythrocytes infected with asexual and sexual stages of Plasmodium falciparum. J Struct Biol. 2012;177:224–32.
49. Boussema T, Okell L, Shekalaghe S, et al. Revisiting the circulation time of plasmodium falciparum gametocytes: molecular detection methods to estimate the duration of gametocyte carriage and the effect of gametocytocidal drugs. Malar J. 2010;9:136.
50. WHO. Guidelines for the treatment of malaria. 2011. p. 194. http://www.who.int/malaria/publications/atoz/9789241547925/en/index.html.
51. Meister S, Plouffe DM, Kuhen KL, et al. Imaging of *Plasmodium* liver stages to drive next-generation anti-malarial drug discovery. Science. 2011; 334(6061):1372–7.

52. Mwakingwe A, Ting L, Hochman S, et al. Noninvasive real-time monitoring of liver-stage development of bioluminescent *Plasmodium* parasites. J Infect Dis. 2009;200:1470–8.
53. Dembele L, Gego A, Zeeman A, et al. Towards an in vitro model of plasmodium hypnozoites suitable for drug discovery. PLoS One. 2011;6:e19162.
54. Peatey CL, Spicer TP, Holder PS, et al. A high-throughput assay for the identification of drugs against late-stage *Plasmodium falciparum* gametocytes. Mol Biochem Parasitol. 2011;180:127–31.
55. D'Alessandro S, Silvestrini F, Dechering K, et al. A *Plasmodium falciparum* screening assay for anti-gametocyte drugs based on parasite lactate dehydrogenase detection. J Antimicrob Chemother. 2013;68:2048–58.
56. Tanaka TQ, Williamson KC. A malaria gametocytocidal assay using oxidoreduction indicator, alamar Blue. Mol Biochem Parasitol. 2011;177:160–3.
57. Delves MJ, Ramakrishnan C, Blacborough AM, et al. A high-throughput assay for the identification of malarial transmission-blocking drugs and vaccines. Int J Parasitol. 2012;42:999–1006.
58. Plouffe DM, Wree M, Du AY, Meister S, et al. High-Throughput Assay and discovery of small molecules that interrupt malaria transmission. Cell Host Microbe. 2016;19:114–26.
59. Atanasov AG, Waltenberger B, Pferschy-Wenzig E, Linder T, Wawrosch C, et al. Discovery and resupply of pharmacologically active plant-derived natural products: a review. Biotechnol Adv. 2015;33(8):1582–614.
60. Winston D, Maimes S. Adaptogens. Herbs for strength, stamina and stress relief. Rochester: Healing Arts Press; 2007. 336.
61. Aguiar AC, da Rocha EM, de Souza NB, França TC, Krettli AU. New approaches in antimalarial drug discovery and development: a review. Mem Inst Oswaldo Cruz Rio de Janeiro. 2012;107(7):831–45.
62. van Dyk S, Griffiths S, van Zyl RL, Malan SF. The importance of including toxicity assays when screening plant extracts for antimalarial activity. Afr J Biotechnol. 2009;8(20):5595–601.
63. O'Brien P, Haskings JR. in vitro cytotoxicity assessment. Methods Mol Biol. 2007;356:415–25.
64. Malinin G. Cytotoxic effect of dimethylsulfoxide on the ultrastructure of cultured rhesus kidney cells. Cryobiology. 1973;10(1):22–32.
65. Szmant HH. Physical properties of dimethyl sulfoxide and its function in biological systems. Ann N Y Acad Sci. 1975;243:20–3.
66. van Tonder JJ, Steenkamp V, Gulumian M. Pre-Clinical Assessment of the Potential Intrinsic Hepatotoxicity of Candidate Drugs, New Insights into Toxicity and Drug Testing, Dr. Sivakumar Gowder (Ed.), InTech; 2013. doi:10.5772/54792. Available from: http://www.intechopen.com.sci-hub.cc/books/new-insights-into-toxicity-and-drug-testing/pre-clinical-assessment-of-the-potential-intrinsic-hepatotoxicity-of-candidate-drugs.
67. Hewitt NJ, Gomez-Lechon MJ, Houston JB, et al. Primary hepatocytes: current understanding of the regulation of metabolic enzymes and transporter proteins and pharmaceutical practice for the use of hepatocytes in metabolism, enzyme induction, transporter, clearance and hepatotoxicity studies. Drug Metab Rev. 2007;39(1):159–234.
68. Chung M, Yu W, Lee J, Lee J. Embryotoxicity and toxicokinetics of the antimalarial artesunate in rats. Toxicol Res. 2013;29(1):27–34.
69. Maurer HH. Toxicokinetics – variations due to genetics and interactions: Basics and examples. www.gtfch.org/cms/images/stories/media/tb/tb2007/s153-155.pdf. Accessed 15 Mar 2016.
70. Gurley BJ. Phytochemical modulators of human drug metabolism: an introduction to clinically relevant herb-drug interactions. Planta Med. 2014; 80:IL27.
71. Williams JA, Hyland R, Jones BC, et al. Drug-drug interactions for UDP-glucuronosyltransferase substrates: a pharmacokinetic explanation of typically observed low exposure (AUCi/AUC ratios). Drug Metab Dispos. 2004;32(11):1201–8.
72. Guengerich FP. Role of cytochrome P450 enzymes in drug-drug interactions. Adv Pharmacol. 1997;43:7–35.
73. Benoit-Vical F, Valentin A, Mallie M, Bastide JM, Bessiere JM. in vitro antimalarial activity and cytotoxicity of *cochlospermum tinctorium* and *C. Planchonii* leaf extracts and essential oils. Planta Med. 1999;65(5):378–81.
74. Ohrt C, Willingmyre CD, Lee P, Knirsch C, Milhous W. Assessment of azithromycin in combination with other antimalarial drugs against *Plasmodium in vitro*. Antimicrob Agents Chemother. 2002;46(8):2518–24.
75. Lima RBS, Silva LFR, Melo MRS, Costa JS, et al. In vitro and in vivo antimalarial activity of plants from Brazilian Amazon. Malar J. 2015;14:508.
76. Soh PN, Benoit-Vical F. Are west African plants a source of future antimalarial drugs? J Ethnopharmacol. 2007;114(2):130–40.
77. Valdes AF, Martinez JM, Lizama RS, Gaiten YG, et al. in vitro antimalarial activity and cytotoxicity of some selected Cuban medicinal plants. Rev Inst Med Trop São Paolo. 2010;52(4):197–201.
78. Pezzuto JM, Angerhofer CK, Mehdi H. In vitro models of human disease states. In: Atta-ur R, editor. Studies in natural products chemistry, Structure and chemistry (Part F). Amsterdam: Elsevier Science B.V; 1998. p. 527.
79. Mojab F. Antimalarial natural products: a review. Avicenna J Phytomed. 2012;2(2):52–62.
80. Ulrich-Merzenich GS. Combination screening of synthetic drugs and plant derived natural compounds-potential and challenges for drug development. Synergy. 2014;1(1):59–69.
81. Peterson JJ, Novick SJ. Nonlinear blending: a useful general concept for the assessment of combination drug synergy. J Recept Signal Transduct Res. 2007;27(2–3):125–46.
82. Cook R, Hennell JR, Lee S, Khoo CS, Carles MC, Higgins VJ, et al. The saccharomyces cerevisiae transcriptome as a mirror of phytochemical variation in complex extracts of equisetum arvense from america, china, Europe and India. BMC Genomics. 2013;14(1):445.
83. Panossian A, Hamm R, Kadioglu O, Wikman G, Efferth T. Synergy and antagonism of active constituents of ADAPT-232 on transcriptional level of metabolic regulation of isolated neuroglial cells. Front Neurosci. 2013;7:16.
84. Tarkang PA, Franzoi KD, Lee S, Lee E, Vivarelli D, Freitas-Junior L, Liuzzi M, et al. in vitro antiplasmodial activities and synergistic combinations of differential solvent extracts of the polyherbal product. Nefang BioMed Res Int. 2014;835013.
85. Berenbaum MC. A method for testing for synergy with any number of agents. J Infect Dis. 1978;137(2):122–30.
86. Tallarida RJ. An overview of drug combination analysis with isobolograms. Perspect Pharmacol. 2006;319(1):1–7.
87. Chou TC. Drug combination studies and their synergy quantification using the chou-talalay method. Cancer Res. 2010;70(2):440–66.
88. Che CT, Wang ZJ, Chow MSS, Lam CWK. Herb-herb combination for therapeutic enhancement and advancement: theory, practice and future perspectives. Molecules. 2013;18(5):5125–41.
89. Foucquier J, Guedj M. Analysis of drug combinations: current methodological landscape. Pharmacol Res Perspect. 2015;3(3):e00149.
90. Zygmunt B, Namiesnik J. Preparation of samples of plant material for chromatographic analysis. J Chromatogr Sci. 2003;41(3):109–16.
91. Sargenti SR, Vichnewski W. Sonication and liquid chromatography as a rapid technique for extraction and fractionation of plant material. Phytochem Anal. 2000;11:69–73.
92. Benthin B, Danz H, Hamburger M. Pressurized liquid extraction of medicinal plants. J Chromatogr A. 1999;837(1–2):211–9.
93. Kim H, Choi Y. Metabolomic analysis of Catharanthus roseus using NMR and principal component analysis. In: Saito K, Dixon RA, Willmitzer L, editors. Plant metabolomics: biotechnology in agricultural and forestry. Berlin: Springer; 2006. p. 261–76.
94. Potterat O, Hamberger M. Combined use of extract libraries and HPLC-based activity profiling for lead discovery: potential challenges and practical considerations. Planta Med. 2014;80(14):1171–81.
95. Potterat O, Hamburger M. Concepts and technologies for tracking bioactive compounds in natural product extracts: generation of libraries and hyphenation of analytical processes with bioassays. Nat Prod Rep. 2013;30(4):546–64.
96. Yen GC, Duh PD. Scavenging effects of methanolic extracts of peanut hulls on free radical and active oxygen species. J Agric Food Chem. 1994;42:629–32.
97. Benzie IFF, Strain JJ. The ferric reducing ability of plasma (FRAP) as a measure of antioxidant power: the FRAP assay. Anal Biochem. 1996;239(1):70–6.
98. Kemal C, Louis-Flamberg P, Krupinsky-Olsen R, Shorter AL. Reductive inactivation of soybean lipoxygenase I by catechols: a possible mechanism for regulation of lipoxygenase activity. Biochemistry. 1987; 26(22):7064–72.
99. Rackova L, Oblozinsky M, Kostalova D, Kettmann V, Bezakova L. Free radical scavenging activity and lipoxygenase inhibition of *Mahonia aquifolium* extract and isoquinoline alkaloids. J Inflam. 2007;4:15–21.
100. Van der Kooy F, Verpoorte R, Marion Meyer JJ. Metabolomic quality control of claimed anti-malarial *Artemisia afra* herbal remedy and *A. afra* and *A. annua* plant extracts. S Afr J Bot. 2008;74:186–9.
101. Adams M, Christen M, Plitzko I, Zimmermann S, Brun R, Kaiser M, Hamburger M. Antiplasmodial lanostanes from the *Ganoderma lucidum* mushroom. J Nat Prod. 2010;73:897–900.

102. Zimmermann S, Thomi S, Kaiser M, Hamburger M, Adams M. Screening and HPLC-based activity profiling for New antiprotozoal leads from european plants. Sci Pharm. 2012;80:205–13.
103. Suberu J, Gromski PS, Nordon A, Lapkin A. Multivariate data analysis and metabolic profiling of artemisinin and related compounds in high yielding varieties of *Artemisia annua* field-grown in Madagascar. J Pharm Biomed Anal. 2016;117:522–31.
104. Allman EL, Painter HJ, Samra J, Carrasquilla M, Llinás M. Metabolomic profiling of the malaria box reveals antimalarial target pathways. Antimicrob Agents Chemother. 2016;60:6635–49.
105. Kafsack BF, Llinas M. Eating at the table of another: metabolomics of host-parasite interactions. Cell Host Microbe. 2010;7:90–9.
106. Salinas JL, Kissinger JC, Jones DP, Galinski MR. Metabolomics for the fight against malaria. Mem Inst Oswaldo Cruz Rio de Janeiro. 2014;109(5):589–97.
107. Butterweck V, Nahrstedt A. What is the best strategy for preclinical testing of botanicals? a critical perspective. Planta Med. 2012;78(8):747–54.
108. Zhang D, Luo G, Ding X, Lu C. Preclinical experimental models of drug metabolism and disposition in drug discovery and development. Acta Pharm Sin B. 2012;2(6):549–61.
109. Alqahtani S, Mohamed LA, Kaddoumi A. Experimental models for predicting drug absorption and metabolism. Expert Opin Drug Metab Toxicol. 2013; 9(10):1241–54.
110. Greek R. Animal Models in Drug Development, New Insights into Toxicity and Drug Testing, Dr. Sivakumar Gowder (Ed.), InTech; 2013. doi:10.5772/53893. Available from: http://www.intechopen.com.sci-hub.cc/books/new-insights-into-toxicity-and-drug-testing/animal-models-in-drug-development.
111. Addae-Mensah I, Fakorede F, Holtel A, Nwaka S. Traditional medicines as a mechanism for driving research innovation in Africa. Malar J. 2011;10 Suppl 1:S9.
112. OECD (Organization for Economic Cooperation Development). Guidance Document on Oral Toxicity Testing 423 and 425. OECD Environment, Health and Safety Publications. Series on testing and assessment No 24. Paris; 2001. Available from: www.oecd.org/ehs/.
113. Lorke D. A new approach to practical acute toxicity testing. Arch Toxicol. 1983;54:275–87.
114. Tarkang PA, Agbor GA, Ayong LS, Okalebo FA, Gauntai AN. Cytotoxicity and in vivo toxicological screening of a polyherbal product. Nefang World J Pharm Res. 2015;4(4):82–101.
115. OECD (Organization for Economic Cooperation Development). Draft guidance on the design and conduct of chronic toxicity and carcinogenicity. In: Series on testing and assessment No 116. 2009.
116. Ifeoma O, Oluwakanyinsola S. Screening of Herbal Medicines for Potential Toxicities, New Insights into Toxicity and Drug Testing, Dr. Sivakumar Gowder (Ed.), InTech; 2013. doi:10.5772/54493. Available from: http://www.intechopen.com.sci-hub.cc/books/new-insights-into-toxicity-and-drug-testing/screening-of-herbal-medicines-for-potential-toxicities.
117. World Health Organization. Global report on antimalarial drug efficacy and drug resistance: 2000–2010. Geneva: WHO; 2010.
118. Waako PJ, Gumede B, Smith P, Folb PI. The in vitro and in vivo antimalarial activity of *Cardiospermum halicacabum* and *Momordica foetida*. J Ethnopharmacol. 2005;99(1):137–43.
119. Peters W, Howells RE, Portus J, Robinson BL, Thomas S, Warhurst DC. The chemotherapy of rodent malaria. XXVII. Studies on mefloquine (WR 142,490). Ann Trop Med Parasitol. 1977;71:407–18.
120. Posner GH, Paik IH, Sur S, McRiner AJ, Borstnik K, Xie S, Shapiro TA. Orally active, antimalarial, anticancer, artemisinin-derived trioxane dimers with high stability and efficacy. J Med Chem. 2003;46(6):1060–5.
121. Fidock DA, Rosenthal PJ, Croft SL, Brun R, Nwaka S. Antimalarial drug discovery: efficacy models for compound screening. Nat Rev Drug Disc. 2004;3(6):509–20.
122. Peter IT, Anatoli VK. The current global malaria situation. Malaria parasite biology, pathogenesis, and protection. Irwin W. Sherman (Ed). Washington, DC: Am Soc Microbiol Press; 1998. p. 11-22. ISBN 1-55581-131-0.
123. Knight DJ, Peters W. The antimalarial action of N-benzyloxy dihydrotriazines. The action of cycloguanil (BRL50216) against rodent malaria and studies on its mode of action. Ann Trop Med Parasitol. 1980;74:393–404.
124. Schmidt LH. Relationships between chemical structures of 8-aminoquinilines and their capacities for radical cure of infections with *Plasmodium cynomolgi* in rhesus monkeys. Antimicrob Agents Chemother. 1983;47:615–52.
125. Miura K, Deng B, Tullo G, et al. Qualification of standard membrane-feeding assay with *Plasmodium falciparum* and potential improvements for future assays. PLoS One. 2013;8:e57909.
126. Blagborough AM, Delves MJ, Ramakrishnan C, et al. Assessing transmission blockade in *Plasmodium* spp. Methods Mol Biol. 2013;923:577–600.
127. Ryley JF, Peters W. The antimalarial activity of some quinone esters. Ann Trop Med Parasitol. 1970;84:209–22.
128. Peters W. Drug resistance in *Plasmodium berghei*. Vincke and lips, 1948; 1 chloroquine resistance. Exp Parasitol. 1965;17:80–9.
129. Wagner H, Ulrich-Merzenich G. Synergy research: approaching a new generation of phytopharmaceuticals. Phytomedicine. 2009;16:97–110.
130. Peters W, Robinson BL. The chemotherapy of rodent malaria. LVI. Studies on the development of resistance to natural and synthetic endoperoxides. Ann Trop Med Parasitol. 1999;93:325–9.
131. Jia W, Fan T, Wang X, Xie G. The polypharmacokinetics of herbal medicines. Science. 2015;350(6262 Suppl):S76–8.
132. Lan K, Xie G, Jia W. Towards polypharmacokinetics: pharmacokinetics of multicomponent drugs and herbal medicines using a metabolomics approach. Evid Based Complement Alternat Med. 2013;2013:819147.
133. Xie G, Zhao A, Zhao L, Chen T, et al. Metabolic fate of tea polyphenols in humans. J Proteome Res. 2012;11(6):3449–57.

11

Circulating micrornas associated with glycemic impairment and progression in Asian Indians

Elena Flowers[1*], Meghana Gadgil[2], Bradley E. Aouizerat[1,3] and Alka M. Kanaya[2,4]

Abstract

Aims/hypothesis: Asian Indians have a high incidence of type 2 diabetes, but factors associated with glycemic progression in this population are not understood. MicroRNAs are emerging as important mediators of glucose homeostasis and have not been previously studied in Asian Indians. We examined microRNA (miR) expression associated with glycemic impairment and progression in Asian Indians from the San Francisco Bay Area. We studied 128 Asian Indians age 45–84 years without known cardiovascular disease and not taking diabetes medications. Oral glucose tolerance tests were performed at baseline and after 2.5 years. We quantified circulating miRs from plasma collected during the enrollment visit using a flow cytometry-based assay.

Results: Glycemic impairment was present in 57 % ($n = 73$) at baseline. MiR-191 was positively associated with glycemic impairment (odds ratio (OR) 1.7 (95 % CI 1.2, 2.4), $p < 0.01$). The prevalence of glycemic progression after 2.5 years was 24 % ($n = 23$). Six miRs were negatively associated with glycemic progression: miR-122 (OR 0.5 (0.2, 0.8), $p < 0.01$), miR-15a (OR 0.6 (0.4, 0.9), $p < 0.01$), miR-197 (OR 0.6 (0.4, 0.9), $p < 0.01$), miR-320a (OR 0.6 (0.4, 0.9), $p < 0.01$), miR-423 (OR 0.6 (0.4, 0.9), $p < 0.01$), and miR-486 (OR 0.5 (0.3, 0.8), $p < 0.01$). Further multivariate adjustment did not attenuate these results.

Conclusions/interpretation: This is the first study to investigate circulating miRs associated with glycemic status among this high-risk ethnic group. Individual miRs were significantly associated with both glycemic impairment and glycemic progression. Further studies are needed to determine whether miR (s) might be useful clinical biomarkers for incident T2D in the Asian Indian population.

Keywords: MicroRNA, Type 2 diabetes, Asian Indians, Glycemic impairment, Biomarkers

Introduction

Asian Indians in the United States have a disproportionately higher prevalence (16–21 %) of type 2 diabetes mellitus (T2D) [1, 2] and associated metabolic conditions [3] compared to other racial groups. The exact biological mechanisms underlying risk in this population compared to other racial/ethnic groups are not well understood. Therefore approaches to risk reduction are limited and show suboptimal efficacy. Current risk screening approaches are limited to the detection of harmful metabolic conditions (i.e., impaired glucose tolerance, impaired fasting glucose). Identification of circulating biomarkers that provide insight about the underlying pathophysiology of T2D in Asian Indians, as well biomarkers associated with incident T2D prior to the onset of impaired glucose metabolism, may allow for earlier detection of the highest risk patients and improved treatments.

MicroRNAs (miRs) are components of an epigenetic mechanism regulating expression of messenger RNAs (mRNAs). Structurally, miRs are 18–24 nucleotide sequences that function by binding to a critical region on mRNA molecules in order to prevent translation into amino acids. More than 2,500 miRs have been identified in humans [4] and approximately 300 of these have been identified in the circulation from both cellular and non-cellular origins. Measurement of miRs captures combined genetic and environmental risk factors to provide a more comprehensive picture of the etiology of complex disease. Recent studies of primarily Caucasian non-Hispanic populations identified differential expression of circulating miRs in individuals with T2D compared to healthy controls [5–8]. MiR-126, which is

* Correspondence: elena.flowers@ucsf.edu
[1]Department of Physiological Nursing, School of Nursing, University of California, 2 Koret Way #N605L, CA 94143 San Francisco, USA

active in endothelial cells, exhibits decreased expression in Caucasian individuals who develop T2D after 10 years compared to those who do not [8]. Cross-sectional studies of miR-126 identified lower expression in individuals with glycemic impairment or T2D. Other studies reported additional individual miRs (e.g., miR-140, miR-155 miR-221, miR-222, miR-320a, miR-375, miR-532) [9, 5, 10–12] that are differentially expressed in T2D and related conditions. These findings support the possibility that circulating miRs may provide novel insight about the biological mechanisms underlying T2D in Asian Indians and function as predictors of incident T2D. This study sought to (1) compare miR expression between Asian Indians with and without prevalent glycemic impairment; and (2) to compare miR expression between Asian Indians who had glycemic progression over 2.5 years to those who remained stable.

Results

We studied 128 participants who were not taking diabetes medications at study enrollment. Of these, 57 % ($n = 73$) exhibited glycemic impairment (i.e., IGT, IFG, T2D). There are more males in this group (29 % vs. 18 %) and higher BMI (26.9 kg/m^2 vs. 24.7 kg/m^2) compared to individuals with normal glycemia ($p < 0.01$ for all, Table 1). The cardiovascular risk profile was worse in the impaired glycemia group with higher systolic (127 mmHg vs. 117 mmHg) and diastolic (75 mmHg vs. 69 mmHg) blood pressure, lower HDL-cholesterol (47 mg/dL vs. 53 mg/dL), and higher triglycerides (146 mg/dL vs. 115 mg/dL) ($p < 0.05$ for all, Table 1). There were no differences in total and LDL-cholesterol. Blood glucose (105 mg/dL vs. 87 mg/dL), insulin (15 μIU/mL vs. 10 μIU/ml), and HOMA-IR (4.1 μIU/mL*mmol/L vs. 2.2 μIU/mL*mmol/L) were all higher in the glycemic impairment group ($p < 0.01$ for all). Additional clinical characteristics were reported previously [13].

Of the 94 participants evaluated after 2.5 years, 24 % ($n = 23$) exhibited glycemic progression. There were no statistically significant differences in baseline clinical characteristics between those who did and did not have incident glycemic impairment (Table 2). In paired analyses, we observed that blood glucose (91 mg/dL vs. 101 mg/dL), insulin (11.5 μIU/mL vs. 17.8 μIU/ml), and HOMA-IR (2.6 μIU/mL*mmol/L vs. 4.5 μIU/mL*mmol/L) increased after 2.5 years in the subset of participants ($n = 23$) whose glycemic impairment worsened (Table 3). However there were no significant changes in cardiovascular risk factors, waist circumference, or BMI.

Of the thirty miRs measured, 6 (i.e., miR-138, miR-192, miR-193b, miR-214, miR-370, miR-375) were below the limit of detection (i.e., 10 AU) and failed to retain a minimum of at least of two of three technical replicates for every participant and were excluded from the analysis. One of the remaining 24 miRs was significantly associated with glycemic impairment at baseline. In unadjusted logistic regression models, miR-191 (odds ratio (OR) 1.7 (1.2, 2.4)) was positively associated with glycemic impairment ($p < 0.05$) (Table 4). In a multivariate adjusted model including age, sex, BMI, and waist circumference, the odds ratio remained statistically significant. Further adjustment for HDL-cholesterol, triglycerides, and blood pressure did not attenuate these effects.

Table 1 Baseline demographic and clinical characteristics in individuals with and without glycemic impairment at baseline

Characteristics Mean ± SD, Median (IQR), or *n* (%)	Glycemic Impairment ($n = 73$)	Normal Glycemia ($n = 55$)	*p*-value
Sex (male)	29 (40)	18 (33)	0.002
Age (years)	56 ± 9	57 ± 7	0.897
Current Smokers	3 (4)	3 (5)	0.386
Physical Activity (MET-minutes/week)	1313 (585, 2940)	1365 (683, 2333)	0.942
Systolic Blood Pressure (mm Hg)	127 ± 15	117 ± 16	<0.001
Diastolic Blood Pressure (mm Hg)	75 ± 12	69 ± 9	0.002
Total Cholesterol (mg/dL)	191 ± 33	194 ± 31	0.683
LDL-c (mg/dL)	116 ± 31	117 ± 27	0.731
HDL-c (md/dL)	47 ± 13	53 ± 15	0.016
Triglycerides (mg/dL)	146 ± 72	115 ± 39	0.006
Fasting Blood Glucose (mg/dL)	105 ± 21	87 ± 6	<0.001
Insulin (μIU/mL)	15 ± 11	10 ± 5	0.001
HOMA-IR (μIU/mL*mmol/L)	4.1 ± 3.4	2.2 ± 1.1	<0.001
Body Mass Index (kg/m^2)	26.9 ± 5.1	24.7 ± 3.6	0.006
Waist Circumference (cm)	98 ± 13	91 ± 11	0.003

cm centimeters, *HDL-c* high density lipoprotein cholesterol, *HOMA-IR* homeostasis model assessment-insulin resistance, *kg/m^2* kg per meter^2, *LDL-c* low density lipoprotein cholesterol, *mcU/mL* microUnit per milliliter, *mg/dL* milligrams per deciliter, *mm Hg* millimeters of mercury, *SD* standard deviation

Table 2 Baseline demographic and clinical characteristics in individuals with progressive glycemic impairment compared to no change at 2.5 years

Characteristics Mean ± SD, Median (IQR), or *n* (%)	Progressive Glycemic Impairment (*n* = 23)	No Change (*n* = 71)	*p*-value
Sex (male)	14 (61)	41 (58)	0.070
Age (years)	55 ± 9	57 ± 9	0.310
Current Smoking	8 (9)	3 (4)	0.705
Physical Activity (MET-minutes/week)	1260 (473, 2100)	1470 (613, 2940)	0.293
Systolic Blood Pressure (mm Hg)	119 ± 20	122 ± 17	0.420
Diastolic Blood Pressure (mm Hg)	71 ± 13	71 ± 10	0.942
Total Cholesterol (mg/dL)	188 ± 39	188 ± 29	0.955
LDL-c (mg/dL)	113 ± 33	112 ± 27	0.872
HDL-c (md/dL)	51 ± 16	50 ± 14	0.780
Triglycerides (mg/dL)	120 ± 65	126 ± 56	0.676
Fasting Blood Glucose (mg/dL)	91 ± 8	91 ± 11	0.813
Insulin (μIU/mL)	11.5 ± 6.2	11.5 ± 6.2	0.807
HOMA-IR (μIU/mL*mmol/L)	2.6 ± 1.5	2.8 ± 2.1	0.715
Body Mass Index (kg/m^2)	25.7 ± 4.7	25.9 ± 4.5	0.878
Waist Circumference (cm)	93 ± 12	94 ± 12	0.856

cm centimeters, *HDL-c* high density lipoprotein cholesterol, *HOMA-IR* homeostasis model assessment-insulin resistance, *kg/m^2* kg per meter^2, *LDL-c* low density lipoprotein cholesterol, *mcU/mL* microUnit per milliliter, *mg/dL* milligrams per deciliter, *mm Hg* millimeters of mercury, *SD* standard deviation

Six miRs were significantly associated with glycemic progression after 2.5 years. These included miR-122 (odds ratio (OR) 0.5 (95 % CI 0.2, 0.8)), miR-15a (OR 0.6 (0.4, 0.9)), miR-197 (OR 0.6 (0.4, 0.9)), miR-320a (OR 0.6 (0.4, 0.9)), miR-423 (OR 0.6 (0.4, 0.9)), and miR-486 (OR 0.5 (0.3, 0.8)), which were all inversely associated with glycemic progression ($p < 0.01$ for all) (Table 4). We adjusted for age, sex, and waist circumference and observed the same significant association with glycemic progression. We then added HDL-cholesterol, triglycerides, and blood pressure to the model and observed the same significant associations. Fold changes are presented in Additional file 1: Table S1.

Discussion

To our knowledge, this is the first study to investigate circulating miRs associated with glycemic impairment in the high risk Asian Indian ethnic group. We evaluated the association between circulating miRs and both prevalent glycemic impairment and glycemic progression after 2.5 years. We found a positive relationship between miR-191 and the presence of glycemic impairment. Six miRs (i.e., miR-122, miR-15a, miR-197, miR-320a, miR-423, miR-486) were differentially expressed between the subset of individuals who had incident glycemic impairment after 2.5 years compared to those who remained stable. All six miRs exhibited an inverse relationship

Table 3 Change in clinical characteristics in individuals with progressive glycemic impairment after 2.5 years (*n* = 23)

Characteristics Mean ± SD or *n* (%)	Baseline	Follow up (2.5 Years)	*p*-value
Systolic Blood Pressure (mm Hg)	119 ± 20	123 ± 13	0.235
Diastolic Blood Pressure (mm Hg)	71 ± 13	76 ± 13	0.081
Total Cholesterol (mg/dL)	188 ± 39	184 ± 30	0.364
LDL-c (mg/dL)	113 ± 33	106 ± 26	0.091
HDL-c (md/dL)	51 ± 16	51 ± 20	0.895
Triglycerides (mg/dL)	120 ± 65	137 ± 69	0.211
Fasting Blood Glucose (mg/dL)	91 ± 8	101 ± 18	0.008
Insulin (μIU/mL)	11.5 ± 6.2	17.8 ± 6.6	<0.001
HOMA-IR (μIU/mL*mmol/L)	2.6 ± 1.5	4.5 ± 2.1	<0.001
Body Mass Index (kg/m^2)	25.7 ± 4.7	26.3 ± 4.9	0.065
Waist Circumference (cm)	93 ± 12	94 ± 13	0.796

cm centimeters, *HDL-c* high density lipoprotein cholesterol, *HOMA-IR* homeostasis model assessment-insulin resistance, *kg/m^2* kg per meter^2, *LDL-c* low density lipoprotein cholesterol, *mcU/mL* microUnit per milliliter, *mg/dL* milligrams per deciliter, *mm Hg* millimeters of mercury, *SD* standard deviation

Table 4 Odds ratios for microRNA expression associated with glycemic impairment

	Unadjusted			Model 1*			Model 2**		
	OR€	95 % CI	*p*-value	OR€	95 % CI	*p*-value	OR€	95 % CI	*p*-value
Prevalent Glycemic Impairment									
hsa-miR-191-5p	1.7	1.2, 2.4	0.002	1.6	1.1, 2.3	0.014	1.5	1.1, 2.2	0.026
Progressive Glycemic Impairment After 2.5 Years									
hsa-miR-122-5p	0.5	0.2, 0.8	0.003	0.4	0.3, 0.8	0.003	0.5	0.3, 0.8	0.003
hsa-miR-15a-5p	0.6	0.4, 0.9	0.040	0.6	0.4, 0.9	0.031	0.6	0.4, 0.9	0.034
hsa-miR-197-3p	0.6	0.4, 0.9	0.020	0.6	0.4, 0.9	0.016	0.6	0.4, 0.9	0.018
hsa-miR-320a	0.6	0.4, 0.9	0.038	0.6	0.4, 0.9	0.045	0.6	0.4, 0.9	0.032
hsa-miR-423-5p	0.6	0.4, 0.9	0.033	0.6	0.4, 0.9	0.039	0.6	0.4, 0.9	0.030
hsa-miR-486-5p	0.5	0.3, 0.8	0.004	0.4	0.3, 0.8	0.003	0.4	0.3, 0.8	0.003

CI confidence interval, *MET* metabolic equivalent
€microRNAs are scaled by quartile
*Model 1 adjusted for age, sex, and waist circumference
**Model 2 adjusted for variables in Model 1 and HDL-cholesterol and triglycerides

with odds for glycemic progression. The addition of clinical covariates (i.e., age, sex, waist circumference, HDL-cholesterol, triglycerides) to logistic regression models did not meaningfully attenuate the association for either glycemic impairment or glycemic progression.

Asian Indians living in the United States have a high prevalence of T2D and related risk factors [3, 14, 1] and the prevalence is increasing drastically in India and other parts of South Asia [15, 16]. While there are some known common risk factors for T2D in this population (i.e., diet, sedentary lifestyle, genetic predisposition), the full etiology is not well understood and therefore approaches to risk reduction have been limited. Identification of circulating miRs associated with glycemic impairment has the potential to provide novel information about the mechanisms underlying T2D. Further, there is the possibility for detection of homogeneous subgroups of individuals at risk based on commonalities in miR expression. In addition, miRs may be useful biomarkers to identify individuals at highest risk for developing T2D who might benefit from aggressive prevention measures.

MiR-486 is inversely associated with risk for glycemic progression. We previously identified that this miR is positively associated with insulin resistance and response to thiazolidenidones, which improve insulin sensitivity, in a multiracial sample [17]. MiR-486 is enriched in muscle tissue where it targets phosphatase and tensin homolog (PTEN) and forkhead box O1a (FOXO1A) and regulates muscle growth and atrophy in mice [18, 19]. In other tissues, PTEN is implicated in insulin signaling and cellular glucose uptake. Inhibition of PTEN decreases blood glucose in rats [20] and mutations in PTEN in humans are associated with insulin sensitivity and glucose tolerance [21]. Peroxisome proliferator-activated receptor γ (PPAR- γ), the primary target of thiazolidenidones, upregulates PTEN, which may lead to changes in insulin sensitivity and blood glucose [22].

MiR-486 has also been implicated in other diseases. Findings from these studies implicate potential mRNAs and biologic pathways targeted by miR-486 that are relevant to a regulatory role in development of risk for T2D. In lung cancer, miR-486 regulates the insulin growth factor signaling pathway by targeting insulin-like growth factor 1 (IGF1), IGF1 receptor (IGF1R), and phosphoinositide-3-kinase, regulatory subunit 1 (alpha) (PIK3R1) [23]. Two prior studies identified low levels of miR-486 in hepatocellular carcinoma cells (HCC) from human biopsy samples and HCC lines *in vitro*. Functional targets of miR-486 in HCC include PIK3R1 [24] and rho-interacting serine/threonine kinase (CITRON) and claudin 10 (CLDN10) [25]. MiR-122, which was negatively associated with glycemic progression in our study and appears to be a target of PPAR- γ [26], is the primary hepatic miR and regulates progression of HCC [27]. Whether miR-486 and miR-122 are co-expressed in hepatocytes and may have related functions in insulin and glucose metabolism in liver or other tissues is not known. Further functional studies are needed to determine if the pathways regulated by miR-486 in other diseases might also be relevant to the development of T2D.

In addition to HCC, associations between miR-122 and other hepatic diseases, including hepatitis, have been well described [28, 29]. Data from *in vitro* studies of hepatic cell lines provide evidence for regulation of hepatic lipid metabolism by miR-122 [30], however our prior study [31] and others [11] found a low level of this miR in individuals free from serious hepatic disease using quantitative polymerase chain reaction-based quantitation.

We found that miR-15 was decreased in individuals who had glycemic progression after 2.5 years. MiR-15a was also decreased in the study of prevalent T2D after 10 years in a Caucasian sample [8]. One *in vitro* study found that miR-15 is increased after 1-h of exposure to glucose but decreased with long-term exposure and may mediate B-cell function and insulin biosynthesis by targeting uncoupling protein-2 (UCP-2) [32]. Several additional studies support a critical role of miR-15a in endothelial cell function and angiogenesis in peripheral vascular, myocardial, and cerebrovascular tissue [33–36]. MiR-15 is increased in the serum of diabetic patients with critical limb ischemia and decreases angiogenesis in pro-angiogenic cells *in vitro* by targeting vascular endothelial growth factor A (VEGFA) [34]. Increased levels of miR-15 are associated with myocardial ischemia/reperfusion injury in mice [33] and suppression of miR-15 by PPAR-γ in cerebral vascular endothelial cells increases pro-angiogenic activity in animal models and *in vitro* studies [35]. We found decreased expression of miR-15 prior to the onset of T2D, which corresponds with pro-angiogenic activity according to data from functional studies. Further research is needed to determine whether there are mechanisms to protect from the long-term vascular consequences of T2D early in the course of the disease.

Consistent with our findings, one prior study identified decreased miR-423 in individuals with T2D and or obesity compared to normal weight non-diabetics [5]. In the same study, neither insulin or treatment with metformin and associated weight loss were associated with any changes in miR-423, though this miR is highly correlated with measures of insulin sensitivity [5]. Only one other study reporting significant findings for miR-423 was identified. In an *in vitro* model of HCC, miR-423 is up-regulated and targets the tumor suppressor gene p21Cip1/Waf1 facilitating oncogenesis [37].

MiR-320, which was decreased in our study, appears to also be enriched in endothelial cells and respond to oxidative stress to regulate cell migration and proliferation [38–41]. Predicted targets of miR-320a from functional studies include IGF1R, polycomb ring finger oncogene (BMI-1), heme-oxygenase 1 (HO-1), glutathione cysteine ligase modifying subunit (GCLM) and oxidative stress induced growth inhibitor 1 (OKL38) and VEGF. Up-regulation of miR-320a results in decreased negative responses to oxidative stress [40, 41] and decreased cellular migration and tumor invasion [38, 39].

Little is known about the function of miR-197. This miR is computationally predicted to target several hundred possible mRNAs, including targets associated with type 2 diabetes (e.g., glucagon (GCG), deiodinase, iodothyronine, type II (DIO2), leptin (LEP), NK2 homeobox 2 (NKX2-2), solute carrier family 30, member 8 (SLC30A8), synapsin I (SYN1), nuclear respiratory factor 1 (NRF1), SHC transforming protein 1 (SHC1), Kruppel-like factor 12 (KLF12), protein kinase C, beta (PRKCB) [42, 43]. Further studies are needed to refine the list of possible mRNA targets and determine the biologic pathways regulated by this miR.

MiR-320a and miR-486 were decreased in individuals who exhibited glycemic progression after 2.5 years. By contrast, our prior study showed a direct relationship with prevalent insulin resistance [17]. The apparent discrepancy in these findings may be the result of the time point at which miRs were measured relative to the progression of disease. In the prior study, we included individuals with confirmed insulin resistance but no diabetes, whereas in this study, we compared individuals who were further along the glycemic spectrum than having isolated insulin resistance without any glycemic impairment. A recent meta-analysis of miRs associated with type 2 diabetes identified similar inconsistencies between studies [11]. Future longitudinal studies relating changes in miRs and progression to T2D are needed in order to understand whether individual miRs are the cause or the consequence of glycemic impairment. A second possible explanation is that our prior study included a multi-racial sample, whereas this study included only Asian Indians.

MiR-126 was associated with risk for type 2 diabetes after 10-years in a primarily Caucasian sample [8], but in our study this miR was one of the least variable and was selected as a normalizer. Similarly to above, possible explanations include the time course of disease compared to when the microRNAs were measured and differences in disease mechanisms between Asian Indians and other racial groups.

The specific biologic mechanisms underlying glycemic impairment and T2D vary between groups and individuals. Identification of circulating miR biomarkers has the possibility to provide information about the specific causal pathways for an individual or group of individuals. Functional studies are needed to identify and validate the exact mRNA targets of the miRs that are differentially expressed in Asian Indians with prevalent or incident glycemic impairment compared to healthy individuals. Future clinical implications include optimization of treatments to target relevant biologic pathways and identification of new pharmacologic targets. Further studies with larger sample sizes and longer follow up are needed to validate the findings for miRs reported here and determine whether there is a set of miRs that significantly improve prodromal risk prediction. Finally, comparisons of circulating miR expression between Asian Indians and other racial groups will provide insight into similarities and differences in the etiology of T2D with future implications for treatments.

There are limitations to this study worthy of consideration. Standardized approaches to normalization of miR expression data from plasma and serum samples are not established. However, consensus is building around normalization approaches that average signals from multiple miRs [44–47]. We used the geNorm algorithm to select the set of three miRs that showed low variability in our sample. These included miR-126, miR-21, and miR-24. Interestingly, miR-126, which showed very little variability in our sample, was previously associated with risk for T2D after 10 years in a primarily Caucasian sample [8]. In a prior study, we showed that MiR-21 is associated with atherogenic dyslipidemia in South Asian men [31]. This miR is also well established in inflammatory pathways [48]. The incongruity of our findings compared with previous studies supports the need to establish standards for data normalization and other methodologic considerations in order to compare findings between studies. Another limitation of this study is the selection of the subset of miRs for which there was some *a priori* evidence to suggest a functional role in glucose metabolism. Future studies should incorporate an agnostic approach to miR detection in order to identify novel targets related to risk for T2D.

We identified individual circulating miRs associated with prevalent glycemic impairment and glycemic progression in the high risk Asian Indian population. Among these are several miRs that have previously been associated with T2D and related conditions in other studies, as well as miRs that are predicted to be implicated in biologically relevant pathways. This is promising evidence to suggest that circulating miRs may be useful for identification of the biologic mechanisms underlying T2D in Asian Indians. Implications include optimization of treatment approaches and new treatment targets. Additional potential clinical applications include improved detection of glycemic impairment and identification of individuals at high risk for progression to T2D.

Methods

Study design, sample, and clinical data collection

We studied participants in the Metabolic syndrome in Asian Indians Living in America (MASALA) Study [13]. Briefly, this is a sample of community-dwelling adults who self-identify as Asian Indian and were free from known cardiovascular disease at baseline. Of 150 participants in the MASALA study, 149 provided complete baseline data. We excluded 21 participants taking diabetes medications at baseline for a sample size for evaluation of prevalent glycemic impairment of 128. After 2.5 years of follow-up, 112 participants completed a second clinical examination. Of these, we excluded 18 participants who had T2D at baseline for a sample size of 94 in the follow-up visit. Participants were sampled by surname from all counties in the San Francisco Bay Area as described previously [13]. Demographic information was collected by self-report. Height, weight, waist circumference, and blood pressure were collected by trained study personnel [13]. Physical activity was assessed using the Typical Week's Physical Activity Questionnaire [49]. Participants were administered 75 g oral glucose and blood glucose measurements were obtained after 120 min. Impaired glucose tolerance (IGT) was defined as 2-h glucose 140–199 mg/dl, impaired fasting glucose (IFG) was defined as fasting glucose 100–125 mg/dl, and T2D was defined as 2-h glucose ≥200 mg/dl, or fasting glucose ≥126 mg/dl. Glycemic impairment was defined as the presence of IGT, IFG, or T2D at baseline. Glycemic progression was defined as (1) progression from normal glycemia to IGT, IFT, or T2D; (2) from IGT to IFG or T2D; or (3) from IFG to T2D after 2.5 years of follow-up. Body mass index (BMI) was calculated using the formula kilograms/meters^2. To estimate insulin sensitivity we calculated homeostasis –model assessment of insulin resistance (HOMA-IR) using the formula I_0 (μIU/mL) * G_0 (mmol/L)/22.5 [50]. Blood used for banking of plasma was collected at baseline into vacutainers containing the preservative EDTA, centrifuged at 4 °C to separate plasma from cellular blood components, and stored at −80 °C. The study was approved by the University of California, San Francisco Institutional Review Board.

Molecular data collection

We selected a panel of 28 miRs (i.e., miR-122-5p, miR-126-3p, miR-138-5p, miR-140-5p, miR-146a-5p, miR-146b-5p, miR-15a-5p, miR-150-5p, miR-191-5p, miR-192-5p, miR-1 93b-3p, miR-195-5p, miR-197-3p, miR-20b-5p, miR-21-59, miR-222-3p, miR-223-3p, miR-24-3p, miR-27a-3p, miR-2 9b-3p, miR-320a, miR-33a-3p, miR-33b-5p, miR-370-3p, miR-375, miR-423-5p, miR-486-5p, miR-503-5p) to measure based on previous data from human studies of blood-based expression of miRs in T2D and related conditions. Two miRs (i.e., miR-214-3p, miR-22-3p) were selected as potential normalizers. MicroRNAs were quantified using the Firefly Circulating miRNA Assay (Firefly BioWorks, Cambridge, MA) providing direct detection of microRNAs from plasma without isolation [51]. MiRs from plasma were hybridized to complementary oligonucleotides covalently attached to encoded hydrogel microparticles. The bound target was ligated to oligonucleotide adapter sequences that serve as universal PCR priming sites. The miR-adapter hybrid molecules were then denatured from the particles at 95 °C and reverse transcription polymerase chain reaction (RT-PCR) was performed using a fluorescent forward primer. Once amplified, the fluorescent target was rehybridized to the original capture particles and scanned on a EMD Millipore Guava 8HT Flow Cytometer (Merck KGaA Darmstadt, Germany). This assay exhibits 90–92 % concordance with other quantitation assays [52] and has been used in previous studies published in peer-reviewed journals [53–55, 17]. Three technical replicate measurements were obtained for each sample and miR target. MiRs that failed to retain at least two of three technical replicates with a robust enough signal for analysis (i.e., 10 AU) for each sample were excluded from analysis.

Statistical analysis

Student's *t*-tests, Pearson's chi-squared tests, and Wilcoxon rank sum tests were used to compare demographic characteristics between groups and paired samples *t*-test were used to compare the sample over time. Normalized expression of each sample for each miR target was calculated using the geometric mean expression of three miRs (i.e., miR-126-3p, miR-21-5p, miR-24-3p) selected using the geNorm algorithm [45]. Logistic regression models were used to determine odds ratios with sequential adjustment for covariates. MiRs were log transformed for logistic regression models. Fold change differential expression of miRs between groups was calculated as the ratio of normalized expression in the group with prevalent glycemic impairment or glycemic progression compared to those who were normoglycemic or stable, respectively. Wilcoxon rank sum tests were used to compare normalized expression of miRs between groups ($\alpha = 0.05$). We used a permutation test to control for the family-wise error rate (FWER) across all miRs.

Abbreviations

miR: MicroRNA; T2D: Type 2 diabetes.

Competing interests

Firefly Bioworks, Inc. provided support for molecular marker measurements but did not contribute to the study design, statistical analysis, or interpretation of the manuscript. The authors declare that they have no competing interests.

Authors' contributions

EF Conceived of the study designed, performed data analysis, and wrote the manuscript. MG contributed to the study design and reviewed and approved the manuscript. BEA contributed to the study design and molecular data collection and reviewed and approved the manuscript. AMK performed clinical data collection, contributed to the study design, and reviewed and approved the manuscript. All authors read and approved the final manuscript.

Funding

Research reported in this publication was supported by the National Center for Advancing Translational Sciences of the NIH under Award Number KL2TR000143, and Resource Centers for Minority Aging Research program Center for Aging in Diverse Communities (CADC) by the National Institute on Aging Award Number P30-AG15272. Its contents are solely the responsibility of the authors and do not necessarily represent the official views of the NIH.

Author details

[1]Department of Physiological Nursing, School of Nursing, University of California, 2 Koret Way #N605L, CA 94143 San Francisco, USA. [2]Division of General Internal Medicine, University of California, San Francisco, USA. [3]Institute for Human Genetics, University of California, San Francisco, USA. [4]Department of Epidemiology and Biostatistics, University of California, San Francisco, USA.

References

1. Karter AJ, Schillinger D, Adams AS, Moffet HH, Liu J, Adler NE, et al. Elevated rates of diabetes in Pacific Islanders and Asian subgroups: The Diabetes Study of Northern California (DISTANCE). Diabetes Care. 2013;36(3):574–9. doi:10.2337/dc12-0722.
2. Kanaya AM, Herrington D, Vittinghoff E, Ewing SK, Liu K, Blaha MJ, et al. Understanding the high prevalence of diabetes in U.S. south Asians compared with four racial/ethnic groups: the MASALA and MESA studies. Diabetes Care. 2014;37(6):1621–8. doi:10.2337/dc13-2656.
3. Kozomara A, Griffiths-Jones S. miRBase: integrating microRNA annotation and deep-sequencing data. Nucleic Acids Res. 2011;39(Database issue):D152–7. doi:10.1093/nar/gkq1027.
4. Kozomara A, Griffiths-Jones S. miRBase: integrating microRNA annotation and deep-sequencing data. Nucleic Acids Res. 2011;39(Database issue):D152–7. doi:10.1093/nar/gkq1027.
5. Ortega FJ, Mercader JM, Moreno-Navarrete JM, Rovira O, Guerra E, Esteve E, et al. Profiling of Circulating MicroRNAs Reveals Common MicroRNAs Linked to Type 2 Diabetes That Change With Insulin Sensitization. Diabetes Care. 2014;37:1375–83. doi:10.2337/dc13-1847.
6. Pescador N, Perez-Barba M, Ibarra JM, Corbaton A, Martinez-Larrad MT, Serrano-Rios M. Serum Circulating microRNA Profiling for Identification of Potential Type 2 Diabetes and Obesity Biomarkers. PLoS One. 2013;8(10):e77251. doi:10.1371/journal.pone.0077251.
7. Wang X, Sundquist J, Zoller B, Memon AA, Palmer K, Sundquist K, et al. Determination of 14 Circulating microRNAs in Swedes and Iraqis with and without Diabetes Mellitus Type 2. PLoS One. 2014;9(1):e86792. doi:10.1371/journal.pone.0086792.
8. Zampetaki A, Kiechl S, Drozdov I, Willeit P, Mayr U, Prokopi M, et al. Plasma microRNA profiling reveals loss of endothelial miR-126 and other microRNAs in type 2 diabetes. Circ Res. 2010;107(6):810–7. doi:10.1161/CIRCRESAHA.110.226357.
9. Liu Y, Gao G, Yang C, Zhou K, Shen B, Liang H, et al. The Role of Circulating MicroRNA-126 (miR-126): A Novel Biomarker for Screening Prediabetes and Newly Diagnosed Type 2 Diabetes Mellitus. Int J Mol Sci. 2014;15(6):10567–77. doi:10.3390/ijms150610567.
10. Wang YT, Tsai PC, Liao YC, Hsu CY, Juo SH. Circulating microRNAs have a sex-specific association with metabolic syndrome. J Biomed Sci. 2013;20:72. doi:10.1186/1423-0127-20-72.
11. Zhu H, Leung SW. Identification of microRNA biomarkers in type 2 diabetes: a meta-analysis of controlled profiling studies. Diabetologia. 2015;58(5):900–11. doi:10.1007/s00125-015-3510-2.
12. Higuchi C, Nakatsuka A, Eguchi J, Teshigawara S, Kanzaki M, Katayama A, et al. Identification of Circulating miR-101, miR-375 and miR-802 as Biomarkers for Type 2 Diabetes. Metabolism. 2015;64(4):489–97. doi:10.1016/j.metabol.2014.12.003.
13. Kanaya AM, Wassel CL, Mathur D, Stewart A, Herrington D, Budoff MJ, et al. Prevalence and correlates of diabetes in South asian indians in the United States: findings from the metabolic syndrome and atherosclerosis in South asians living in america study and the multi-ethnic study of atherosclerosis. Metab Syndr Relat Disord. 2010;8(2):157–64. doi:10.1089/met.2009.0062.
14. Misra R, Patel T, Kotha P, Raji A, Ganda O, Banerji M, et al. Prevalence of diabetes, metabolic syndrome, and cardiovascular risk factors in US Asian Indians: results from a national study. J Diabetes Complications. 2009. doi:10.1016/j.jdiacomp.2009.01.003.
15. Federation ID. IDF Diabetes Atlas. Internaional Diabetes Federation, Brussels, Belgium. 2013. http://www.idf.org/diabetesatlas. Accessed March 5 2015.
16. Gujral UP, Narayan KM, Pradeepa RG, Deepa M, Ali MK, Anjana RM, et al. Comparing Type 2 Diabetes, Prediabetes, and Their Associated Risk Factors in Asian Indians in India and in the U.S.: The CARRS and MASALA Studies. Diabetes Care. 2015;38(7):1312–8. doi:10.2337/dc15-0032.
17. Flowers E, Aouizerat BE, Abbasi F, Lamendola C, Grove KM, Fukuoka Y et al. Circulating microRNA-320a and microRNA-486 predict thiazolidinedione response: Moving towards precision health for diabetes prevention. Metabolism. 2015. doi:10.1016/j.metabol.2015.05.013
18. Small EM, O'Rourke JR, Moresi V, Sutherland LB, McAnally J, Gerard RD, et al. Regulation of PI3-kinase/Akt signaling by muscle-enriched microRNA-486. Proc Natl Acad Sci U S A. 2010;107(9):4218–23. doi:10.1073/pnas.1000300107.
19. Xu J, Li R, Workeneh B, Dong Y, Wang X, Hu Z. Transcription factor FoxO1, the dominant mediator of muscle wasting in chronic kidney disease, is inhibited by microRNA-486. Kidney Int. 2012;82(4):401–11. doi:10.1038/ki.2012.84.

20. Butler M, McKay RA, Popoff IJ, Gaarde WA, Witchell D, Murray SF, et al. Specific inhibition of PTEN expression reverses hyperglycemia in diabetic mice. Diabetes. 2002;51(4):1028–34.
21. Pal A, Barber TM, Van de Bunt M, Rudge SA, Zhang Q, Lachlan KL, et al. PTEN mutations as a cause of constitutive insulin sensitivity and obesity. N Engl J Med. 2012;367(11):1002–11. doi:10.1056/NEJMoa1113966.
22. Tamguney T, Stokoe D. New insights into PTEN. J Cell Sci. 2007;120(Pt 23):4071–9. doi:10.1242/jcs.015230.
23. Peng Y, Dai Y, Hitchcock C, Yang X, Kassis ES, Liu L, et al. Insulin growth factor signaling is regulated by microRNA-486, an underexpressed microRNA in lung cancer. Proc Natl Acad Sci U S A. 2013;110(37):15043–8. doi:10.1073/pnas.1307107110.
24. Huang XP, Hou J, Shen XY, Huang CY, Zhang XH, Xie YA, et al. MicroRNA-486-5p, which is downregulated in hepatocellular carcinoma, suppresses tumor growth by targeting PIK3R1. FEBS J. 2015;282(3):579–94. doi:10.1111/febs.13167.
25. Sun H, Cui C, Xiao F, Wang H, Xu J, Shi X et al. MiR-486 regulates metastasis and chemosensitivity in hepatocellular carcinoma by targeting CLDN10 and CITRON. Hepatology research : the official journal of the Japan Society of Hepatology. 2015. doi:10.1111/hepr.12500
26. Song K, Han C, Zhang J, Lu D, Dash S, Feitelson M, et al. Epigenetic regulation of MicroRNA-122 by peroxisome proliferator activated receptor-gamma and hepatitis b virus X protein in hepatocellular carcinoma cells. Hepatology. 2013;58(5):1681–92. doi:10.1002/hep.26514.
27. Coulouarn C, Factor VM, Andersen JB, Durkin ME, Thorgeirsson SS. Loss of miR-122 expression in liver cancer correlates with suppression of the hepatic phenotype and gain of metastatic properties. Oncogene. 2009;28(40):3526–36. doi:10.1038/onc.2009.211.
28. Hu J, Xu Y, Hao J, Wang S, Li C, Meng S. MiR-122 in hepatic function and liver diseases. Protein Cell. 2012;3(5):364–71. doi:10.1007/s13238-012-2036-3.
29. Jopling C. Liver-specific microRNA-122: Biogenesis and function. RNA Biol. 2012;9(2):137–42. doi:10.4161/rna.18827.
30. Flowers E, Froelicher ES, Aouizerat BE. MicroRNA regulation of lipid metabolism. Metabolism. 2013;62(1):12–20. doi:10.1016/j.metabol.2012.04.009.
31. Flowers E, Singh K, Molina C, Mathur A, Aouizerat BE. MicroRNA associated with atherogenic dyslipidemia in South Asian men. Int J Cardiol. 2013;168(5):4884–5. doi:10.1016/j.ijcard.2013.07.029.
32. Sun LL, Jiang BG, Li WT, Zou JJ, Shi YQ, Liu ZM. MicroRNA-15a positively regulates insulin synthesis by inhibiting uncoupling protein-2 expression. Diabetes Res Clin Pract. 2011;91(1):94–100. doi:10.1016/j.diabres.2010.11.006.
33. Liu LF, Liang Z, Lv ZR, Liu XH, Bai J, Chen J, et al. MicroRNA-15a/b are up-regulated in response to myocardial ischemia/reperfusion injury. J Geriatr Cardiol. 2012;9(1):28–32. doi:10.3724/sp.j.1263.2012.00028.
34. Spinetti G, Fortunato O, Caporali A, Shantikumar S, Marchetti M, Meloni M, et al. MicroRNA-15a and microRNA-16 impair human circulating proangiogenic cell functions and are increased in the proangiogenic cells and serum of patients with critical limb ischemia. Circ Res. 2013;112(2):335–46. doi:10.1161/circresaha.111.300418.
35. Yin KJ, Deng Z, Hamblin M, Xiang Y, Huang H, Zhang J, et al. Peroxisome proliferator-activated receptor delta regulation of miR-15a in ischemia-induced cerebral vascular endothelial injury. J Neurosci. 2010;30(18):6398–408. doi:10.1523/jneurosci.0780-10.2010.
36. Yin KJ, Olsen K, Hamblin M, Zhang J, Schwendeman SP, Chen YE. Vascular endothelial cell-specific microRNA-15a inhibits angiogenesis in hindlimb ischemia. J Biol Chem. 2012;287(32):27055–64. doi:10.1074/jbc.M112.364414.
37. Lin J, Huang S, Wu S, Ding J, Zhao Y, Liang L, et al. MicroRNA-423 promotes cell growth and regulates G(1)/S transition by targeting p21Cip1/Waf1 in hepatocellular carcinoma. Carcinogenesis. 2011;32(11):1641–7. doi:10.1093/carcin/bgr199.
38. Guo T, Feng Y, Liu Q, Yang X, Jiang T, Chen Y, et al. MicroRNA-320a suppresses in GBM patients and modulates glioma cell functions by targeting IGF-1R. Tumour Biol. 2014;35(11):11269–75. doi:10.1007/s13277-014-2283-4.
39. Qi X, Li J, Zhou C, Lv C, Tian M. MicroRNA-320a inhibits cell proliferation, migration and invasion by targeting BMI-1 in nasopharyngeal carcinoma. FEBS Lett. 2014;588(20):3732–8. doi:10.1016/j.febslet.2014.08.021.
40. Schrottmaier WC, Oskolkova OV, Schabbauer G, Afonyushkin T. MicroRNA miR-320a modulates induction of HO-1, GCLM and OKL38 by oxidized phospholipids in endothelial cells. Atherosclerosis. 2014;235(1):1–8. doi:10.1016/j.atherosclerosis.2014.03.026.
41. Tang H, Lee M, Sharpe O, Salamone L, Noonan EJ, Hoang CD, et al. Oxidative stress-responsive microRNA-320 regulates glycolysis in diverse biological systems. FASEB J. 2012;26(11):4710–21. doi:10.1096/fj.11-197467.
42. Wong N, Wang X. miRDB: an online resource for microRNA target prediction and functional annotations. Nucleic Acids Res. 2015;43(Database issue):D146–52. doi:10.1093/nar/gku1104.
43. Lagana A, Forte S, Giudice A, Arena MR, Puglisi PL, Giugno R et al. miRo: a miRNA knowledge base. Database : the journal of biological databases and curation. 2009;2009:bap008. doi:10.1093/database/bap008.
44. Farina NH, Wood ME, Perrapato SD, Francklyn CS, Stein GS, Stein JL, et al. Standardizing Analysis of Circulating MicroRNA: Clinical and Biological Relevance. J Cell Biochem. 2013;115:805–11. doi:10.1002/jcb.24745.
45. Mestdagh P, Van Vlierberghe P, De Weer A, Muth D, Westermann F, Speleman F, et al. A novel and universal method for microRNA RT-qPCR data normalization. Genome Biol. 2009;10(6):R64. doi:10.1186/gb-2009-10-6-r64.
46. Meyer SU, Kaiser S, Wagner C, Thirion C, Pfaffl MW. Profound effect of profiling platform and normalization strategy on detection of differentially expressed microRNAs–a comparative study. PLoS One. 2012;7(6):e38946. doi:10.1371/journal.pone.0038946.
47. Qureshi R, Sacan A. A novel method for the normalization of microRNA RT-PCR data. BMC Med Genet. 2013;6 Suppl 1:S14. doi:10.1186/1755-8794-6-S1-S14.
48. Kumarswamy R, Volkmann I, Jazbutyte V, Dangwal S, Park DH, Thum T. Transforming growth factor-beta-induced endothelial-to-mesenchymal transition is partly mediated by microRNA-21. Arterioscler Thromb Vasc Biol. 2012;32(2):361–9. doi:10.1161/ATVBAHA.111.234286.
49. Ainsworth BE, Irwin ML, Addy CL, Whitt MC, Stolarczyk LM. Moderate physical activity patterns of minority women: the Cross-Cultural Activity Participation Study. J Womens Health Gend Based Med. 1999;8(6):805–13. doi:10.1089/152460999319129.
50. Matthews DR, Hosker JP, Rudenski AS, Naylor BA, Treacher DF, Turner RC. Homeostasis model assessment: insulin resistance and beta-cell function from fasting plasma glucose and insulin concentrations in man. Diabetologia. 1985;28(7):412–9.
51. Chapin SC, Appleyard DC, Pregibon DC, Doyle PS. Rapid microRNA profiling on encoded gel microparticles. Angew Chem Int Ed Engl. 2011;50(10):2289–93. doi:10.1002/anie.201006523.
52. Firefly Bioworks, Inc. http://fireflybio.com/sites/default/files/Documentation/TechNotes/Pregibon_miRNAProfiling_2012.pdf. Accessed July 14 2015.
53. Le MT, Hamar P, Guo C, Basar E, Perdigao-Henriques R, Balaj L, et al. miR-200-containing extracellular vesicles promote breast cancer cell metastasis. J Clin Invest. 2014;124(12):5109–28. doi:10.1172/jci75695.
54. Hoss AG, Labadorf A, Latourelle JC, Kartha VK, Hadzi TC, Gusella JF, et al. miR-10b-5p expression in Huntington's disease brain relates to age of onset and the extent of striatal involvement. BMC Med Genet. 2015;8(1):10. doi:10.1186/s12920-015-0083-3.
55. Ren Z, Ambros VR. Caenorhabditis elegans microRNAs of the let-7 family act in innate immune response circuits and confer robust developmental timing against pathogen stress. Proc Natl Acad Sci U S A. 2015;112(18):E2366–75. doi:10.1073/pnas.1422858112.

12

Critical appraisal of the role of serum albumin in cardiovascular disease

Shih-Chieh Chien[1,2], Chun-Yen Chen[2], Chao-Feng Lin[2] and Hung-I Yeh[2*]

Abstract

Concentration of serum albumin (SA), a multifunctional circulatory protein, is influenced by several factors, including its synthesis rate, catabolism rate, extravascular distribution, and exogenous loss. Moreover, both nutritional status and systemic inflammation affect the synthesis of SA. Determining SA concentration aids in risk prediction in various clinical settings. It is of interest to understand the prognostic value of SA in the full spectrum of cardiovascular disease (CVD) in the era of newly developed pharmacological and interventional treatments. Proper interpretation of SA in addition to established risk factors potentially provides a better risk discrimination and thereby presents an option to modify therapeutic strategies accordingly. In this narrative review, we summarize the basic features of SA and its associated physiological functions contributing to its prognostic impacts on CVD. Finally, we discuss the prognostic role of SA in CVDs based on existing evidence.

Keywords: Serum albumin, Cardiovascular disease, Prognosis, Literature review

Background

The properties and role of albumin have been explored for more than five centuries, since it was first precipitated from urine by Paracelsus [1]. Nowadays, we already have clarity on much of the information about albumin from studies carried out. Serum albumin (SA), the most abundant circulatory protein, is associated with several vital physiological functions, such as maintaining oncotic pressure and microvascular integrity, regulating metabolic and vascular functions, providing binding ligands for substances, antioxidant activities, and anticoagulant effects. Furthermore, SA is inversely related to inflammatory processes by modulating neutrophil adhesion and cell signaling moieties [2, 3].

SA is traditionally regarded as a biomarker for reliable risk prediction in various clinical settings. An increased risk in all-cause mortality and cardiovascular (CV) mortality has been shown to be associated with low SA concentration [4]. In the current era, innovative revascularization procedures and emerging medical therapies have altered the clinical features of cardiovascular disease (CVD) and its prognosis. Hence, identifying new biomarkers and re-evaluating the significance of traditional risk factors are important [5]. It is also interesting to understand the prognostic value of SA in the full spectrum of CVD so that the physicians can employ SA for risk prediction among selected populations and thereby offer an optimal therapeutic strategy accordingly.

This article reviews the basic concepts and the proposed functions of albumin, focusing on the link between SA and CVD based on existing evidence.

Structure and biochemistry of albumin

Albumin is a member of the albumin superfamily, which also includes the transport proteins α-fetoprotein, vitamin D -binding protein (Gc-globulin), and afamin (α-albumin). Albumin is an aglycosylated, negatively charged protein consisting of 585 amino acids forming a single polypeptide chain of molecular weight 66.5 kDa [6, 7]. The chain is composed of abundant charged residues such as lysine and aspartic acid and has no prosthetic groups or carbohydrate attached to it. Structurally, albumin has a heart shape in x-ray crystallography (measuring 80 × 30 Å) but in solution its conformation is ellipsoid [3]. The mature, circulating molecule is arranged in a series of α-helices, stabilized by 17 disulfide bonds, and comprises three homologous domains (I–III). Each of these domains has two subdomains (A and B) composed of 4 and 6

* Correspondence: hiyeh@mmh.org.tw
[2]Cardiovascular Division, Department of Internal Medicine, MacKay Memorial Hospital, Mackay Medical College, No. 92, Sec. 2, Zhongshan N. Rd, Taipei City 10449, Taiwan, Republic of China

α-helices, respectively. Albumin in solution is characterized by a flexible texture, owing to the presence of disulfide bonds between domains that confer ability to change between different conformational states. One unbound cysteine residue (Cys-34) in subdomain IA is a redox active thiol (–SH) group. The thiol moiety is capable of thiolation (HSA-S-R) and nitrosylation (HSA-S-NO) as well as binding of substances [7].

Metabolism and distribution of albumin

The total albumin pool is about 3.5–5 g/kg body weight, of which 40–45% is present in the intravascular space and the remaining is present in the interstitial space [2]. The reference range for albumin concentrations in serum is approximately 3.5–5.0 g/dL and the cases with the concentration less than 3.5 g/dL is usually referred as hypoalbuminemia [8]. Albumin changes from intravascular to extravascular compartment at a rate of 5%/hour and the degradation corresponds to 5% of the daily whole-body protein turnover [2, 3] The transcapillary escape rate is increased in a variety of diseases [9]. In general, SA excretion via urine is minimal. This could be explained from its size and charge as well as its active reabsorption in renal tubuli [10]. Albumin is degraded into amino acids in all parts of the body. The biological half-life of SA is almost three weeks [10]. The amount of albumin metabolized, approximately 10% of the concentration per day under normal physiological conditions [9].

Synthesis of albumin occurs in the liver and is influenced by several factors, including diet and nutrition, colloidal oncotic pressure, exposure to hormones, and disease states (Table 1). Albumin synthesis may be suppressed by fasting or consumption of a protein-deficient diet [11], exogenous supply of substances raising colloidal oncotic pressure [12, 13], and comorbid diabetes or hepatic disease [14, 15]. Conversely, albumin synthesis increase by consumption of a high-protein (amino acid) diet [11] and exposure to growth hormones, corticosteroids as well as insulin [14, 16, 17].

Biological functions of albumin

Colloid oncotic pressure

Albumin has lower molecular weight than the average of serum globulins but its concentration is higher conferring major osmotic significance, contributing to 80% of total plasma colloid oncotic pressure. The osmotic pressure from SA concentration alone accounts for approximately 60% of the total oncotic pressure and the remaining 40% is attributed to the negative charges surrounding the protein, which attract and retain cations, particularly Na + in the vascular compartment. This effect is so called the Gibbs–Donnan effect, which retains water and enhances the oncotic pressure [2].

Table 1 Factors influencing albumin synthesis

Factors that increase synthesis	Factors that decrease synthesis
High-protein diet [11]	Protein-deficient diet [11]
High calories [11]	Fasting [11]
COP↓ [12, 13]	COP↑ [12, 13]
Growth hormone [15]	Diabetes [14]
Corticosteroids [16]	Hepatic disease [17]
Insulin [14]	Sepsis, trauma [2]

Abbreviation: *COP* colloidal oncotic pressure

Binding capacities of albumin

The presence of a net charge and the ligand-binding sites enable SA to bind to and transport various substances, either endogenous or exogenous, such as inorganic ions, trace elements, vitamins, fatty acids, bilirubin, hormones, thyroxine, steroids, and drugs. These important binding sites for different substances have been well studied [7]. The binding capacities are influenced by several factors such as SA concentration, comorbidities, or presence of competitive compounds [2].

Blood viscosity and vascular function

An animal study showed that lack of albumin reduced erythrocyte deformability and subsequently increased blood viscosity [18]. This phenomenon of low SA and high blood viscosity is also observed in patients with nephrotic syndrome [19]. Moreover, SA is suggested to maintain the permeability of the capillary membrane [20]. Furthermore, it is proposed that hypoalbuminemia impairs the vasodilatory response to nitric oxide (NO) [21].

Antioxidant effects

Oxidative stress, due to reactive oxygen species (ROS) or reactive nitrogen species (RNS), can inflict damage on molecules, leading to the accumulation of toxic end products causing cellular dysfunction. This has been implicated in the pathogenesis of inflammation and atherosclerosis. Physiologically, SA contains abundant thiol groups, accounting for 80% of the total thiols in plasma scavenging ROS or RNS [3]. Moreover, a number of albumin-bound substances, such as NO and bilirubin, possess antioxidant properties, contributing to additional protection from oxidative stress [22, 23].

Anticoagulant effects

Investigations have demonstrated that low SA concentration is related to attenuated fibrinolysis [24]. The bioavailability of prostacyclin (PGI2), a naturally occurring vasodilator and a potent inhibitor of platelet aggregation, is dependent on the albumin concentration [25]. SA is also proposed to have a heparin-like activity. This effect is possibly explained by the similarities in structure and net charge with heparin [2].

Inflammatory responses of serum albumin

The activation of inflammatory response leads to a relevant change in plasma proteins, cytokines, and complements. SA is a negative-phase protein whose concentration decreases in response to inflammation. Although the mechanisms are not completely clear, it is presumed that a large proportion of amino acid is utilized to synthesize positive-phase proteins rather than albumin in the liver during an inflammatory response [26]. This hypothesis is supported by the investigations on sialylated glycoproteins in serum. Some of the sialylated glycoproteins rapidly increase in response to the onset of inflammation and are regarded as an index of acute phase response [27].

Regulating cholesterol transport

Although albumin does not have specific binding sites for cholesterol, it is considered to be a regulator of cholesterol transport. Aqueous transfer is an important mechanism contributing to cellular cholesterol efflux and SA acts as a shuttle, enhancing aqueous diffusion. [28] Moreover, SA is showed specific binding to vesicles which contained cholesterol [29]. Study showed that cholesterol efflux reduced approximately 40% from fibroblasts in the absence of plasma albumin by immunoaffinity chromatography [30]. It is proposed that cholesterol flux between numerous cholesterol pools would be enhanced by SA, thereby facilitating the restoration of steady-state levels as cholesterol is metabolized [28]. This effect possibly aids in explaining the relationship between SA and CVD.

Serum albumin and prognosis in cardiovascular disease

SA concentration serves as a reliable prognostic factor for CVD since a serendipitous finding in 1989 [8]. Numerous studies were designed and performed with the purpose of explaining the mechanisms, verifying the relationship, and extending the applications to relevant fields (Fig. 1) (Table 2). In general, the association of low SA concentration and adverse outcomes is thought to be multifactorial. All the above mentioned biological functions of SA, including the maintenance of vascular integrity [20], vasodilatory effects [21], binding ability for toxins [22, 23], regulating cholesterol transport [28–30], anticoagulant effects [2, 24, 25], and antioxidant capacities [2, 3, 22, 23], are implicated in the pathogenesis. Moreover, reduced SA concentration can also be the result of inflammatory conditions [26] or inadequate nutritional intake [11], rendering potential implications on the prognosis of CVD (Fig. 2).

Albumin and mortality in the general population

The majority of studies supported that lower SA concentration is associated with an increased risk of mortality. Phillips et al. first conducted a population-based, prospective cohort study (British Regional Heart Study), involving 7735 middle-aged men with or without a preexisting disease to evaluate the correlation between SA concentration and mortality. As a result of an average 9.2 years of follow-up, SA concentration was found to be inversely correlated with all-cause mortality, CV mortality, cancer mortality in both the groups with or without a preexisting disease [8]. This result was further supported by another longitudinal analysis from National Health and Nutrition Examination Survey Epidemiologic Follow-up Study (NHEFS). SA concentration of ≥4.5 g/dL was associated with a reduced risk of all-cause mortality (RR: 0.73, 95% CI: 0.62–0.85 for men and RR: 0.71, 95% CI: 0.59–0.85 for women), CV mortality (RR: 0.69, 95% CI: 0.55–0.85 for men and RR: 0.74, 95% CI: 0.58–0.96 for women) and non-CV mortality (RR: 0.77, 95% CI: 0.61–0.97 for men and RR: 0.66, 95% CI: 0.50–0.88 for women) [31] Kuller et al. reported that SA concentration could be an independent predictor of mortality and morbidity in middle-aged men with a high risk of coronary heart events. The association was stronger for coronary heart disease deaths than for nonfatal myocardial infarction (MI) [32]. In the Paris Health Study, there was a significant inverse association observed between SA concentration and all-cause mortality in men, but not in women [33]. This result was contrary to that of the Framingham Offspring Study, which reported an inverse relation between SA concentration and mortality in women but not in men [34]. Results from a meta-analysis, including 8 prospective studies, have shown that subjects with SA levels in the bottom third (estimated 3.8 g/dL) have a 1.9-fold increased risk for all-cause mortality and 2.0-fold increased risk for CV mortality, compared with those in the top third (estimated 4.2 g/dL) [4]. All the aforementioned studies were published before or around 2000. In a recent Japanese cohort study, low SA concentration independently predicted all-cause and cause-specific (cancer, infection and CVD) mortality after a long-term (15 years) follow-up [35].

Albumin and coronary heart events in the general population

Whether SA concentration could predict nonfatal coronary heart events is an interesting but controversial issue. In the Multiple Risk Factor Intervention trial and the Framingham Offspring study, there was a significant inverse relationship between SA concentration and risk of MI [32, 34]. In the Atherosclerosis Risk In Communities (ARIC) Study, low SA concentration was only associated with incident MI in individuals who were current smokers [36]. Moreover, low SA did not provide adequate predictive power for incident coronary heart events in the older populations (aged 65–74 years) in

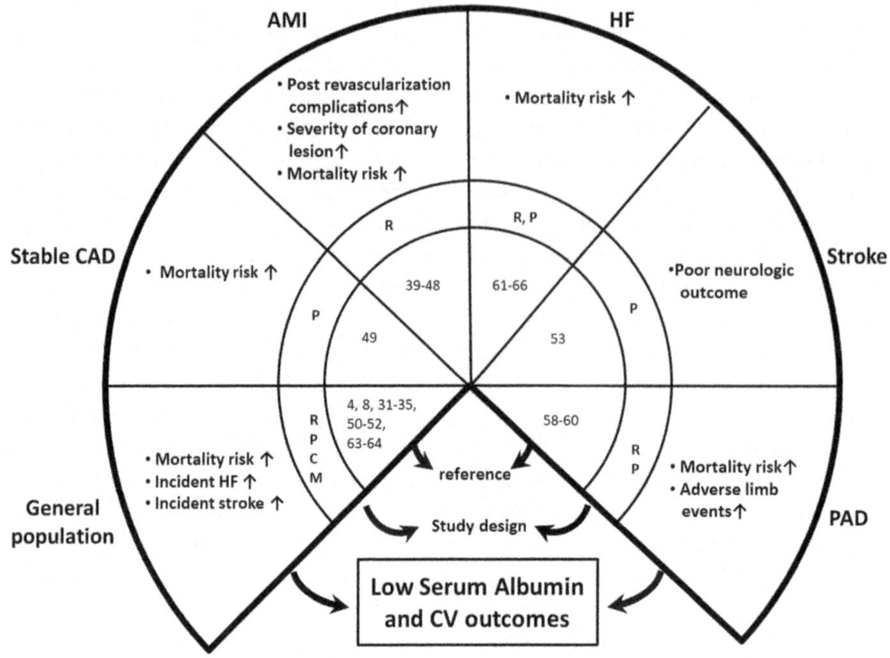

Fig. 1 Serum albumin and prognosis across the cardiovascular continuum. Abbreviation: CAD: coronary artery disease; AMI: acute myocardial infarction, HF: heart failure; PAD: peripheral arterial disease

NHEFS [31]. From a prospective study on the elderly (aged 65 years and older), low SA concentration was identified with a high risk for coronary heart events in women but not in men [37]. In Zutphen Elderly Study, SA only predicted the incidences of coronary heart events among men with elevated total cholesterol [38]. Thus, the risk discrimination of incident coronary heart events using SA concentration is not consistent and varies with different designs of studies. It is possible that low SA concentration does have a direct causative role for incident coronary heart events but could be an indicator of an underlying condition [34]. Similar to the previous section, all the data reviewed here were derived from studies published before or around 2000.

Albumin and prognosis in coronary artery disease

In the presence of effective pharmacological and interventional treatments for coronary artery disease (CAD) after the millennium, the prognostic value of SA has been emphasized further. Among individuals with an acute phase of CAD, SA is also reported as a strong prognostic factor [39–41]. Hartopo et al. evaluated small number patients with acute coronary syndrome (ACS) from a single center. Hypoalbuminemia (< 3.5 g/dL) measured upon admission was associated with in-hospital adverse events, including death, acute heart failure, cardiogenic shock, and reinfarction. This association, however, is not significant by adjusting other risk factors (OR: 2.8, 95% CI: 0.7–9.5) [42] Oduncu et al. retrospectively analyzed 1706 patients with ST-segment elevation myocardial infarction (STEMI) treated with primary percutaneous coronary intervention (PCI), and reported that hypoalbuminemia is associated with both in-hospital mortality and long-term mortality, with a median follow-up of 40 months (23.3 vs. 8.4%, $P < 0.001$). In a multivariate model, hypoalbuminemia independently predicted long-term mortality (HR: 2.98, 95% CI: 1.35–6.58) [39]. The importance of SA in the older patients with STEMI was also demonstrated [40] Plakht et al. categorized SA concentration more delicately in patients with acute MI. They found that SA concentration upon admission provided clear risk discrimination for 10-year mortality [41].

Among patients undergoing isolated coronary artery bypass graft, higher preoperative SA concentration reduced the 30-day and/or in-hospital mortality and major complications [43]. Similar prognostic impacts were also reported among those undergoing PCI [44]. SA could be used as an important indicator of angiographic finding or adverse events associated with PCI. ACS patients with hypoalbuminemia had higher frequencies of multivessel disease, a higher thrombus burden, and a longer lesion length [39]. Low SA concentration(< 3.65 g/dL) was proposed as an independent predictor of high SYNTAX score (≥33) and both factors, SA and SYNTAX score, were linked with the outcomes [45]. Moreover, SA

Table 2 Clinical studies investigating the relation between serum albumin and cardiovascular disease

Study	Year	Number	Characteristics of patients	Albumin cut-off value	Outcomes
Coronary artery disease (CAD)					
Hartopo et al. [42]	2010	82	ACS	< 3.5 g/dL	↑In-hospital adverse event[a]
Bhamidipati et al. [43]	2011	2794	CAD undergoing CABG	< 3 g/dL	↑Mortality and post-operative complications
Oduncu et al. [39]	2013	1706	STEMI undergoing primary PCI	< 3.5 g/dlL	↑3.5-year all mortality and advanced HF
Sujino et al. [40]	2015	62	Age ≧ 85 years, STEMI	Continuous variable	↑In-hospital mortality
Murat et al. [46]	2015	890	ACS undergoing PCI	Continuous variable	↑Contrast induced acute kidney injury and in-hospital mortality
Kurtul et al. [47]	2015	536	STEMI undergoing PCI	< 3.75 g/dL	↑Risk of no-reflow after PCI
Plakht et al. [41]	2016	8750	AMI	categorize albumin level by 3.4, 3.7, 3.9, 4.1 g/dL	↑10-year all mortality
Kurtul et al. [45]	2016	1303	ACS undergoing coronary angiography	< 3.3 g/dL	↑SYNTAX score and in-hospital mortality
Celik et al. [48]	2016	341	PCI with a BMS	< 3.81 g/dL	↑Risk of in-stent restenosis after PCI
Wada et al. [44]	2017	2860	CAD undergoing PCI	3.8 g/dL; 4.1 g/dL	↑MACE and 10-year all mortality[b]
Chien et al. [49]	2017	734	Stable CAD	< 3.5 g/dL	↑1.5-year MACE and mortality[c]
Ischemic stroke					
Gillum et al. [50]	1994	4897	White men aged 65–74 years; Blacks aged 45–74 years	< 4.2 vs > 4.4 g/dL	↑14-year stroke incidence and stroke mortality
Dziedzic et al. [53]	2004	759	Acute ischemic stroke	< 4.9 g/dL	Poor 3-month neurologic outcome[d]
Hostmark et al. [52]	2006	5071	30–75 years	< 4.7 g/dL	↑(self-reported) Stroke incidence
Xu et al. [51]	2014	2986	>40 years old	< 4.2 vs > 4.6 g/dL	↑12-year stroke incidence
Peripheral Arterial Disease (PAD)					
O'Hare et al. [56]	2002	14,427	Hemodialysis patients	Continuous variable	↑PAD incidence
Beddhu et al. [57]	2002	1411	Hemodialysis patients	< 3.6 g/dL	↑PAD incidence
Schillinger et al. [60]	2004	702	PAD patients with less than 2 traditional risk factors	< 3.85 g/dL	↑1-year MACE[f]
Ishii et al. [59]	2013	450	Hemodialysis patients undergoing endovascular therapy	< 3.6 g/dL	↑3-year major adverse limb event[e]
Tsai et al. [58]	2015	444	Hemodialysis patients	Continuous variable	↑4-year all or CV mortality
Heart failure (HF)					
Horwich et al. [61]	2008	1726	Systolic HF	≦ 3.4 g/dl	↑1- and 5- year all mortality ↑Urgent heart transplant
Kinugasa et al. [63]	2009	349	Age ≧ 65, Acute HF	< 3.2 g/dL	↑In-hospital mortality
Uthamalingam et al. [64]	2010	438	Acute, systolic HF	< 3.4 g/dL	↑1-year cardiac mortality
Gopal et al. [67]	2010	2907	Aged 70–79 years without HF	< 4.0 g/dl	↑6-year HF risk but the risk declined annually
Filippatos et al. [68]	2011	5450	Aged ≥65 years, without HF	≦ 3.5 mg/dL	↑10-year HF incidence
Liu et al. [62]	2012	576	Acute HF, preserved EF	≦ 3.4 g/dl	↑1-year all mortality
Polat et al. [65]	2014	135	Acute, systolic HF	< 3.1 g/dL	↑1-year mortality
Bonilla-Palomas et al. [66]	2014	362	Acute HF	≦ 3.4 g/dL	↑In-hospital and 1-year all mortality

Abbreviation: *STEMI* ST-segment elevation myocardial infarction, *HF* heart failure, *PCI* percutaneous coronary intervention, *AMI* acute myocardial infarction, *ACS* acute coronary syndrome, *CAD* coronary artery disease, *CABG* coronary artery bypass graft, *CV* cardiovascular, *MACE* major adverse cardiac event, *BMS* bare-metal stent, *PAD* peripheral arterial disease, *EF* left ventricular ejection fraction

Continuous variable is addressed if studies analyzed the influence of serum albumin with a manner of continuous variable instead of a definite cut-off value

[a]In-hospital adverse events include mortality, acute heart failure, cardiogenic shock, and reinfarction

[b]MACE include nonfatal myocardial infarction and mortality

[c]MACE include nonfatal myocardial infarction, nonfatal stroke and cardiovascular mortality

[d]Poor neurologic outcome was defined as modified Rankin Scale >3 or mortality

[e]Major adverse limb event was defined as a composite of target lesion revascularization, amputation and all-cause mortality

[f]MACE include a composite of nonfatal MI, coronary revascularization, and all-cause mortality

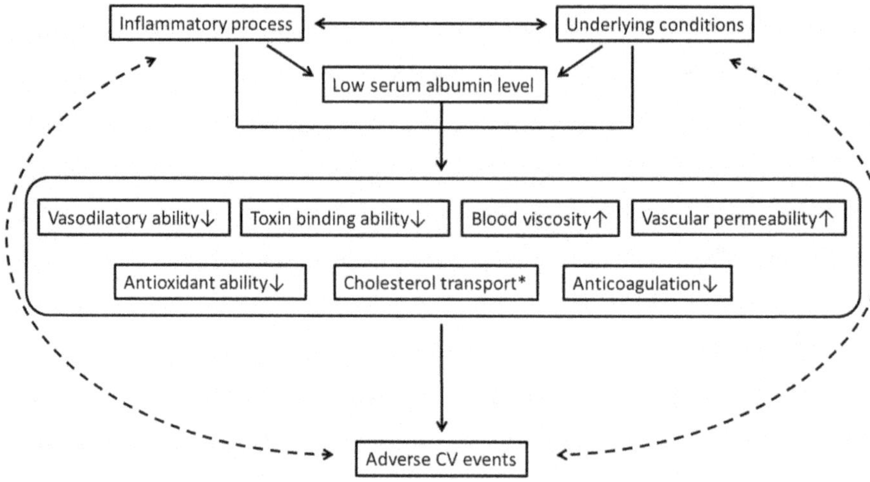

Fig. 2 Proposed interaction between serum albumin and CV outcomes. Abbreviation: CV: Cardiovascular. * Serum albumin is proposed to enhance cholesterol transport between numerous cholesterol pools, facilitating the restoration of steady-state levels as cholesterol is metabolized [28]

concentration on admission is inversely associated with post-PCI contrast-induced acute kidney injury in patients with acute coronary syndrome [46]. Furthermore, SA concentration is an important predictor of no-reflow phenomenon following primary PCI and in-stent restenosis rate after bare-metal stent implantation [47, 48].

We have recently reported the results of hypoalbuminemia and adverse CV outcomes in the Biosignature study, which enrolled CAD patients in stable condition at baseline prospectively. Patients with hypoalbuminemia had an increased risk of 1.5-year in major adverse CV events and in all-cause mortality (major adverse CV events, HR: 3.68, 95% CI: 1.03–13.19; all-cause mortality, HR: 6.81, 95% CI: 1.01–45.62) [49]. This study unequivocally confirms the important association between SA and individuals with chronic stable CAD.

Albumin and prognosis in ischemic stroke

Data from the First National Health and Nutrition Examination Survey (NHANES I) Epidemiologic Follow-up Study suggested that SA concentration < 4.2 g/dL was associated with an increased risk of stroke incidence and death compared with SA >4.4 g/dL in middle-aged white men and black men [50]. The inverse relation of reduced SA and incident stroke was also observed in two studies (the Northern Manhattan Study and the cross-sectional Norwegian Oslo Health Study) [51, 52]. Dziedzic et al. investigated 759 patients with acute ischemic stroke. The reduced risk of poor outcome, defined as modified Rankin Scale >3, or death was observed within the upper quartile of SA (OR: 0.43, 95% CI: 0.26–0.7) [53]. Despite the apparent relations between higher SA concentration and better outcome from epidemiologic evidence, active therapy with albumin solution in acute ischemic stroke did not improve the outcome. This was true also for intracerebral hemorrhage and pulmonary edema where increased risk rates were identified [54, 55].

Albumin and prognosis in peripheral arterial disease

A cross-section investigation suggested SA concentration is also inversely associated with the incidence of peripheral artery disease (PAD) among patients undergoing hemodialysis [56]. Moreover, data from the HEMO study, enrolling 1411 patients undergoing hemodialysis, suggested that the risk for CVD linearly increased as albumin level decreased in patients with SA concentration ≥ 3.6 g/dL. The odds ratio with each 1 g/dL increase in SA decreased by 61% for PAD, 68% for CAD, 67% for CVD, and 77% for all atherosclerotic diseases [57].

Low SA concentration is associated with an increased risk of all-cause mortality among hemodialysis patients with PAD in a single center retrospective study [58]. It was also proposed as a single or add-on predictor of major adverse limb events, a composite of target lesion revascularization, amputation and all-cause mortality in hemodialysis patients undergoing endovascular intervention [59]. However, a prospective study enrolling angiographically proven PAD patients suggested that the prognostic value of SA in major adverse cardiac events, a composite of MI, coronary revascularization, and all-cause mortality was limited to the subjects who had only two traditional risk factors or less [60]. The prognostic effect of SA in PAD is attenuated when the severity or the complexity of comorbidities increases, contributing to a major impact on the outcomes.

Albumin and prognosis in heart failure

The development of heart failure (HF) can be the result of a sole cardiac disorder or, rather more often, the results from other CVD and impaired cardiac function and structure. Hence, the relationship between SA and HF is liable to be considered here. Hypoalbuminemia is prevalent in HF patients, in approximately one-third of those in chronic state and in up to half of all hospitalized patients [61, 62]. Hypoalbuminemia (≤ 3.2 g/dL) is an important predictor of in-hospital mortality among elderly patients who were admitted for acute HF [63]. Hypoalbuminemia appears to be reliable in predicting mortality among individuals with HF and a reduced ejection fraction (< 40%), both in acute [64–66] and chronic states [61]. However, results from individuals of HF and preserved ejection fraction (HFpEF) in two retrospective studies differed. Uthamalingam et al. evaluated 37 HFpEF patients who were admitted for acute decompensated HF; hypoalbuminemia was not found to be clearly associated with 1-year mortality [64]. In another study conducted by Liu et al. enrolling more participants, i. e. 611 individuals consecutively admitted for acute decompensated HF with preserved ejection fraction, hypoalbuminemia was found to be useful in predicting 1-year all-cause mortality after adjusting the baseline factors [62].

SA and HF risk association was investigated in elderly patients. A community-based cohort study investigated 2907 healthy individuals aged between 70 and 79. Those with low baseline SA concentrations were at risk for developing HF, but this risk declined over time [67]. In the Cardiovascular Health Study, enrolling 5450 healthy individuals aged ≥65 years, hypoalbuminemia was found to be significantly associated with incident HF in 10 years by using propensity matched analysis [68]. Since the established study reported a significant association between echocardiographic parameters and HF, the impact of SA on cardiac dysfunction should be investigated [69]. This would not only elucidate the link between SA and HF but also aid early detection of subclinical cardiac dysfunction in healthy individuals.

Conclusions

The measurement of SA is widely available and popular in current medical institutes because of its perceived reliability and low cost. Since SA implicates several important physiological functions, the determined SA concentration reflects physical or healthy status and thereby predicts the prognosis. It is clear that an improvement in risk-specific approaches, which can provide robust and accurate risk prediction, are needed to curb the ongoing burden of CVD [70]. We have to be acquainted with applications of albumin in comprehensive CV fields. Tailored therapies, such as nutritional intervention and direct albumin administration, in individuals with low SA concentration, considered as high-risk groups, should be investigated with randomized placebo-controlled trials to understand its clinical efficacy and safety [71]. In addition, it is warranted to continue exploring the additional roles of albumin in CVD.

Abbreviations

ARIC: Atherosclerosis Risk In Communities Study; CAD: Coronary artery disease; CV: Cardiovascular; CVD: Cardiovascular disease; HF: Heart failure; HFpEF: Heart failure with preserved ejection fraction; MI: Myocardial infarction; NHEFS: National Health and Nutrition Examination Survey Epidemiologic Follow-up Study; NO: Nitric oxide; PAD: Peripheral artery disease; PCI: Percutaneous coronary intervention; RNS: Reactive nitrogen species; ROS: Reactive oxygen species

Acknowledgments

All authors acknowledge the support from MacKay Memorial Hospital (MMH-E-106-03).

Funding

This review received no specific funding from any agency in the public, commercial, or not-for-profit sectors.

Authors' contributions

SCC drafted the manuscript. CYC had made substantial contributions to the section on albumin and prognosis in coronary artery disease of this review. CFL participated in editing table and graph of the prognostic value of serum albumin. HIY reviewed and edited the manuscript. All authors read and approved the final manuscript.

Competing interests

All authors have no competing interests to be declared.

Author details

[1]Department of Critical Care Medicine, MacKay Memorial Hospital, No. 92, Sec. 2, Zhongshan N. Rd, Taipei City 10449, Taiwan, Republic of China. [2]Cardiovascular Division, Department of Internal Medicine, MacKay Memorial Hospital, Mackay Medical College, No. 92, Sec. 2, Zhongshan N. Rd, Taipei City 10449, Taiwan, Republic of China.

References

1. Peters T Jr. 1 - Historical Perspective. In: All about albumin. San Diego: Academic Press; 1995. p. 1–8.
2. Nicholson JP, Wolmarans MR, Park GR. The role of albumin in critical illness. Br J Anaesth. 2000;85(4):599–610.
3. Quinlan GJ, Martin GS, Evans TW. Albumin: biochemical properties and therapeutic potential. Hepatology. 2005;41(6):1211–9.
4. Danesh J, Collins R, Appleby P, Peto R. Association of fibrinogen, C-reactive protein, albumin, or leukocyte count with coronary heart disease: meta-analyses of prospective studies. JAMA. 1998;279(18):1477–82.
5. Beatty AL, IA K, Bibbins-Domingo K, Christenson RH, DeFilippi CR, Ganz P, et al. Traditional risk factors versus biomarkers for prediction of secondary events in patients with stable coronary heart disease: from the heart and soul study. J Am Heart Assoc. 2015;4(7):e001646.
6. Peters T Jr. 2 - The Albumin Molecule: Its Structure and Chemical Properties. In: All About Albumin. San Diego: Academic Press; 1995. p. 9–II.
7. Kragh-Hansen U. Human Serum Albumin: A Multifunctional Protein. In: Otagiri M, Chuang VTG, editors. Albumin in medicine: pathological and clinical applications. Singapore: Springer Singapore; 2016. p. 1–24.
8. Phillips A, Shaper AG, Whincup PH. Association between serum albumin and mortality from cardiovascular disease, cancer, and other causes. Lancet. 1989; 2(8677):1434–6.
9. Boldt J. Use of albumin: an update. BJA. Br J Anaesth. 2010;104(3):276–84.
10. Bern M, Sand KM, Nilsen J, Sandlie I, Andersen JT. The role of albumin receptors in regulation of albumin homeostasis: implications for drug delivery. J Control Release. 2015;211:144–62.
11. Arnal M, Obled C, Attaix D, Patureau-Mirand P, Bonin D. Dietary control of protein turnover. Diabete Metab. 1987;13(6):630–42.
12. Dich J, Hansen SE, Thieden HI. Effect of albumin concentration and colloid osmotic pressure on albumin synthesis in the perfused rat liver. Acta Physiol Scand. 1973;89(3):352–8.

13. Oratz M, Rothschild MA, Schreiber SS. Effect of dextran infusions on protein synthesis by hepatic microsomes. Am J Phys. 1970;218(4):1108–12.
14. De Feo P, Gaisano MG, Haymond MW. Differential effects of insulin deficiency on albumin and fibrinogen synthesis in humans. J Clin Invest. 1991;88(3):833–40.
15. Tessari P. Protein metabolism in liver cirrhosis: from albumin to muscle myofibrils. Curr Opin Clin Nutr Metab Care. 2003;6(1):79–85.
16. Johnson TR, Rudin SD, Blossey BK, Ilan J, Ilan J. Newly synthesized RNA: simultaneous measurement in intact cells of transcription rates and RNA stability of insulin-like growth factor I, actin, and albumin in growth hormone-stimulated hepatocytes. Proc Natl Acad Sci U S A. 1991;88(12):5287–91.
17. Nawa K, Nakamura T, Kumatori A, Noda C, Ichihara A. Glucocorticoid-dependent expression of the albumin gene in adult rat hepatocytes. J Biol Chem. 1986; 261(36):16883–8.
18. Joles JA, Willekes-Koolschijn N, Koomans HA. Hypoalbuminemia causes high blood viscosity by increasing red cell lysophosphatidylcholine. Kidney Int. 1997;52(3):761–70.
19. McGinley E, Lowe GD, Boulton-Jones M, Forbes CD, Prentice CR. Blood viscosity and haemostasis in the nephrotic syndrome. Thromb Haemost. 1983;49(3):155–7.
20. Demling RH. Effect of plasma and interstitial protein content on tissue edema formation. Curr Stud Hematol Blood Transfus. 1986;53:36–52.
21. Keaney JF Jr, Simon DI, Stamler JS, Jaraki O, Scharfstein J, Vita JA, et al. NO forms an adduct with serum albumin that has endothelium-derived relaxing factor-like properties. J Clin Invest. 1993;91(4):1582–9.
22. Rubbo H, Parthasarathy S, Barnes S, Kirk M, Kalyanaraman B, Freeman BA. Nitric oxide inhibition of lipoxygenase-dependent liposome and low-density lipoprotein oxidation: termination of radical chain propagation reactions and formation of nitrogen-containing oxidized lipid derivatives. Arch Biochem Biophys. 1995;324(1):15–25.
23. Stocker R, Glazer AN, Ames BN. Antioxidant activity of albumin-bound bilirubin. Proc Natl Acad Sci U S A. 1987;84(16):5918–22.
24. Gandrille S, Aiach M. Albumin concentration influences fibrinolytic activity in plasma and purified systems. Fibrinolysis. 1990;4(4):225–32.
25. Mikhailidis DP, Mikhailidis AM, Dandona P. Effect of human plasma proteins on stabilisation of platelet anti-aggregatory activity of prostacyclin. Ann Clin Biochem. 1982;19(Pt 4):241–4.
26. Gabay C, Kushner I. Acute-phase proteins and other systemic responses to inflammation. N Engl J Med. 1999;340(6):448–54.
27. Varma R, Michos GA, Varma RS, Brown RD Jr. The protein-bound carbohydrates of seromucoid from normal human serum. J Clin Chem Clin Biochem. 1983;21(5):273–7.
28. Sankaranarayanan S, De la Llera-Moya M, Drazul-Schrader D, Phillips MC, Kellner-Weibel G, Rothblat GH. Serum albumin acts as a shuttle to enhance cholesterol efflux from cells. J Lipid Res. 2013;54(3):671–6.
29. Meierhofer T, van den Elsen JM, Cameron PJ, Munoz-Berbel X, Jenkins AT. The interaction of serum albumin with cholesterol containing lipid vesicles. J Fluoresc. 2010;20(1):371–6.
30. Fielding CJ, Moser K. Evidence for the separation of albumin- and apo A-I-dependent mechanisms of cholesterol efflux from cultured fibroblasts into human plasma. J Biol Chem. 1982;257(18):10955–60.
31. Gillum RF, Makuc DM. Serum albumin, coronary heart disease, and death. Am Heart J. 1992;123(2):507–13.
32. Kuller LH, Eichner JE, Orchard TJ, Grandits GA, McCallum L, Tracy RP. The relation between serum albumin levels and risk of coronary heart disease in the multiple risk factor intervention trial. Am J Epidemiol. 1991;134(11):1266–77.
33. Darne B, Ducimetiere P, Guize L. Serum albumin and mortality. (letter). Lancet. 1990;335(8685):350–1.
34. Djousse L, Rothman KJ, Cupples LA, Levy D, Ellison RC. Serum albumin and risk of myocardial infarction and all-cause mortality in the Framingham offspring study. Circulation. 2002;106(23):2919–24.
35. Umeki Y, Adachi H, Enomoto M, Fukami A, Nakamura S, Nohara Y, et al. Serum albumin and Cerebro-cardiovascular mortality during a 15-year study in a community-based cohort in Tanushimaru, a cohort of the seven countries study. Intern Med. 2016;55(20):2917–25.
36. Nelson JJ, Liao D, Sharrett AR, Folsom AR, Chambless LE, Shahar E, et al. Serum albumin level as a predictor of incident coronary heart disease: the atherosclerosis risk in communities (ARIC) study. Am J Epidemiol. 2000;151(5):468–77.
37. Corti MC, Salive ME, Guralnik JM. Serum albumin and physical function as predictors of coronary heart disease mortality and incidence in older persons. J Clin Epidemiol. 1996;49(5):519–26.
38. Weijenberg MP, Feskens EJ, Souverijn JH, Kromhout D. Serum albumin, coronary heart disease risk, and mortality in an elderly cohort. Epidemiology. 1997;8(1):87–92.
39. Oduncu V, Erkol A, Karabay CY, Kurt M, Akgun T, Bulut M, et al. The prognostic value of serum albumin levels on admission in patients with acute ST-segment elevation myocardial infarction undergoing a primary percutaneous coronary intervention. Coron Artery Dis. 2013;24(2):88–94.
40. Sujino Y, Tanno J, Nakano S, Funada S, Hosoi Y, Senbonmatsu T, et al. Impact of hypoalbuminemia, frailty, and body mass index on early prognosis in older patients (>/=85 years) with ST-elevation myocardial infarction. J Cardiol. 2015; 66(3):263–8.
41. Plakht Y, Gilutz H, Shiyovich A. Decreased admission serum albumin level is an independent predictor of long-term mortality in hospital survivors of acute myocardial infarction. Soroka acute myocardial infarction II (SAMI-II) project. Int J Cardiol. 2016;219:20–4.
42. Hartopo AB, Gharini PP, Setianto BY. Low serum albumin levels and in-hospital adverse outcomes in acute coronary syndrome. Int Heart J. 2010;51(4):221–6.
43. Bhamidipati CM, LaPar DJ, Mehta GS, Kern JA, Upchurch Jr GR, Kron IL, et al. Albumin is a better predictor of outcomes than body mass index following coronary artery bypass grafting. Surgery. 2011;150(4):626–34.
44. Wada H, Dohi T, Miyauchi K, Shitara J, Endo H, Doi S, et al. Impact of serum albumin levels on long-term outcomes in patients undergoing percutaneous coronary intervention. Heart Vessel. 2017;32(9):1085-92.
45. Kurtul A, Murat SN, Yarlioglues M, Duran M, Ocek AH, Koseoglu C, et al. Usefulness of serum albumin concentration to predict high coronary SYNTAX score and in-hospital mortality in patients with acute coronary syndrome. Angiology. 2016;67(1):34–40.
46. Murat SN, Kurtul A, Yarlioglues M. Impact of serum albumin levels on contrast-induced acute kidney injury in patients with acute coronary syndromes treated with percutaneous coronary intervention. Angiology. 2015;66(8):732–7.
47. Kurtul A, Ocek AH, Murat SN, Yarlioglues M, Demircelik MB, Duran M, et al. Serum albumin levels on admission are associated with angiographic no-reflow after primary percutaneous coronary intervention in patients with ST-segment elevation myocardial infarction. Angiology. 2015;66(3):278–85.
48. Celik IE, Yarlioglues M, Kurtul A, Duran M, Koseoglu C, Oksuz F, et al. Preprocedural albumin levels and risk of in-stent restenosis after coronary stenting with bare-metal stent. Angiology. 2016;67(5):478–83.
49. Chien SC, Chen CY, Leu HB, CH S, Yin WH, Tseng WK, et al. Association of low serum albumin concentration and adverse cardiovascular events in stable coronary heart disease. Int J Cardiol. 2017;241:1–5.
50. Gillum RF, Ingram DD, Makuc DM. Relation between serum albumin concentration and stroke incidence and death: the NHANES I epidemiologic follow-up study. Am J Epidemiol. 1994;140(10):876–88.
51. WH X, Dong C, Rundek T, Elkind MS, Sacco RL. Serum albumin levels are associated with cardioembolic and cryptogenic ischemic strokes: northern Manhattan study. Stroke. 2014;45(4):973–8.
52. Hostmark AT, Tomten SE. Serum albumin and self-reported prevalence of stroke: a population-based, cross-sectional study. Eur J Cardiovasc Prev Rehabil. 2006;13(1):87–90.
53. Dziedzic T, Slowik A, Szczudlik A. Serum albumin level as a predictor of ischemic stroke outcome. Stroke. 2004;35(6):e156–8.
54. Hill MD, Martin RH, Palesch YY, Moy CS, Tamariz D, Ryckborst KJ, et al. Albumin Administration in Acute Ischemic Stroke: safety analysis of the ALIAS part 2 multicenter trial. PLoS One. 2015;10(9):e0131390.
55. Martin RH, Yeatts SD, Hill MD, Moy CS, Ginsberg MD, Palesch YY, ALIAS. (Albumin in acute ischemic stroke) trials: analysis of the combined data from parts 1 and 2. Stroke. 2016;47(9):2355–9.
56. O'Hare AM, Hsu CY, Bacchetti P, Johansen KL. Peripheral vascular disease risk factors among patients undergoing hemodialysis. J Am Soc Nephrol. 2002;13(2):497–503.
57. Beddhu S, Kaysen GA, Yan G, Sarnak M, Agodoa L, Ornt D, et al. Association of serum albumin and atherosclerosis in chronic hemodialysis patients. Am J Kidney Dis. 2002;40(4):721–7.
58. Tsai MH, Liou HH, Leu JG, Yen MF, Chen HH. Sites of peripheral artery occlusive disease as a predictor for all-cause and cardiovascular mortality in chronic hemodialysis. PLoS One. 2015;10(6):e0128968.
59. Ishii H, Aoyama T, Takahashi H, Kamoi D, Tanaka M, Yoshikawa D, et al. Serum albumin and C-reactive protein levels predict clinical outcome in hemodialysis patients undergoing endovascular therapy for peripheral artery disease. Atherosclerosis. 2013;227(1):130 4.

60. Schillinger M, Exner M, Mlekusch W, Amighi J, Sabeti S, Schlager O, et al. Serum albumin predicts cardiac adverse events in patients with advanced atherosclerosis - interrelation with traditional cardiovascular risk factors. Thromb Haemost. 2004;91(3):610–8.
61. Horwich TB, Kalantar-Zadeh K, MacLellan RW, Fonarow GC. Albumin levels predict survival in patients with systolic heart failure. Am Heart J. 2008; 155(5):883–9.
62. Liu M, Chan CP, Yan BP, Zhang Q, Lam YY, Li RJ, et al. Albumin levels predict survival in patients with heart failure and preserved ejection fraction. Eur J Heart Fail. 2012;14(1):39–44.
63. Kinugasa Y, Kato M, Sugihara S, Hirai M, Kotani K, Ishida K, et al. A simple risk score to predict in-hospital death of elderly patients with acute decompensated heart failure–hypoalbuminemia as an additional prognostic factor. Circ J. 2009; 73(12):2276–81.
64. Uthamalingam S, Kandala J, Daley M, Patvardhan E, Capodilupo R, Moore SA, et al. Serum albumin and mortality in acutely decompensated heart failure. Am Heart J. 2010;160(6):1149–55.
65. Polat N, Aydin M, Yildiz A, Acet H, Akil MA, Bilik MZ, et al. The prognostic significance of serum albumin in patients with acute decompensated systolic heart failure. Acta Cardiol. 2014;69(6):648–54.
66. Bonilla-Palomas JL, Gamez-Lopez AL, Moreno-Conde M, Lopez-Ibanez MC, Anguita-Sanchez M, Gallego de la Sacristana A, et al. Hypoalbuminemia in acute heart failure patients: causes and its impact on hospital and long-term mortality. J Card Fail. 2014;20(5):350–8.
67. Gopal DM, Kalogeropoulos AP, Georgiopoulou VV, Tang WW, Methvin A, Smith AL, et al. Serum albumin concentration and heart failure risk the health, aging, and body composition study. Am Heart J. 2010;160(2):279–85.
68. Filippatos GS, Desai RV, Ahmed MI, Fonarow GC, Love TE, Aban IB, et al. Hypoalbuminaemia and incident heart failure in older adults. Eur J Heart Fail. 2011;13(10):1078–86.
69. Hung C-L, Wu Y-J, Liu C-C, Hou CJ-Y, Hung T-C, Yeh H-I, et al. Age-related ventricular remodeling is an independent risk for heart failure symptoms in subjects with preserved systolic function. International Journal of Gerontology. 2011;5(1):17–24.
70. Lloyd-Jones DM. Cardiovascular risk prediction: basic concepts, current status, and future directions. Circulation. 2010;121(15):1768–77.
71. Lim S-L, Lye J. Nutritional intervention incorporating expedited 10 g protein counter (EP-10) to improve the albumin and transferrin of chronic hemodialysis patients. ISRN Nutrition. 2013;2013:396570.

13

Dental implant bioactive surface modifications and their effects on osseointegration

Hsiu-Wan Meng[1], Esther Yun Chien[2] and Hua-Hong Chien[3*]

Abstract

Background: The purpose of this article is to review and update the current developments of biologically active dental implant surfaces and their effect on osseointegration.

Methods: PubMed was searched for entries from January 2006 to January 2016. Only in-vivo studies that evaluated the effects of biomolecular coatings on titanium dental implants inserted into the bone of animals or humans were included.

Results: Thirty four non-review studies provided data and observations were included in this review. Within the criteria, four categories of biomolecular coatings were evaluated. The potential biomolecules include bone morphogenetic proteins in 8 articles, other growth factors in 8 articles, peptides in 5 articles, and extracellular matrix in 13 articles. Most articles had a healing period of 1 to 3 months and the longest time of study was 6 months. In addition, all studies comprised of implants inserted in animals except for one, which evaluated implants placed in both animals and humans. The results indicate that dental implant surface modification with biological molecules seem to improve performance as demonstrated by histomorphometric analysis (such as percentage of bone-to-implant contact and peri-implant bone density) and biomechanical testing (such as removal torque, push-out/pull-out tests, and resonance frequency analysis).

Conclusions: Bioactive surface modifications on implant surfaces do not always offer a beneficial effect on osseointegration. Nevertheless, surface modifications of titanium dental implants with biomolecular coatings seem to promote peri-implant bone formation, resulting in enhanced osseointegration during the early stages of healing. However, long-term clinical studies are needed to validate this result. In addition, clinicians must keep in mind that results from animal experiments need not necessarily reflect the human clinical reality.

Keywords: Dental implant, Bioactive surface modification, Osseointegration

Background

Osseointegrated implants have been used to replace missing teeth and as an anchorage for orthodontic tooth movement with direct bone contact [1]. The concept of osseointegration was originally introduced by Brånemark et al. [2] in 1969. Albrektsson et al. [3] suggested that this was "a direct functional and structural connection between living bone and the surface of a load carrying implant." Another clinical definition provided by Zarb and Albrektsson [4] proposed that osseointegration was "a process whereby clinically asymptomatic rigid fixation of alloplastic materials is achieved and maintained in bone during functional loading."

Surface modifications of titanium dental implants have been studied and applied to improve biological surface properties, which favors the mechanism of osseointegration. Machined implant surfaces, representing the starting point of implant surface design, were used for decades according to the classic protocols in which several months were essential to achieve osseointegration [5]. Consequently, topographic and chemical surface modifications replaced machined surfaces to a

* Correspondence: chien.60@osu.edu
[3]Division of Periodontology, College of Dentistry, The Ohio State University, 305 West 12th Avenue, Columbus, OH 43210, USA

great extent in clinical application [6]. Various methods have been developed to increase the surface roughness of dental implants, including blasting with ceramic particles/acid etching [7, 8], titanium plasma spraying [9, 10], electrochemical anodization [11, 12], and calcium phosphate coatings [13, 14].

Furthermore, a novel research field investigating the addition of bioactive molecules to titanium implant surfaces has emerged in implant dentistry. A bioactive molecule is a material having an effect on or eliciting a response from living tissue [15]. Molecules with potential to be applied for bioactive purposes include bioceramics, ions, and biomolecules [16–19]. In this review article, the research interest was limited to titanium dental implants coated with a biomolecule, an organic molecule that is produced by a living organism.

Several reviews have been conducted to assess the effects of different implant surface modifications on peri-implant bone formation and osseointegration [20, 21]. Although it has been reported that the use of bioactive molecules represents a growing area of research in implant dentistry with an aim of achieving quicker osseointegration [22, 23], there are questions that have not previously been answered: (1) which type of biomolecular coatings are presently studied? and (2) what can we expect as the possible effects of biomolecular coatings? Consequently, these display the need for a broad review focused on current developments of biologically active dental implant surfaces. Therefore, the aim of this article is to review and update the current developments of biologically active dental implant surfaces and their impact on osseointegration.

Materials and methods

Criteria for Considering Studies for This Review

Inclusion criteria

- Current developments published during January 2006 to January 2016
- In vivo study
- Titanium implant surfaces coated with biomolecules
- Threaded screw-type implants or implants with recessions or indentations
- Evaluation of the effect of biomolecular coatings on bone formation or osseointegration

Exclusion criteria

- In vitro study
- Use of biomolecules to fill the defect before or after implant placement
- Cylindrical, non-threaded implants
- Intentional creation of peri-implant defects
- Evaluation of the effect of biomolecular coatings on soft tissue, regeneration, ridge augmentation or sinus floor elevation
- Implants that were loaded

Search Methods for Identification of Studies

Electronic searching

PubMed (January 2006 to January 2016) was searched using the keywords "biologically active dental implant surface," "bioactive dental implant surface," "dental implant surface modification," "bone morphogenetic proteins (BMPs)," "growth factor," "peptide," "Arg-Gly-Asp (RGD)," or "collagen." Papers were limited to those articles published in English.

Hand searching

Reference lists of any potential studies were examined in an attempt to identify any other studies.

Results

Among the available literature, 4 categories of biomolecular coatings were outlined and assessed in this review: (1) BMPs, (2) non-BMP growth factors, (3) peptides, and (4) extracellular matrix (ECM).

Modification of dental implant surfaces with BMPs (Table 1)

Becker et al. [24] investigated bone formation onto sand-blasted and acid-etched (control group), chromosulfuric acid surface-enhanced (CSA group), and recombinant human BMP-2 (rhBMP-2) biocoated CSA [BMP-A group: non-covalently immobilized rhBMP-2 (596 ng/cm^2); BMP-B group: covalently immobilized rhBMP-2 (819 ng/cm^2)] implants after placement in the mandibles and tibiae of dogs. After 4 weeks of healing, bone to implant contact (BIC) values appeared to be highest for the BMP-B group, followed by BMP-A, CSA and the control in both the mandible and the tibia. Bone density measured at a distance of less than 1 mm adjacent to each implant revealed a similar pattern of difference between groups as to that of BIC; however, no differences between groups were observed at a distance greater than 1 mm. It was concluded that rhBMP-2 immobilized by covalent and noncovalent methods on CSA-treated implant surfaces appeared to be stable and stimulated direct bone apposition in a concentration-dependent manner.

Lan et al. [25] investigated the influence of rhBMP-2 on bone-implant osseointegration in the femurs of rabbits. Thirty-two implants were evenly divided into 2 groups. Implants in group A were coated with 1.0 mg rhBMP-2 and implants in group B were not coated with rhBMP-2. Twelve weeks after implantation, the pull-out binding strengths of group A were significantly greater than that of group B. Scanning electronic microscopy

Table 1 Surface modification of dental implants with BMPs

Author	Animal – bone site	Mode of surface modification	Length of study	Findings
Becker et al. [24]	Dog – mandible and tibia	1. C: sand-blasted and acid-etched 2. CSA 3. BMP-A: non-covalently immobilized rhBMP-2 (596 ng/cm^2) 4. BMP-B: covalently immobilized rhBMP-2 (819 ng/cm^2)	4 weeks	BIC and BD: BMP-B > BMP-A > CSA > C
Lan et al. [25]	Rabbit - femur	1. A: with rhBMP-2 2. B: without rhBMP-2	12 weeks	- Pull-out strength: A (36.5 N) > B (27.6 N) - Bone formation: A > B
Liu et al. [26]	Pig – maxilla	1. Ti + CaP + BMP-2 inc 2. Ti + CaP + BMP-2 ads 3. Ti + CaP + BMP-2 ads + inc 4. Ti + CaP 5. Ti + BMP-2 ads 6. Ti	3 weeks	- Bone volume was highest for Ti & CaP and lowest for CaP/BMP-2 ads - Bone-interface coverage of the implant surface was highest for CaP and lowest for Ti/BMP-2 ads
Wikesjo et al. [27]	Dog - mandible	1. TPO + rhBMP-2 (0.2 mg/ml) ads 2. TPO + rhBMP-2 (4.0 mg/ml) ads 3. TPO (control)	8 weeks	% of BIC: - TPO surfaces coated with 0.2 mg/ml rhBMP-2: 43.3% vs. TPO control: 71.7% - TPO surfaces coated with 4 mg/ml rhBMP-2: 35.4% vs. TPO control: 68.2%
Wikesjo et al. [28]	Monkey - maxilla	1. TPO + rhBMP-2 (2.0 mg/ml) ads 2. TPO + rhBMP-2 (0.2 mg/ml) ads 3. TPO (control)	16 weeks	% of BIC - Uncoated TPO surfaces: 74 - 75% - TPO surfaces coated with 2.0 mg/ml rhBMP-2: 43% - TPO surfaces coated with 0.2 mg/ml rhBMP-2: 37%
Huh et al. [29]	Dog - mandible	1. rhBMP-2 coated implants 2. uncoated anodized implants (control)	8 weeks	% of BIC - Uncoated control: 40.16% - rhBMP-2 coated: 41.88% Implant stability test - Uncoated control: ISQ = 74.27 - rhBMP-2 coated: ISQ = 79.21
Hunziker et al. [30]	Pig - maxilla	1. Ti 2. Ti + CaP 3. Ti + rhBMP-2 (10 μg) ads 4. Ti + CaP + rh BMP-2 (10 μg) ads 5. Ti + CaP + rh BMP-2 (12.95 μg) inc 6. Ti + CaP + rhBMP-2 ads + inc	1, 2, and 3 weeks	Volume fraction of total bone - Ti + CaP + BMP-2, with either ads or inc or both, have the highest values at 1 week - Ti + CaP + BMP-2 inc and Cap groups have the highest values at 2 weeks - Ti + CaP + BMP-2 inc and Cap groups have the highest values at 3 weeks
Kim et al. [31]	Dog - mandible	1. SLA (control) 2. SLA + rhBMP-2 (0.1 mg/mL) 3. SLA + rhBMP-2 (0.5 mg/mL) 4. SLA + rhBMP-2 (1 mg/mL)	8 weeks	% of BIC - Control: Buccal: 0.67%; Lingual: 23.37% - rhBMP-2 (0.1 mg/mL): Buccal: 10.24%; Lingual: 26.50% - rhBMP-2 (0.5 mg/mL): Buccal: 24.47%; Lingual: 35.45% - rhBMP-2 (1 mg/mL): Buccal: 18.42%; Lingual: 33.43% BV - Control: Buccal: 2.77%; Lingual: 46.50% - rhBMP-2 (0.1 mg/mL): Buccal: 13.30%; Lingual: 60.50% - rhBMP-2 (0.5 mg/mL): Buccal: 33.67%; Lingual: 66.17% - rhBMP-2 (1 mg/mL): Buccal: 35.67%; Lingual: 65.00% Implant stability test - Control: ISQ = 60.17 - rhBMP-2 (0.1 mg/mL): ISQ = 64.83 - rhBMP-2 (0.5 mg/mL): ISQ = 71.67 - rhBMP-2 (1 mg/mL): ISQ = 72.00

CSA chromosulfuric acid surface-enhanced; *BIC* bone to implant contact; *BD* bone density; *Ti* titanium; *CaP* calcium phosphate; *BMP* bone morphogenetic protein; *inc* incorporated; *ads* adsorbed; *TPO* titanium porous oxide; *SLA* sandblasted and acid-etched surface

showed extensive mineralized matrixes on the surface of the implants in group A but not B. Under confocal laser scanning microscopy, there was significantly more percentage of marked bone adjacent to the implant surface in group A compared to group B at both 4 and 8 weeks. The authors concluded that rhBMP-2 improves the quantity and quality of implant-bone osseointegration.

In the maxillae of adult miniature pigs, Liu et al. [26] assessed the influence of BMP-2 and its mode of delivery on the osteoconductivity of dental implants with 6 different types of surfaces, including uncoated titanium (Ti) surfaces, BMP-2 adsorbed to uncoated Ti (Ti/BMP-2 ads), calcium phosphate (CaP)-coated Ti surfaces (CaPTi), BMP-2 adsorbed to CaPTi (CaPTi/BMP-2 ads),

BMP-2 incorporated into CaPTi (CaPTi/BMP-2 inc), and BMP-2 adsorbed to and incorporated into CaPTi (CaP/BMP-2 ads + inc). After 3 weeks, the volume of bone deposited within the osteoconductive space was highest for coated and uncoated implants with no BMP-2, while the lowest value was achieved with coated implants bearing only adsorbed BMP-2. Bone coverage of the implant surface was highest for CaPTi, while the lowest amount of bone coverage was observed for Ti/BMP-2 ads. It was concluded that the osteoconductivity of implant surfaces can be negatively modulated by BMP-2 and its method of delivery.

Wikesjo et al. [27] studied whether adsorbing rhBMP-2 onto a titanium porous oxide (TPO) implant surface might increase or accelerate local bone formation and support osseointegration in the posterior mandible (type II bone) in dogs. Implants with a TPO surface were adsorbed with rhBMP-2 at 0.2 mg/ml or 4.0 mg/ml, whereas TPO implants without rhBMP-2 served as controls. After 8 weeks of healing, implants coated with rhBMP-2 (4.0 mg/ml) exhibited markedly increased bone formation and bone metabolic activity compared with that observed for implants coated with rhBMP-2 (0.2 mg/ml) and controls. BIC appeared significantly lower for rhBMP-2-coated implants when compared to the control, however, the BIC in BMP-2 coated implants is clinically respectable. Finally, it was concluded that rhBMP-2 adsorbed onto TPO implant surfaces is able to induce dose-dependent peri-implant bone remodeling, resulting in the formation of normal, physiologic bone and clinically applicable osseointegration within 8 weeks.

A similar study conducted by Wikesjo et al. [28] to evaluate local bone formation and osseointegration in the posterior maxillae (type IV bone) was analyzed in 8 adult monkeys. Each animal received three TPO implants adsorbed with either rhBMP-2 at 2.0 mg/ml or 0.2 mg/ml in one quadrant and three TPO implants without rhBMP-2 in the contra-lateral quadrant as control. After 16 weeks, BIC was significantly higher for uncoated TPO surfaces versus TPO surfaces coated with either 2 mg/ml or 0.2 mg/ml rhBMP-2. Additionally, rhBMP-2 coated TPO implants exhibited a pinpoint BIC pattern regardless of rhBMP-2 concentrations; on the other hand, the controls exhibited a thin layer of bone covering most of the implant threads, resulting in higher BIC. Sites receiving 2.0 mg/ml of rhBMP-2 implants exhibited new peri-implant bone formation, while contralateral controls exhibited residual native bone close to the implant surface. The authors concluded that rhBMP-2-coated TPO surfaces enhanced local bone formation in type IV bone in a dose-dependent fashion in non-human primates, resulting in significant osseointegration.

Huh et al. [29] investigated anodized implants coated with rhBMP-2 on the effect of bone formation in dogs. Eighteen uncoated and 18 rhBMP-2 coated implants were randomly installed into the mandibular alveolar ridge of 6 young adult dogs for 8 weeks. The implant stability quotient (ISQ) and histometric analysis were examined to evaluate the effect of rhBMP-2 on the stimulation of bone formation. The BMP group showed significantly higher ISQ values than the control group at 8 weeks after implant placement. Similarly, histometric analysis indicated that the changes of bucco-lingual alveolar bone level were significantly higher in the BMP group than in the control group. However, the differences in mean percentage of BIC and bone density were not statistically significant. It was concluded that the rhBMP-2 coated implants can enhance bone formation and increase implant stability in dogs.

In the maxillae of adult miniature pigs, Hunziker et al. [30] studied whether the capacity of BMP-2 to induce peri-implant bone formation can be influenced by its mode of delivery. Six different implant surfaces: (1) Ti implant surface as control; (2) CaP coated Ti implant; (3) BMP-2 (10 μg) adsorbed onto Ti implant; (4) BMP-2 (10 μg) adsorbed onto CaP coated Ti implant; (5) BMP-2 (12.95 μg) incorporated into CaP coated Ti implant; and (6) BMP-2 (10 μg + 12.95 μg) adsorbed onto and incorporated into CaP coated Ti implant were established and tested in the maxillae of 18 adult miniature pigs. The histomorphometric analysis of bone formation was at 1, 2, and 3 weeks after implant placement. The incorporated or adsorbed BMP-2 on CaP coated Ti implant surface did not benefit peri-implant bone formation compared to the CaP coated Ti implant surface. However, the osteoinductive efficacy of BMP-2 can be influenced by its mode of delivery.

A study was conducted to investigate the effects of rhBMP-2 on osseointegration in dogs [31]. Three different concentrations of rhBMP-2 (0.1, 0.5, and 1 mg/mL) were applied to sandblasted and acid etched (SLA) implants and served as an experimental group, while SLA implants were used as a control group. Two months after tooth extraction, four animals received implants coated with 3 different concentrations of rhBMP-2 in one side of the mandible while the contralateral site received SLA implants. BIC, bone volume (BV) and implant stability were analyzed at 8 weeks after implant placement. The mean BIC and BV were greater in the 0.5 and 1.0 mg/mL rhBMP-2 groups than in the 0.1 mg/mL and control groups. Furthermore, the ISQ values were highest in the 1.0 mg/mL group. It was concluded that the SLA implants coating with 0.5 and 1.0 mg/mL of rhBMP-2 was more effective in enhancing osseointegration.

Modification of dental implant surfaces with non-BMP growth factors (Table 2)

Anitua [32] compared BIC of titanium implant surface (Ti) to human autologous plasma-rich growth factor-coated titanium implants (PRGF) in the tibiae and radii of goats. Histomorphometry analysis performed after 8 weeks showed that titanium implant surfaces with PRGF demonstrated significantly higher percentage of BIC. Every biopsy of the implants made with PRGF revealed bone surrounding the entire implant; whereas non-PRGF-coated implants were surrounded by cortical bone only in the middle third. Furthermore, 1391 implants were bioactivated with PRGF and installed in 295 patients. The author reported that 99.6% of the implants treated with PRGF were well osseointegrated. It was concluded that osseointegration was enhanced by covering the implant surface with PRGF before insertion into the alveolar bone.

Lan et al. [33] studied the effect of combining rhBMP-2 and recombinant human basic fibroblast growth factor (rhbFGF) or recombinant human insulin-like growth factor-1 (rhIGF-1) on bone-implant osseointegration in rabbits. Sixty-four implants were coated with polylactic acid and equally divided into 4 groups. Implants in group 1 were applied with 1.0 mg rhBMP-2 and 200 μg rhbFGF, group 2 with 1.0 mg rhBMP-2 and 250 μg rhIGF-1, group 3 with only 1.0 mg rhBMP-2, and group 4 were used as controls and had no growth factors applied. During the healing period, fluorescent bone markers were administered at 4 and 8 weeks. Twelve weeks after the implantation in the femurs of rabbits, implants and surrounding bone were collected and prepared for confocal laser scanning microscopy analysis. There was a statistical difference in bone formation between rhBMP-2 and non-rhBMP-2 groups at 4 or 8 weeks. The new bone formation in groups 1 and 2 was greater than that of group 3 at 8 weeks. It was concluded that rhBMP-2 could increase new bone formation and was able to act synergistically with rhbFGF and rhIGF-1 to improve osseointegration.

In a rabbit tibia model, Park et al. [34] evaluated the bone response around anodized titanium implants coated with fibroblast growth factor-fibronectin (FGF-FN) fusion protein. Twenty implants were evenly divided into 2 groups. Implants in group 1 were anodized under a constant voltage of 300 V, whereas implants in group 2 were anodized under a constant voltage of 300 V and then soaked in a solution containing FGF-FN (65 μg/mL) for 24 h. After 12 weeks of healing, the mean removal torque value for group 2 was significantly greater than that of group 1. Under histomorphometric analysis, the percentage of BIC was significantly higher in group 2 than in group 1. The authors concluded that the FGF-FN fusion protein coating on anodized implants may enhance osseointegration.

Nikolidakis et al. [35] examined the effect of transforming growth factor β1 (TGF-β1) on the early bone healing around dental implants installed into the femoral condyle of goats. Eight healthy female goats were used in this study, and each animal received 3 implants: one Ti (control), one Ti loaded with 0.5 μg TGF-β1 (Ti-$TGF_{0.5}$), and one Ti loaded with 1.0 μg TGF-β1 (Ti-$TGF_{1.0}$). Six weeks after implantation, an intervening fibrous tissue layer occurred around approximately half of the TGF-β1 loaded implants. Ti implants without TGF-β1 treatment demonstrated the highest percentage of BIC, while implants with 1.0 μg TGF-β1 showed the lowest amount. The difference between the two aforementioned groups was statistically significant. The authors concluded that a low dose of TGF-β1 has a negative influence on the integration of oral implants in trabecular bone during the early post-implantation healing phase.

Schouten et al. [36] investigated the effect of implant design, surface properties, and TGF-β1 on peri-implant bone response. Two geometrically different implant types, screw type (St) and push-in type (Pi), were used. Additionally, the implant surfaces were modified with an electrosprayed CaP coating, either enriched or not enriched with TGF-β1. A total of 54 implants, equally divided into six groups, were installed into the femoral condyles of nine goats for 12 weeks. With respect to implant geometry, St implants showed an overall better biological healing process than Pi implants. In term of surface properties, the deposition of CaP coating significantly increased percentage of BIC for both implant types. The enrichment of CaP-coated implants with TGF-β1, however, did not significantly improve peri-implant bone response. The authors concluded that an extensive improvement of the bone response to titanium implants can be obtained by adding an electrosprayed CaP coating. The supplementation of a 1 μg TGF-β1 coating has only a marginal effect.

Lee et al. [37] analyzed the effect of poly(lactide-co-glycolide) (PLGA) in combination with bFGF coating on an anodized titanium implant surface by electrospray. Forty-eight implants were equally divided into 4 groups and inserted into rabbit tibiae. Group 1 implants were anodized under 300 V; group 2 implants were anodized and then coated with 0.02 ml PLGA; group 3 implants were anodized and then coated with 0.02 ml PLGA/bFGF (10 ng bFGF); and group 4 implants were anodized and then coated with 0.2 ml PLGA/bFGF (100 ng bFGF). Histomorphometric analysis was performed via light microscopy and computerized image analysis of the implants that had been in situ for 12 weeks. Implants in group 4 (44.7%) had significant higher mean BIC percentage than that seen in groups 1 (31.4%) and 2 (33.6%). It was suggested that coating a titanium implant with PLGA incorporated with bFGF by electrospray

Table 2 Surface modification of dental implants with other growth factors

Author	Animal – bone site	Mode of surface modification	Length of study	Findings
Anitua [32]	Goat – tibia and radius	1. Ti (control) 2. Ti + PRGF	8 weeks	% of BIC - Ti + PRGF: 51% - Ti: 22%
Lan et al. [33]	Rabbit - femur	1. Group 1: rhBMP-2 (1.0 mg) + rhbFGF (200 μg) 2. Group 2: rhBMP-2 (1.0 mg) + rhIGF-1 (250 μg) 3. Group 3: rhBMP-2 (1.0 mg) 4. Group 4: no growth factor (control)	4 and 8 weeks	% of new bone formation - Group 1: 7.0% at 4 weeks, 10.0% at 8 weeks - Group 2: 7.6% at 4 weeks, 9.9% at 8 weeks - Group 3: 6.2% at 4 weeks, 8.0% at 8 weeks - Group 4: 5.0% at 4 weeks, 6.0% at 8 weeks
Park et al. [34]	Rabbit - tibia	1. Group 1: anodized under constant 300 voltage 2. Group 2: anodized under constant 300 voltage + FGF-FN fusion protein (65 μg/mL)	12 weeks	Mean removal torque value - Group 1: 37.6 Ncm - Group 2: 44.8 Ncm % of BIC - Group 1: 76.4% - Group 2: 88.0%
Nikolidakis et al. [35]	Goat – femoral condyle	1. Control: Ti 2. Ti-TGF(0.5): Ti + 0.5 μg TGF-β1 3. Ti-TGF(1.0): Ti + 1.0 μg TGF-β1	6 weeks	% of BIC - Ti: 65% - Ti-TGF(0.5): 48% - Ti-TGF(1.0): 45%
Schouten et al. [36]	Goat – Femoral condyle	1. Screw type implant: St 2. St + CaP 3. St + CaP + TGF-β1 (1.0 μg) 4. Push-in type implant: Pi 5. Pi + CaP 6. Pi + CaP + TGF-β1 (1.0 μg)	12 weeks	% of BIC - St: 44% - St + CaP: 58% - St + CaP + TGF-β1: 64% - Pi : 23% - Pi + CaP: 46% - Pi + CaP + TGF-β1: 52%
Lee et al. [37]	Rabbit – tibia	1. Group 1: anodized (under 300 voltage) 2. Group 2: anodized + 0.02 ml PLGA 3. Group 3: anodized + 0.02 ml PLGA/bFGF (10 ng bFGF) 4. Group 4: anodized + 0.2 ml PLGA/bFGF (100 ng bFGF)	12 weeks	% of BIC - Groups 1: 31.4% - Group 2: 33.6% - Group 3: around 37% - Group 4: 44.7%
Ramazanoglu et al. [38]	Pig – frontal skull	1. AE (control) 2. CaP coated 3. CaP + rhBMP-2 inc 4. CaP + $rhVEGF_{165}$ inc 5. CaP + rhBMP-2 inc + $rhVEGF_{165}$ inc	1, 2, and 4 weeks	% of BIC for ROI 1 + 4 - AE: 3.4% at 1 week; 11.5% at 2 weeks; 16.1% at 4 weeks - CaP: 5.2% at 1 week; 19.2% at 2 weeks; 23.5% at 4 weeks - CaP + BMP-2: 1.8% at 1 week; 15.5% at 2 weeks; 21.6% at 4 weeks - CaP + VEGF: 3.1% at 1 week; 15.2% at 2 weeks; 22.6% at 4 weeks - CaP + BMP-2 + VEGF: 3.3% at 1 week; 22.1% at 2 weeks; 23.2% at 4 weeks % of BIC for ROI 2 + 3 - AE: 10.6% at 1 week; 14.6% at 2 weeks; 20.1% at 4 weeks - CaP: 15.4% at 1 week; 22.6% at 2 weeks; 24.9% at 4 weeks - CaP + BMP-2: 8.2% at 1 week; 27.3% at 2 weeks; 23.6% at 4 weeks - CaP + VEGF: 8.5% at 1 week; 23% at 2 weeks; 24.4% at 4 weeks - CaP + BMP-2 + VEGF: 9.6% at 1 week; 31.7% at 2 weeks; 31.8% at 4 weeks
Schliephake et al. [39]	Rat - tibia	1. SAE (control) 2. SAE + OAS 3. SAE + OAS + rhVEGF-conjugated to complementary oligonucleotide strands	1, 4, and 13 weeks	% of BIC for 1 and 4 weeks - SAE: 14.5% at 1 week; 40.6% at 4 weeks - SAE + OAS: 14.1% at 1 week; 40.2% at 4 weeks - SAE + OAS + VEGF: 15.1% at 1 week; 60.1% at 4 weeks % of BIC for 13 weeks All groups were between 75% to 80% with no significantly differences between groups

Ti titanium implant surface; *BIC* bone to implant contact; *PRGF* human plasma-rich growth factor; *hrBMP-2* recombinant human bone morphogenetic protein-2; *rhbFGF* recombinant human basic fibroblast growth factor; *rhIGF-1* recombinant human insulin-like growth factor; *FGF-FN* fibroblast growth factor-fibronectin; *TGF-β1* transforming growth factor β1; *St* screw type implant; *Pi* push-in type implant; *CaP* calcium phosphate coating; *PLGA* poly(lactide-co-glycolide); *bFGF* basic fibroblast growth factor; *AE* acid-etched; *VEGF* vascular endothelial growth factor; *CaP* calcium phosphate; *SAE* sandblasted and acid-etched; *OAS* DNA oligonucleotide anchor strands may enhance bone formation near the surface of an implant installed in bone.

Ramazanoglu et al. [38] studied whether coating implant surfaces with rhBMP-2 and recombinant human vascular endothelial growth factor I65 (rhVEGFI65) affects osseointegration in pigs. Five different groups of implants: (1) acid-etched surface (AE; control group); (2) CaP coated surface (CaP group); (3) CaP bearing incorporated rhBMP-2 (BMP group); (4) CaP bearing incorporated rhVEGFI65 (VEGF group); and (5) CaP bearing incorporated rhBMP-2 + rhVEGFI65 (BMP + VEGF group) were established and tested in the frontal skulls of 9 pigs. Osseointegration was assessed by histomorphometric analysis of bone formation at 1, 2, and 4 weeks. At 2 weeks, the BMP and BMP + VEGF groups showed significant enhancement in BV density compared to the AE control group. All implants with CaP coating demonstrated significant enhanced BIC rates compared with the AE controls at 2 weeks. However, the BMP + VEGF group did not significantly enhance BIC at 4 weeks. It was concluded that the biomimetic CaP coated implant surfaces with both BMP and VEGF enhances BV density, but not BIC.

Schliephake et al. [39] tested whether rhVEGF stimulates peri-implant bone formation in rats. Three different implant surfaces: (1) sandblasted acid-etch (SAE) implants; (2) SAE implants coated with DNA oligonucleotide anchor strands (SAE + OAS); and (3) SAE + OAS hybridized with rhVEGF-conjugated to complementary oligonucleotide strands, were studied in the tibiae of 36 rats. The BIC and BD were assessed 1, 4, and 13 weeks after implant placement. Implant surfaces with rhVEGF hybridization showed the highest BIC 1 month after implant placement. It was concluded that rhVEGF can accelerate BIC to a certain extent.

Modification of dental implant surfaces with peptides (Table 3)

Germanier et al. [40] investigated whether implant surfaces with Arg-Gly-Asp (RGD)-peptide-modified polymer could enhance early bone apposition in the maxillae of miniature pigs. Test and control implants had the same microrough structure identical to SLA surfaces, but differed in their surface chemistry coating. Four different implant surfaces: (1) SLA without

Table 3 Surface modification of dental implants with peptides

Author	Animal – bone site	Surface modification	Length of study	Findings
Germanier et al. [40]	Pig – maxilla	1. SLA (control) 2. SLA + PLL-*g*-PEG 3. SLA + PLL-*g*-PEG/PEG-RDG 4. SLA + PLL-*g*-PEG/PEG-RGD	2 and 4 weeks	% of BIC - SLA: 43.6% at 2 weeks, 62.5% at 4 weeks - SLA + PLL-*g*-PEG: 55.9% at 2 weeks, 67.4% at 4 weeks - SLA + PLL-*g*-PEG/PEG-RDG: 48.5% at 2 weeks, 75.5% at 4 weeks - SLA + PLL-*g*-PEG/PEG-RGD: 61.7% at 2 weeks, 62.5% at 4 weeks
Barros et al. [41]	Dog – mandible	1. A: microstructured + HA + low concentrated (20 µg/ml) peptide 2. B: microstructured + HA 3. C: microstructured 4. D: microstructured + HA + high concentrated (200 µg/ml) peptide	12 weeks	% of BIC - A: 60.4% - B: 62.4% - C: 58.0% - D: 65.4% BD - A: 54.7% - B: 46.0% - C: 45.3% - D: 40.7%
Yang et al. [42]	Rabbit – femur and tibia	1. Control: uncoated 2. RGD-coated	4, 8, and 12 weeks	% of BIC - Control: 50.2%, 58.5%, and 60.9% at 4, 8, and 12 weeks, respectively - RGD-coated: 70.0%, 74.9%, and 82.2% at 4, 8, and 12 weeks, respectively
Lutz et al. [43]	Pig – forehead	1. Group A: HA 2. Group B: HA + P-15 (20 µg/ml) 3. Group C: HA + P-15 (200 µg/ml)	14 and 30 days	% of BIC for ROI A and ROI B, respectively - A: 63.8 & 76.7% at 14 days, 70.9 & 75.8% at 30 days - B: 72.1 & 72.5% at 14 days, 69.9 & 74.6% at 30 days - C: 88.2 & 88.7% at 14 days, 80.5 & 88.5% at 30 days BD for ROI A and ROI B, respectively - A: 49.5 & 36.2% at 14 days, 38.4 & 28.7% at 30 days - B: 44.0 & 31.6% at 14 days, 45.7 & 42.9% at 30 days - C: 44.9 & 36.1% at 14 days, 47.2 & 44.5% at 30 days
Yoo et al. [44]	Rabbit - tibia	1. Anodized Ti implant (control) 2. PLGA/rhBMP-2 coated	3 and 7 weeks	% of BIC (total) - Control: 27.26% at 3 weeks; 31.47% at 7 weeks - PLGA/rhBMP-2: 34.69% at 3 weeks; 35.32% at 7 weeks

SLA sandblasted and acid-etched surface; *PLL-g-PEG* poly(L-lysine)-graft-poly(ethylene glycol); *RDG* Arg-Asp-Gly; *RGD* Arg-Gly-Asp; *BIC* bone to implant contact; *BD* bone density; *HA* hydroxyapatite; *P-15* P-15 peptide; *ROI* region of interest coating as control; and coating with (2) poly(L-lysine)-graft-poly(ethylene glycol) (PLL-*g*-PEG); (3) PLL-*g*-PEG/PEG-RGD; or (4) PLL-*g*-PEG/PEG-Arg-Asp-Gly(RDG) were examined histomorphometrically for osteoblastic activity and bone apposition. The RGD-modified implants demonstrated significant increase in BIC apposition at 2 weeks as compared with the controls. However, no further significant increase in percentage of BIC was observed in RGD-coated implants at 4 weeks as compared to the controls. On the contrary, the PEG and PEG/RDG groups did show significantly higher BIC than the control group at 4 weeks. It was concluded that the PLL-*g*-PEG/PEG-RGD coatings may stimulate greater bone apposition in the very early stages of bone healing following implant placement.

Barros et al. [41] analyzed the effect of a biofunctionalized implant surface on osseointegration in the mandibles of dogs for 12 weeks. All implants were lined by the same microrough surface topography provided by the grit-blasting/acid-etching process to create a micro-structured surface. For biofunctionalization of the implant surface, a low or high concentration of bioactive peptide was absorbed to hydroxyapatite (HA) coatings. Thus, 4 different types of implant surfaces were tested: (1) micro-structured + HA + a low concentration of bioactive peptide (20 μg/mL); (2) micro-structured + HA; (3) micro-structured; and (4) micro-structured + HA + a high concentration of bioactive peptide (200 μg/mL). Implants with 200 μg/mL peptide had the highest mean value of direct BIC, but no statistically significant differences were detected between the groups. In addition, bone density analysis revealed that implant surfaces with 20 μg/mL peptide provided a higher adjacent bone density when compared to the other groups. Nevertheless, the differences between the groups were also not statistically significant. The authors concluded that biofunctionalization of the implant surface might interfere in the bone apposition around implants, especially regarding the aspect of bone density.

Yang et al. [42] compared the ability of uncoated titanium implant surfaces with RGD-coated surfaces to bond to bone in the femurs and tibiae of rabbits. Sixty implants (30 uncoated control and 30 RGD-coated) were inserted into the femurs of 30 rabbits, and 30 implants (15 control and 15 RGD-coated) were installed into the tibias of 15 rabbits. The RGD-coated implants exhibited significantly greater percentages of BIC than those of the control implants at 4, 8, and 12 weeks after implantation. In addition, the RGD-coated implants revealed statistically significant higher removal torque values at 8 and 12 weeks. It was concluded that RGD-coated implants have a positive effect on bone-bonding ability by producing higher BIC and removal torque values.

Lutz et al. [43] studied the influence of a P-15 peptide coated implant on early implant osseointegration in adult pigs for a period of 14 and 30 days. All surfaces of dental implants were grit-blasted and acid-etched followed by HA coating. For the implants in the test group, two concentrations of P-15 (20 μg/ml and 200 μg/ml) were bound to the HA surface. Implants without P-15 coating served as the control group. Implants with the 200 μg/ml P-15 had significantly higher value of BIC at 14 and 30 days compared with the other groups. Both concentrations of P-15 revealed better peri-implant bone density compared to the control group at 30 days. It was concluded that biofunctionalization of the implant surface with a biomimetic active peptide has a positive effect on osseointegration by creating higher percentages of BIC at 14 and 30 days and greater peri-implant bone density at 30 days.

Yoo et al. [44] examined whether biochemical coating of anodized Ti implant surface with poly(lactide-co-glycolide) (PLGA) and BMP-2 stimulates bone growth in rabbits. Eighteen of each group – anodized Ti implants (control group) and implants coated with 80 μL of PLGA and 50 μg/mL of rhBMP-2 (experimental group) – were placed in the tibiae of 8 rabbits for 3 and 7 weeks. Under histomorphometric analysis, the BIC was significantly higher in the PLGA/BMP-2 group than those of the control group at 3 weeks. However, the significant difference disappeared at 7 weeks. The authors concluded that PLGA/BMP-2 coated implants facilitated osseointegration during early healing.

Modification of dental implant surfaces with ECM (Table 4)

Morra et al. [45] investigated whether biochemical modification of the anodized titanium surfaces with collagen (ColpTi) has a positive effect on osseointegration in rabbit femur trabecular bone. Histomorphometric analysis revealed that a higher amount of bone inside the screw threads and in contact with the surface was observed on ColpTi implants at 4 weeks. ColpTi had a significantly higher percentage of BIC compared to the control anodized titanium surface. They concluded that osseointegration in trabecular bone can be enhanced by biochemical surface modification with collagen.

Schliephake et al. [46] examined whether a composite coating of calcium phosphate and mineralized collagen I could enhance peri-implant bone formation. Four types of implants were evaluated in the mandibles of dogs for 3 months by measuring BIC and BV density (BVD). The control group comprised of implants with an uncoated machined titanium surface. The modified groups included implants coated with HA, collagen I, or a composite coating of HA and mineralized collagen I. After 1 month, the percentage of BIC was significantly higher only in the group of implants with the composite

Table 4 Modification of dental implant surfaces with ECM

Author	Animal – bone site	Surface modification	Length of study	Findings
Morra et al. [45]	Rabbit – femur	1. pTi: anodization of titanium implant 2. ColpTi: collagen coated titanium implant	4 weeks	% of BIC - pTi: 36.9% - ColpTi: 63.7% % of bone ingrowth - pTi: 29.0% - ColpTi: 43.3%
Schliephake et al. [46]	Dog - mandible	1. Machined titanium surface (control) 2. Machine + Collagen I (collagen only) 3. Machine + calcium phosphate (HA-only) 4. Machine + calcium phosphate + Collagen I (composite)	1 and 3 months	% of BIC - Control: 31.5% at 1 month, 41.2% at 3 months - Collagen-only: 41.9% at 1 month, 60.2% at 3 months - HA-only: 45.2% at 1 month, 61.7% at 3 months - Composite: 62.6% at 1 month, 59.0% at 3 months BVD - Control: 16.1% at 1 month, 40.6% at 3 months - Collagen-only: 22.9% at 1 month, 62.6% at 3 months - HA-only: 33.0% at 1 month, 58.5% at 3 months - Composite: 40.9% at 1 month, 67.3% at 3 months
Stadlinger et al. [47]	Pig – mandible	1. Coll: collagen type I 2. Coll/CS: collagen type I + chondroitin sulfate 3. Coll/CS/BMP: collagen type I + chondroitin sulfate + BMP-4	22 weeks	% of BIC - Coll: 45% - Coll/CS: 55% - Coll/CS/BMP: 41% Implant stability test at 22 weeks - Coll: ISQ = 73 - Coll/CS: ISQ = 69 - Coll/CS/BMP: ISQ = 67
Ferguson et al. [48]	Sheep – pelvis	1. Ti: sandblasted and acid-etched titanium 2. Zir: sandblasted and etched zirconia 3. CaP: Ti coated with calcium phosphate 4. APC: Ti modified via anodic plasma-chemical treatment 5. Bisphos: bisphosphonate coated Ti 6. Coll/CS: Ti coated with collagen containing chondroitin sulfate	8 weeks	Removal torque values at 8 weeks (N-mm) - Ti: 1,884 - Zir: 1,005 - CaP: 1,683 - APC: 919 - Bisphos: 1,835 - Coll/CS: 1,593
Stadlinger et al. [49]	Pig – mandible	1. Coll: collagen coated Ti 2. Coll/DC: collagen + DC 3. Coll/CS: collagen + CS 4. Coll/DC/TGF: collagen + DC + TGF- β1 5. Coll/CS/BMP: collagen + CS + BMP-4 6. Coll/DC/CS/BMP/TGF: collagen + DC + CS + BMP-4 + TGF- β1	3, 4, 5 and 6 weeks	% of BIC at 3, 4, 5, and 6 weeks Total - Coll: 12.45% - Coll/DC: 12.65% - Coll/CS: 28.28% - Coll/DC/TGF: 16.27% - Coll/CS/BMP: 22.92% - Coll/DC/CS/BMP/TGF: 11.43%
Stadlinger et al. [50]	Pig – mandible	1. Coll: collagen 2. Coll/CS: collagen + CS 3. Coll/CS/BMP-4: collagen + CS + rhBMP-4	6 months	% of BIC - Coll: 30% - Coll/CS: 40% - Coll/CS/rhBMP-4: 27%
Langhoff et al. [51]	Sheep – pelvis	1. Control: sandblasted and acid-etched Ti 2. CaP: calcium phosphate coated 3. APC: plasma anodized 4. Coll/CS: collagen + CS coated 5. Bisphos: bisphosphonate coated 6. Zir: sandblasted and etched zirconia	8 weeks	- All implants were well osseointegrated - No significant differences in % of BIC
Schliephake et al. [52]	Dog – mandible	1. MS: machined surface 2. DAE: dual acid-etched surface 3. RGD: RGD + DAE 4. Coll: collagen I + DAE 5. Coll/CS: collagen I + CS + DAE 6. Coll/CS/BMP-2: collagen I + CS + BMP-2 + DAE	4 and 12 weeks	% of BIC - MS: 25.4% at 4 weeks, 37.7% at 12 weeks - DAE: 40.9% at 4 weeks, 57.6% at 12 weeks - RGD: 41.4% at 4 weeks, 59.4% at 12 weeks - Coll: 40.4% at 4 weeks, 56.3% at 12 weeks - Coll/CS: 31.1% at 4 weeks, 66.4% at 12 weeks - Coll/CS/BMP-2: 43.7% at 4 weeks, 60.6% at 12 weeks
Stadlinger et al. [53]	Pig – mandible	1. Control: sandblasted and acid-etched Ti 2. Coll/CS1: Ti + collagen + low dose CS 3. Coll/CS2: Ti + collagen + high dose CS	1 and 2 months	% of BIC for the entire implant at 1 and 2 months - Control: 51.6% at 1 month, 62.7% at 2 months - Coll/CS1: 68.4% at 1 month, 71% at 2 months - Coll/CS2: 63.1% at 1 month, 67.9% at 2 months

Table 4 Modification of dental implant surfaces with ECM *(Continued)*

Morra et al. [54]	Rabbit – femur and tibia	1. Ti: acid-etched titanium 2. CollTi: collagen type I + Ti	2 and 4 weeks	% of BIC was significantly higher around CollTi when compared with Ti both in femur and tibia at 2 weeks. No significant differences were observed at 4 weeks.
Alghamdi et al. [55]	Dog - mandible	1. Ti (control) 2. Nano-CaP-coated 3. Type I collagen coated	4 and 12 weeks	Overall BV - Ti: 47.5% at 4 weeks; 65.1% at 12 weeks - Nano-CaP: 49.5% at 4 weeks; 67.2% at 12 weeks - Collagen: 61.4% at 4 weeks; 72.7 at 12 weeks Inner zone BV - Ti: 10.5% at 4 weeks; 37.5% at 12 weeks - Nano-CaP: 23.1% at 4 weeks; 38.2% at 12 weeks - Collagen: 28.4% at 4 weeks; 52.4 at 12 week
Stadlinger et al. [56]	Pig - maxilla	1. SAE 2. Collagen type I coating (Coll) 3. Coll + CS (low amount) 4. Coll + CS (high amount) 5. Coll + high-SH 6. Coll + low-SH	4 and 8 weeks	% of BIC - SAE: 56% at 4 weeks; 66.4% at 8 weeks - Coll: 36.8% at 4 weeks; 68.7% at 8 weeks - Coll + CS (low): 70.4% at 4 weeks; 74.7% at 8 weeks - Coll + CS (high): 51.2% at 4 weeks; 63.5% at 8 weeks - Coll + high-SH: 50.3% at 4 weeks; 64.3% at 8 weeks - Coll + low-SH: 53.9% at 4 weeks; 65.5% at 8 weeks BVD - SAE: 23.2% at 4 weeks; 45.2% at 8 weeks - Coll: 26.2% at 4 weeks; 48.9% at 8 weeks - Coll + CS (low): 28.1% at 4 weeks; 54.9% at 8 weeks - Coll + CS (high): 27.4% at 4 weeks; 45.2% at 8 weeks - Coll + high-SH: 23.6% at 4 weeks; 42.9% at 8 weeks - Coll + low-SH: 21.8% at 4 weeks; 46.9% at 8 weeks
Lee et al. [57]	Rabbit - tibia	1. AE (control) 2. HA coating 3. Coll + HA coating 4. Coll + HA + BMP-2 coating	6 weeks	% of BIC - AE: 21.38% - HA coating: 24.18% - Coll + HA coating: 41.45% - Coll + HA + BMP-2 coating: 30.72%

ECM extracellular matrix; *HA* hydroxyapatite; *BVD* newly formed peri-implant bone; *BMP-4* bone morphogenetic protein-4; *Ti* titanium implant; *ISQ* implant stability quotient; *CaP* calcium phosphate; *Bisphos* bisphosphonate; *CS* chondroitin sulfate; *DC* decorin; *TGF-β1* transforming growth factor β1; *rhBMP-4* recombinant human bone morphogenetic protein-4; *RGD* RGD peptide; *SH* sulfate hyaluronan; *AE* acid-etched

coating of calcium phosphate and mineralized collagen I. All coated implants showed significantly higher BVD of newly formed peri-implant bone after 1 month. Both BIC and BVD were significantly greater in all coated implants compared to the controls after 3 months. The authors concluded that coating an implant by biomimetically combining collagen I and HA can enhance BIC and peri-implant bone formation.

Stadlinger et al. [47] studied whether the application of chondroitin sulfate in combination with type I collagen, with or without BMP-4, can augment ossification and thus improve implant stability. One hundred and twenty implants were placed in the mandibles of 20 miniature pigs for 6 months. Three different surface coatings were produced: (1) collagen type I (coll); (2) coll/chondroitin sulfate (coll/CS); and (3) coll/CS/BMP-4 (coll/CS/BMP). Six implants (2 of each type of surface) were randomly installed on either side of the mandible in each minipig. The histomorphometry results demonstrated that the percentage of BIC was highest for coll/CS, followed by coll and coll/CS/BMP. The implant stability, as measured by resonance frequency analysis (RFA), was highest in the coll group. Although statistically significant differences were not observed in both BIC and RFA, coll and coll/CS implant coatings had a positive trend in beneficial characteristics for osseointegration, compared with the further integration of BMP-4.

Using a sheep pelvis model, Ferguson et al. [48] tested 6 different implant surface modifications and their effect on implant osseointegration at 2, 4, and 8 weeks after implantation. Peri-implant bone density and removal torque were analyzed on 6 different implant surfaces: (1) sandblasted and acid-etched titanium (Ti), (2) sandblasted and acid-etched zirconia, (3) Ti coated with calcium phosphate (CaP), (4) Ti modified via anodic plasma-chemical treatment (APC), (5) bisphosphonate-coated Ti (Bisphos), and (6) Ti coated with collagen containing chondroitin sulfate (Coll/CS). No significant differences in peri-implant bone density were identified between groups. Removal torque values for Ti, CaP, Bisphos and Coll/CS were significantly higher than those for zirconia and APC at 8 weeks after implant placement. The authors suggested that biofunctional coating of the implant surface with calcium phosphate, bisphosphonate or collagen containing chondroitin sulfate seems to have the potential to enhance peri-implant bone healing, but no additional benefit can be shown when compared to the effectiveness of SLA surface modification.

Stadlinger et al. [49] examined whether implants coated with extracellular matrix (ECM) components could improve osseointegration in pigs. The 6 surface coatings tested in this study were: (1) collagen (coll); (2) collagen and decorin (coll/DC); (3) collagen and chondroitin sulfate (coll/CS); (4) coll/DC and TGF-β1 (coll/DC/TGF); (5) coll/CS and BMP-4 (coll/CS/BMP); and (6) coll/CS/DC, TGF-β1 and BMP-4 (coll/CS/DC/BMP/TGF). Eight miniature pigs each received 6 implants in the mandible. The highest BIC was observed in coll/CS or coll/CS/BMP coated implants during the 6 weeks of healing, and was statistically higher at weeks 5 and 6 compared to other coatings. The authors implied that implant surfaces coated with coll/CS and coll/CS/BMP could lead to a higher degree of bone formation compared to other ECM components.

Stadlinger et al. [50] tested whether the addition of chondroitin sulfate (CS) and rhBMP-4 on a collagen-coated (coll) implant could further improve osseointegration in pigs. One hundred and twenty implants with 3 distinct surface coatings (coll, coll/CS, and coll/CS/rhBMP-4) were placed into the mandibles of 20 minipigs. The percentage of BIC was measured 6 months after implantation by histomorphometric analysis. The highest percentage of BIC was observed in coll/CS (40%), followed by coll (30%) and coll/CS/rhBMP-4 (27%). The authors suggested that the addition of CS to a collagen coated implant could promote osseointegration. However, further inclusion of a fairly low amount of rhBMP-4 had a negative effect on bone formation compared to coll/CS.

Langhoff et al. [51] compared 6 modified implant surfaces for osseointegration in a sheep pelvis model for 8 weeks. The six types of dental implant surfaces tested in this study were: (1) sandblasted and acid-etched (control), (2) calcium phosphate (CaP), (3) plasma anodized (APC), (4) type I collagen + chondroitin sulfate (coll/CS), (5) bisphosphonate (BisP), and (6) zirconia (Zr). All tested implants revealed decent osseointegration with only slight differences compared to the control implant surfaces. New bone formation was observed around all tested implants in the cancellous bone by 2 weeks and built up steadily until 8 weeks. The authors concluded that there were no significant differences in osseointegration between the six different implant surfaces. However, there was a clear tendency for col/CS, CaP and BisP to show better BIC values at 8 weeks compared to APC or Zr.

In the mandibles of foxhounds, Schliepake et al. [52] evaluated whether organic coatings on an implant surface could enhance peri-implant bone formation. Six types of implants were examined histomorphometrically in each foxhound: (1) machined surface (MS), (2) dual acid-etched surface (DAE), (3) DAE coated with RGD (RGD), (4) DAE coated with type I collagen (coll), (5) DAE coated with coll and chondroitin sulfate (coll/CS), and (6) coll/CS and rhBMP-2 (coll/CS/BMP-2). After 1 month, all coated implant groups exhibited significantly higher BIC values than that of the MS group, but not from that of the DAE group. After 3 months, with the exception of the coll group, the same held true for the mean BIC of all coated DAE groups. The mean BVD of the newly formed peri-implant bone did not reach a significant difference among any of the surfaces in 1 and 3 months. The authors concluded that organic coatings with coll, RGD, or CS with or without rhBMP-2 on DAE implant surface did not enhance peri-implant BV density when compared with the DAE surfaces, but did improve BIC when compared with the MS surfaces. It appears that the organic coatings did not offer further benefits than the benefits of DAE surfaces.

Stadlinger et al. [53] investigated whether coating an implant surface with collagen and chondroitin sulfate would enhance bone formation and implant stability, compared with an uncoated control. Three different implant surfaces, (1) sandblasted acid-etched implants (control), (2) collagen with low dose chondroitin sulfate (CS1), and (3) collagen with high dose chondroitin sulfate (CS2), were tested in the mandibles of 20 minipigs. Bone formation was determined by the percentage of BIC and relative peri-implant BV density (rBVD) after 1 and 2 months of healing, whereas implant stability was measured by RFA. Coated implants had significantly higher BIC compared with controls after 1 month of healing, but no significant difference could be found between CS1 and CS2. The percentage of BIC was increased for all surfaces after 2 months of healing; however, no significant differences were identified among the three groups. Similarly, no statistical differences in rBVD and RFA were found. It was concluded that collagen/CS has an encouraging effect on bone formation in short-term healing.

Morra et al. [54] investigated the effect of collagen covalently linked to acid-etched implants on peri-implant bone formation. Implants were installed in rabbit femurs and tibiae for up to 4 weeks. Histomorphometric analysis at 2 weeks revealed that significantly higher BIC was observed in collagen coated implants both in femurs and tibiae. On the other hand, no significant differences in BIC were detected at 4 weeks. The authors concluded that type I collagen covalently linked to acid-etched Ti implant surfaces could enhance peri-implant bone formation during early healing.

In the mandibles of dogs, Alghamdi et al. [55] evaluated whether type I collagen improves peri-implant bone formation. Three types of implants: (1) non-coated Ti implants; (2) nano-CaP-coated Ti implants; and (3) type I collagen-coated implants were placed in the mandibles of 16 beagle dogs 3 months after tooth extraction. Both histomorphometry and micro-CT were measured to evaluate peri-implant bone formation at 4 and 12 weeks after implant placement. Three different zones (inner: 0-300 μm; middle: 300-600 μm; and outer: 600-1000 μm) of bone around the implant surfaces were assessed. Nano-CaP and collagen-coated implants demonstrated a significantly higher BV in the inner zone compared to non-coated implants at 4 weeks. However, no significant difference was identified in the BV between all groups at 12 weeks as indicated by both histomorphometric and micro-CT analysis. It was concluded that collagen modification of implant surfaces did not improve peri-implant bone formation.

Stadlinger et al. [56] evaluated whether extracellular matrix coating on implant surfaces increases bone formation in minipigs. Six different implant surfaces were created and tested in the maxillae of 20 minipigs: (1) SAE Ti implant; (2) collagen type I coated implants; (3) collagen type I + low amount of CS ; (4) collagen type I + high amount of CS; (5) collagen type I + high-sulfate hyaluronan; and (6) collagen type I + low-sulfate hyaluronan. The BIC and BV density were measured using histomorphometric analysis at 4 and 8 weeks after implant placement. ISQ values were obtained for implant stability. Implants coated with the lower CS and collagen showed significantly more BIC compared to all other groups at 4 weeks. However, the only significant difference in BIC at 8 weeks was found between the lower CS group and the control group. The differences in BV density and ISQ value were not statistically significant at both 4 and 8 weeks. In addition, a higher concentration of CS and the application of sulfate hyaluronan exhibited no increase in BIC. It was concluded that the coating of extracellular matrix exhibited no beneficial effect in the aspect of BV density and ISQ value.

In the tibiae of rabbits, Lee et al. [57] studied whether implant surfaces coated with HA and type I collagen influence peri-implant bone formation. Four different implant surfaces were prepared and tested in 12 New Zealand rabbits: (1) uncoated control (acid-etched); (2) HA coated; (3) collagen + HA coated; and (4) collagen + HA + BMP-2. Peri-implant bone formation and BIC were assessed by histomorphometric analysis 6 weeks after implant placement. Under the histomorphometric analysis, only the collagen + HA coating surfaces displayed significantly greater peri-implant bone formation and BIC. Furthermore, adding BMP-2 to the implant surface did not show any advantage compared to the collagen + HA coating surface. It was concluded that collagen and HA coatings significantly increased new bone formation and BIC compared to the other coatings, and the additional BMP-2 coating did not display further benefits.

Discussion

The primary intention of endosseous implant surface modifications is to absolutely modulate the implant and host tissue response and accomplish better osseointegration. This review evaluated whether bioactive surface modifications are capable of enhancing osseointegration in comparison to uncoated titanium surfaces in animals. This review has identified 34 research articles that used histomorphometric analysis to evaluate peri-implant bone formation in animals. Four categories of biomolecular coatings, including BMP, non-BMP growth factors, peptides, and ECM, were established in this review. Several different animal models were used in these 34 studies, suggesting different dynamics of bone formation especially in early healing times [58]. These factors may influence for the observed BIC values.

Four out of 8 BMP coating studies reported a positive effect on implant osseointegration [25, 26, 30, 31]. Among those 4 studies, two studies demonstrated a positive effect only with higher concentrations of BMP. Five out of 8 of the other growth factor coating studies reported an encouraging effect on peri-implant bone formation [32–34, 37, 39]. Whereas, 4 out of 5 studies in the peptide coating category exhibited a promising effect on osseointegration [40, 42–44]. Among those 4 studies, two of them reported a positive effect only at the early healing stage. Finally, there were 7 out of 13 studies for the ECM coating group that revealed a positive effect on bone formation. Two of the 7 studies showed that osseointegration was enhanced when two types of ECM were coated on implant surfaces. Therefore, bioactive surface modifications on implant surfaces do not always offer a beneficial effect on osseointegration. This review is partially in line with the systematic review and meta-analysis conducted by Jenny et al. [59]

One reason for the observed BIC variances in different animals could be the overall faster bone regeneration in dogs compared to pigs [59]. Therefore, the observed BIC may not reflect the actual effect of the specific type of surface modification on osseointegration in different animal models. Another factor that may influence peri-implant bone formation is the anatomic location of the implant placement as the dynamics of bone formation differ in different locations. It was reported that the percentage of BIC for implants coated with growth factors increased in extraoral locations and decreased in intraoral ones [59]. Furthermore, the time of healing in different animals may also play a critical role in the aspect of osseointegration. Implant healing time showed large variation ranging from 1 week to 6 months. However, some studies assessed a single time point, while others evaluated up to four time points.

In summary, the present review assessed the impact of bioactive surface modifications on implant osseointegration.

It was difficult to conclude that biological implant surface coating offers a beneficial effect on peri-implant bone formation. Readers must keep in mind that all these factors make the inter-study comparison more difficult and further complicate the interpretation of results. Furthermore, long-term prospective clinical studies in humans are required to verify whether a positive effect in animals will translate to humans.

Conclusions

Bioactive surface modifications on implant surfaces do not always offer a beneficial effect on osseointegration. Nevertheless, surface modifications of titanium dental implants with biomolecular coatings seem to promote peri-implant bone formation, resulting in enhanced osseointegration during the early stages of healing. Several factors make the inter-study comparison more difficult and further complicate the interpretation of results in peri-implant bone formation. However, long-term clinical studies are needed to validate the long-term success of biomolecular coated implants. Furthermore, it must be kept in mind that results of animal experiments need not necessarily reflect the human clinical reality.

Abbreviations

APC: Anodic plasma-chemical; BIC: Bone to implant contact; Bisphos: Bisphosphonate-coated; BMPs: Bone morphogenetic proteins; BVD: Bone volume density; CaP: Calcium phosphate; CaP/BMP-2 ads + inc: Bone morphogenetic protein-2 adsorbed to and incorporated into calcium phosphate-coated titanium surfaces; CaPTi: Calcium phosphate-coated titanium surfaces; CaPTi/BMP-2 ads: Bone morphogenetic protein-2 adsorbed to calcium phosphate-coated titanium surfaces; CaPTi/BMP-2 inc: Bone morphogenetic protein-2 incorporated into calcium phosphate-coated titanium surfaces; Coll: Collagen type I; Coll/CS: Collagen type I/chondroitin sulfate; Coll/CS/BMP: Collagen/chondroitin sulfate/bone morphogenetic protein; Coll/CS/BMP-4: Collagen type I/chondroitin sulfate/bone morphogenetic protein-4; Coll/CS/DC/BMP/TGF: Collagen/chondroitin sulfate/decorin/ bone morphogenetic protein/ transforming growth factor; Coll/CS/rhBMP-4: Collagen/chondroitin sulfate/bone morphogenetic protein-4; Coll/DC: Collagen/decorin; Coll/DC/TGF: Collagen/decorin/transforming growth factor; ColpTi: Anodized titanium surfaces with collagen; CSA: Chromosulfuric acid; DAE: Dual acid-etched; ECM: Extracellular matrix; FGF-FN: Fibroblast growth factor-fibronectin; HA: Hydroxyapatite; MS: Machined surface; Pi: Push-in type; PLGA: Poly(lactide-co-glycolide); PLL-g-PEG: Poly(L-lysine)-graft-poly(ethylene glycol); PRGF: Plasma-rich growth factor; rBVD: Relative peri-implant bone volume density; RDG: (Arg-Asp-Gly) peptide; RFA: Resonance frequency analysis; RGD: (Arg-Gly-Asp) peptide; rhbFGF: Recombinant human basic fibroblast growth factor; rhBMP-2: Recombinant human bone morphogenetic protein-2; rhIGF-1: Recombinant human insulin-like growth factor-1; SLA: Sandblasted and acid-etched; St: Screw type; TGF-β1: Transforming growth factor β1; Ti: Titanium surfaces; Ti/BMP-2 ads: Bone morphogenetic protein-2 adsorbed to uncoated titanium surfaces; TPO: Titanium porous oxide; Zr: Zirconia

Acknowledgements

Not applicable.

Funding

This study is self-funded.

Authors' contributions

HM participated in the design of the study, carried out the literature search and drafted the manuscript. EC conceived of the study, and participated in its design and helped to draft the manuscript. HC critically reviewed and edited this manuscript. All authors read and approved the final manuscript.

Competing interests

The authors declare that they have no competing interests.

Author details

[1]Department of Periodontics, University of Texas School of Dentistry at Houston, Houston, TX, USA. [2]College of Dentistry, The Ohio State University, Columbus, OH, USA. [3]Division of Periodontology, College of Dentistry, The Ohio State University, 305 West 12th Avenue, Columbus, OH 43210, USA.

References

1. Sohn D, Lee JK, An K. Minor tooth movements using microimplant anchorage: case reports. Implant Dent. 2008;17:32–9.
2. Brånemark P, Adell R, Breine U, Hansson B, Lindström J, Ohlsson A. Intra-osseous anchorage of dental prostheses. I. Experimental studies. Scand J Plast Reconstr Surg. 1969;3:81–100.
3. Albrektsson T, Brånemark P, Hansson H, Lindström J. Osseointegrated titanium implants. Requirements for ensuring a long-lasting, direct bone-to-implant anchorage in man. Acta Orthop Scand. 1981;52:155–70.
4. Zarb G, Albrektsson T. Osseointegration: A requiem for the periodontal ligament? Int J Periodontics Restorative Dent. 1991;11:81–91.
5. Albrektsson T, Sennerby L. State of the art in oral implants. J Clin Periodontol. 1991;18:474–81.
6. Albrektsson T, Wennerberg A. Oral implant surfaces: part I. review focusing on topographic and chemical properties of different surfaces and in vivo responses to them. Int J Prosthodont. 2004;17:536–43.
7. Novaes A, Papalexiou V, Grisi M, Souza S, Taba M, Kajiwara J. Influence of implant microstructure on the osseointegration of immediate implants placed in periodontally infected sites. A histomorphometric strudy in dogs. Clin Oral Implants Res. 2004;15:34–43.
8. Buser D, Nydegger T, Oxland T, et al. Interface shear strength of titanium implants with a sandblasted and acid-etched surface: a biomechanical study in the maxilla of miniature pigs. J Biomed Mater Res A. 1999;45:75–83.
9. Al-Nawas B, Groetz K, Goetz H, Duschner H, Wagner W. Comparative histomorphometry and resonance frequency analysis of implants with moderately rough surfaces in a loaded animal model. Clin Oral Implants Res. 2008;19:1–8.
10. Klokkevold P, Johnson P, Dadgostari S, Caputo A, Davies J, Nishimura R. Early endosseous integration enhanced by dual acid etching of titanium: a torque removal study in the rabbit. Clin Oral Implants Res. 2001;12:350–7.
11. Burgos P, Rasmusson L, Meirelles L, Senerby L. Early bone tissue response to turned and oxidized implants in a rabbit tibia. Clin Implant Dent Relat Res. 2008;10:181–90.
12. Huang Y, Xiropaidis A, Sorensen R, Albandar J, Hall J, Wikesjo U. Bone formation of titanium porous oxide (TiUnite) oral implants in type IV bone. Clin Oral Implants Res. 2005;16:105–11.
13. Mendes V, Moineddin R, Davies J. The effect of discrete calcium phosphate nanocrystals on bone-bonding to titanium surfaces. Biomaterials. 2007;28:4748–55.
14. Mendes V, Moineddin R, Davies J. Discrete calcium phosphate nanocrystalline deposition enhances osteoconduction on titanium based implant surfaces. J Biomed Mater Res A. 2009;90:577–85.
15. The American Academy of Periodontology. Glossary of Periodontal Terms, 4th ed. Chicago: The American Academy of Periodontology; 2001.
16. Badr N, Hadary A. Hydroxyapatite-electroplated cp-titanium implant and its bone integration potentiality: an in vivo study. Implant Dent. 2007;16:297–308.
17. Zagury R, Harari N, Conz M, Soares A, Vidigal G. Histomorphometric analyses of bone interface with titanium-aluminum-vanadium and hydroxyapatite-coated implants by biomimetic process. Implant Dent. 2007;16:290–6.
18. Cooper L, Zhou Y, Takebe J. Fluoride modification effects on osteoblast behavior and bone formation at TiO_2 grit-blasted c.p. titanium endosseous implants. Biomaterials. 2006;27:926–36.

19. Ellingsen J, Johansson C, Wennerberg A, Holmén A. Improved retention and bone-to-implant contact with fluoride-modified titanium implants. Int J Oral Maxillofac Implants. 2004;19:659–66.
20. Novaes A, Souza S, Barros R, Pereira K, Iezzi G, Piattelli A. Influence of implant surfaces on osseointegration. Braz Dent J. 2010;21:471–81.
21. Stanford C. Surface modification of biomedical and dental implants and the processes of inflammation, wound healing and bone formation. Int J Mol Sci. 2010;11:354–69.
22. Kim TI, Jang JH, Kim HW, Knowles JC, Ku Y. Biomimetic approach to dental implants. Curr Pharm Des. 2008;14:2201–11.
23. Junker R, Dimakis A, Thoneick M, Jansen JA. Effects of implant surface coatings and composition on bone integration: a systematic review. Clin Oral Implants Res. 2009;20:185–206.
24. Becker J, Kirsch A, Schwarz F, et al. Bone apposition to titanium implants biocoated with recombinant human bone morphogenetic protein-2 (rhBMP-2). A pilot study in dogs. Clin Oral Investig. 2006;10:217–24.
25. Lan J, Wang ZF, Shi B, Xia HB, Cheng XR. The influence of recombinant human BMP-2 on bone-implant osseointegration: biomechanical testing and histomorphometric analysis. Int J Oral Maxillofac Surg. 2007;36:345–9.
26. Liu Y, Enggist L, Kuffer AF, Buser D, Hunziker EB. The influence of BMP-2 and its mode of delivery on the osteoconductivity of implant surfaces during the early phase of osseointegration. Biomaterials. 2007;28:2677–86.
27. Wikesjo UM, Xiropaidis AV, Qahash M, et al. Bone formation at recombinant human bone morphogenetic protein-2-coated titanium implants in the posterior mandible (Type II bone) in dogs. J Clin Periodontol. 2008;35:985–91.
28. Wikesjo U, Huang Y, Xiropaidis A, et al. Bone formation at recombinant human bone morphogenetic protein-2-coated tetanium implants in the posterior maxilla (Type IV bone) in non-human promates. J Clin Periodontol. 2008;35:992–1000.
29. Huh JB, Kim SE, Kim HE, et al. Effects of anodized implants coated with Escherichia coli-derived rhBMP-2 in beagle dogs. Int J Oral Maxillofac Surg. 2012;41:1577–84.
30. Hunziker EB, Enggist L, Küffer A, Buser D, Liu Y. Osseointegration: the slow delivery of BMP-2 enhances osteoinductivity. Bone. 2012;51:98–106.
31. Kim NH, Lee SH, Ryu JJ, Choi KH, Huh JB. Effects of rhBMP-2 on sandblasted and acid etched titanium implant surfaces on bone regeneration and osseointegration: Spilt-mouth designed pilot study. Biomed Res Int. 2015;Article ID:459393.
32. Anitua E. Enhancement of osseointegration by generating a dynamic immplant surface. J Oral Implantol. 2006;32:72–6.
33. Lan J, Wang Z, Wang Y, Wang J, Cheng X. The effect of combinant human bone morphogenetic protein-2 and basic fibroblast growth factor or insulin-like growth factor-I on dental implant osseointegration by confocal laser scanning microscopy. J Periodontol. 2006;77:357–63.
34. Park JM, Koak JY, Jang JH, Han CH, Kim SK, Heo SJ. Osseointegration of anodized titanium implants coated with fibrobalst growth factor-fibronectin (FGF-FN) fusion protein. Int J Oral Maxillofac Implants. 2006;21:859–66.
35. Nikolidakis D, Meijer GJ, Oortgiesen DA, Walboomers XF, Jansen JA. The effect of a low dose of transforming growth factor β1 (TFG-β1) on the early bone-healing around oral implants inserted in trabecular bone. Biomaterials. 2009;30:94–9.
36. Schouten C, Meijer GJ, van den Beucken JJ, Spauwen PH, Jansen JA. Effects of implant geometry, surface properties, and TFG-β1 on peri-implant bone response: an experimental study in goats. Clin Oral Implants Res. 2009;20:421–9.
37. Lee SY, Koak JY, Heo SJ, Kim SK, Lee SJ, Nam SY. Osseointegration of anodized titanium implants coated with poly(lactide-co-glycolide)/basic fibrobalst growth factor by electrospray. Int J Oral Maxillofac Implants. 2010;25:315–20.
38. Ramazanoglu M, Lutz R, Ergun C, von Wilmowsky C, Nkenke E, Schlegel KA. The effect of combined delivery of recombinant human bone morphogenetic protein-2 and recombinant human vascular endothelial growth factor 165 from biomimetic calcium-phosphate-coated implants on osseointegration. Clin Oral Implants Res. 2011;22:1433–9.
39. Schliephake H, Rublack J, Förster A, Schwenzer B, Reichert J, Scharnweber D. Functionalization of titanium implants using a modular system for binding and release of VEGF enhances bone-implant contact in a rodent model. J Clin Periodontol. 2015;42:302–10.
40. Germanier Y, Tosatti S, Broggini N, Textor M, Buser D. Enhanced bone apposition around biofunctionalized sandblasted and acid-etched titanium implant surfaces. A histomorphometric study in miniature pigs. Clin Oral Implants Res. 2006;17:251–7.
41. Barros RR, Novaes Jr AB, Papalexiou V, et al. Effect of biofunctionalized implant surface on osseointegration: a histomorphometric study in dogs. Braz Dent J. 2009;20:91–8.
42. Yang GL, He FM, Yang XF, Wang XX, Zhao SF. In vivo evaluation of bone-bonding ability of RGD-coated porous implant using layer-by-layer electrostatic self-assembly. J Biomed Mater Res A. 2009;90:175–85.
43. Lutz R, Srour S, Nonhoff J, Weisel T, Damien CJ, Schlegel KA. Biofunctionalization of titanium implants with a biomimetic active peptide (P-15) promotes early osseointegration. Clin Oral Implants Res. 2010;21:726–34.
44. Yoo SY, Kim SK, Heo SJ, Koak JY, Lee JH, Heo JM. Biochemical responses of anodized titanium implants with a Poly(lactide-co-glycolide)/Bone Morphogenetic Protein-2 submicron particle coating. Part 2: an in vivo study. Int J Oral Maxillofac Implants. 2015;30:754–60.
45. Morra M, Cassinelli C, Cascardo G, et al. Collagen I-coated titanium surfaces: mesenchymal cell adhesion and in vivo evaluation in trabecular bone implants. J Biomed Mater Res A. 2006;78:449–58.
46. Schliephake H, Scharnweber D, Roesseler S, Dard M, Sewing A, Aref A. Biomimetic calcium phosphate composite coating of dental implants. Int J Oral Maxillofac Implants. 2006;21:738–46.
47. Stadlinger B, Pilling E, Huhle M, et al. Influence of extracellular matrix coatings on implant stability and osseointegration: an animal study. J Biomed Mater Res B Appl Biomater. 2007;83:222–31.
48. Ferguson SJ, Langhoff JD, Voelter K, et al. Biomechanical comparison of different surface modifications for dental implants. Int J Oral Maxillofac Implants. 2008;23:1037–46.
49. Stadlinger B, Pilling E, Mai R, et al. Effect of biological implant surface coatings on bone formation, applying collagen, proteoglycans, glycosaminoglycans and growth facotrs. J Mater Sci Mater Med. 2008;19:1043–9.
50. Stadlinger B, Pilling E, Huhle M, et al. Evaluation of osseointegration of dental implants coated with collagen, chondroitin sulphate and BMP-4: an animal study. Int J Oral Maxillofac Surg. 2008;37:54–9.
51. Langhoff D, Voelter K, Scharnweber D, et al. Comparison of chemically and pharmaceutically modified titanium and zirconia implant surfaces in dentistry: a study in sheep. Int J Oral Maxillofac Surg. 2008;37:1125–32.
52. Schliephake H, Aref A, Scharnweber D, Bierbaum S, Sewing A. Effect of modifications of dual acid-etched implant surfaces on peri-implant bone formation. Part I: organic coatings. Clin Oral Implants Res. 2009;20:31–7.
53. Stadlinger B, Bierbaum S, Grimmer S, et al. Increased bone formation around coated implants. J Clin Periodontol. 2009;36:698–704.
54. Morra M, Cassinelli C, Cascardo G, Bollati D, Rodriguez Y, Baena R. Multifunctional implant surfaces: surface characterization and bone response to acid-etched Ti implants surface-modified by fibrillar collagen I. J Biomed Mater Res A. 2010;94:271–9.
55. Alghamdi HS, van Oirschot BA, Bosco R, et al. Biological response to titanium implants coated with nanocrystals calcium phosphate or type 1 collagen in a dog model. Clin Oral Implants Res. 2013;24:475–83.
56. Stadlinger B, Hintze V, Bierbaum S, et al. Biological functionalization of dental implants with collagen and glycosaminoglycans - a comparative study. J Biomed Mater Res B Appl Biomater. 2012;100:331–41.
57. Lee SW, Hahn BD, Kang TY, et al. Hydroxyapatite and collagen combination-coated dental implants display better bone formation in the peri-implant area than the same combination plus bone morphogenetic protein-2-coated implants, hydroxyapatite only coated implants, and uncoated implants. J Oral Maxillofac Surg. 2014;72:53–60.
58. Pearce AI, Richards RG, Milz S, Schneider E, Pearce SG. Animal models for implant biomaterial research in bone: a review. Eur Cell Mater. 2007;13:1–10.
59. Jenny G, Jauernik J, Bierbaum S, et al. A systematic review and meta-analysis on the influence of biological implant surface coatings on periimplant bone formation. J Biomed Mater Res A. 2016;104:2898–910.

14

c-MYB is a transcriptional regulator of *ESPL1*/ Separase in *BCR-ABL*-positive chronic myeloid leukemia

Wiltrud Prinzhorn*, Michael Stehle, Helga Kleiner, Sabrina Ruppenthal, Martin C. Müller, Wolf-Karsten Hofmann, Alice Fabarius and Wolfgang Seifarth

Abstract

Background: Genomic instability and clonal evolution are hallmarks of progressing chronic myeloid leukemia (CML). Recently, we have shown that clonal evolution and blast crisis correlate with altered expression and activity of Separase, a cysteine endopeptidase that is a mitotic key player in chromosomal segregation and centriole duplication. Hyperactivation of Separase in human hematopoietic cells has been linked to a feedback mechanism that posttranslationally stimulates Separase proteolytic activity after imatinib therapy-induced reduction of Separase protein levels.

Methods and Results: In search for potential therapy-responsive transcriptional mechanisms we have investigated the role of the transcription factor c-MYB for Separase expression in CML cell lines (LAMA-84, K562, BV-173) and in clinical samples. Quantitative RT-PCR and Western blot immunostaining experiments revealed that c-MYB expression levels are decreased in an imatinib-dependent manner and positively correlate with Separase expression levels in cell lines and in clinical CML samples. RNA silencing of c-MYB expression in CML cell lines resulted in reduced Separase protein levels. Gelshift and ChIP assays confirmed that c-MYB binds to a putative c-MYB binding sequence located within the ESPL1 promoter.

Conclusions: Our data suggest that *ESPL1*/Separase is a regulatory target of c-MYB. Therefore, c-MYB, known to be required for BCR-ABL-dependent transformation of hematopoietic progenitors and leukemogenesis, may also control the Separase-dependent fidelity of mitotic chromosomal segregation and centriole duplication essential for maintenance of genomic stability.

Keywords: *ESPL1*/Separase, c-MYB, CML, Imatinib, BCR-ABL, Genomic stability

Background

ESPL1/Separase, a cysteine endopeptidase, is a key player of chromosomal segregation and centrosome duplication. In mitotic anaphase, it accomplishes proteolytic cleavage of Cohesin, a "glue" multi-protein complex that is responsible for cohesion of sister chromatids and of mother and daughter centrioles, the perpendicular oriented core structures of centrosomes [1–3]. Proper temporal and spatial activation of Separase proteolytic activity warrants chromosomal fidelity by establishing an accurate chromosomal segregation [4]. Furthermore, it is an essential prerequisite for semiconservative centriole duplication as the disengagement of mother and daughter centrioles licenses the cell cycle-associated duplication of centrosomes [5]. Failure to do so will result in premature segregation of chromatids and/or formation of anaphase bridges from lagging chromosomes [6]. Moreover, unscheduled (cell cycle uncoupled) activation of Separase can lead to aberrant high numbers of centrosomes (i.e. centrosome amplification) and subsequently to a defective mitotic spindle apparatus [7]. Both defects cause the emergence of aberrant karyotypes (aneuploidy), a hallmark of most advanced human malignancies [8–10]. In non-malignant cells where chromosome segregation

* Correspondence: wiltrud.haass@medma.uni-heidelberg.de
III. Medizinische Klinik (Hämatologie und Onkologie), Wissenschaftliches Labor, Medizinische Fakultät Mannheim der Universität Heidelberg, Pettenkofer Str. 22, 68169 Mannheim, Germany

and centrosomal duplication are tightly coupled to the cell cycle, Separase is temporary activated on metaphase to anaphase transition [11, 12]. Separase is tightly regulated on both translational and posttranslational levels. The latter includes multiple inhibitory mechanisms combining Securin binding, specific serine residue phosphorylation (pSer1126) by CyclinB1/CDK1, autocatalytic cleavage, and PP2A-dependent stabilization of Separase-bound Securin. All these mechanisms work together to prevent ectopic and unscheduled activation of intracellular Separase molecules [13–16].

In human cancer, *ESPL1*/Separase is frequently overexpressed and the resulting deregulated proteolytic activity is associated with the occurrence of supernumerary centrosomes, chromosomal missegregation and aneuploidy [6, 9, 13, 17]. Overexpression of Separase in the mammary gland of a MMTV-*ESPL1* mouse model led to the development of highly aneuploid mammary carcinomas with high levels of chromosomal instability and aggressive disease phenotypes [18]. Consequently, Separase has been identified as an aneuploidy promoter that, when overexpressed and hyperactive, functions as an oncogene and renders cells susceptible not only for chromosomal missegregation-induced aneuploidy but also for DNA damage and loss of key tumor suppressor gene loci associated with tumorigenesis and disease progression [18–20].

This holds true for chronic myeloid leukemia (CML) as well, a clonal neoplastic disorder of hematopoietic stem cells caused by the genomic reciprocal translocation t(9;22)(q34;q11), which results in the formation of the Philadelphia chromosome. The fusion product, a BCR-ABL tyrosine kinase (TK) with deregulated TK activity, is the key player in CML pathogenesis. It affects various downstream signaling pathways by reprogramming the prior lineage commitment of hematopoietic stem and early progenitor cells [21]. Compromising multiple aspects of cellular behavior, including proliferation, apoptosis, cell to cell signaling and differentiation, the BCR-ABL oncoprotein triggers aberrant clonal hematopoiesis and drives disease progression from chronic phase (CP) toward the fully transformed phenotype of blast crisis (BC) [22]. Imatinib (IM) is a selective TK inhibitor (TKI) and presents one of the current first line treatments for CML [23, 24]. Despite significant decreases in BCR-ABL mRNA levels in the bone marrow compartment under IM long-term therapy, persistence of residual CML clones with low BCR-ABL expression and insensitivity to IM treatment makes disease eradication by TKI treatment unlikely [13, 25, 26]. Recent evidence suggests that kinase activity of BCR-ABL oncoprotein in CML stem cells is inhibited by TKI treatment without affecting CML stem cell survival [27, 28]. Obviously, additional cellular mechanisms promote CML stem cell survival and maintenance, rendering these cells TKI resistant and eventually promote relapse [29, 30]. About 35 % of patients in CP develop resistance or intolerance to IM and frequently undergo clonal evolution [31]. Clonal evolution denotes a heterogeneous entity of clonal molecular changes in BCR-ABL-positive hematopoietic stem/progenitor cells and has been described in about 30 % and 80 % of patients in accelerated phase (AP) and BC, respectively [32]. Emergence of altered chromosome numbers, collectively termed aneuploidy, involves an additional derivative chromosome 22, chromosome 17 abnormalities, trisomy 8, and are associated with poor prognosis [33, 34].

Recently, we have reported that enhanced rates of acquired chromosomal aberrations, clonal evolution and fast disease progression (time to BC) in CML patients undergoing long-term IM treatment correlate with enhanced proteolytic activity of Separase in the respective *in vitro* models [35]. Mechanistically, this was linked to a BCR-ABL-dependent regulatory feedback mechanism that posttranslationally stimulates Separase proteolytic activity after IM-induced decreases of Separase expression in b3a2 BCR-ABL fusion type CML cell lines [35]. To date, it was unclear what underlying transcriptional or translational mechanism may be involved in the IM-dependent regulation of Separase expression in BCR-ABL-positive cells.

The transcription factor c-MYB is known to play an important role in BCR-ABL-dependent leukemogenesis. The expression of c-MYB is enhanced by BCR-ABL [36–38]. C-MYB is a 75 KDa nuclear protein and a leucine zipper transcription factor encoded by the proto-oncogene *c-MYB*. It plays a pivotal role in proliferation, survival and differentiation of normal myeloid progenitors [39]. Conditional knockout of *c-MYB* expression in adult hematopoietic stem cells causes loss of self-renewal due to impaired proliferation and accelerated differentiation [40]. On the other hand, overexpression of *c-MYB* in myeloid and erythroid cell lines has been demonstrated to block differentiation and prevents maturation-associated growth arrest [41]. Aberrant (enhanced) *c-MYB* expression has been found in various human malignancies including T-cell leukemia and acute and chronic myeloid leukemias [42]. Moreover, various genetic lesions affecting c-MYB activity in human leukemias, such as chromosomal translocation, gene duplication and truncations have been reported [39, 43, 44]. However, in CML cells, the *c-MYB* gene has been reported to be intact but protein levels are often increased, in part, due to enhanced protein stability via BCR-ABL-regulated activation of PI-3 K/Akt/GSKIIIß dependent pathways [36]. This altered regulatory mechanism has been considered to explain why leukemic blast cells appear to depend on high c-MYB expression levels more than their normal counterparts [45]. Functional studies of c-MYB by ChIP-Seq experiments revealed that c-MYB functions as a hematopoietic master regulator [46]. It binds directly near or within 793 genes thereby affecting more than 2300 genes that make up the gene signatures for normal and leukemic stem/progenitor cells and myeloid development. Despite being usually considered as a transactivator, c-MYB is also able to directly repress many target genes pointing to an important role for myelopoiesis and leukemogenesis through both positive and negative transcriptional regulation [47]. For example, c-MYB modulates the expression of *CD34, c-Kit, c-Myc, Flt-3 and Bcl-2* all playing important roles for proliferation and survival of hematopoietic cells [38]. Moreover, c-MYB directly regulates CyclinB1 expression and contributes to the control of the G2/M cell cycle phase [48, 49], thereby directly controlling one of the key posttranslational inhibitors of Separase [13, 14].

In this study, we set out to investigate the role of c-MYB for the regulation of *ESPL1*/Separase expression in CML. We report that c-MYB binds to a c-MYB binding motif located within the *ESPL1* promoter and functions as a positive regulator of *ESPL1*/Separase expression as demonstrated by *c-MYB*-directed siRNA silencing. Moreover, IM treatment led to equally decreased c-MYB and *ESPL1*/Separase expression levels in CML cell lines and primary cells.

Results

In search for transcriptional mechanisms that could explain the IM-associated downregulation of Separase protein levels we analyzed the conditional context between c-MYB expression, Separase and IM treatment. Confirming and expanding previously published work we performed cell culture experiments on four human cell lines [13, 35]. Of these, U937 cells served as model for leukemic but BCR-ABL-negative cells. All cell lines were treated with therapeutic doses of IM (1 to 5 μM) as performed in our previous studies [13, 50–52]. In accordance with data from extensive studies on the dose-dependent effects and time kinetics of IM we applied lower IM doses (range: 1 to 2.5 μM) for leukemia-derived p210BCR-ABL-positive cells (LAMA-84 and K562) than for p210BCR-ABL-negative cells (U937, 5 μM) [53, 54]. Treating CML cell lines with IM doses higher than 2.5 μM for a longer period than 24 h impeded the collection of sufficient viable cells for Western blot analysis (data not shown).

Concerted decrease of c-MYB and ESPL1 expression levels under IM treatment

Treatment of the CML cell lines LAMA-84 and K562 with therapeutic IM doses for 24 h revealed decreased expression levels for c-MYB and *ESPL1*/Separase on both transcriptional and protein levels as shown on representative Western blot composite images (Fig. 1, Table 1). It should be emphasized that the weak treatment schedule (≤2.5 μM IM for 24 h) still enabled CrkL phosphorylation (Fig. 1, lower panel). Thus, when compared to the respective untreated cells, the decreasing c-MYB protein levels in LAMA-84 (−25.7 ± 9.6 %) and K562 (−37.1 ±

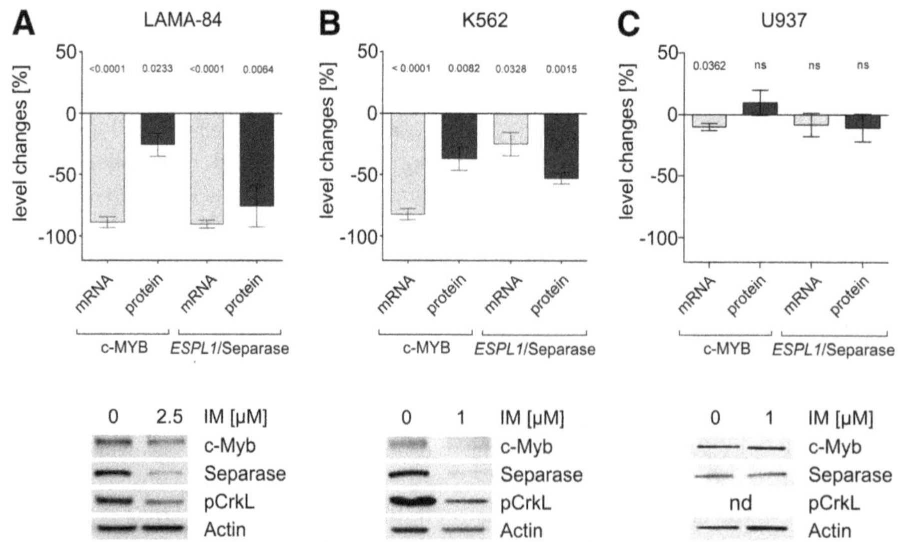

Fig. 1 Analysis of *c-MYB* and *ESPL1* transcript levels, c-MYB and Separase protein levels in LAMA-84 (**a**), K562 (**b**) and BCR-ABL-negative control cells (U937) (**c**) upon IM treatment. Treatment (dose, period) was performed as noted in Table 1. Level changes (Δ-values in %) are shown as calculated from comparison with the corresponding untreated cells. Upper panel. Transcript levels were analyzed by qRT-PCR, protein levels by Western blot immunostaining densitometry. Representative Western blot images are shown in the lower panel. In all qRT-PCR experiments the housekeeping gene *Gus* (beta-glucuronidase) served as internal standard. For Western blot immunostaining experiments Actin was used as loading control and reference parameter. Densitometric data are derived from at least triplicate experiments and are denoted in Table 1. P-values are given above the respective column. Abbreviations: ns, not significant; nd, not determined

Table 1 Percent changes (Δ-values are differences between means) in *c-MYB* and *ESPL1*/Separase transcript and protein levels under IM treatment when compared to corresponding untreated cells

Cell line, dose and period of treatment	*c-MYB* transcript levels[a]	c-MYB protein levels[b]	*ESPL1* transcript levels[a]	Separase protein levels[b]
LAMA-84, 2.5 μM IM, 24 h	−88.8 ± 4.4, $p < 0.0001$	−25.7 ± 9.6, $p = 0.0233$	−90.3 ± 3.3, $p < 0.0001$	−75.8 ± 16.8, $p = 0.0064$
K562, 1 μM IM, 24 h	−82.4 ± 4.4, $p < 0.0001$	−37.1 ± 9.6, $p = 0.0082$	−25.0 ± 9.7, $p = 0.0328$	−53.1 ± 4.4, $p = 0.0015$
U937, 5 μM IM, 48 h	−9.1 ± 2.9, $p = 0.0363$	+9.8 ± 10.2, $p = 0.3942$	−8.1 ± 9.5, $p = 0.4198$	−10.5 ± 11.2, $p = 0.3775$

[a] Δ-values [%] were calculated from at least triplicate qRT-PCR experiments and were normalized to the housekeeping gene *Gus*
[b] Δ-values [%] are derived from at least triplicate Western blot immunostaining experiments. All protein values were normalized to Actin as loading control
Abbreviations: *d* days, *h* hours, *IM* imatinib; + increase, − decrease

9.6 %) cells concurred with decreased *ESPL1* transcript levels of −90 ± 3.3 % and −25.0 ± 9.7 %, respectively. One might argue that the observed decline may be due to IM-related changes in the cell cycle. However, FACS analysis of tested cells revealed no differences neither in G2/M cell proportion nor in the apoptotic cell fraction (<12 %) that could clarify the observed decreases in c-MYB and *ESPL1*/Separase expression levels (compare Fig. 3b in Ref. [13]). Treatment of BCR-ABL-negative control cells (U937) with IM revealed no changes in c-MYB protein and *ESPL1*/Separase expression levels (Table 1, Fig. 1).

Similar results were obtained when paired clinical samples ($n = 5$), each pair derived from the same CML patient before (at diagnosis) and during IM therapy were comparatively monitored for *c-MYB* and *ESPL1* transcript levels (Fig. 2). Two female and three male patients, all with b3a2 *BCR-ABL* fusion type, were analyzed. The median age was 58 years (range, 47 to 78). Mean time between diagnosis and sampling of the second specimen from the same patient after achievement of MMR under IM treatment was 3.6 years (range, 2 to 6.5). These experiments suggest synchronous regulatory mechanisms for c-MYB and *ESPL1*/Separase expression upon IM treatment *in vitro* and *in vivo*.

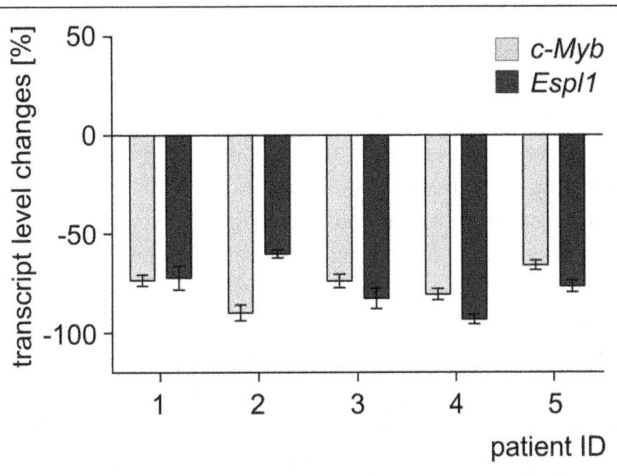

Fig. 2 Comparative analysis of *c-MYB* and *ESPL1* transcript levels in paired cDNA samples of CML patients ($n = 5$) before and under IM therapy. Percent changes (Δ-values are differences between means) are shown corresponding to expression level changes within paired samples, each pair derived from the same patient at differing time points (sample at diagnosis (before IM treatment) vs. sample after major molecular response (MMR) achievement under IM therapy). All transcript levels were normalized to *Gus* and represent mean values of triplicate qRT-PCR assays

Decreased Separase expression levels after c-*MYB* silencing in CML cell lines

To test the direct regulatory influence of c-MYB on Separase expression we silenced *c-Myb* transcription in LAMA-84 and BV-173 cells and monitored the influence of the resulting decline in c-MYB protein levels on Separase expression (Fig. 3). The siRNA-induced decrease in available c-MYB molecules resulted in decreased c-MYB protein levels in BV-173 (−49 ± 13.6 %) and LAMA-84 cells (−47.6 ± 7.9 %). This suggests a direct regulatory relationship between c-MYB and *ESPL1*/Separase.

c-MYB binds to a putative c-MYB recognition site located within the *ESPL1* promoter

The *ESPL1* promoter features two hormone responsive elements and two TP53 binding sites that are located 12,777 and 16,059 bases upstream of the predicted transcription start site (TSS) [20]. For details go to the Human Genome Browser (http://www.ncbi.nlm.nih.gov/gene?cmd=Retrieve&dopt=Graphics&list_uids=9700) and find the TSS at position 53,662,083 (+ strand) of the NC_000012.11 Chromosome 12 Reference GRCh37.913 Primary Assembly. The Champion ChIP Transcription Factor Search Portal based on SABiosciences' proprietary database known as DECODE (DECipherment Of DNA Elements) was used to identify the putative c-MYB binding site within the *Espl1* promoter (for more information see http://www.sabiosciences.com/chipqpcrsearch.php?app=TFBS). A hypothetical c-MYB binding site was found 15,623 bases upstream of the TSS (53,646,460 - 53,646,470) and thus, is located between both TP53 sites (see Fig. 4a). In order to determine whether the putative c-MYB binding site of the *ESPL1* promoter can actually bind the c-MYB protein, we performed electrophoretic mobility shift assays (EMSA). Native nuclear extracts prepared from exponentially growing BV-173 cells were incubated with a FITC-labeled double stranded oligonucleotide (Fig. 4b lane 1) featuring the c-MYB binding site of the *ESPL1* promoter. As shown in Fig. 4b left panel, addition of nuclear extract to the

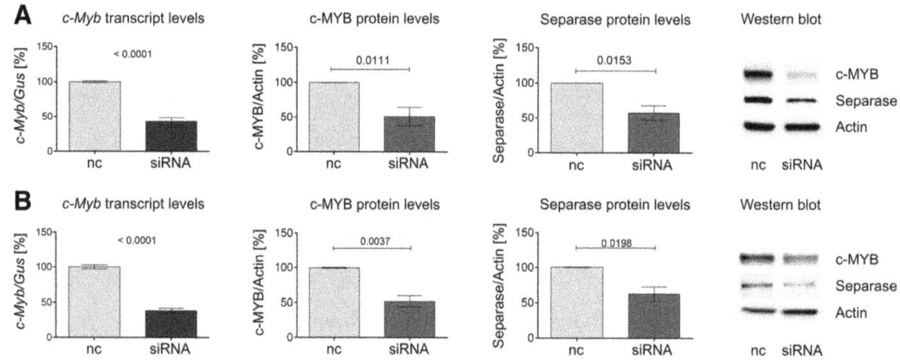

Fig. 3 Separase expression after *c-MYB* silencing by RNAi in BV-173 and LAMA-84 cells. BV-173 (panel **a**) and LAMA-84 cells (panel **b**) were treated with negative control siRNA (nc) and *c-MYB*-specific siRNA (siRNA). *C-MYB* transcript levels are measured by qRT-PCR (left column). The house-keeping gene *Gus* (beta-glucuronidase) served as internal standard. C-MYB and Separase regulation on protein levels were determined by quantitative Western blot immunostaining experiments 48 h post transfection (middle and right columns, respectively). Corresponding representative Western blot images are shown in the very right panels of A and B. Actin served as loading control for Western blot immunostaining. All densitometric data are derived from at least triplicate experiments

FITC-labeled oligonucleotide (lane 2) led to the formation of an oligo/protein complex with retarded electrophoretic migration (shift). Addition to the incubation mix of a 100fold molar excess of unlabeled c-MYB binding site oligonucleotide successfully competed with the formation of the shifted signal (lane 3). For corroboration of c-MYB protein binding, the native agarose gel was blotted under denaturing conditions followed by immunostaining with an anti-c-MYB antibody (right panel). The contribution of c-MYB to the shift signal (lane 2) was confirmed. In addition, the unlabeled competitor oligonucleotide (lane 3) appeared as shifted signal as well confirming specific abrogation of the FITC signal (left panel, lane 3) by the unlabeled competitor DNA. The second and lower band may be due altered electrophoretic mobility of at least some of the native oligo/c-MYB complexes after addition of 100fold excess of the unlabelled competitor. To demonstrate *in vivo* binding of c-MYB protein to the putative c-MYB recognition site located within the *ESPL1* promoter we performed ChIP experiments on BV-173 cells. As shown in Fig. 4c a significant enrichment of ESPL1 promoter-related target DNA was observed when using a c-MYB-specific IgG antibody for chromatin immunoprecipitation when compared to the unspecific IgG antibody control. In summary, our *in vitro* and *in vivo* data suggest that c-MYB directly binds to the *ESPL1* promoter and positively regulates *ESPL1*/Separase expression.

Discussion

In search for transcriptional mechanisms that may explain the previously observed IM-associated downregulation of Separase protein levels in CML [13] followed by posttranslational hyperactivation of Separase proteolytic activity, we have analyzed the conditional context between c-MYB expression, Separase and IM treatment. We found that the transcription factor c-MYB, known to play a pivotal role in proliferation, survival and differentiation of normal myeloid progenitors, is a direct positive regulator of Separase expression. Specifically, we demonstrated by EMSA (Fig. 4b) and ChIP that c-MYB interacts with a putative c-MYB binding motif located within the *ESPL1* promoter. In fact, in all tested CML cell lines (K562, LAMA-84, BV-173) and in primary cells from CML patients coinciding c-MYB and *ESPL1*/Separase expression levels irrespective to therapeutic treatment (IM) and silencing (siRNA) conditions (Figs. 1, 2 and 3) were observed. This suggests that the *ESPL1* promoter is under transcriptional control of the transcription factor c-MYB concurring with former results of Kohmura and coworkers who found a downregulation of c-MYB mRNA levels in K562 cells after incubation with IM [55].

Our results further coincide with previous studies reporting that p210BCR-ABL functions as enhancer of c-MYB expression and plays an important role in BCR-ABL-dependent leukemogenesis as the leukemic blast cells appear to rely on high levels of c-MYB protein more than normal progenitors [37, 45]. Moreover, c-MYB promotes centriole duplication and, when mutated, can lead to centrosome amplification as demonstrated in mouse and Drosophila model systems [56, 57]. Previous microarray data point to c-MYB as part of the regulatory network associated with CML progression including clonal evolution and genetic instability [58, 59].

The positive regulatory impact of c-MYB on *ESPL1*/Separase expression explains well the observations of Patel and Gordon who found abnormally high Separase expression levels in CML cells of chronic and blast phase when compared to normal CD34+ cells. It was then speculated that BCR-ABL expression may

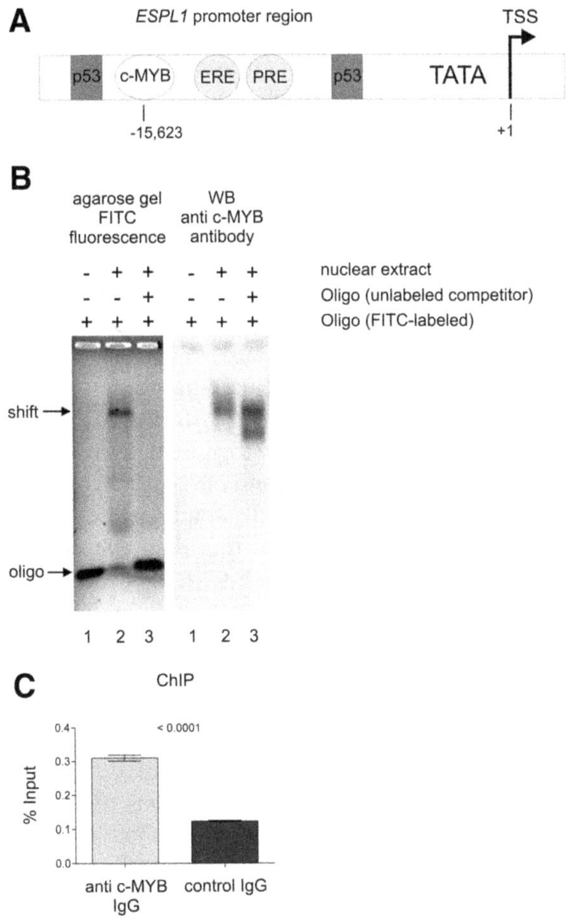

Fig. 4 Electrophoretic mobility shift assay (EMSA) using synthetic *ESPL1* promoter-derived c-MYB binding site probes and Chromatin immunoprecipitation (ChIP). **a** Schematic drawing depicting the *ESPL1* Separase promoter and location of predicted regulatory DNA motifs (drawing not to scale) (Pati 2008). The arrow shows the predicted transcription start site (TSS). Abbreviations: TATA, TATA box; PRE, progesterone responsive element; ERE, estrogen responsive element; p53, p53 binding element; c-MYB, predicted c-MYB binding element. Numbers denote upstream distances with respect to the TSS. **b** A FITC-labeled double stranded DNA oligonucleotide corresponding to the putative c-MYB binding site of the *ESPL1* promoter was incubated with native BV-173 nuclear extract. DNA/protein complexes were resolved on a 0.5 % TBE 1.0 % native LE/GTG agarose gel. The left panel (tonal inversion) shows FITC-related fluorescence signaling of the gel before blotting, the right panel depicts the corresponding anti-c-MYB Western blot immunostaining. The lanes represent: lane 1, DNA target (FITC-labeled oligonucleotide) without nuclear extract; lane 2, DNA target with nuclear extract; lane 3, DNA target with nuclear extract and with 100fold molar excess of analogous unlabeled oligonucleotide as binding competitor. **c** ChIP analysis of BV-173 cells. DNA fragments immunoprecipitated by anti-c-MYB IgG and a non-binding control IgG were amplified by qRT-PCR. Results are expressed as percentage of input (average). ChIP results are derived from at least triplicate qRT-PCR measurements

upregulate *ESPL1*/Separase and influence the occurrence of centrosomal aberrations [60].

Our data provide the first proof of direct regulatory relationship between BCR-ABL, c-MYB and *ESPL1*/Separase and give a plausible mechanistic explanation on how BCR-ABL may trigger dislocation between the centrosome-centriole cycle and the cell cycle in CML contributing to clonal evolution and genomic instability. The therapeutic administration of IM "normalizes" c-MYB protein levels - as shown in LAMA-84 and K562 cells (Fig. 1) - either by slowing down the transcriptional rate of *c-MYB* or by antagonizing enhanced c-MYB protein stability elicited by BCR-ABL via the PI-3 K/AKT pathway [36, 55]. The anticipated decrease of c-MYB protein levels after IM treatment is also in line with data of Flamant and coworkers who demonstrated that the drug results in a rapid increase in the expression of regulatory microRNAs such as miR-150 that is a strong negative regulator of c-MYB protein expression [61, 62].

Conclusions

In conclusion, our data suggest that *ESPL1*/Separase is a regulatory target of c-MYB and that c-MYB expression is modulated by IM treatment. Therefore, c-MYB, known to be required for BCR-ABL-dependent transformation of hematopoietic progenitors and leukemogenesis, may also influence Separase-related proteolytic events such as chromosomal segregation and centriole duplication, the ordered course of which is essential for maintenance of centrosomal and genomic stability.

Methods

Cell lines and culture conditions

Four human cell lines (K562, LAMA-84, BV-173, U937) were investigated. Of these, K562, LAMA-84 and BV-173 are BCR-ABL-positive IM responsive CML cell lines. U937 cells served as BCR-ABL-negative control cells. All cell lines were obtained from the DSMZ (German Collection of Microorganisms and Cell Cultures, Braunschweig, Germany) and were cultured in RPMI-1640 medium supplemented with 10 % fetal bovine serum and 1 % penicillin-streptomycin (Gibco/Invitrogen, Karlsruhe, Germany) at 37 °C in 5 % CO_2 atmosphere. Exponentially growing cells were used in at least triplicate experiments.

Patients and ethics statement

Paired cDNA samples of randomly chosen CML patients ($n = 5$) from the German CML-Study IV (registered at www.clinicaltrials.gov as # NCT00055874) were investigated by qRT-PCR. Each sample pair was derived from peripheral blood of the same patient at the time point of diagnosis (before IM treatment) and after achievement of major molecular response (MMR) under IM therapy. Blood sampling was performed in the context of regular therapeutic monitoring. The procedure followed the declaration of Helsinki and was approved by the IRB/Medizinische Ethikkommision II der Medizinischen Fakultät Mannheim der Ruprecht-Karls-Universität Heidelberg. (http://www.umm.uni-heidelberg.de/inst/ethikkommission, # 2013-509 N-MA from 2013-02-21). Written informed consent was obtained from all patients. Two female and three male patients, all with b3a2 *BCR-ABL* fusion type, were analyzed. The median age was 58 years (range, 47 to 78). Mean time between diagnosis and sampling of the second specimen from the same patient after achievement of MMR under IM treatment was 3.6 years (range, 2 to 6.5).

IM treatment

Cells were treated with IM (Biomol GmbH, Hamburg, Germany) in concentrations of 1 to 5 µM for 24 h (K562, LAMA-84) and 48 h (U937) according to the rationale pointed out in references [13, 35]. Untreated cells served as controls.

Western blot analysis, antibodies

Western blot immunostaining of Separase and Actin was performed as described previously [13]. For c-MYB detection, an anti-c-MYB monoclonal rabbit antibody (ab45150; Abcam, Cambridge, UK) at a dilution of 1:10,000 was used. Signals were visualized with a ChemiDoc™ XRS+ System (BIO-RAD, München, Germany) after secondary antibody staining (goat anti-rabbit IgG HRP conjugated antibody (1:10,000; Santa Cruz Biotechnology Inc., Heidelberg, Germany) utilizing SuperSignal West Femto Maximum Sensitivity Substrate (Thermo Fisher Scientific, Bonn, Germany). Image acquisition and densitometric analysis was performed using Image Lab Software (version 3.0.1, BIO-RAD). All values were normalized with Actin as loading control. Image cropping and tonal adjustments across the entire image were performed with Adobe Photoshop CS4 (Adobe Systems Inc., San Jose, CA, USA).

RNA extraction and quantification of *ESPL1* and *c-MYB* transcripts by qRT-PCR

Total RNA was extracted using RNeasy kit (Qiagen, Hilden, Germany) and reverse transcribed using Superscript II kit (Gibco/Invitrogen). For quantification of *ESPL1* and *c-MYB* transcript levels, the commercial Hs_MYB_1_SG and Hs_ESPL1_1_SG QuantiTect Primer Assays (Qiagen) were employed according to the instructions (two-step Light Cycler 480 protocol) of the manufacturer, respectively. For normalization, the housekeeping gene beta-glucuronidase (*Gus*, NM_000181, GUSB, primer set Hs_GUSB_1_SG, QuantiTect Primer Assay, Qiagen) was amplified. QRT-PCR was performed with the Roche LightCycler 480 System, using LC480 DNA Master SYBR Green and the standard LightCycler protocol (Roche Diagnostics, Mannheim, Germany). Relative transcript levels calculated from triplicate measurements were calculated by the $2^{-\Delta\Delta CT}$ method with values normalized to *Gus* and relative to transcription in untreated control cells [63].

***C-MYB* silencing by siRNA**

C-MYB-specific siRNA (FlexiTube GeneSolution GS4602 for *c-MYB*) was purchased from Qiagen. As negative controls the same cells were transfected with AllStars Negative Control siRNA (Qiagen), a nonsilencing siRNA with no homology to any known mammalian gene. Transfection was accomplished using the Nucleofector manual (program T016, Lonza GmbH, Köln, Germany). For siRNA treatment, 1.5×10^6 cells were resuspended in 100 µl Cell Line Nucleofector Solution V (Lonza) containing 18 µl Supplement S Solution (Lonza). The siRNA was added to a final concentration of 0.01 nmol per 10^6 cells. 24 h after transfection *c-MYB* transcript levels were analyzed by qRT-PCR. Protein lysates for Western blot immunostaining experiments were prepared 48 h after transfection.

***ESPL1* promoter electrophoretic mobility shift assay (EMSA)**

Native nuclear extracts were prepared from BV-173 cells according to a rapid micropreparation method [64]. FITC-labeled oligonucleotides (32mers) corresponding to the c-MYB-binding site sequence in the human *ESPL1* promoter (Human genome browser http://www.ncbi.nlm.nih.gov/gene?cmd=Retrieve&dopt=Graphics&list_uids=9700), NC_000012.11 chromosome 12 reference GRCh37.p13 primary assembly; c-MYB binding position: chr12: 53,646,460 - 53,646,470) were synthesized by Sigma GmbH (Rödermark, Germany). Oligonucleotide sequences (c-MYB binding sequence underlined) were: MYB_sense, FITC-CTCCCA CCCACCCAACTGGTCCCTCCGGTCTG; MYB_antisense, FITC-CAGACCGGAGGGACCAGTTGGGTGGGT GGGAG. EMSA was performed using the EMSA kit (order no. E33075) of Life Technologies GmbH (Darmstadt, Germany) according to the instructions of the manufacturer. In brief, 2 µg of nuclear extract were mixed with binding buffer prior to addition of 30 ng of annealed double stranded oligonucleotide corresponding to the c-MYB binding site within the *ESPL1* promoter. After incubation for 20 min at RT, 2 µl of EMSA loading dye was added and the DNA/protein complexes were resolved by electrophoresis (80 V for 90 min) on a 0.5 % TBE 1.0 % native LE/GTG agarose gel. Detection of FITC-labeled DNA oligonucleotides was performed using a ChemiDoc™ XRS+ System (BIO-RAD). Consecutively, the same agarose gel was blotted onto Immobilon-P membrane (Millipore, Bedford, USA) using a Trans Blot SD semi-dry electrophoretic transfer cell (BIO-RAD) at 15 V (current limit at 5 mA/cm^2) for

30 min. C-MYB Protein detection was performed as described in the Western blot analysis section.

Chromatin immunoprecipitation (ChIP)

ChIP was performed using the EpiTect ChIP OneDay Kit (#334471, Qiagen, Hilden) according to the instructions of the manufacturer. In brief, $1.5x10^6$ BV-173 cells per sample were lysed and sonicated (5 times 6 s, 0.5 W) using the Vibra-Cell™ system (Sonics, Newtown, USA). Immunoprecipitation was performed with an anti-c-MYB antibody (ab17851, Abcam, Cambridge, UK) and an unspecific control IgG1 control antibody (ab91353, Abcam) according to the manual. For quantification of the immunoprecipitated DNA target, the ChIP qPCR Primer Assay GPH1003144(+)02A (Sabioscience/Qiagen) was applied employing the Roche LightCycler 480 System, using LC480 DNA Master SYBR Green and the standard LightCycler protocol as already described (Roche Diagnostics, Mannheim, Germany). Results derived from triplicate experiments were expressed as percentage of input sample taken before immunoprecipitation during the ChIP procedure. Therefore, the Ct values of the IP fractions were normalized to the input fraction.

Statistical analysis

Statistical significance of unpaired data was analyzed by the Student's *t*-test using the GraphPad Prism software version 6.0 (GraphPad Inc., La Jolla, USA). Values of $p < 0.05$ were considered significant.

Abbreviations

AP: accelerated phase; BC: blast crisis; ChIP: chromatin immunoprecipitation; CML: chronic myeloid leukemia; CP: chronic phase; EMSA: electrophoretic mobility shift assay; ERE: estrogen responsive element; IM: imatinib; PRE: progesterone responsive element; qRT-PCR: quantitative reverse transcription-PCR; RNAi: RNA-interference; TK: tyrosine kinase; TSS: transcription start site.

Competing interests

The authors declare that they have no competing interests.

Authors' contributions

WP and WS contributed to the experimental design, analyzed and interpreted the data, and wrote the manuscript. WP HK MS performed the experiments. WP SR HK MS MCM WKH AF WS provided expertise and editing. All authors read and approved the final manuscript.

Acknowledgements

We thank Susanne Brendel for excellent technical assistance.

Support and funding

WS received a grant from the Deutsche Krebshilfe (www.krebshilfe.de, no. 110625) and from the Deutsche José Carreras Leukämie-Stiftung e.V. (www.carreras-stiftung.de/, no. DJCLS R 14/11). The funders had no role in study design, data collection and analysis, interpretation of data and in writing the manuscript.

References

1. Chestukhin A, Pfeffer C, Milligan S, DeCaprio JA, Pellman D. Processing, localization, and requirement of human separase for normal anaphase progression. Proc Natl Acad Sci U S A. 2003;100(8):4574–9. doi:10.1073/pnas.0730733100.
2. Schockel L, Mockel M, Mayer B, Boos D, Stemmann O. Cleavage of cohesin rings coordinates the separation of centrioles and chromatids. Nat Cell Biol. 2011;13(8):966–72. doi:10.1038/ncb2280.
3. Simmons-Kovacs LA, Haase SB. Cohesin: it's not just for chromosomes anymore. Cell Cycle. 2010;9(9):1750–3.
4. Uhlmann F. Secured cutting: controlling separase at the metaphase to anaphase transition. EMBO Rep. 2001;2(6):487–92. doi:10.1093/embo-reports/kve113.
5. Nigg EA. Centrosome duplication: of rules and licenses. Trends Cell Biol. 2007;17(5):215–21. doi:10.1016/j.tcb.2007.03.003.
6. Zhang N, Ge G, Meyer R, Sethi S, Basu D, Pradhan S, et al. Overexpression of Separase induces aneuploidy and mammary tumorigenesis. Proc Natl Acad Sci U S A. 2008;105(35):13033–8. doi:10.1073/pnas.0801610105.
7. Nigg EA, Raff JW. Centrioles, centrosomes, and cilia in health and disease. Cell. 2009;139(4):663–78. doi:10.1016/j.cell.2009.10.036.
8. Chan JY. A clinical overview of centrosome amplification in human cancers. Int J Biol Sci. 2011;7(8):1122–44.
9. Meyer R, Fofanov V, Panigrahi A, Merchant F, Zhang N, Pati D. Overexpression and mislocalization of the chromosomal segregation protein separase in multiple human cancers. Clin Cancer Res. 2009;15(8):2703–10. doi:10.1158/1078-0432.CCR-08-2454.
10. Mitelman F, Levan G, Nilsson PG, Brandt L. Non-random karyotypic evolution in chronic myeloid leukemia. Int J Cancer. 1976;18(1):24–30.
11. Agircan FG, Schiebel E. Sensors at centrosomes reveal determinants of local separase activity. PLoS Genet. 2014;10(10):e1004672. doi:10.1371/journal.pgen.1004672.
12. Shindo N, Kumada K, Hirota T. Separase sensor reveals dual roles for separase coordinating cohesin cleavage and cdk1 inhibition. Dev Cell. 2012;23(1):112–23. doi:10.1016/j.devcel.2012.06.015.
13. Haass W, Stehle M, Nittka S, Giehl M, Schrotz-King P, Fabarius A, et al. The proteolytic activity of separase in BCR-ABL-positive cells is increased by imatinib. PLoS One. 2012;7(8):e42863. doi:10.1371/journal.pone.0042863.
14. Holland AJ, Taylor SS. Cyclin-B1-mediated inhibition of excess separase is required for timely chromosome disjunction. J Cell Sci. 2006;119(Pt 16):3325–36. doi:10.1242/jcs.03083.
15. Waizenegger I, Gimenez-Abian JF, Wernic D, Peters JM. Regulation of human separase by securin binding and autocleavage. Curr Biol. 2002;12(16):1368–78.
16. Yim H, Erikson RL. Regulation of the final stage of mitosis by components of the pre-replicative complex and a polo kinase. Cell Cycle. 2011;10(9):1374–7.
17. Basu D, Zhang N, Panigrahi AK, Horton TM, Pati D. Development and validation of a fluorogenic assay to measure separase enzyme activity. Anal Biochem. 2009;392(2):133–8. doi:10.1016/j.ab.2009.05.046.
18. Mukherjee M, Byrd T, Brawley VS, Bielamowicz K, Li XN, Merchant F, et al. Overexpression and constitutive nuclear localization of cohesin protease Separase protein correlates with high incidence of relapse and reduced overall survival in glioblastoma multiforme. J Neurooncol. 2014. doi:10.1007/s11060-014-1458-6.
19. Mukherjee M, Ge G, Zhang N, Edwards DG, Sumazin P, Sharan SK, et al. MMTV-Espl1 transgenic mice develop aneuploid, estrogen receptor alpha (ERalpha)-positive mammary adenocarcinomas. Oncogene. 2013. doi:10.1038/onc.2013.493.
20. Pati D. Oncogenic activity of separase. Cell Cycle. 2008;7(22):3481–2.
21. Sawyers CL. Chronic myeloid leukemia. N Engl J Med. 1999;340(17):1330–40. doi:10.1056/NEJM199904293401706.
22. Calabretta B, Perrotti D. The biology of CML blast crisis. Blood. 2004;103(11):4010–22. doi:10.1182/blood-2003-12-4111.
23. Druker BJ, Guilhot F, O'Brien SG, Gathmann I, Kantarjian H, Gattermann N, et al. Five-year follow-up of patients receiving imatinib for chronic myeloid leukemia. N Engl J Med. 2006;355(23):2408–17. doi:10.1056/NEJMoa062867.
24. Hochhaus A, Schenk T, Erben P, Ernst T, La Rosee P, Muller MC. Cause and management of therapy resistance. Best Pract Res Clin Haematol. 2009;22(3):367–79. doi:10.1016/j.beha.2009.05.004.
25. Bolton-Gillespie E, Schemionek M, Klein HU, Flis S, Hoser G, Lange T, et al. Genomic instability may originate from imatinib-refractory chronic myeloid leukemia stem cells. Blood. 2013;121(20):4175–83. doi:10.1182/blood-2012-11-466938.
26. Kumari A, Brendel C, Hochhaus A, Neubauer A, Burchert A. Low BCR-ABL expression levels in hematopoietic precursor cells enable persistence of

chronic myeloid leukemia under imatinib. Blood. 2012;119(2):530–9. doi:10.1182/blood-2010-08-303495.
27. Hamilton A, Helgason GV, Schemionek M, Zhang B, Myssina S, Allan EK, et al. Chronic myeloid leukemia stem cells are not dependent on Bcr-Abl kinase activity for their survival. Blood. 2012;119(6):1501–10. doi:10.1182/blood-2010-12-326843.
28. Perl A, Carroll M. BCR-ABL kinase is dead; long live the CML stem cell. J Clin Invest. 2011;121(1):22–5. doi:10.1172/JCI43605.
29. Morotti A, Panuzzo C, Fava C, Saglio G. Kinase-inhibitor-insensitive cancer stem cells in chronic myeloid leukemia. Expert Opin Biol Ther. 2014;14(3):287–99. doi:10.1517/14712598.2014.867323.
30. Naka K, Hoshii T, Hirao A. Novel therapeutic approach to eradicate tyrosine kinase inhibitor resistant chronic myeloid leukemia stem cells. Cancer Sci. 2010;101(7):1577–81. doi:10.1111/j.1349-7006.2010.01584.x.
31. Schnittger S, Bacher U, Dicker F, Kern W, Alpermann T, Haferlach T, et al. Associations between imatinib resistance conferring mutations and Philadelphia positive clonal cytogenetic evolution in CML. Genes Chromosomes Cancer. 2010;49(10):910–8. doi:10.1002/gcc.20801.
32. Cortes J, O'Dwyer ME. Clonal evolution in chronic myelogenous leukemia. Hematol Oncol Clin North Am. 2004;18(3):671–84. doi:10.1016/j.hoc.2004.03.012.
33. O'Dwyer ME, Mauro MJ, Kurilik G, Mori M, Balleisen S, Olson S, et al. The impact of clonal evolution on response to imatinib mesylate (STI571) in accelerated phase CML. Blood. 2002;100(5):1628–33. doi:10.1182/blood-2002-03-0777.
34. Verma D, Kantarjian H, Shan J, O'Brien S, Estrov Z, Garcia-Manero G, et al. Survival outcomes for clonal evolution in chronic myeloid leukemia patients on second generation tyrosine kinase inhibitor therapy. Cancer. 2010; 116(11):2673–81. doi:10.1002/cncr.25015.
35. Haass W, Kleiner H, Weiss C, Haferlach C, Schlegelberger B, Muller MC, et al. Clonal evolution and blast crisis correlate with enhanced proteolytic activity of separase in BCR-ABL b3a2 fusion type CML under imatinib therapy. PLoS One. 2015;10(6):e0129648. doi:10.1371/journal.pone.0129648.
36. Corradini F, Cesi V, Bartella V, Pani E, Bussolari R, Candini O, et al. Enhanced proliferative potential of hematopoietic cells expressing degradation-resistant c-Myb mutants. J Biol Chem. 2005;280(34):30254–62. doi:10.1074/jbc.M504703200.
37. Lidonnici MR, Corradini F, Waldron T, Bender TP, Calabretta B. Requirement of c-Myb for p210(BCR/ABL)-dependent transformation of hematopoietic progenitors and leukemogenesis. Blood. 2008;111(9):4771–9. doi:10.1182/blood-2007-08-105072.
38. Manzotti G, Mariani SA, Corradini F, Bussolari R, Cesi V, Vergalli J, et al. Expression of p89(c-Mybex9b), an alternatively spliced form of c-Myb, is required for proliferation and survival of p210BCR/ABL-expressing cells. Blood Cancer J. 2012;2(5):e71. doi:10.1038/bcj.2012.16.
39. Greig KT, Carotta S, Nutt SL. Critical roles for c-Myb in hematopoietic progenitor cells. Semin Immunol. 2008;20(4):247–56. doi:10.1016/j.smim.2008.05.003.
40. Lieu YK, Reddy EP. Conditional c-myb knockout in adult hematopoietic stem cells leads to loss of self-renewal due to impaired proliferation and accelerated differentiation. Proc Natl Acad Sci U S A. 2009;106(51):21689–94. doi:10.1073/pnas.0907623106.
41. Selvakumaran M, Liebermann DA, Hoffman-Liebermann B. Deregulated c-myb disrupts interleukin-6- or leukemia inhibitory factor-induced myeloid differentiation prior to c-myc: role in leukemogenesis. Mol Cell Biol. 1992; 12(6):2493–500.
42. Pattabiraman DR, Gonda TJ. Role and potential for therapeutic targeting of MYB in leukemia. Leukemia. 2013;27(2):269–77. doi:10.1038/leu.2012.225.
43. Clappier E, Cuccuini W, Kalota A, Crinquette A, Cayuela JM, Dik WA, et al. The C-MYB locus is involved in chromosomal translocation and genomic duplications in human T-cell acute leukemia (T-ALL), the translocation defining a new T-ALL subtype in very young children. Blood. 2007;110(4):1251–61. doi:10.1182/blood-2006-12-064683.
44. Tomita A, Watanabe T, Kosugi H, Ohashi H, Uchida T, Kinoshita T, et al. Truncated c-Myb expression in the human leukemia cell line TK-6. Leukemia. 1998;12(9):1422–9.
45. Calabretta B, Sims RB, Valtieri M, Caracciolo D, Szczylik C, Venturelli D, et al. Normal and leukemic hematopoietic cells manifest differential sensitivity to inhibitory effects of c-myb antisense oligodeoxynucleotides: an in vitro study relevant to bone marrow purging. Proc Natl Acad Sci U S A. 1991; 88(6):2351–5.
46. Lorenzo PI, Brendeford EM, Gilfillan S, Gavrilov AA, Leedsak M, Razin SV, et al. Identification of c-Myb target genes in K562 cells reveals a role for c-Myb as a master regulator. Genes Cancer. 2011;2(8):805–17. doi:10.1177/1947601911428224.
47. Zhao L, Glazov EA, Pattabiraman DR, Al-Owaidi F, Zhang P, Brown MA, et al. Integrated genome-wide chromatin occupancy and expression analyses identify key myeloid pro-differentiation transcription factors repressed by Myb. Nucleic Acids Res. 2011;39(11):4664–79. doi:10.1093/nar/gkr024.
48. Deng QL, Ishii S, Sarai A. Binding site analysis of c-Myb: screening of potential binding sites by using the mutation matrix derived from systematic binding affinity measurements. Nucleic Acids Res. 1996;24(4):766–74.
49. Nakata Y, Shetzline S, Sakashita C, Kalota A, Rallapalli R, Rudnick SI, et al. c-Myb contributes to G2/M cell cycle transition in human hematopoietic cells by direct regulation of cyclin B1 expression. Mol Cell Biol. 2007;27(6):2048–58. doi:10.1128/MCB.01100-06.
50. Fabarius A, Giehl M, Rebacz B, Kramer A, Frank O, Haferlach C, et al. Centrosome aberrations and G1 phase arrest after in vitro and in vivo treatment with the SRC/ABL inhibitor dasatinib. Haematologica. 2008;93(8):1145–54. doi:10.3324/haematol.12793.
51. Giehl M, Fabarius A, Frank O, Erben P, Zheng C, Hafner M, et al. Expression of the p210BCR-ABL oncoprotein drives centrosomal hypertrophy and clonal evolution in human U937 cells. Leukemia. 2007;21(9):1971–6. doi:10.1038/sj.leu.2404834.
52. Fabarius A, Giehl M, Frank O, Duesberg P, Hochhaus A, Hehlmann R, et al. Induction of centrosome and chromosome aberrations by imatinib in vitro. Leukemia. 2005;19(9):1573–8. doi:10.1038/sj.leu.2403861.
53. Deininger M, Buchdunger E, Druker BJ. The development of imatinib as a therapeutic agent for chronic myeloid leukemia. Blood. 2005;105(7):2640–53. doi:10.1182/blood-2004-08-3097.
54. Di Gion P, Kanefendt F, Lindauer A, Scheffler M, Doroshyenko O, Fuhr U, et al. Clinical pharmacokinetics of tyrosine kinase inhibitors: focus on pyrimidines, pyridines and pyrroles. Clin Pharmacokinet. 2011;50(9):551–603. doi:10.2165/11593320-000000000-00000.
55. Kohmura K, Miyakawa Y, Kawai Y, Ikeda Y, Kizaki M. Different roles of p38 MAPK and ERK in STI571-induced multi-lineage differentiation of K562 cells. J Cell Physiol. 2004;198(3):370–6. doi:10.1002/jcp.10426.
56. Fung SM, Ramsay G, Katzen AL. Mutations in Drosophila myb lead to centrosome amplification and genomic instability. Development. 2002; 129(2):347–59.
57. Tan FE, Vladar EK, Ma L, Fuentealba LC, Hoh R, Espinoza FH, et al. Myb promotes centriole amplification and later steps of the multiciliogenesis program. Development. 2013;140(20):4277–86. doi:10.1242/dev.094102.
58. Oehler VG, Yeung KY, Choi YE, Bumgarner RE, Raftery AE, Radich JP. The derivation of diagnostic markers of chronic myeloid leukemia progression from microarray data. Blood. 2009;114(15):3292–8. doi:10.1182/blood-2009-03-212969.
59. Zheng C, Li L, Haak M, Brors B, Frank O, Giehl M, et al. Gene expression profiling of CD34+ cells identifies a molecular signature of chronic myeloid leukemia blast crisis. Leukemia. 2006;20(6):1028–34. doi:10.1038/sj.leu.2404227.
60. Patel H, Gordon MY. Abnormal centrosome-centriole cycle in chronic myeloid leukaemia? Br J Haematol. 2009;146(4):408–17. doi:10.1111/j.1365-2141.2009.07772.x.
61. Flamant S, Ritchie W, Guilhot J, Holst J, Bonnet ML, Chomel JC, et al. Micro-RNA response to imatinib mesylate in patients with chronic myeloid leukemia. Haematologica. 2010;95(8):1325–33. doi:10.3324/haematol.2009.020636.
62. Lu J, Guo S, Ebert BL, Zhang H, Peng X, Bosco J, et al. MicroRNA-mediated control of cell fate in megakaryocyte-erythrocyte progenitors. Dev Cell. 2008;14(6):843–53. doi:10.1016/j.devcel.2008.03.012.
63. Livak KJ, Schmittgen TD. Analysis of relative gene expression data using real-time quantitative PCR and the 2(–Delta Delta C(T)) Method. Methods. 2001;25(4):402–8. doi:10.1006/meth.2001.1262.
64. Andrews NC, Faller DV. A rapid micropreparation technique for extraction of DNA-binding proteins from limiting numbers of mammalian cells. Nucleic Acids Res. 1991;19(9):2499.

15

Update on the first-line treatment for *Helicobacter pylori* infection

Chih-Chieh Huang[1], Kuo-Wang Tsai[2], Tzung-Jiun Tsai[1,3] and Ping-I Hsu[1,3,4*]

Abstract

Because the prevalence of antibiotic resistance markedly increases with time worldwide, anti-*H. pylori* treatment is continuing to be a great challenge forsphysicians in clinical practice. The Real-world Practice & Expectation of Asia-Pacific Physicians and Patients in *Helicobacter Pylori* Eradication (REAP-HP) Survey demonstrated that the accepted minimal eradication rate of anti-*H. pylori* regimen in *H. pylori*-infected patients was 91%. The Kyoto Consensus Report on *Helicobacter Pylori* Gastritis also recommended that, within any region, only regimens which reliably produce eradication rates of ≥90% in that population should be used for empirical treatment. This article is aimed to review current first-line eradication regimens with a per-protocol eradication rate exceeding 90% in most geographic areas. In regions with low (≦15%) clarithromycin resistance, 14-day hybrid (or reverse hybrid), 10 ~ 14-day sequential, 7 ~ 14-day concomitant, 10 ~ 14-day bismuth quadruple or 14-day triple therapy can achieve a high eradication rate in the first-line treatment of *H. pylori* infection. However, in areas with high (>15%) clarithromycin resistance, standard triple therapy should be abandoned because of low eradication efficacy, and 14-day hybrid (or reverse hybrid), 10 ~ 14-day concomitant or 10 ~ 14-day bismuth quadruple therapy are the recommended regimens. If no recent data of local antibiotic resistances of *H. pylori* strains are available, universal high efficacy regimens such as 14-day hybrid (or reverse hybrid), concomitant or bismuth quadruple therapy can be adopted to meet the recommendation of consensus report and patients' expectation.

Keywords: *Helicobacter pylori*, First-line, Therapy, Hybrid therapy, Sequential therapy, Concomitant therapy, Triple therapy

Background

Helicobacter pylori (*H. pylori*) infect more than 50% of humans globally. It is the major cause of chronic gastritis, peptic ulcer, gastric mucosa-associated lymphoid tissue lymphoma (MALToma), and gastric adenocarcinoma [1, 2]. Eradication of *H. pylori* can effectively prevent the recurrence of peptic ulcer disease [3, 4]. Anti- *H. pylori* therapy is currently recommended in the treatment of *H pylori*-related gastric MALToma [5]. Additionally, eradication of *H pylori* is advocated as a preventative method in regions with high incidence of gastric adenocarcinoma [6, 7].

A recent survey for *H. pylori* eradication therapy revealed that 7-day standard triple therapy remained the most popular regimen in the Asia-Pacific region [8]. However, the eradication rate of 7-day standard triple therapy has declined to less than 80% in most countries worldwide owing to increasing resistance rate to antibiotics [9–12]. The Kyoto Consensus Report on *Helicobacter Pylori* Gastritis recommends that, within any region, only regimens which reliably produce eradication rates of ≥90% in that population should be used for empirical treatment [13]. Current medicine practice emphasizes shared decision making with patients. It is therefore important for physicians to know the expectations of patients and try to meet patients' expectations on eradication therapy when they prescribe anti-*H. pylori* regimen. The survey for the Real-world Practice & Expectation of Asia-Pacific Physicians and Patients in

* Correspondence: williamhsup@yahoo.com.tw
[1]Division of Gastroenterology, Department of Internal Medicine, Kaohsiung Veterans General Hospital and National Yang-Ming University, Kaohsiung, Taiwan
[3]Taiwan Acid-related Disease (TARD) Study Group, Kaohsiung, Taiwan

Helicobacter Pylori Eradication (REAP-HP) showed that the expected minimal eradication rate in patients was 91.4% [8]. Hence, physicians should prescribe an eradication regimen with cure rate exceeding 90% to treat their *H. pylori*-infected patients. This article is aimed to review current novel first-line eradication regimens with a per-protocol (PP) eradication rate exceeding 90% in most geographic areas.

Current antibiotic resistance

The main reasons for eradication failure of standard triple therapy include antibiotic resistance, poor compliance and rapid metabolism of proton pump inhibitor (PPI) [10, 14, 15]. Clarithromycin resistance has been identified as the main reason for the failure of standard triple therapy [16, 17]. Pooled data from 20 studies involving 1975 patients treated with standard triple therapy showed an eradication rate of 88% in clarithromycin-sensitive strains versus 18% in clarithromycin-resistant strains [10]. Therefore, the background rate of clarithromycin resistance is critically important for the efficacy of standard triple therapy.

The prevalence of antibiotic resistance varies in different geographic regions and appears to be increasing with time in most countries worldwide [18–24]. For example, an increase in clarithromycin resistance was observed in Korea from 7.0% in 2009 to 16.0% in 2011 [23]. The resistance rate of *H. pylori* to clarithromycin in Japan had increased gradually from 2% in 1996 to approximately 30% in 2004 [22]. In China, a marked increase of clarithromycin resistance was seen from 8.6% in 2000 to 20.7% in 2009 [21]. The recent clarithromycin resistance rates of *H. pylori* in China, Taiwan, Japan, Turkey, Italy and the United States are approximately 50, 15, 30, 40, 30 and 13%, respectively [20]. The prevalence of metronidazole resistance quite varies in different countries. The resistance rate of *H. pylori* to metronidazole remains high in China (41.6 - 67.4% between 2008 and 2015). In contrast, the prevalence of metronidazole resistance is extremely low in Japan [22]. Nishizawa et al. described an overall resistance rate of 2.1% in patients studied from 2012 to 2104 [24]. In Korea, the prevalence of metronidazole resistance had increased from 45.1% in 2009 to 56.3% in 2011 [23]. Besides clarithromycin and metronidazole, amoxicillin is also one of the most commonly used antibiotics in first-line anti-*H. pylori* therapy. However, resistance to amoxicillin remains extremely low (less than 5%) in most countries [16, 20, 23, 24].

Updated *H. pylori* therapy

With the rising prevalence of antimicrobial resistance, standard triple therapy is no longer effective in most countries [15–17]. The eradication rate of the 7-day standard triple therapy in 14 hospitals over the Tokyo metropolitan area in 2010 was only 66.5 and 378.7% by intention-to-treat (ITT) and per-protocol (PP) analyses, respectively [25]. The regimen achieved a success rate of 68.5% by PP analysis in Korea [26]. Clinicians should therefore avoid triple therapies unless it has been proven to achieve an adequate success rate locally. Currently, several strategies including bismuth quadruple, non-bismuth quadruple (i.e., sequential, concomitant and hybrid) and high-dose dual therapies have proposed to increase the eradication rate [27–32]. Figure 1 summaries the regimens of these new therapies.

Sequential therapy

Sequential therapies developed by Zullo et al. consists of a 5-day dual therapy with a PPI (standard dose, b.i.d.) and amoxicillin (1 g, b.i.d.) followed by a 5-day triple therapy with a PPI (standard dose, b.i.d.), clarithromycin (500 mg, b.i.d.) and metronidazole (500 mg, b.i.d.) [27]. Clarithromycin resistance also reduces the efficacy of sequential therapy. However, the impact of clarithromycin

Standard triple therapy				
PPI	1#	bid	7-14d	
Amoxicillin	1g	bid	7-14d	
Clarithromycin	500mg	bid	7-14d	
Bismuth quadruple therapy				
PPI	1#	bid	7-14d	
Bismuth	120mg	qid	7-14d	
Metronidazole	250mg	qid	7-14d	
Tetracycline	500mg	qid	7-14d	
Sequential therapy				
PPI	1#	bid	10d	
Amoxicillin	1g	bid	5d	
Clarithromycin	500mg	bid		5d
Metronidazole	250mg	qid		5d
Concomitant therapy				
PPI	1#	bid	7-14d	
Amoxicillin	1g	bid	7-14d	
Clarithromycin	500mg	bid	7-14d	
Metronidazole	250mg	qid	7-14d	
Hybrid therapy				
PPI	1#	bid	14d	
Amoxicillin	1g	bid	14d	
Clarithromycin	500mg	bid		7d
Metronidazole	250mg	qid		7d
Reverse hybrid therapy				
PPI	1#	bid	14d	
Amoxicillin	1g	bid	14d	
Clarithromycin	500mg	bid	7d	
Metronidazole	250mg	qid	7d	
High-dose therapy				
PPI	1#	qid	14d	
Amoxicillin	750g	qid	14d	

Fig. 1 Current anti-*H pylori* regimens

resistance on sequential therapy is markedly less than that on standard triple therapy because sequential therapy contains metronidazole as an additional antibiotic [16]. A randomized, double-blind, placebo-controlled trial demonstrated that the PP eradication rates of sequential therapy and standard triple therapy for clarithromycin-resistant strains were 89 and 29%, respectively [33]. The eradication rate of 10-day sequential therapy was superior to that of 7-day standard triple therapy in several randomized controlled trials [16, 33]. However, meta-analysis revealed that 10-day sequential therapy was not superior to 14-day standard triple therapy [34]. Either clarithromycin or metronidazole resistance can undermine the efficacy of sequential therapy [16, 35]. The eradication rates of 10-day sequential therapy for the strains with non-resistance, single clarithromycin resistance, single metronidazole resistance and dual resistances were 95, 70, 78, and 43%, respectively, in a recent prospective randomized controlled trial [35]. In addition, this therapy is more complex and requires changing antibiotics during the treatment course which may reduce the treatment compliance of patients.

Concomitant therapy

Concomitant therapy is another novel regimen proven successful in the presence of clarithromycin resistance [16, 30]. It is a 4-drug regimen containing a PPI (standard dose, b.i.d.), clarithromycin (500 mg, b.i.d.), amoxicillin (1 g, b.i.d.) and metronidazole (500 mg, b.i.d.) which are all given for the entire duration of therapy (Fig. 1). Meta-analysis demonstrated that concomitant therapy is more effective than standard triple therapy (90% versus 78% by ITT analysis) [36]. Dual clarithromycin and metronidazole resistance undermines the efficacy of concomitant therapy. A recent randomized controlled trial revealed that the eradication rates of 7-day concomitant therapy for the *H pylori* strains with nonresistance, single clarithromycin resistance, single metronidazole resistance, and dual clarithromycin and metronidazole resistance were 100.0, 100.0, 100.0, and 66.7%, respectively [16].

The efficacy of concomitant therapy was also related to the duration of treatment [37]. A tendency toward better results with longer treatments (7–10 days versus 3–5 days) has been observed [37]. Concomitant therapy is less complex than sequential therapy as this regimen does not involve changing drugs halfway through.

Hybrid and reverse hybrid therapies

Hybrid therapy was introduced by Hsu et al. in Taiwan in 2011 [29]. This regimen consists of a dual therapy with a proton pump inhibitor (PPI) and amoxicillin for 7 days followed by a quadruple regimen with a PPI, amoxicillin, clarithromcyin and metronidazole for 7 days. It produced an eradication rate of 99.1% by PP analysis and 97.4% by ITT analysis in Taiwan [16]. A systemic review showed that the eradication rates of hybrid therapy for clarithromycin-sensitive and resistant strains were 99.1 and 85.7%, respectively [38]. The impact of metronidazole resistance on the efficacy of the new therapy also appeared minor (susceptible strains: 100% [68/68]; resistant strains: 94.2% [49/52]) [38]. Several randomized controlled trials demonstrated that hybrid regimens were comparable with or more effective than sequential regimens [38–42]. A recent large multicentre randomized controlled trial demonstrated that both 14-day hybrid and 14-day concomitant therapies cured more than 90% of patients with *H pylori* infections in areas of high clarithromycin and metronidazole resistance [43]. However, significantly more patients were compliant with hybrid therapy (98.8%) than concomitant therapy (95.2%) [43]. Meta-analysis revealed that hybrid therapy and concomitant therapy achieved comparable eradication rate [38]. Recently, the Taiwan *H pylori* Consensus Report recommends 14-day hybrid, concomitant and bismuth quadruple therapies as choices of anti-*H pylori* treatment in areas with either high or low clarithromycin resistance [44].

Switching drugs halfway through the course increases the complexity of an anti-*H pylori* regimen. Reversing the sequence of drug administration (a quadruple regimen followed by a dual regimen) may simplify hybrid therapy (a one-step two-phase therapy; Fig. 1). A pilot multicenter, randomized trial demonstrated that reverse hybrid therapy was highly effective in Taiwan (eradication rate by PP analysis: 96%) and superior to standard triple therapy [43]. A retrospective cohort study demonstrated that reverse hybrid therapy yielded a similar eradication rate as standard hybrid therapy [45]. The new therapy appears to be a simple, highly effective, and well-tolerated treatment for *H pylori* infection in the era of increasing antibiotic resistance.

High-dose dual therapy

High-dose dual therapy developed by Yang et al. is another emerging treatment for *H pylori* infection [32]. The new therapy consists of high-dose PPI (one tablet q.i.d) and amoxicillin (750 mg q.i.d), which may keep the intragastric pH at a value higher than 6.5 regardless of *CYP2C19* genotype [46] and maintain steady plasma concentration of amoxicillin above the minimal inhibitory concentration for *H pylori* [47]. The efficacy of the new therapy was significantly higher than that of standard triple therapy in Taiwan [42]. However, it was less effective as the first-line therapy for eradicating *H pylori* in Korea [48]. Currently, data on high-dose dual therapy are scarce, and further studies to investigate the simple regimens are needed.

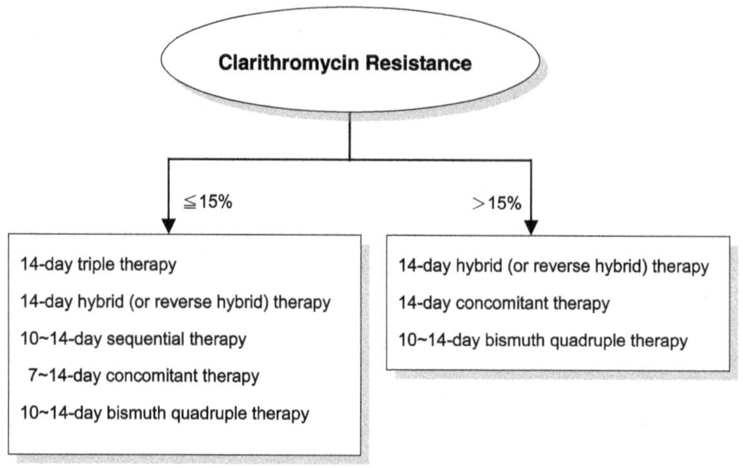

Fig. 2 Recommended anti-*H pylori* regimens in regions with different clarithromycin resistant rates

Bismuth quadruple therapy

Bismuth-containing quadruple therapy containing a PPI, bismuth, metronidazole and tetracycline is recommended as the choice treatment for *H pylori* infection in areas of either low or high clarithromycin resistance in the Maastricht V/Florence Consensus Report [49]. The optimal treatment duration of bismuth-containing quadruple therapy remains unclear. However, the efficacy of bismuth quadruple therapy for 1–3 days, 4 days or 7 days was less effective than when given for 10–14 days [50]. Bismuth quadruple therapy for 10–14 days achieved ≧ 85% eradication rate, even in areas with a high prevalence of metronidazole resistance [50]. However, 14-day bismuth quadruple therapy had a much higher frequency of adverse events than 14-day hybrid therapy (55.5% vs 15.7%, $P < 0.001$) [51].

Quinolone-containing triple therapy

A quinolone-containing triple therapy is effective as the first-line therapy for *H pylori* infection. Its cure rates range from 72 to 96% [52]. The regimen might be considered in populations with clarithromycin resistance greater than 15–20% and quinolone resistance less than 10% [53]. Nonetheless, a quinolone-based triple therapy is not generally recommended as a first-line therapy due to concerns of the rising prevalence of quinolone-resistant strains. Additionally, the increased use of quinolone would likely lead to the development of more quinolone-resistant pathogens for respiratory and urogenital tract infection.

Conclusion

Current consensus report on *H. pylori* eradication therapy recommends that only regimens that reliably produce eradication rates of ≥90% should be used for empirical treatment. The REAP-HP Survey also revealed that the accepted minimal eradication rate of anti-*H. pylori* therapy in infected patients was 91%. To meet the recommendation of the consensus report and patients' expectation, 14-day triple, 14-day hybrid (or reverse hybrid), 10 ~ 14-day sequential, 7 ~ 14-day concomitant or 10 ~ 14-day bismuth quadruple therapy can be adopted as the first-line treatment for *H. pylori* infection in areas with low (≦15%) clarithromycin resistance (Fig. 2). In areas with high (>15%) clarithromycin resistance, standard triple therapy should be abandoned, and 14-day hybrid (or reverse hybrid), 10 ~ 14-day concomitant or 10 ~ 14-day bismuth quadruple therapy can be used to treat *H. pylori* infection. If no recent data of local antibiotic resistances of *H. pylori* strains are available, universal high efficacy regimens such as 14-day hybrid (or reverse hybrid), concomitant or bismuth quadruple therapy can be adopted to meet the recommendation of consensus report and patients' expectation.

Abbreviations

H. pylori: *Helicobacter pylori*; ITT: Intention to treat; MALToma: Mucosa-associated lymphoid tissue lymphoma; PP: Per protocol; PPI: Proton pump inhibitor; REAP-HP: Real-world practice & expectation of Asia-Pacific physicians and patients in *Helicobacter pylori* eradication

Acknowledgements

The authors are indebted to Miss Joyce Chen for figure preparation.

Funding

The study was funded by the Kaohsiung Veterans General Hospital (Grant Numbers: VGHKS106-091 and VGHKS105-81) and the Ministry of Science and Technology, Exacutive Yuan, ROC, Taiwan (Grant Number: MOST 104-2314-B-075B-001-MY2). The grant from the Kaohsiung Veterans General Hospital was contributed to English revision, and the grant from the Ministry of Science and Technology, Executive Yuan, ROC, Taiwan was contributed to reference search.

Authors' contributions

CCH and PIH worked equally in study design, data analysis, and drafting of manuscript. KWT and TJT performed reference search and revised the manuscript. All authors read and approved the final manuscript.

Consent for publication

Not applicable.

Competing interests

The authors declare that they have no competing interests.

Author details

[1]Division of Gastroenterology, Department of Internal Medicine, Kaohsiung Veterans General Hospital and National Yang-Ming University, Kaohsiung, Taiwan. [2]Department of Medical Education and Research, Kaohsiung Veterans General Hospital, Kaohsiung, Taiwan. [3]Taiwan Acid-related Disease (TARD) Study Group, Kaohsiung, Taiwan. [4]Division of Gastroenterology, Department of Internal Medicine, Kaoshiung Veterans General Hospital, 386 Ta Chung 1st Road, Kaohsiung 813, Taiwan, ROC.

References

1. Vakil N, Megraud F. Eradication therapy for helicobacter pylori. Gastroenterology. 2007;133:985–1001.
2. Malfertheiner P, Chan FK, McColl KE. Peptic ulcer disease. Lancet. 2009;374: 1449–61.
3. Graham DY, Lew GM, Klein PD, Evans DG, Evans DJ Jr, Saeed ZA, et al. Effect of treatment of helicobacter pylori infection on the long-term recurrence of gastric or duodenal ulcer. A randomized controlled study. Ann Intern Med. 1992;116:705–8.
4. Sung JJ, Chung SC, Ling TK, Yung MY, Leung VK, Ng EK, et al. Antibacterial treatment of gastric ulcer associated with helicobacter pylori. N Engl J Med. 1995;332:139–42.
5. Zucca E, Dreyling M. Gastric marginal zone lymphoma of MALT type: ESMO clinical recommendations for diagnosis, treatment and follow-up. Ann Oncol. 2009;200(Suppl 4):113–4.
6. Asaka M. A new approach for elimination of gastric cancer deaths in Japan. Int J Cancer. 2013;132:1272–6.
7. Fock KM, Katelaris P, Sugano K, Ang TL, Hunt R, Talley NJ, et al. Second Asia-Pacific consensus guidelines for helicobacter pylori infection. J Gastroenterol Hepatol. 2009;24:1587–600.
8. Chuah Y-Y, Wu D-C, Chuah S-K, Yang J-C, Lee T-H, Yeh H-Z, et al. The survey for Real-World-Practice & Expectation of Asia-Pacific physicians and patients in *Helicobacter Pylori* eradication (REAP-HP survey). Helicobacter. 2017; in press
9. Gumurdulu Y, Serin E, Ozer B, Kayaselcuk F, Ozsahin K, Cosar AM, et al. Low eradication rate of helicobacter pylori with triple 7–14 days and quadruple therapy in Turkey. World J Gastroenterol. 2004;10:668–71.
10. Megraud F. H pylori antibiotic resistance: prevalence, importance, and advances in testing. Gut. 2004;53:1374–84.
11. Kim JS, Kim BW, Hong SJ, Kim JI, Shim KN, Kim JH, et al. Sequential therapy versus triple therapy for the first line treatment of helicobacter pylori in Korea: a Nationwide randomized trial. Gut Liver. 2016;10:556–61.
12. De Francesco V, Margiotta M, Zullo A, Hassan C, Troiani L, Burattini O, et al. Clarithromycin-resistant genotypes and eradication of helicobacter pylori. Ann Intern Med. 2006;144:94–100.
13. Sugano K, Tack J, Kuipers EJ, Graham DY, El-Omar EM, Miura S, et al. Kyoto global consensus report on helicobacter pylori gastritis. Gut. 2015;64: 1353–67.
14. Graham DY, Akiko S. New concepts of resistance in the treatment of helicobacter pylori infections. Nat Clin Pract Gastroenterol Hepatol. 2008;5: 321–31.
15. Graham DY, Lee YC, Wu MS. Rational helicobacter pylori therapy: evidence-based medicine rather than medicine-based evidence. Clin Gastroenterol Hepatol. 2014;12:177–86.
16. Hsu PI, Wu DC, Chen WC, Tseng HH, Yu HC, Wang HM, et al. Randomized controlled trial comparing 7-day triple, 10-day sequential, and 7-day concomitant therapies for helicobacter pylori infection. Antimicrob Agents Chemother. 2014;58:5936–42.
17. Houben MH, van de Beek D, Hensen EF, de Craen AJ, Rauws EA, Tytgat GN. A systemic review of helicobacter pylori therapy – the impact of antimicrobial resistance on eradication rates. Aliment Pharmacol Ther. 1999; 13:1047–55.
18. Gatta L, Vakil N, Vaira D, Scarpignato C. Global eradication rates for helicobacter pylori infection: systematic review and meta-analysis of sequential therapy. BMJ. 2013;347:f4587. doi:10.1136/bmj.f4587.
19. Meyer JM, Silliman NP, Wang W, Siepman NY, Sugg JE, Morris D, et al. Risk factors for helicobacter pylori resistance in the UnitedStates: the surveillance of H. Pylori antimicrobial resistance partnership (SHARP) study, 1993–1999. Ann Intern Med. 2002;136:13–24.
20. Thung I, Aramin H, Vavinskaya V, Gupta S, Park JY, Crowe SE, et al. Review article:the global emergence of helicobacter pylori antibiotic resistance. Aliment Pharmacol Ther. 2016;43:514–33.
21. Sun QJ, Liang X, Zheng Q, Gu WQ, Liu WZ, Xiao SD, et al. Resistance of helicobacter pylori to antibiotics from 2000 to 2009 in shanghai. World J Gastroenterol. 2010;16:5118–21.
22. Horiki N, Omata F, Uemura M, Suzuki S, Ishii N, Iizuka Y, et al. Annual change of primary resistance to clarithromycin among helicobacter pylori isolates from 1996 through 2008 in Japan. Helicobacter. 2009;14:86–90.
23. An B, Moon BS, Kim H, Lim HC, Lee YC, Lee G, et al. Antibiotic resistance in helicobacter pylori strains and its effect on H. Pylori eradication rates in a single center in Korea. Ann Lab Med. 2013;33:415–9.
24. Nishizawa T, Maekawa T, Watanabe N, Harada N, Hosoda Y, Yoshinaga M, et al. Clarithromycin versus Metronidazole as first-line helicobacter pylori eradication: a multicenter, prospective, randomized controlled study in Japan. J Clin Gastroenterol. 2015;49:468–71.
25. Kawai T, Takahashi S, Suzuki H, Sasaki H, Nagahara A, Asaoka D, et al. Changes in the first line helicobacter pylori eradication rates using the triple therapy-a multicenter study in the Tokyo metropolitan area (Tokyo helicobacter pylori study group). J Gastroenterol Hepatol. 2014;29(Suppl 4): 29–32.
26. Chung JW, Jung YK, Kim YJ, Kwon KA, Kim JH, Lee JJ, et al. Ten-day sequential versus triple therapy for helicobacter pylori eradication: a prospective, open-label, randomized trial. J Gastroenterol Hepatol. 2012;27: 1675–80.
27. Zullo A, De Francesco V, Hassan C, Morini S, Vaira D. The sequential therapy regimen for helicobacter pylori eradication: a pooled-data analysis. Gut. 2007;56:1353–7.
28. Song ZQ, Zhou LY. Hybrid, sequential and concomitant therapies for Helciobacter pylori eradication: A systemic review and meta-analysis. World J Gastroenterol 2016;22:4766–75.
29. Hsu PI, Wu DC, Wu JY, Graham DY. Modified sequential helicobacter pylori therapy: proton pump inhibitor and amoxicillin for 14 days with clarithromycin and metronidazole added as a quadruple (hybrid) therapy for the final 7 days. Helicobacter. 2011;16:139–45.
30. Wu DC, Hsu PI, Wu JY, Opekun AR, Kuo CH, Wu IC, et al. Sequential and concomitant therapies with 4 drugs are equally effective for eradication of H pylori infection. Clin Gastroenterol Hepatol. 2010;8:36–41.
31. Malfertheiner P, Bazzoli F, Delchier JC, Celiñski K, Giguère M, Rivière M, et al. Helicobacter pylori eradication with a capsule containing bismuth subcitrate potassium, metronidazole, and tetracycline given with omeprazole versus clarithromycin-based triple therapy: a randomised, open-label, non-inferiority, phase 3 trial. Lancet. 2011;377:905–13.
32. Yang JC, Lin CJ, Wang HL, Chen JD, Kao JY, Shun CT, et al. High-dose dual therapy is superior to standard first-line or rescue therapy for helicobacter pylori infection. Clin Gastroenterol Hepatol. 2015;13:895–905.
33. Vaira D, Zullo A, Vakil N, Gatta L, Ricci C, Perna F, et al. Sequential therapy versus standard triple-drug therapy for helicobacter pylori eradication: a randomized trial. Ann Intern Med. 2007;146:556–63.
34. Gatta L, Vakil N, Leandro G, Di Mario F, Vaira D. Sequential therapy or triple therapy for helicobacter pylori infection: systematic review and meta-analysis of randomized controlled trials in adults and children. Am J Gastroenterol. 2009;104:3069–79.
35. Liou JM, Chen CC, Chen MJ, Chen CC, Chang CY, Fang YJ, et al. Sequential versus triple therapy for the first-line treatment of helicobacter pylori: a multicentre, open-label, randomised trial. Lancet. 2013;381:205–13.
36. Essa AS, Kramer JR, Graham DY, Treiber G. Meta-analysis: four-drug, three-antibiotic, non-bismuth-containing "concomitant therapy" versus triple therapy for helicobacter pylori eradication. Helicobacter. 2009;14:109 18.

37. Kongchayanun C, Vilaichone RK, Pornthisarn B, Amornsawadwattana S, Mahachai V. Pilot study to identify the optimum duration of concomitant helicobacter pylori eradication therapy in Thailand. Helicobacter. 2012;17: 282–5.
38. Hsu PI, Lin PC, Graham DY. Hybrid therapy for helicobacter pylori infection: a systemic review and meta-analysis. World J Gastroenterol. 2015;21:12954–62.
39. Sardarian H, Fakheri H, Hosseini V, Taghvaei T, Maleki I, Mokhtare M. Comparison of hybrid and sequential therapies for helicobacter pylori eradication in Iran: a prospective randomized trial. Helicobacter. 2013;18: 129–34.
40. Chen KY, Lin TJ, Lee HC, Wang CK, Wu DC. Hybrid vs sequential therapy for eradication of helicobacter pylori in Taiwan: a prospective randomized trial. World J Gastroenterol. 2015;21:10435–42.
41. De Francesco V, Hassan C, Ridola L, Giorgio F, Ierardi E, Zullo A. Sequential, concomitant and hybrid first-line therapies for helicobacter pylori eradication: a prospective randomized study. J Med Microbiol. 2014;63:748–52.
42. Oh DH, Lee DH, Kang KK, Park YS, Shin CM, Kim N, et al. Efficacy of hybrid therapy as first-line regimen for helicobacter pylori infection compared with sequential therapy. J Gastroenterol Hepatol. 2014;29:1171–6.
43. Molina-Infante J, Romano M, Fernandez-Bermejo M, Federico A, Gravina AG, Pozzati L, et al. Optimized nonbismuth quadruple therapies cure most patients with helicobacter pylori infection in populations with high rates of antibiotic resistance. Gastroenterology. 2013;145:121–128.e1.
44. Sheu BS, Wu MS, Chiu CT, Lo JC, Wu DC, Liou JM, et al. Consensus on the clinical management, screening-to-treat, and surveillance of helicobacter pylori infection to improve gastric cancer control on a nationwide scale. Helicobacter. 2017; doi:10.1111/hel.12368.
45. Hsu PI, Wu DC. Reverse hybrid therapy achieves a similar eradication rate as hybrid therapy in the treatment of *Helicobacter pylori* infection. Gastroenterology. 2016;150(Suppl 1):S73.
46. Sugimoto M, Furuta T, Shirai N, Kajimura M, Hishida A, Sakurai M, et al. Different dosage regimens of rabeprazole for nocturnal gastric acid inhibition in relation to cytochrome P450 2C19 genotype status. Clin Pharmacol Ther. 2004;76:290–301.
47. Craig WA. Pharmacokinetic/pharmacodynamic parameters: rationale for antibacterial dosing of mice and men. Clin Infect Dis. 1998;26:1–10.
48. Kwack W, Lim Y, Lim C, Graham DY. High dose Ilaprazole/amoxicillin as first-line regimen for helicobacter pylori infection in Korea. Gastroenterol Res Pract. 2016;2016:1648047.
49. Malfertheiner P, Megraud F, O'Morain CA, Gisbert JP, Kuipers EJ, Axon AT, et al. Management of Helicobacter pylori infection — the Maastricht V/ Florence consensus report. Gut. 2017;66:6–30.
50. Fischbach L, Evans EL. Meta-analysis: the effect of antibiotic resistance status on the efficacy of triple and quadruple first-line therapies for helicobacter pylori. Aliment Pharmacol Ther. 2007;26:343–57.
51. Hsu PI, Wu DC, Tsay FW. Both 14-day hybrid and bismuth containing quadruple therapies cure most patients with *Helicobacter pylori* infection in populations with moderate antibiotic resistance: a randomized controlled trial. Gastroenterology. 2016;150(Suppl 1):S72–3.
52. Berning M, Krasz S, Miehlke S. Should quinolones come first in helicobacter pylori therapy? Therap Adv Gastroenterol. 2011;4:103–14.
53. Hsu PI, Kao SS. Therapy of helicobacter pylori infection: many drugs for which association? In: Manfredi M, Luigi De'Angelis G, editors. Helicobacter pylori. New York: Nova Science Publishers, Inc; 2013. p. 347–62.

16

The effect of n-3 polyunsaturated fatty acids on incidence and severity of oxaliplatin induced peripheral neuropathy

Ali Esfahani[1], Mohammad hossein Somi[1], Hormoz Ayromlou[2], Alireza Nikanfar[3], Mohammad Asghari Jafarabadi[4], Bina Eftekhar Sadat[5] and Zohreh Ghoreishi[6*]

Abstract

Background: Oxaliplatin induced peripheral neurotoxicity (OXIPN) is the major dose-limiting and long-lasting side effect of oxaliplatin. N-3 PUFAs have neuroprotective property via their effects on voltage-gated ion channels and by reducing the production of proinflammatory cytokines that causes neuropathy. This study was a randomized double blind placebo controlled trial to find the possible advantages of n-3 PUFAs for preventing and reducing the severity of OXIPN in patients with colon cancer.

Methods: Eligible patients with colon cancer randomly allocated to take n-3 PUFAs pearls, 640 mg t.i.d during chemotherapy with oxaliplatin and one month after the cessation of the treatment or placebo. All patients were evaluated for incidence and severity of OXIPN based on "reduced Total Neuropathy Score" in which clinical and electrophysiological assessments were included.

Results: Seventeen patients (47 %) of the n-3 PUFA supplemented group ($n = 36$) did not develop PN while it was 11 %(4 patients) in the placebo group ($n = 35$). There was a significant difference in PN incidence (OR = 0.14, .95 % CI = (0.04 to 0.49), $p = 0.002$). The difference of OXIPN severity was significant between the two study groups (B = −1.61, 0.95 % CI = (−2.59 to −0.62), $p = 0.001$).

Conclusions: N-3 PUFAs may have neuroprotective effect for reducing the incidence and severity of OXIPN. Finding an effective prophylactic or symptomatic therapy for OXIPN would significantly improve the patients' quality of life.

Keywords: Colon cancer, n-3 polyunsaturated fatty acids, Oxaliplatin, Neuropathy

Background

Colorectal cancer (CRC) is one of the most common cancers in the world with a considerable mortality rate and rising incidence during the last decades [1]. Oxaliplatin is now a central choice for treatment of advanced CRC [2] as the first line chemotherapy regimen [3] and as adjuvant therapy [4]. However, it induces a peripheral neuropathy which is the major dose-limiting side effect of this chemotherapeutic agent. Oxaliplatin-induced peripheral neuropathy (OXIPN) results in an acute transient syndrome, and a chronic sensory-motor axonal peripheral neuropathy. It may be a dose-limiting and disabling neurotoxicity that continues for a long time [5–8].

Eicosapentaenoic acid (EPA) and docosahexaenoic acid (DHA) are two main forms of n-3 polyunsaturated fatty acids (PUFAS). They are structural components of cell phospholipid membranes including those of the nervous system [9]. They have beneficial effects on a number of psychiatric and neurodegenerative diseases [9–11]. At present, there is no neuroprotective agent for prophylaxis and treatment of OXIPN [5, 12, 13], although several compounds have been proposed to have some effects on acute form of OXIPN. We previously reported

* Correspondence: zohreh_ghoreishy@yahoo.com
[6]Nutrition Research Center, Tabriz University of Medical Sciences, Tabriz, Iran

the efficacy of n-3 PUFAs for prophylaxis against paclitaxel-induced peripheral neuropathy in patients with breast cancer [14].

The possible advantages of n-3 PUFAs for preventing and reducing the severity of OXIPN in patients with colon cancer were assessed in the present study that is the first attempt in this area. As CRC survivors are the third largest population of cancer survivors [2, 5, 13], attenuating the risk of OXIPN- the major factor that decreases their quality of life- is now a major concern. Moreover, the serum level of proinflammatory cytokines was measured for assessing their changes during supplementation with n-3 PUFAs.

Methods

Primary outcome

This randomized double-blind placebo-controlled trial was conducted to assess the effect of n-3 PUFAs on incidence and severity of OXIPN in patients with colon cancer undergoing chemotherapy with oxaliplatin.

Patients

From February 2012 to January 2015, male or female patients with confirmed stage III colon cancer, aged between 20 and 85 years, and treated at Sheikhorrais University Clinic with oxaliplatin, 130 mg/m^2 IV, administered over 2 h infusion in day 1 and oral capecitabine (1000 mg/m^2, b.i.d) on days 1–4, to be repeated every 3 weeks for 8 cycles, were enrolled. Other inclusion criteria of the study were WHO performance status score of 0-1, and normal kidney and liver function.

Patients were excluded from the study if they had pre-existing peripheral neuropathy (PN) due to diabetes mellitus, alcoholic disease, HIV, and inherited PN- associated disorders. Patients who received other neurotoxic drugs prior to oxaliplatin therapy or those who were on any form of supplement therapy (fish oil, vitamins and minerals) were also excluded from the study.

Intervention and randomization

Eligible patients were randomly allocated in a 1:1 ratio to receive n-3 PUFAs pearls (Mor DHA Mini I.Q. Minami Nutrition NV, Drie Eikenstraat 661, 2650 Edegem, Belgium) at a dose of 640 mg (54 % DHA, 10 % EPA) three times a day coinciding with the start of chemotherapy until one month after the end of treatment or placebo pearls containing sun flower oil (Dana Pharma, Tabriz, Iran). Placebo and n-3 PUFAs pearls were similar in appearance and color and administered based on the same protocol.

Random allocation software (RAS) version 1.0.0. (Esfahan, Iran) was used for Permuted block randomization to assign patients to either the n-3 PUFAs supplemented group or the control group. Only the randomization coordinator of the study was aware of the patients' allocations.

Neurologic evaluation

All patients were evaluated prior to chemotherapy and one month after the cessation of treatment (about 25 weeks) by the same neurologist who carried out both clinical and electrophysiological assessments. He was blinded to the patient's allocation to study groups.

The presence of chronic OXIPN and grading of its severity was ascertained by reduced Total Neuropathy Score (TNSr) as the primary outcome measures. TNSr is an easy to use composite scale for assessing chemotherapy-induced peripheral neuropathy (CIPN) [15]. Subjective sensory symptoms, pin sensibility, deep tendon reflexes, and sural and peroneal amplitude (a total of 7 parameters) are all included in TNSr. Each parameter has a score from 0 to 4, based on the measured severity; then the total score ranges from 0 to 28 that grades OXIPN as follows: grade 0, no OXIPN, 1–10, mild; 11–19, moderate; and 20–28, severe OXIPN [14].

Secondary outcome

a) Nerve conduction studies (NCVs)
   Electrophysiological studies were carried out unilaterally (right side) under a uniform protocol using a Nicolet/VIASYS Viking Quest EMG Machine [16]. Thirty-two to 34°C was set as the distal skin temperature. The estimated parameters included: Distal motor latency (DML), peak to baseline amplitude of compound muscle action potential (a-CMAP), and motor conduction velocity for tibial, Peroneal and ulnar nerves. Moreover, peak-to-peak amplitude of sensory action potentials (a-SAP) and sensory conduction velocity (antidromic technique) of sural and ulnar nerves were also measured.
b) Proinflammatory cytokines
   Serum levels of proinflammatory cytokines: interleukin-6 (IL-6), tumor necrosis factor alpha (TNF-α), and high-sensitivity C-reactive Protein (hs-CRP) were measured before the onset of chemotherapy and one month after the cessation of treatment by Human IL-6 Platinum ELISA, Human TNF alpha Platinum ELISA (eBioscience, INC. San Diego, CA 92121, USA) and Minineph™ Human kits (Birmingham, UK) respevtively.

Protocol approvals and patient consent

This study (IRCT201112158397N2) was approved by the Ethics Committee of Tabriz University of Medical Sciences (No: 5/4/10130) and informed consent was obtained from all the study subjects before any intervention.

Statistical analysis

Data have been shown using mean (SD) and frequency (percent) for quantitative and qualitative variables respectively. To define the differences of nerve conduction measurements, analysis of covariance was used adjusting baseline measurements. Logistic regression analysis was performed to find the difference of OXIPN incidence between the two groups, estimating the odds ratio. Ordinal regression analysis was done to compare the severity of OXIPN. All tests were two-tailed and significance level was determined 0.05. For analyzing the results on an intention to treat (ITT) basis, multiple imputation was performed by related variables. Statistical power of the study was 80 % and all analysis was done using spss software, (spss Inc., Chicago, IL).

Sample size

To determine the sample size, primary information was obtained from the study by Ghoreishi et al. In this study, the protective effect of n-3 PUFAs against paclitaxel-induced neuropathy in patients with breast cancer was assessed. Using odds ratio (OR) = 0.3, $\alpha = 0.05$, a power of 80 %, and two-tailed analysis and G Power software (Franz Foal, Kiel University, Germany), the minimum sample size was estimated 38 subjects and after considering 30 % lost to follow up, it was increased to 50.

Results

Patients

Among the 84 recruited patients, 13 patients were excluded from the study due to diabetes mellitus, declined to participate, and taking some kinds of oral supplements (Fig. 1). Therefore, 71 patient were randomly allocated to receive n-3 PUFAs ($n = 36$, 50 % male with the average of age and BMI as: 54.14 ± 10.53 & 23.47 ± 3.40 kg/m^2 respectively) or placebo ($n = 35$, 60 % male, with the average of age and BMI as: 53.40 ± 15.70 & 23.22 ± 4.77 kg/m^2 respectively). There was not any statistical difference between two groups in terms of gender, age, and BMI ($P = .477$, .816, and .806 respectively, Table 1). The rate of drop out was 5 patients in n-3 PUFAs supplemented group and 7 patients in the placebo group (Fig. 1), so the response rate was 80.09 %. Data of the main outcome (incidence and severity of OXIPN), was divided into 2 categories: code 1 allocated to missing and code 2 allocated to valid observations. Then demographic variables were compared between ITT patients and efficacy population. Accordingly, they were not statistically different in terms of age ($P = 0.658$), BMI ($P = 0.224$) and gender ($P = 0.354$).

All patients suffered from metastatic colon cancer (stage III) and they treated with oxaliplatin, 130 mg/m^2 IV, administered over 2 h infusion in day 1 and oral capecitabine (1000 mg/m^2, b.i.d) on days 1–4, to be repeated every 3 weeks for 8 cycles. No patient received radiation therapy. The patients of the two groups were equivalent regarding the treatment protocol.

Assessment of OXIPN

One month after the cessation of chemotherapy, 17 patients (47 %) did not develop OXIPN in n-3 PUFAs supplemented group while the remaining 19 patients manifested some grade of neurotoxicity based on TNSr: mild OXIPN in 15(42 %) patients; moderate and severe OXIPN in 1(3 %) and 3(8 %) patients respectively. In placebo group, OXIPN was disclosed in 31 (88 %) of the patients: mild OXIPN in 20 patients (57 %), moderate and severe OXIPN in 7 patients (20 %) and 4 patients (12 %) respectively (Fig. 2). A significant difference was observed between the two groups in OXIPN incidence (OR = 0.14, .95 % CI = (0.04 to 0.49), $p = 0.002$). So group I had 86 % lower risk of PN incidence. The number needed to treat (NNT) to prevent one PN event was 2, and absolute risk reduction(ARR) for supplemented group compared with the control group was 0.41(0.16 to 0.59). Remarkably, there were a statistically significant difference in severity of OXIPN between these two groups (B = −1.61, .95 % CI = (−2.59 to −.62), $p = 0.001$). Adjusting for age, the differences between incidence and severity of OXIPN were more significant [(OR = 0.11, .95 % CI = (0.27 to 0.42), $p = 0.001$); (B = −1.74, .95 % CI = (−2.74 to − .75), $p = 0.001$)].

Nerve conduction studies

Significant statistical changes were observed between two study groups in terms of tibial and ulnar motor a-CMAP at one month after the cessation of chemotherapy (Table 2). However, the percent change measured (final measures versus the baseline values) showed that the deterioration of tibial, and ulnar a-CMAP was considerable in placebo group while they were increased in the. Moreover, the increase of peroneal nerve a-CMAP in the n-3 PUFAs group was much more than the increase in the placebo group (Table 2).

There was not a statistically difference between the two study groups according to sensory conduction studies, although a considerable trend for the differences of sural a-SAPs was observed between the two groups. The percent change of both sural and ulnar nerves' a-SAP showed a considerable decrease however, the decrease of the a-SAPs was strongly more pronounced in the placebo group at one month after the cessation of chemotherapy (Table 3).

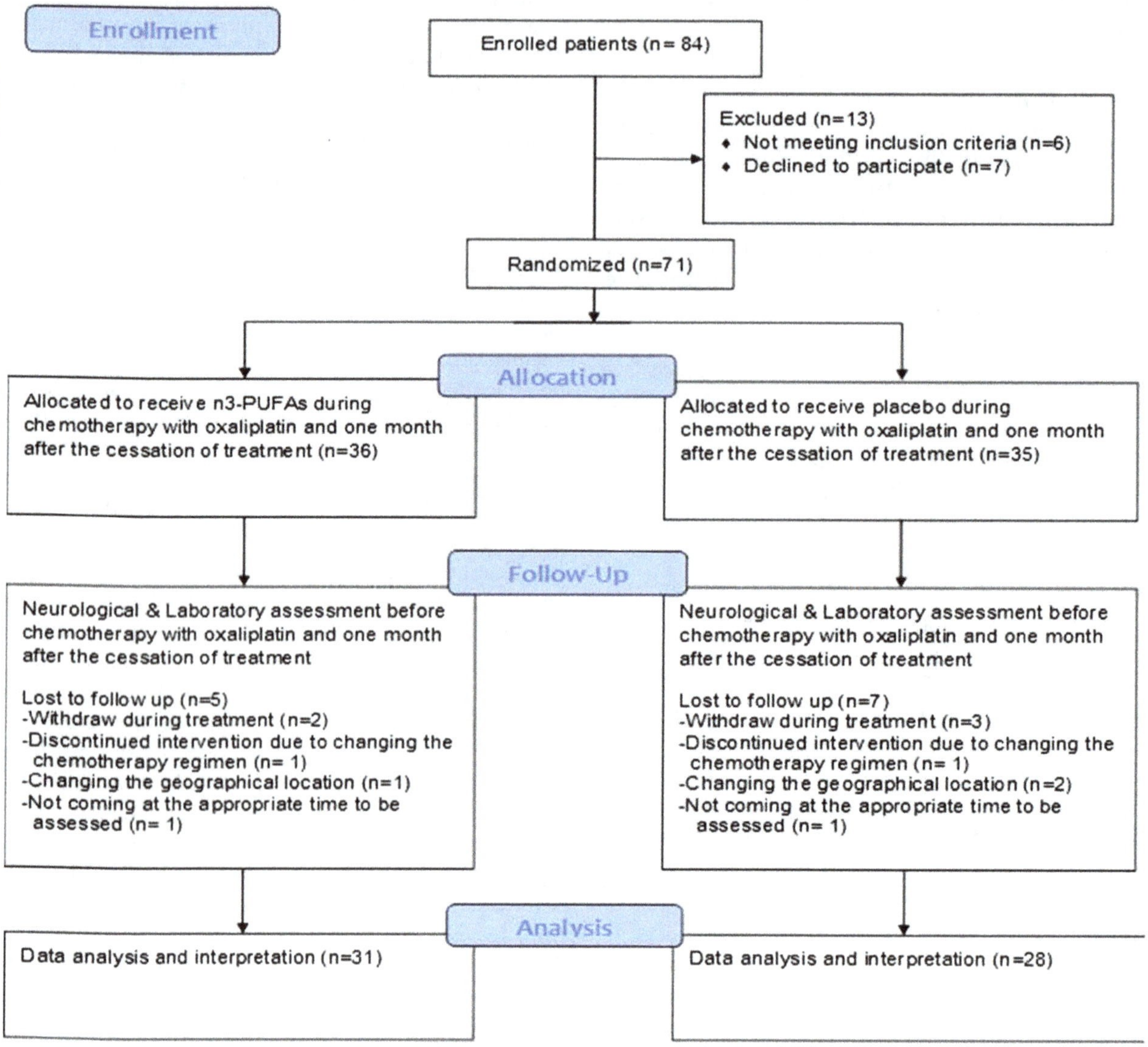

Fig. 1 Flowdiagram of the study

Proinflammatory cytokines

At the end of supplementation period (one month after the cessation of chemotherapy), the serum levels of IL-6 and TNF-α decreased 20.91 and 12.50 % respectively in the n-3 PUFAs group while they were increased in the placebo group without statistically significant differences. The serum level of hs-CRP was decreased in both groups although it was further reduced in the placebo group (61.02 % vs. 55.21 %, Table 4).

Discussion

We assessed the efficacy of n-3 PUFAs, mainly DHA, for preventing and reducing the severity of OXIPN in patients with colon cancer. Patients undergoing chemotherapy with oxaliplatin (XELOX regimen) randomly assigned to receive n-3 PUFAs pearls or placebo during the treatment courses and one month after the cessation of therapy (about 25 weeks) while incidence and severity of OXIPN were assessed in both time. This study showed that n3- PUFAs are protective against OXIPN in patients with colon cancer. Here we focused solely on chronic OXIPN that is a sensory- motor axon loss and the major dose-limiting side effect of oxaliplatin. It begins at a cumulative dose of 750–850 mg/m^2 and may be continued for a long time after the end of treatment [7, 17].

Clinical and electrophysiological finding were summarized by TNSr [15, 18] (ranging 0 to 28). It can be easily used for determining the incidence and severity of CIPN and it has a significant correlation with the known oncologic toxicity scales such as NCI-CTC, Ajani and ECOG scales, and the complete version of TNS as

Table 3 Comparing the sensory nerve conduction measurements between the two study groups

	n-3 PUFAs (Mean ± SD)	Placebo (Mean ± SD)	Mean Difference	95 % CI *P*-value
Sural nerve				
aSAP1(μV)	9.95 (5.52–16.40)	5.50 (3.40–14.10)	-	.033***
aSAP 2[a]	6.30 (4.60–10.30)	.00 (.00–7.32)		.052[b]
%Change[c]	− 36.68	− 100.00		
SCV1(m/s)	43.99 ± 15.17	44.82 ± 6.27	−.83	−6.44 to 4.78, .766*
SCV 2	42.29 ± 15.51	29.67 ± 13.01	12.24	2.22 to 22.26, .018**
% Change	−3.84	− 33.80		
Ulnar nerve				
aSAP1(μV)	27.90 (16.82–42.77)	17.50 (12.40–35.50)	-	.144***
a- SAP 2	22.80 (6.20–27.30)	10.14 (2.70–18.60)		.430[b]
% Change	− 18.28	− 42.06		
SCV1(m/s)	51.66 ± 8.34	50.15 ± 8.23	1.50	−2.51 to 5.52, .457*
SCV 2	44.08 ± 11.14	42.62 ± 7.26	.98	−4.61 to 6.57, .726**
% Change	− 14.66	− 15.01		

a-SAP sensory action potential amplitude, *SCV* sensory conduction velocity
**P* value is reported based on Independent-Samples *T*-Test
***P* value is reported based on the analysis of covariance, adjusted for baseline values
****P* value is reported based on the Mann–Whitney *U* Test
[a]One month after the cessation of chemotherapy
[b]*P* value is reported based on the Mann–Whitney *U* Test (for changes of values during the intervention period)
[c]Percent change in proportion to the baseline values

taste, and were well tolerated by the patients. The US Food and Drug Administration (FDA) recommended maximum levels of 3 g per day of n-3 PUFAs supplementation [31]. In the current study, the total dose of n-3 PUFAs administered was 1244.1 mg per day (640 mg: 54%DHA, 10 % EPA, t.i.d) which was far below the maximum FDA recommended for more prudence. No considerable side effects were reported by the patients.

Among a wide variety of compounds assessed for the prevention or treatment of chemotherapy-induced neuropathy, including vitamin E [32], Ca- Mg infusion [33–35], amifostine, glutamine, and glutathione [36], the Ca- Mg infusion was effective in this field. There is a concern, however of interference with the clinical efficacy of chemotherapy. Other compounds such as antidepressants, anticonvulsants [36] and green tea [37] had limited effects or they were not studied in RCTs.

Lack of long-term follow up of the patients due to high cost needed was one of the limitations of this study. Therefore, coasting phenomenon and self-improvement after the cessation of chemotherapy was not compared between the two study groups. Moreover, placebo did not smell fish oil and it may be considered as another limitation of this study. Despite the relatively small

Table 4 Serum levels of proinflammatory cytokines in two groups of patients

	n-3 PUFAs (Median, percentile 25–75)	Placebo (Median, percentile 25-75)	*P*-value
IL-6[a] 1(pg/ml)	28.70 (20.50–42.60)	21.50 (15.20–51.10)	.194*
IL-6 2	22.70 (17.10–30.45)	25.50 (16.80–55.40)	.396**
% Change	−20.91	18.60	
TNF-α[b] 1(pg/ml)	4.00 (3.60–5.25)	4.30 (3.60–5.60)	.218*
TNF-α 2	3.50 (3.15–4.97)	4.35 (3.15–4.97)	.097**
% Change	−12.50	1.16	
hs-CRP 1(mg/l)	2.95 (.92–7.30)	2.88 (1.31–15.40)	.505*
hs-CRP 2	1.15 (.82–2.32)	1.29 (.82–2.90)	.390**
% Change	−61.02	−55.21	

**P* value is reported based on the Mann–Whitney *U* Test
***P* value is reported based on the Mann–Whitney *U* Test (for changes of values during the intervention period)
[a]Interleukin-6
[b]Tumor necrosis factor-α

sample size of this study (we could not run a multicenter RCT, because of some problems in coordination between centers), the incidence and severity of OXIPN was different between the n-3 PUFAs and placebo groups, maybe due to the strong effect of DHA on the peripheral nervous system of the patients through the different mechanisms pointed out here and other presently unknown reasons, as the precise mechanism of OXIPN is not clear.

Conclusions

OXIPN will continue for a long time in patients who received oxaliplatin and it has a remarkable influence on the patients' quality of life [1, 7]. As the survival of this group of patients is increased significantly worldwide, finding an effective prophylactic or symptomatic therapy for OXIPN should be of special interest [2, 5]. In this study, n-3 PUFAs supplementation could reduce the incidence and severity of OXIPN in patients with colon cancer. It is well tolerated by patients because of few if any complications. Therefore, given the low-cost and safety of DHA, it can be recommended as a prophylactic and therapeutic agent for OXIPN. Further studies with larger sample size and longer follow-up are needed to confirm these findings.

Abbreviations

a-CMAP, amplitude of compound muscle action potential; a-SAP, sensory action potentials; CIPN, chemotherapy-induced peripheral neuropathy; CRC, colorectal cancer; DHA, docosahexaenoic acid; DML, distal motor latency; EPA, eicosapentaenoic acid; MCV, motor conduction velocity; NCVs, the nerve conduction studies; OXIPN, oxaliplatin-induced peripheral neuropathy; PUFAS, n-3 polyunsaturated fatty acids; TNSr, reduced total neuropathy score

Acknowledgements

The authors thank "Sanofi - IRAN" that was the financial sponsor of this research, grant number: Oxali_L_06172. The authors are also grateful to Minami Nutrition Company, for kind help to provide n-3 PUFAs pearls. We also thank Dana Pharma Pharmaceutical Company that provided us with placebo pearls.

Funding

This study was funded by "Sanofi" in IRAN.

Authors' contributions

Ali Esfahani, Mohammad hossein Somi, Alireza Nikanfar, and Zohreh Ghoreishi were involved in the study design and concept. Ali Esfahani was responsible for data collection. Hormoz Ayromlou and Bina Eftekhar Sadat were responsible for neurologic assessment and interpretation, Mohammad Asghari Jafarabadi carried out the statistical analysis and interpretation, Zohreh Ghoreishi was responsible for interpretation of the data and preparing the manuscript. All authors reviewed the manuscript. All authors read and approved the final manuscript.

Competing interests

The authors declare that they have no competing interests.

Author details

[1]Gastroenterology, Liver & Gastrointestinal Diseases Research Center, Tabriz University of Medical Sciences, Tabriz, Iran. [2]Neurosciences Research Center, Tabriz University of Medical Sciences, Tabriz, Iran. [3]Hematology and Oncology Research Center, Tabriz University of Medical Sciences, Tabriz, Iran. [4]Tabriz Health Services Management Research Center and Department of Statistics and Epidemiology, Faculty of Health and Nutrition, Tabriz University of Medical sciences, Tabriz, Iran. [5]Physical Medicine & Rehabilitation Research Center, Tabriz University of Medical Sciences, Tabriz, Iran. [6]Nutrition Research Center, Tabriz University of Medical Sciences, Tabriz, Iran.

References

1. Argyriou AA, Polychronopoulos P, Iconomou G, Koutras A, Makatsoris T, Gerolymos MK, Gourzis P, Assimakopoulos K, Kalofonos HP, Chroni E. Incidence and characteristics of peripheral neuropathy during oxaliplatin-based chemotherapy for metastatic colon cancer. Acta Oncol. 2007;46(8):1131–7.
2. Burakgazi AZ, Messersmith W, Vaidya D, Hauer P, Hoke A, Polydefkis M. Longitudinal assessment of oxaliplatin-induced neuropathy. Neurology. 2011;77(10):980–6.
3. de Gramont A, Figer A, Seymour M, Homerin M, Hmissi A, Cassidy J, Boni C, Cortes-Funes H, Cervantes A, Freyer G. Leucovorin and fluorouracil with or without oxaliplatin as first-line treatment in advanced colorectal cancer. J Clin Oncol. 2000;18(16):2938–47.
4. André T, Boni C, Mounedji-Boudiaf L, Navarro M, Tabernero J, Hickish T, Topham C, Zaninelli M, Clingan P, Bridgewater J. Oxaliplatin, fluorouracil, and leucovorin as adjuvant treatment for colon cancer. N Engl J Med. 2004; 350(23):2343–51.
5. Bennett BK, Park SB, Lin CSY, Friedlander ML, Kiernan MC, Goldstein D. Impact of oxaliplatin-induced neuropathy: a patient perspective. Support Care Cancer. 2012;20(11):2959–67.
6. Gamelin E, Gamelin L, Bossi L, Quasthoff S. Clinical aspects and molecular basis of oxaliplatin neurotoxicity: current management and development of preventive measures. In: Seminars in oncology: 2002. Elsevier; 2002: 21–33.
7. Mols F, Beijers T, Lemmens V, van den Hurk CJ, Vreugdenhil G, van de Poll-Franse LV. Chemotherapy-induced neuropathy and its association with quality of life among 2-to 11-year colorectal cancer survivors: results from the population-based PROFILES registry. J Clin Oncol. 2013. doi: 10.1200/JCO.2013.49.1514.
8. Ventzel L, Jensen AB, Jensen AR, Jensen TS, Finnerup NB. Chemotherapy-induced pain and neuropathy: A prospective study in patients treated with adjuvant oxaliplatin or docetaxel. Pain. 2016;157(3):560-68.
9. Shapiro H. Could n-3 polyunsaturated fatty acids reduce pathological pain by direct actions on the nervous system? Prostaglandins Leukot Essent Fatty Acids. 2003;68(3):219–24.
10. Mazza M, Pomponi M, Janiri L, Bria P, Mazza S. Omega-3 fatty acids and antioxidants in neurological and psychiatric diseases: an overview. Prog Neuro-Psychopharmacol Biol Psychiatry. 2007;31(1):12–26.
11. Coste TC, Gerbi A, Vague P, Pieroni G, Raccah D. Neuroprotective effect of docosahexaenoic acid-enriched phospholipids in experimental diabetic neuropathy. Diabetes. 2003;52(10):2578–85.
12. Visovsky C, Collins M, Abbott L, Aschenbrenner J, Hart C. Putting Evidence Into Practice®: Evidence-based interventions for chemotherapy-induced peripheral neuropathy. Clin J Oncol Nurs. 2007;11(6):901–13.
13. Park SB, Lin CSY, Krishnan AV, Goldstein D, Friedlander ML, Kiernan MC. Long-term neuropathy after oxaliplatin treatment: challenging the dictum of reversibility. Oncologist. 2011;16(5):708–16.
14. Ghoreishi Z, Esfahani A, Djazayeri A, Djalali M, Golestan B, Ayromlou H, Hashemzade S, Jafarabadi MA, Montazeri V, Keshavarz SA. Omega-3 fatty acids are protective against paclitaxel-induced peripheral neuropathy: a randomized double-blind placebo controlled trial. BMC Cancer. 2012;12(1):355.
15. Cavaletti G, Bogliun G, Marzorati L, Zincone A, Piatti M, Colombo N, Parma G, Lissoni A, Fei F, Cundari S. Grading of chemotherapy-induced peripheral neurotoxicity using the Total Neuropathy Scale. Neurology. 2003;61(9):1297–300.
16. Kimura J. Electrodiagnosis in diseases of nerve and muscle: principles and practice. Oxford University Press; 2001.
17. Serenoa M, Gutiérrez-Gutiérrezb G, Gómez-Raposoa C, Miriam López-Gómeza MM-S, Tébara FZ, Rodriguez-Antonac C, Casadod E.

Oxaliplatin induced-neuropathy in digestive tumors. Crit Rev Oncol Hematol. 2014;89(1):166–78.
18. Argyriou AA, Polychronopoulos P, Koutras A, Iconomou G, Iconomou A, Kalofonos HP, Chroni E. Peripheral neuropathy induced by administration of cisplatin-and paclitaxel-based chemotherapy. Could it be predicted? Support Care Cancer. 2005;13(8):647–51.
19. Argyriou AA, Polychronopoulos P, Chroni E. The usefulness of nerve conduction studies in objectively assessing oxaliplatin-induced peripheral neuropathy. Oncologist. 2007;12(11):1371–2.
20. Park SB, Krishnan AV, Lin C, Goldstein D, Friedlander M, Kiernan MC. Mechanisms underlying chemotherapy-induced neurotoxicity and the potential for neuroprotective strategies. Curr Med Chem. 2008;15(29):3081–94.
21. Fossat P, Dobremez E, Bouali-Benazzouz R, Favereaux A, Bertrand SS, Kilk K, Léger C, Cazalets J-R, Langel U, Landry M. Knockdown of L calcium channel subtypes: differential effects in neuropathic pain. J Neurosci. 2010;30(3): 1073–85.
22. Tatsushima Y, Egashira N, Narishige Y, Fukui S, Kawashiri T, Yamauchi Y, Oishi R. Calcium channel blockers reduce oxaliplatin-induced acute neuropathy: a retrospective study of 69 male patients receiving modified FOLFOX6 therapy. Biomed Pharmacother. 2013;67(1):39–42.
23. Ferrier GR, Redondo I, Zhu J, Murphy MG. Differential effects of docosahexaenoic acid on contractions and L-type Ca2+ current in adult cardiac myocytes. Cardiovasc Res. 2002;54(3):601–10.
24. Vreugdenhil M, Bruehl C, Voskuyl RA, Kang JX, Leaf A, Wadman WJ. Polyunsaturated fatty acids modulate sodium and calcium currents in CA1 neurons. Proc Natl Acad Sci. 1996;93(22):12559–63.
25. Tonini G, Santini D, Vincenzi B, Borzomati D, Dicuonzo G, La Cesa A, Onori N, Coppola R. Oxaliplatin may induce cytokine-release syndrome in colorectal cancer patients. J Biol Regul Homeost Agents. 2001;16(2):105–9.
26. Boyette-Davis JA, Walters ET, Dougherty PM. Mechanisms involved in the development of chemotherapy-induced neuropathy. Pain Manag. 2015;5(4): 285–96.
27. Binshtok AM, Wang H, Zimmermann K, Amaya F, Vardeh D, Shi L, Brenner GJ, Ji R-R, Bean BP, Woolf CJ. Nociceptors are interleukin-1beta sensors. J Neurosci. 2008;28(52):14062–73.
28. Bazan NG, Molina MF, Gordon WC. Docosahexaenoic acid signalolipidomics in nutrition: significance in aging, neuroinflammation, macular degeneration, Alzheimer's, and other neurodegenerative diseases. Annu Rev Nutr. 2011;31:321.
29. Xu Z-Z, Liu X-J, Berta T, Park C-K, Lu N, Serhan CN, Ji R-R. Neuroprotectin/ protectin D1 protects against neuropathic pain in mice after nerve trauma. Ann Neurol. 2013;74(3):490–5.
30. Bazan NG. The docosanoid neuroprotectin D1 induces homeostatic regulation of neuroinflammation and cell survival. Prostaglandins Leukot Essent Fatty Acids. 2013;88(1):127–9.
31. Lee JH, O'Keefe JH, Lavie CJ, Marchioli R, Harris WS. Omega-3 fatty acids for cardioprotection. In: Mayo Clinic Proceedings: 2008. Elsevier; 2008: 324–332.
32. Kottschade LA, Sloan JA, Mazurczak MA, Johnson DB, Murphy BP, Rowland KM, Smith DA, Berg AR, Stella PJ, Loprinzi CL. The use of vitamin E for the prevention of chemotherapy-induced peripheral neuropathy: results of a randomized phase III clinical trial. Support Care Cancer. 2011;19(11):1769–77.
33. Wen F, Zhou Y, Wang W, Hu QC, Liu YT, Zhang PF, Du ZD, Dai J, Li Q. Ca/ Mg infusions for the prevention of oxaliplatin-related neurotoxicity in patients with colorectal cancer: a meta-analysis. Ann Oncol. 2013. doi: 10. 1093/annonc/mds211.
34. Grothey A, Nikcevich DA, Sloan JA, Kugler JW, Silberstein PT, Dentchev T, Wender DB, Novotny PJ, Chitaley U, Alberts SR. Intravenous calcium and magnesium for oxaliplatin-induced sensory neurotoxicity in adjuvant colon cancer: NCCTG N04C7. J Clin Oncol. 2011;29(4):421–7.
35. Pachman DR, Ruddy K, Sangaralingham LR, Grothey A, Shah ND, Beutler AS, Hubbard JM, Loprinzi CL. Calcium and Magnesium Use for Oxaliplatin-Induced Neuropathy: A Case Study to Assess How Quickly Evidence Translates Into Practice. J Natl Compr Canc Netw. 2015;13(9):1097–101.
36. Piccolo J, Kolesar JM. Prevention and treatment of chemotherapy-induced peripheral neuropathy. Am J Health Syst Pharm. 2014;71(1):19–25.
37. Lee JS, Kim YT, Jeon EK, Won HS, Cho Y-S, Ko YH. Effect of green tea extracts on oxaliplatin-induced peripheral neuropathy in rats. BMC Complement Altern Med. 2012;12(1):124.

17

Evaluation of two high-throughput proteomic technologies for plasma biomarker discovery in immunotherapy-treated melanoma patients

Su Yin Lim[1,2], Jenny H. Lee[1,2], Sarah J. Welsh[1,2], Seong Beom Ahn[1], Edmond Breen[3], Alamgir Khan[3], Matteo S. Carlino[2,4,5], Alexander M. Menzies[2,4,6], Richard F. Kefford[1,2,5], Richard A. Scolyer[2,4], Georgina V. Long[2,4,6] and Helen Rizos[1,2,7*]

Abstract

Background: Selective kinase and immune checkpoint inhibitors, and their combinations, have significantly improved the survival of patients with advanced metastatic melanoma. Not all patients will respond to treatment however, and some patients will present with significant toxicities. Hence, the identification of biomarkers is critical for the selection and management of patients receiving treatment. Biomarker discovery often involves proteomic techniques that simultaneously profile multiple proteins but few studies have compared these platforms.

Methods: In this study, we used the multiplex bead-based Eve Technologies Discovery assay and the aptamer-based SomaLogic SOMAscan assay to identify circulating proteins predictive of response to immunotherapy in melanoma patients treated with combination immune checkpoint inhibitors. Expression of four plasma proteins were further validated using the bead-based Millipore Milliplex assay.

Results: Both the Discovery and the SOMAscan assays detected circulating plasma proteins in immunotherapy-treated melanoma patients. However, these widely used assays showed limited correlation in relative protein quantification, due to differences in specificity and the dynamic range of protein detection. Protein data derived from the Discovery and Milliplex bead-based assays were highly correlated.

Conclusions: Our study highlights significant limitations imposed by inconsistent sensitivity and specificity due to differences in the detection antibodies or aptamers of these widespread biomarker discovery approaches. Our findings emphasize the need to improve these technologies for the accurate identification of biomarkers.

Keywords: Cytokines, Multiplexing, Luminex, Aptamers, SOMAscan, Biomarkers, Liquid biopsies, Immune checkpoint inhibitors, Melanoma

Background

The identification and validation of biomarkers for monitoring disease progression, and predicting response to therapy and patient outcome is a rapidly growing field in cancer research. Cancer patients are currently being treated with new generations and combinations of targeted drugs [1, 2] and immunotherapy [3, 4] but, the activity of these drugs is hampered by variable response rates and the development of treatment resistance [5–7]. For example, approximately 60% of patients with advanced melanoma respond to the combination of the cytotoxic T lymphocyte antigen-4 (CTLA-4) inhibitor, ipilimumab, with an inhibitor of the programmed death-1 (PD-1) receptor (pembrolizumab or nivolumab). However, the benefit of this drug combination comes with significant toxicity and 40% of patients will show no response to therapy [8, 9]. As a result, the identification

* Correspondence: Helen.rizos@mq.edu.au
[1]Faculty of Medicine and Health Sciences, Macquarie University, Sydney, Australia
[2]Melanoma Institute Australia, Sydney, Australia

and validation of reliable, sensitive and accurate predictive biomarkers is necessary for the improved selection and management of cancer patients.

Circulating biomarkers, identified in liquid biopsies such as serum and plasma, can provide an accurate and minimally invasive means for monitoring disease progression, tumor heterogeneity and treatment response. Analysis of certain circulating biomarkers has already yielded important prognostic and diagnostic information, such as prostate-specific antigen (PSA) in prostate cancer [10] and carcinoembryonic antigen (CEA) in colorectal cancer [11], while others have assisted assessment of treatment response and resistance, including circulating tumor DNA (ctDNA) [12, 13] and cancer antigen CA125 [14].

Biomarker discovery using proteomic analysis of liquid biopsies usually involves bead-based multiplex Luminex assays, aptamer-based assays or unbiased mass spectrometry. A literature search using the terms "cancer biomarker" and "liquid biopsy" (August 1, 2017) for publications reporting on liquid biomarker discovery in cancer found 62 publications applying the bead-based system, 36 publications using aptamer-based assays and 252 publications based on mass spectrometry. Although significant attention has focused on cancer biomarker discovery, few studies have compared commonly used protein detection and quantitation platforms.

In this study, we compared a bead-based multiplex assay (Eve Technologies 65-plex Human Cytokine/-Chemokine Discovery assay) and an aptamer-based technology (SomaLogic SOMAscan assay) for biomarker discovery in 47 plasma samples derived from 24 melanoma patients treated with combination pembrolizumab and ipilimumab therapy. We show that these widely used assays have limited correlation in relative protein quantification, and this was largely due to differences in specificity and the dynamic range of protein detection. Further, we found that discrepancies in protein quantification and detection were more apparent when two different detection reagents (i.e. antibodies vs. aptamers) were used. Our findings highlight significant limitations in two common approaches for biomarker discovery, and underscore the need for robust method validation and independent assay assessment for blood-based biomarker discovery.

Methods

Patients, treatment and clinical assessment

This study included 24 metastatic melanoma patients treated with immunotherapy at Westmead Hospital and Melanoma Institute Australia between July 2014 and December 2015. Patients were treated with pembrolizumab in combination with ipilimumab, administered according to the schedule in the MK3475–029 clinical trial (NCT02089685). Informed consent was obtained from all patients under approved human research ethics committee protocols from the Royal Prince Alfred Hospital.

Investigator-determined objective response was assessed radiologically with computed tomography scans 12 weeks after start of treatment. Patients were divided into responders (Response Evaluation Criteria In Solid Tumor; RECIST CR and PR) and non-responders (RECIST SD and PD) based on RECIST 1.1 guidelines [15] (Fig. 1).

Patient characteristics, clinicopathologic and demographic information including mutation status, lactate dehydrogenase (LDH) levels, disease distribution and American Joint Committee on Cancer (AJCC) M stage (7th edition) were collected (Table 1).

Plasma samples

Peripheral blood samples (~10 ml) were collected from patients in EDTA vacutainer tubes (BD Vacutainer Blood Collection Tubes) before treatment (baseline biopsy) and early during therapy (EDT; collected between 1 to 6 weeks after treatment initiation). All patients had an available EDT sample and 23 patients also had a matched baseline biopsy. Blood samples were centrifuged at 1500 rpm (800 x g) for 15 min at room temperature to separate plasma. Approximately 3–4 ml plasma were collected and centrifuged again at 4100 rpm (1600 x g) for 10 min at room temperature. Clarified plasma samples (1 ml aliquots) were stored at −80 °C, and the plasma volume required for the Discovery (155 μl), SOMAscan (130 μl) and Milliplex (50 μl) assays were obtained from the same plasma aliquot.

Proteomic assays

Undiluted baseline and EDT plasma samples from 24 patients were profiled using the 65-plex Discovery assay

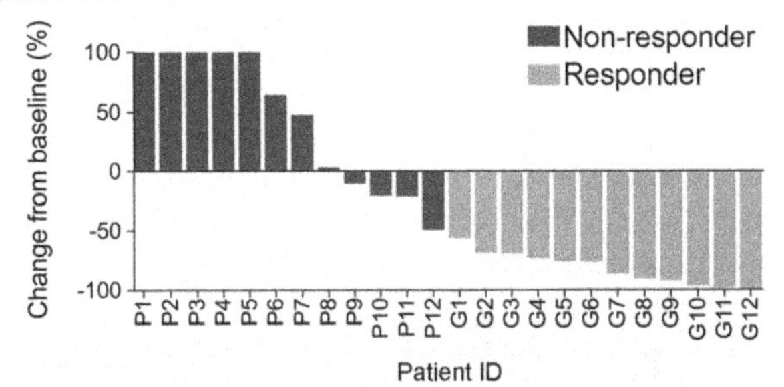

Fig. 1 RECIST response of melanoma patients. Melanoma patients were divided into responding (n = 12) or non-responding (n = 12) groups based on RECIST 1.1 (response evaluation criteria in solid tumor) guidelines following the Week 12 computed tomography scan. Patients in the responding group showed RECIST CR (complete response) or PR (partial response) while those in the non-responding group had RECIST SD (stable disease) or PD (progressive disease). The percentage of change in target lesions from baseline to Week 12 is shown

Table 1 Patient characteristics and treatment outcomes

Patient ID	RECIST at Week 12	Baseline LDH (U/L)	PFS (months)[a]	OS (months)[a]
Responders				
G1	PR	167	Response ongoing	Alive
G2	PR	215	Response ongoing	Alive
G3	PR	159	Response ongoing	Alive
G4	PR	217	Response ongoing	Alive
G5	PR	185	Response ongoing	Alive
G6	PR	206	Response ongoing	Alive
G7	PR	268	Response ongoing	Alive
G8	PR	167	Response ongoing	Alive
G9	PR	227	Response ongoing	Alive
G10	PR	187	Response ongoing	Alive
G11	PR	140	Response ongoing	Alive
G12	CR	150	Response ongoing	Alive
Non-responders				
Patient ID	RECIST at Week 12	Baseline LDH (U/L)	PFS (months)[a]	OS (months)[a]
P1	PD	303	2.7	5.8
P2	PD	568	2.7	5.1
P3	PD	329	2.7	3.1
P4	PD	300	1.1	Alive
P5	PD	271	0.5	Alive
P6	PD	267	2.7	Alive
P7	PD	169	2.8	Alive
P8	SD	226	4	Alive
P9	SD	269	4.1	Alive
P10	SD	176	2.7	21.7
P11	SD	195	Response ongoing	Alive
P12	SD	402	5.5	8.3

Abbreviations: *PR* partial response, *SD* stable disease, *PD* progressive disease, *CR* complete response, *LDH* lactate dehydrogenase, *PFS* progression free survival, *OS* overall survival, *U/L* units per liter

[a]Data cut off on 30th April, 2017. 11 out of 24 patients had progressed at time of analysis, all of whom were in the non-responders group. Median follow-up for these patients is 24.3 months. Normal range of LDH is 120–250 U/L

(Human Cytokine Array/Chemokine Array 65-Plex Panel; Cat no: HD65, Eve Technologies, Alberta, Canada) and the 1310 protein SOMAscan assay (SomaLogic, Inc. CO, USA).

The 65-plex Discovery assay is based on the Luminex technology and utilizes the Millipore assay that comprises of fluorescent color-coded beads pre-coated with capture antibodies targeting 65 specific cytokines. Plasma samples were incubated with the beads before the addition of biotinylated detection antibodies followed by phycoerythrin (PE)-conjugated streptavidin. Bound cytokines were identified and quantitated using the Bio-Rad BioPlex 200 bead analyzer consisting of a dual-laser system which i) activates the fluorescent beads to identify the specific cytokine and, ii) excites the PE conjugate to determine the magnitude of fluorescence, which is in direct proportion to reflect the amount of bound cytokine. This assay utilized 150 μl of plasma per run and each run was performed in duplicate; duplicates did not vary by more than 4%.

The SOMAscan assay uses SOMAmer (Slow Off-rate Modified Aptamer) reagents, which consist of modified short DNA sequences that bind specific protein analytes [16]. Plasma samples were incubated with SOMAmer reagents and protein analytes bound to SOMAmer reagents were then biotinylated before capturing the SOMAmer-protein complexes with streptavidin beads. The SOMAmer-protein complexes were detached, and SOMAmer reagents collected and hybridized to complementary sequences on a microarray chip and quantified by fluorescence, which directly correlates with protein amount in the plasma samples. This assay utilized 130 μl of plasma sample per assay run singly. Five patient plasma samples were run in different batches and data showed high concordance ($r = 0.99$, $p < 0.0001$) between batch runs.

Expression of IL-1α, IL-1RA, TNFα and IL-6 in 13 baseline and 15 EDT plasma samples were further validated using the Luminex technology (Milliplex MAP Human Cytokine/Chemokine Panel; Cat no: HCYTOMAG-60 K, Millipore, St. Charles, MO). This bead-based assay is similar to the 65-plex Discovery assay and utilizes fluorescent color-coded beads pre-coated with capture antibodies targeting 4 specific cytokines. Plasma samples were filtered through 0.22 μm spin filters and 25 μl of undiluted plasma was run in duplicates per assay. Duplicates did not vary by more than 5%. Samples were assayed on a robotic liquid handling workstation (epMotion 5075, Eppendorf, Germany) and read with the BioPlex Systems 100 (Bio-Rad) as previously reported [17].

Fluorescence intensity values derived from the Discovery, SOMAscan and Milliplex assays were reported as relative fluorescent units (RFU). Additionally, for the Discovery and Milliplex assays, a protein standard consisting of purified cytokines at known concentrations was included in each batch run; absolute protein concentrations were calculated from the standard curve and reported as pg/ml. Protein standards were not included in the SOMAscan assay and as such, absolute protein concentrations were not determined.

Statistical analysis

Differential protein expression analysis was performed using the limmaGP module in GenePattern [18]. Comparison between two groups was performed using Mann-Whitney test, correlation analysis using Spearman's correlation coefficient, and patient characteristics compared using a Chi square test in GraphPad Prism (version 7.02). Principal Component Analysis (PCA) was performed using the ClutVis program [19].

Results

Patient response

Twelve patients responded to pembrolizumab in combination with ipilimumab with a complete response (CR, n = 1) or a partial response (PR, n = 11) and twelve patients had no objective response, i.e. stable (SD, n = 5) or progressive disease (PD, n = 7). Clinical characteristics across these two response groups were similar for age, sex and disease volume but were significantly different in the known prognostic factors of baseline LDH and AJCC tumor stage (Tables 1 and 2); earlier AJCC stage and normal LDH are associated with good response to combination immunotherapy.

Comparison of assay performance

Baseline and EDT plasma samples from the responding and non-responding patients were analyzed for expression of multiple proteins using the 65-plex Discovery assay (Eve Technologies; 65 proteins detected) and the SOMAscan assay (SomaLogic; 1310 detected proteins).

The 65-plex Discovery assay has a reported dynamic range of 0.64 pg/ml to 10,000 pg/ml, comparable to other Luminex assays, and a minimal limit of detection (sensitivity) ranging from 0.1 pg/ml to 55.8 pg/ml while the inter-assay variability (coefficient of variation; CV) was between 3.5–18.9% for the 65 cytokines included in the panel [20]. Fluorescence intensity values were detected for every protein in all plasma samples in the Discovery assay, and varied from 46.26 RFU to 13,069 RFU, with a median of 184.7 RFU (Fig. 2a). However, despite a dynamic range across five orders of magnitude, absolute protein concentrations could not be calculated for 15 of the 65 cytokines in more than 75% of plasma samples, as the fluorescence values were below the standard curve (Table 3).

Fluorescence intensity values have been shown to be more robust indicators of protein expression compared to absolute concentrations in terms of reproducibility, and for statistical differential analysis [21, 22]. Boxplot graphs showed median fluorescence intensity distributions of the plasma samples were within the range of the standard curve for most of the 65 cytokines in the Discovery assay (Standard 1–7; Additional file 1: Figure S1a and b). However, five of the 65 cytokines (Eotaxin-3, IL-21, IL-3, IL-9 and TSLP) had median fluorescence distributions that were below the standard curve range (Additional file 1: Figure S1b). Detailed analysis of these 5 cytokines showed a symmetrical distribution of RFU (Additional file 1: Figure S2), suggesting that these fluorescence values are unlikely to be background artefacts

Table 2 Summary of patient characteristics

Characteristics	Responders (n = 12)	Non-responders (n = 12)	P value
Age – no. (%)			
> 65	6 (50%)	2 (17%)	0.083
≤ 65	6 (50%)	10 (83%)	
Sex – no. (%)			
Male	9 (75%)	9 (75%)	>0.999
Female	3 (25%)	3 (25%)	
LDH – no. (%)			
> 1× ULN	1 (8%)	8 (67%)	0.0032
≤ 1× ULN	11 (92%)	4 (33%)	
Disease volume – no. (%)			
SPOD > 1000 mm^2	7 (58%)	10 (83%)	0.178
SPOD ≤ 1000 mm^2	5 (42%)	2 (17%)	
AJCC tumor stage – no. (%)			
M1a or M1b	6 (50%)	1 (8%)	0.025
M1c	6 (50%)	11 (92%)	
Mutation – no. (%)			
$BRAF^{V600E/K}$	3 (25%)	5 (42%)	0.3865
Non-$BRAF^{V600E/K}$	9 (75%)	7 (58%)	

Abbreviations: *LDH* lactate dehydrogenase, *SPOD* sum of product of diameters, *AJCC* American Joint Committee on Cancer, *ULN* upper limit of normal. The p value was calculated using the Chi square test for a two by two contingency table

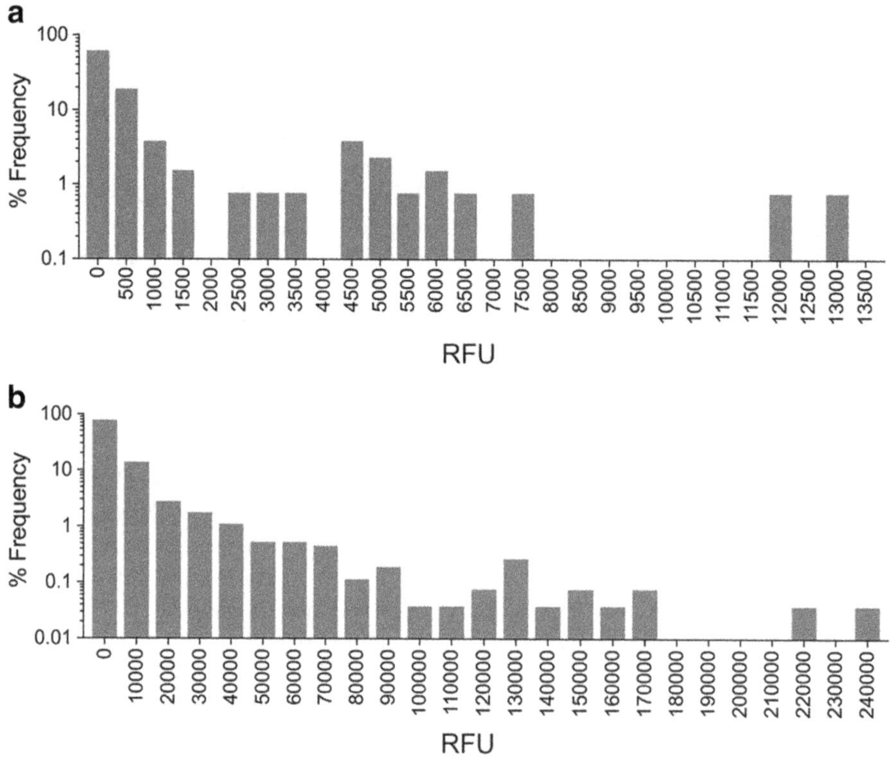

Fig. 2 Density distribution of fluorescence intensity values. The distribution, range and frequency of relative fluorescence intensity units (RFU) of proteins detected in all 47 patient samples in the (**a**). Discovery assay and (**b**). SOMAscan assay are shown

despite the low readings. As such, fluorescence intensity readings for all 65 cytokines were used in our analyses instead of derived concentrations.

The SOMAscan assay has a larger dynamic range compared to the Discovery assay, detecting protein level from fM to μM across eight orders of magnitude. The average minimal limit of detection is 1.6 pg/ml and the CV varied between 2.9–12.6% for all 1310 protein analytes [23]. Fluorescence data for all 1310 proteins were detected in all plasma samples, and ranged from 45.33 RFU to 238,857 RFU, with a median of 1254 RFU (Fig. 2b). Protein standards of known concentrations were not included for the analytes in the SOMAscan assay, thus absolute protein concentrations could not be calculated and fluorescence data were used instead.

It is important to mention that although fluorescence intensity readings reflect relative protein quantity, they are not directly comparable across different analytes in the SOMAscan assay. For example, a two fold increase in RFU values does not indicate a two fold increase in protein quantity.

Comparison of protein identification and quantification

The Discovery and SOMAscan assays have 49 proteins in common (Fig. 3a) and the fluorescence intensity values for each of these 49 proteins were median collapsed and analyzed for correlation.

As shown in Fig. 3b, the Discovery and SOMAscan median expression data for the 49 shared proteins in the PRE and EDT clinical samples were weakly correlated ($r = 0.309$, $p = 0.0308$, $n = 47$ plasma samples). However, when compared individually, only 12 of the 49 shared proteins showed significant positive correlation between these two assays (both PRE and EDT samples were compared; Table 4). The lack of correlation did not appear to reflect relative fluorescence readings as both high (CTACK and Eotaxin-1) and low level (IL-7 and I-309) proteins were not significantly correlated in these assays (Additional file 1: Figure S3). We noted that nearly all of the 37 proteins that did not correlate between the two assays showed one of two features. The proteins had low RFU in the Discovery assay ($p < 0.01$, Fig. 4a) and/or the proteins showed limited range of RFU in the SOMAscan assay when compared to the equivalent RFU range of the Discovery assay (Fig. 4b). For instance, 30 out of the 37 proteins (81%) that were not correlated had a median RFU of less than 100 in the Discovery assay, and in the SOMAscan assay, 27 out of the 37 proteins (73%) that were not correlated showed limited RFU distribution compared to the Discovery assay.

Table 3 Detection limits of the Discovery assay

Cytokine	Samples within standard curve[a]	Cytokine	Samples within standard curve[a]	Cytokine	Samples within standard curve[a]
BCA-1	47/47 (100%)	IL-6	43/47 (91%)	**MCP-3**	20/47 (43%)
CTACK	47/47 (100%)	**IL-7**	26/47 (55%)	MCP-4	46/47 (98%)
EGF	38/47 (81%)	IL-8	39/47 (83%)	MDC	47/47 (100%)
ENA-78	47/47 (100%)	IL-9	47/47 (100%)	**MIP-1α**	34/47 (72%)
Eotaxin-1	47/47 (100%)	IL-10	42/47 (89%)	MIP-1β	44/47 (94%)
Eotaxin-2	45/47 (96%)	**IL-12P40**	27/47 (57%)	MIP-1d	47/47 (100%)
Eotaxin-3	47/47 (100%)	IL-12P70	41/47 (87%)	PDGF-AA	47/47 (100%)
FGF-2	47/47 (100%)	**IL-13**	22/47 (47%)	PDGF-BB	46/47 (98%)
Flt-3 Ligand	20/47 (43%)	IL-15	46/47 (98%)	RANTES	37/47 (79%)
Fractalkine	42/47 (89%)	IL-16	47/47 (100%)	sCD40L	47/47 (100%)
G-CSF	40/47 (85%)	IL-17A	39/47 (83%)	**SCF**	20/47 (43%)
GM-CSF	40/47 (85%)	IL-18	43/47 (91%)	SDF-1	46/47 (98%)
GRO pan	45/47 (96%)	IL-20	45/47 (96%)	TARC	47/47 (100%)
IFNα2	42/47 (89%)	**IL-21**	22/47 (47%)	TGF-a	36/47 (77%)
IFNγ	36/47 (77%)	IL-23	45/47 (96%)	TNFα	47/47 (100%)
IL-1α	46/47 (98%)	IL-28A	46/47 (98%)	**TNFβ**	22/47 (47%)
IL-1B	35/47 (74%)	**IL-33**	29/47 (62%)	TPO	39/47 (83%)
IL-1RA	40/47 (85%)	IP-10	47/47 (100%)	TRAIL	47/47 (100%)
IL-2	28/47 (60%)	I-309	47/47 (100%)	TSLP	42/47 (89%)
IL-3	47/47 (100%)	**LIF**	33/47 (70%)	**VEGF-A**	32/47 (68%)
IL-4	19/47 (40%)	MCP-1	47/47 (100%)	6CKINE	47/47 (100%)
IL-5	36/47 (77%)	MCP-2	47/47 (100%)		

[a]Percentage of the 47 plasma samples with target protein fluorescence intensity values within the protein standard curve. Absolute cytokine concentration for 15/65 cytokines (shown in bold) could not be calculated in more than 75% of plasma samples because fluorescence intensity values were below the standard curve

To validate the protein data, we assessed expression of four proteins (IL-1RA, IL-1A, TNFα and IL-6) that were measured in both the Discovery and SOMAscan assays, and showed variable expression and correlation data (i.e. only TNFα was highly expressed in the Discovery and SOMAscan assays, whereas IL-1RA, IL-1A and IL-6 were not correlated and showed moderate to low expression). These four circulating proteins were assessed in 28 plasma samples from a subset of the same patients (n = 15) using the MAP Human Cytokine/Chemokine Milliplex assay. Fluorescence intensity values for each of the 4 proteins were analyzed for correlation between all three assays. Only TNFα was significantly correlated between all assays while IL-1RA, IL-1A and IL-6 showed significant positive correlation between the Milliplex assay and the Discovery assay but not the SOMAscan assay (Fig. 5a).

Because absolute protein concentrations could be derived for the four proteins from the Discovery and Milliplex assays, we additionally correlated these values and found significant positive correlation for TNFα, IL-1RA and IL-6 (Fig. 5b). Absolute concentration values of IL-1A from the Discovery and Milliplex assays were not significantly correlated, however, it is important to point out that these values could not be calculated from the Milliplex assay in more than 65% of plasma samples as their fluorescence intensities were below the standard curve.

Identification of differentially expressed proteins in immunotherapy response

We performed differential expression analyses to identify circulating proteins predictive of response to immunotherapy. The PRE and EDT plasma samples were grouped into either response (n = 12 for PRE, n = 12 for EDT samples) or non-response (n = 11 for PRE, n = 12 for EDT samples) groups and differential expression between the two groups was analyzed using LimmaGP. From the 1310 proteins in the SOMAscan assay, 178 were differentially expressed in EDT plasma samples ($q < 0.25$, $p < 0.05$), whereas no proteins were differentially expressed in the baseline samples between the two response groups. 175 out of the 178 differentially expressed proteins were expressed higher in the non-

a

CTACK	GRO pan	IL-9	IFNγ	sCD40L
EGF	IL-1A	IL-10	MCP-1	TARC
ENA-78	IL-1B	IL-13	MCP-2	TNFα
Eotaxin-1	IL-2	IL-16	MCP-3	TNFß
Eotaxin-2	IL-3	IL-17	MCP-4	TPO
Eotaxin-3	IL-4	IL-20	MDC	TSLP
Flt-3 ligand	IL-5	IL-23	PDGF-AA	VEGF
Fractalkine	IL-6	IL-1RA	PDGF-BB	6CKine
G-CSF	IL-7	IP-10	RANTES	MIP-1α
GM-CSF	IL-8	I-309	SDF-1	

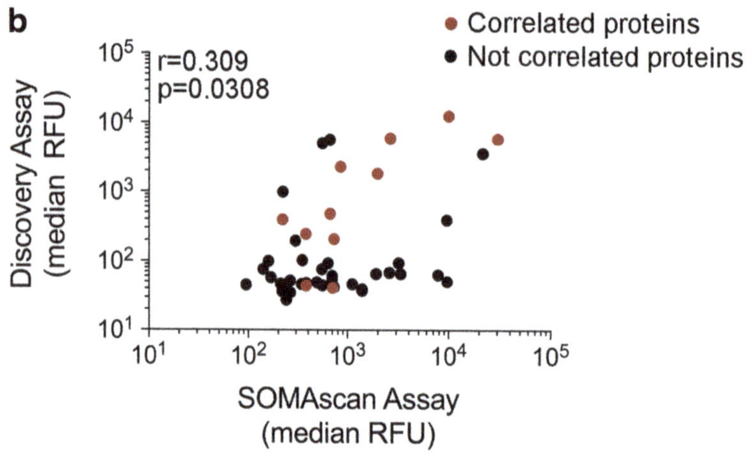

Fig. 3 Correlation of common protein targets. **a** List of the 49 proteins shared by the SOMAscan and Discovery Assays. **b** The median relative fluorescence units (RFU) of each of the 49 proteins in all 47 patient samples were derived from the SOMAscan and Discovery assays and tested for correlation (Spearman's rank correlation coefficient; $r = 0.3165$, $p = 0.0267$). Twelve of the 49 proteins (represented in red) showed significant positive correlation between the two assays when tested individually using Spearman's rank correlation coefficient (results of the statistical analysis shown in Table 4)

response group and PCA analysis of the differentially expressed proteins indicated clear separation of the EDT plasma samples between the two groups (Fig. 6a). In contrast, comparison of the fluorescence intensity values of the 65 cytokines from the Discovery assay did not reveal any significant differences at baseline or EDT. Of the 178 differentially expressed proteins in EDT samples from the SOMAscan assay, five were part of the Discovery assay panel. However, the five proteins (EGF, SDF-1, CTACK, IL-20 and IL-6) were not positively correlated between the two assays (Table 4).

We also compared changes in proteins in response to therapy and assessed whether these changes predicted response. For this analysis, EDT RFU values were subtracted from the matched baseline RFU data. None of the 65 cytokines from the Discovery assay showed significant differences between the two patient groups in response to therapy. However, we found that 32 SOMAscan proteins were differentially altered on therapy in the response versus non-response groups ($q < 0.25$, $p < 0.05$). These 32 proteins were all higher (i.e. upregulated on therapy) in the non-response group and PCA analysis of the differentially regulated proteins showed some separation between the two response groups (Fig. 6b). Of the 32 SOMAscan proteins that were significantly altered in response to therapy, MIP-1α and IL-3 were included in the Discovery assay panel, but expression data of these from the two assays did not show significant correlation (Table 4).

Discussion

Despite advances in proteomic technologies and high-throughput analyte detection systems, successful identification and validation of new biomarkers for cancer diagnosis, and for predicting treatment response has been poor. A significant challenge lies in the limitations of current proteomic techniques. For example, mass spectrometry, although offering more accurate identification of proteins, is limited by interference from high abundance proteins. Other technologies such as multiplex bead-based and aptamer-based assays also have limitations imposed by the specificity and potential cross-reactivity of the capture antibodies or aptamers.

Table 4 Correlation analysis of Discovery and SOMAScan assays

Cytokine	*r* value	*P* value[a]	Cytokine	*r* value	*P* value[a]	Cytokine	*r* value	*P* value[a]
CTACK	0.0242	0.8719	IL-4	0.1467	0.3252	MCP-4	0.1200	0.4218
EGF	0.2815	0.0553	IL-5	0.1427	0.3387	**MDC**	0.5461	<0.0001
ENA-78	0.2833	0.0536	IL-6	0.2487	0.0918	MIP-1α	−0.0028	0.9852
Eotaxin-1	0.2312	0.1179	IL-7	−0.0071	0.9618	**PDGF-AA**	0.7951	<0.0001
Eotaxin-2	0.1752	0.2388	**IL-8**	0.4526	0.0014	**PDGF-BB**	0.6449	<0.0001
Eotaxin-3	0.5295	0.0001	IL-9	0.1587	0.2866	RANTES	−0.0445	0.7664
Flt-3 Ligand	0.4585	0.0012	IL-10	−0.2023	0.1727	**sCD40L**	0.4882	0.0005
Fractalkine	−0.4095	0.0043	IL-13	0.0454	0.7619	SDF-1	0.2765	0.0599
G-CSF	0.0897	0.5486	IL-16	−0.2042	0.1686	**TARC**	0.8669	<0.0001
GM-CSF	0.1330	0.3727	IL-17A	0.1628	0.2743	**TNFα**	0.3373	0.0204
GROpan	0.4460	0.0017	IL-20	−0.3942	0.0061	**TNFβ**	0.3215	0.0275
IFNγ	−0.0659	0.6595	IL-23	−0.1467	0.3252	TPO	0.1433	0.3366
IL-1A	−0.0624	0.6767	**IP-10**	0.5764	<0.0001	TSLP	−0.0460	0.7587
IL-1B	0.1263	0.3975	I-309	−0.1289	0.3877	VEGF	−0.1383	0.3539
IL-1RA	0.0253	0.8661	MCP-1	0.0614	0.6818	6CKine	0.1104	0.4602
IL-2	−0.467	0.0009	MCP-2	−0.2492	0.0912			
IL-3	0.1065	0.4761	MCP-3	−0.2023	0.1728			

[a]Spearman's rank correlation coefficient test. Only 12 (shown in bold) of the 49 common proteins showed significant positive correlation between the Discovery and SOMAScan assays ($p < 0.05$)

In this study, we compared two proteomic techniques widely used in biomarker discovery. We found that the Discovery and SOMAscan assays showed poor correlation in fluorescence data for 49 shared proteins, and as such, these assays did not detect any proteins in common that identified melanoma patients likely to respond to immunotherapy. The lack of correlation appears to be associated with low detection levels in the Discovery assay and/or restricted range of detection for the SOMAscan platform. To gain further insights into the variability between these assays, we re-quantitated four common cytokines using the Milliplex assay, which also utilizes the bead-based Luminex technology. As expected, all four re-tested cytokines were significantly correlated between the Milliplex and Discovery assays. In contrast, three of four re-tested cytokines (i.e. IL-1RA, IL-1α and IL-6) were not correlated between the Luminex and SomaLogic platforms, and importantly these three cytokines showed a limited range of RFU in the SOMAscan assays. These data strongly suggest that the variability between the Discovery and SOMAscan assays reflect poor specificity and sensitivity of many of the capture antibodies or aptamers.

Our analysis of the data from the Discovery assay did not yield any proteins reflective of response to immunotherapy. However, from the SOMAscan assay, 178 proteins were differentially expressed early during therapy in plasma of patients who responded to treatment compared to those who did not respond, and 32 proteins were upregulated upon treatment in patients who did not respond to immunotherapy. These differentially expressed proteins could represent potential predictive biomarkers of immunotherapy response but given the poor concordance between the Discovery and SOMAscan assays, these targets need to be further validated using separate proteomic approaches and in a larger patient cohort. The complete list and analysis of differentially expressed proteins will be reported as part of another study.

It is also worth noting that there may be more value in using the fluorescence intensity data to identify potential targets during differential expression analysis. To support this, we observed that the mean fluorescence values of the lower standards (S1 and S2, Additional file 1: Figure S1) of some cytokines (i.e. SDF-1 and MIP-1a) did not separate well. This suggests decreased sensitivity in detection of these low-level cytokines, and in turn, may contribute to errors in absolute concentration calculation for each of these cytokines as their standard curve will be skewed. However, this effect will not impact analysis using fluorescence values alone.

Conclusions

Our study highlights inadequacies in two proteomic platforms commonly used for biomarker discovery, which up till now, have not been evaluated extensively side by side. We show that each technique had specific limitations including sensitivity and specificity of the

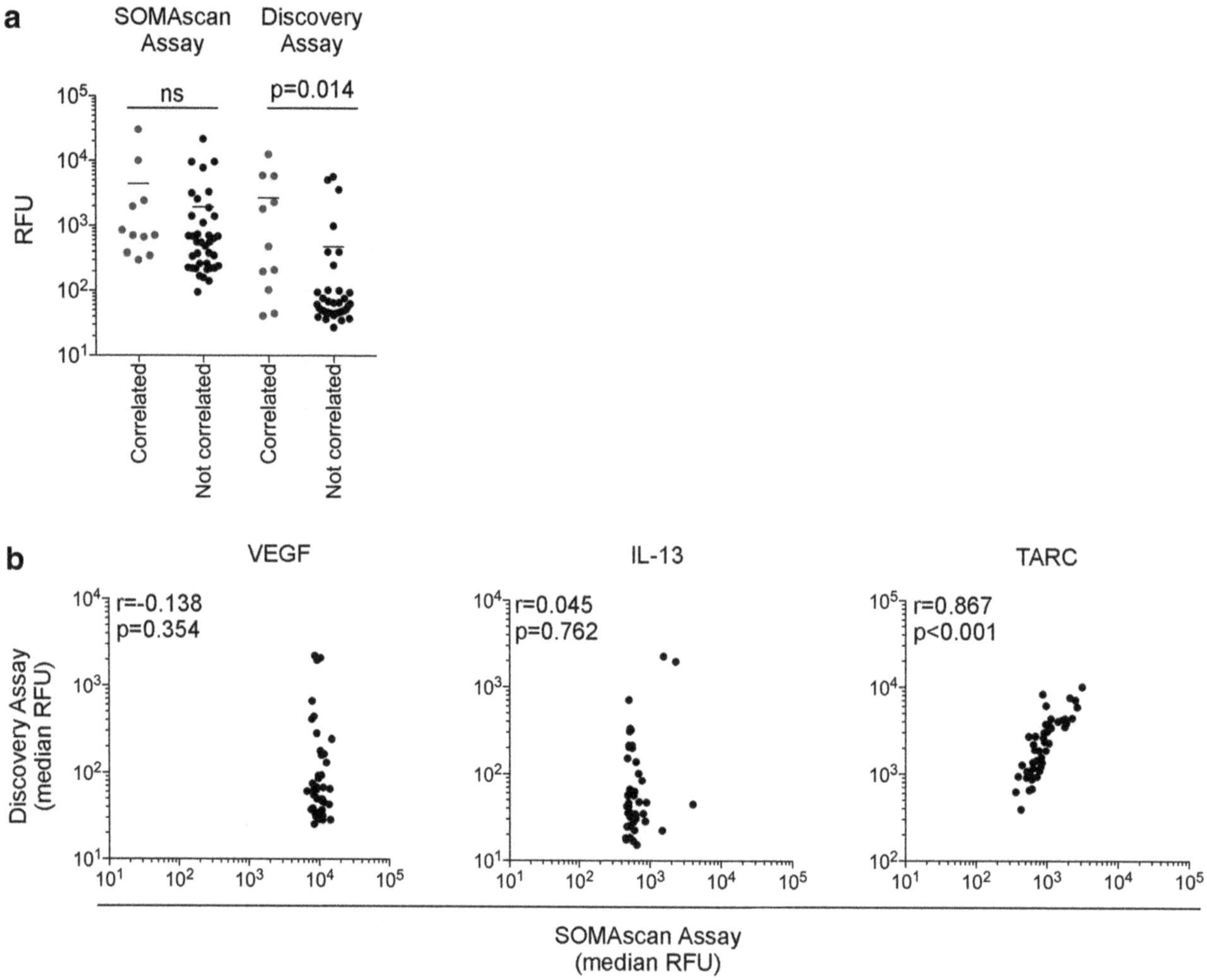

Fig. 4 Sensitivity and range of detection of the protein assays. **a** Scatter plot of RFU values for the 49 shared proteins comparing correlated and non-correlated proteins in the Discovery and SOMAscan assays. The RFU values between the correlated and non-correlated proteins in each assay were compared using a Mann-Whitney test (**b**). Median RFU of VEGF, IL-13 and TARC from the SOMAscan and Discovery assays were tested for correlation using Spearman's rank correlation coefficient; only TARC showed significant positive correlation (r = 0.867, p < 0.001). Correlation graphs of the non-correlated, high abundance VEGF and low abundance IL-13 showed limited range of RFU in the SOMAscan assay compared to the Discovery assay, in contrast to the correlated TARC protein

aptamers and antibodies, which may impede biomarker discovery, and this is particularly relevant as these two assays are routinely applied for this purpose. Our findings underscore the critical need for sensitive, accurate and reproducible protein detection systems, and although the application of multiple, independent detection platforms could be beneficial for discovery, this is not always possible or practical. In particular, the proteomic approaches described in this report are expensive and it is not always possible to apply multiple detection methods when analyzing limited and unique patient biopsies. Further, discordant results between assays, as shown in this study, may necessitate additional measurements of the target proteins.

Method development and validation is essential for the field of biomarker discovery. For instance, the identification of all plasma proteins bound to each SOMAmer reagent by liquid chromatography and tandem mass spectroscopy is an ongoing process that will validate the specificity of the aptamers. Indeed, this has recently resulted in the removal of five aptamer reagents due to non-specific protein enrichment from human plasma and protein preparations. Similarly, although individual detection antibodies used in bead-based assays are tested for cross-reactivity, this is limited to reactivity against a restricted panel of antigens. At present, we rely on a series of modern proteomic methods each with significant limitations that hamper the rapid and accurate identification of novel biomarkers. Investment in improving and advancing these technologies is critical to increasing the effectiveness and value of proteomic biomarker discovery.

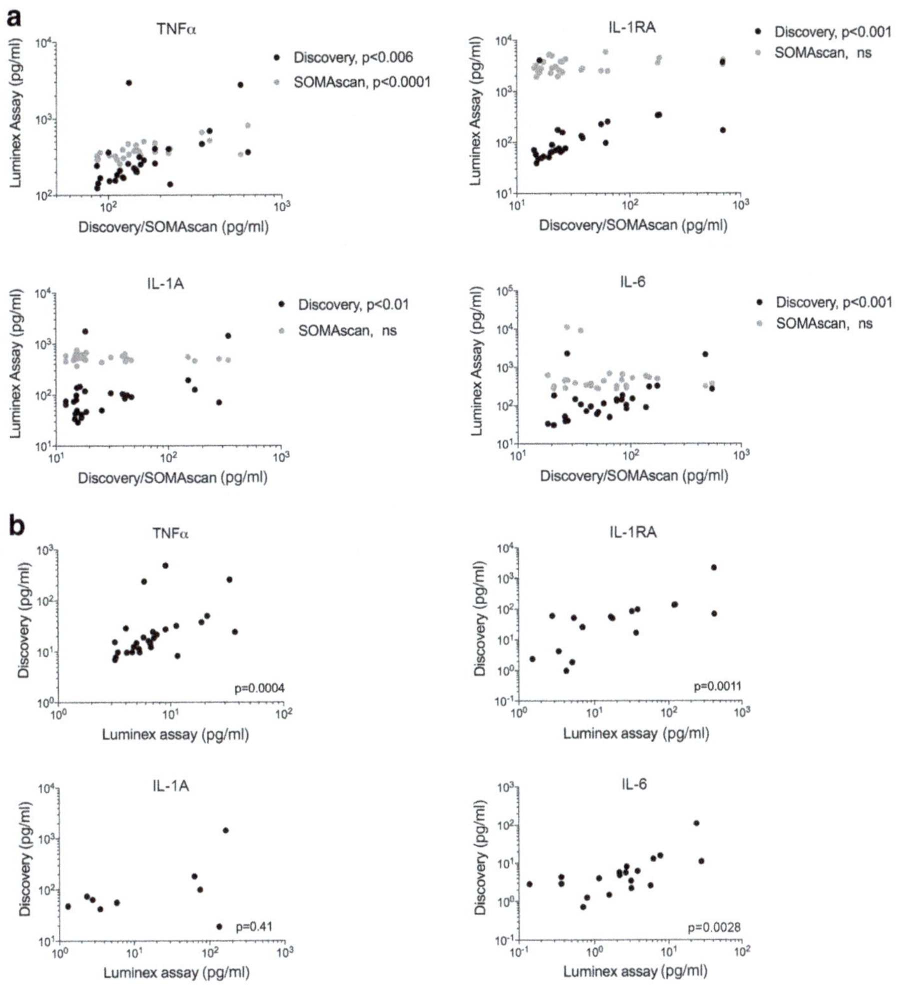

Fig. 5 Correlation of four protein targets in bead-based and aptamer-based assays. **a** The relative fluorescence units (RFU) of each of the 4 proteins (IL-1A, IL-1RA, TNFα and IL-6) in 28 plasma samples were derived from the Milliplex, SOMAscan and Discovery assays and tested for correlation (Spearman's rank correlation coefficient). **b** The absolute protein concentrations (pg/ml) of each of the 4 proteins (IL-1A, IL-1RA, TNFα and IL-6) in 28 plasma samples were derived from the Milliplex and Discovery assays and tested for correlation (Spearman's rank correlation coefficient)

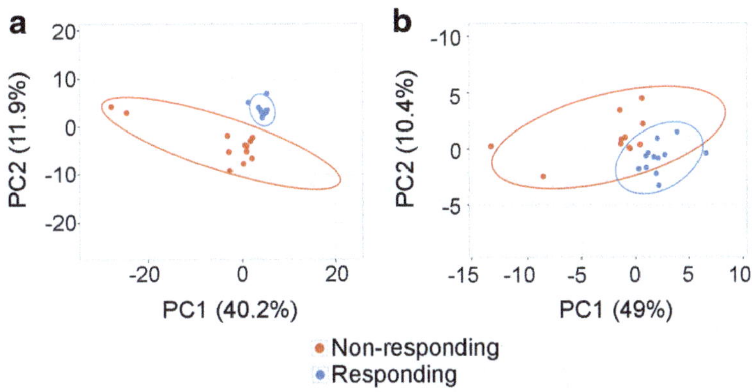

Fig. 6 Principal Component Analysis (PCA) of differentially expressed proteins. PCA plots of the (**a**) 178 differentially expressed protein in EDT plasma samples and (**b**) 32 differentially expressed proteins altered in response to immunotherapy showed good separation between the responding (blue) and non-responding (red) patients

Abbreviations
AJCC: American Joint Committee on Cancer; CEA: Carcinoembryonic antigen; CR: Complete response; ctDNA: circulating tumor DNA; CTLA-4: Cytotoxic T lymphocyte antigen 4; EDT: Early during therapy; IL: Interleukin; PCA: Principle component analysis; PD: Progressive disease; PD-1: Programmed cell death 1; PR: Partial response; PRE: Baseline; PSA: Prostate specific antigen; RECIST: Response evaluation criteria in solid tumors; RFU: Relative fluorescence unit; SD: Stable disease; TNF: Tumor necrosis factor

Acknowledgements
We would like to thank the biobanking staff at the Melanoma Institute Australia, Royal Prince Alfred and Westmead Hospitals.

Funding
This work was supported by funding from NHMRC project grants #1130423 and #1093017.
SYL is supported by grant #1123911, awarded through the Priority-driven Collaborative Cancer Research Scheme and co-funded by Cancer Australia and Cure Cancer Australia Foundation. AMM is supported by a Cancer Institute NSW Fellowship. RS is supported by an NHMRC Practitioner Fellowship. GVL and HR are supported by NHMRC Research Fellowships.

Authors' contributions
SYL and HR analyzed and interpreted the protein and clinical data and wrote the manuscript. JHL, MSC, AMM, RFK, RAS and GVL provided the clinical samples and data. SBA, EB and AG acquired and processed protein data. All authors read, revised and approved the final manuscript.

Competing interests
MSC has been on advisory boards for MSD, Novartis, BMS, Amgen and Pierre Fabre. AMM has been on advisory boards for MSD, Novartis, Pierre Fabre and Chugai and has received honoraria from BMS and Roche. RFK has been on advisory boards for Roche, Amgen, BMS, Merck, Novartis and TEVA and has received honoraria from Merck, BMS and Novartis. GVL has been on advisory boards for Array, Amgen, BMS, Novartis, Merck and Pierre Fabre and has received honoraria from Roche and Merck. The remaining authors declare no conflict of interest.

Author details
[1]Faculty of Medicine and Health Sciences, Macquarie University, Sydney, Australia. [2]Melanoma Institute Australia, Sydney, Australia. [3]Australian Proteome Analysis Facility, Macquarie University, Sydney, Australia. [4]Sydney Medical School, University of Sydney, Sydney, Australia. [5]Westmead Hospital, Sydney, Australia. [6]Royal North Shore and Mater Hospitals, Sydney, Australia. [7]Department of Biomedical Sciences, Faculty of Medicine and Health Sciences, 2 Technology Place, Macquarie University, Sydney, NSW 2109, Australia.

References
1. Holderfield M, Deuker MM, McCormick F, McMahon M, Targeting RAF. Kinases for cancer therapy: BRAF-mutated melanoma and beyond. Nat Rev Cancer. 2014;14:455–67.
2. Hu-Lieskovan S, Robert L, Homet Moreno B, Ribas A. Combining targeted therapy with immunotherapy in BRAF-mutant melanoma: promise and challenges. J Clin Oncol. 2014;32:2248–54.
3. Sharma P, Allison JP. Immune checkpoint targeting in cancer therapy: toward combination strategies with curative potential. Cell. 2015;161:205–14.
4. Mahoney KM, Rennert PD, Freeman GJ. Combination cancer immunotherapy and new immunomodulatory targets. Nat Rev Drug Discov. 2015;14:561–84.
5. Restifo NP, Smyth MJ, Snyder A. Acquired resistance to immunotherapy and future challenges. Nat Rev Cancer. 2016;16:121–6.
6. Sullivan RJ, Flaherty KT. Resistance to BRAF-targeted therapy in melanoma. Eur J Cancer. 2013;49:1297–304.
7. Kelderman S, Schumacher TN, Haanen JB. Acquired and intrinsic resistance in cancer immunotherapy. Mol Oncol. 2014;8:1132–9.
8. Larkin J, Hodi FS, Wolchok JD. Combined Nivolumab and Ipilimumab or monotherapy in untreated melanoma. N Engl J Med. 2015;373:1270 1.
9. Hodi FS, Chesney J, Pavlick AC, Robert C, Grossmann KF, McDermott DF, Linette GP, et al. Combined nivolumab and ipilimumab versus ipilimumab alone in patients with advanced melanoma: 2-year overall survival outcomes in a multicentre, randomised, controlled, phase 2 trial. Lancet Oncol. 2016;17:1558–68.
10. Hernandez J, Thompson IM. Prostate-specific antigen: a review of the validation of the most commonly used cancer biomarker. Cancer. 2004;101: 894–904.
11. Grunnet M, Sorensen JB. Carcinoembryonic antigen (CEA) as tumor marker in lung cancer. Lung Cancer. 2012;76:138–43.
12. Alix-Panabieres C, Pantel K. Clinical applications of circulating tumor cells and circulating tumor DNA as liquid biopsy. Cancer Discov. 2016;6:479–91.
13. Lee JH, Long GV, Boyd S, Lo S, Menzies AM, Tembe V, Guminski A, et al. Circulating tumour DNA predicts response to anti-PD1 antibodies in metastatic melanoma. Ann Oncol. 2017;
14. Bast RC, Jr., Badgwell D, Lu Z, Marquez R, Rosen D, Liu J, Baggerly KA, et al. New tumor markers: CA125 and beyond. Int J Gynecol Cancer 2005;15 Suppl 3:274–281.
15. Eisenhauer EA, Therasse P, Bogaerts J, Schwartz LH, Sargent D, Ford R, Dancey J, et al. New response evaluation criteria in solid tumours: revised RECIST guideline (version 1.1). Eur J Cancer. 2009;45:228–47.
16. Gold L, Ayers D, Bertino J, Bock C, Bock A, Brody EN, Carter J, et al. Aptamer-based multiplexed proteomic technology for biomarker discovery. PLoS One. 2010;5:e15004.
17. Khan A. Detection and quantitation of forty eight cytokines, chemokines, growth factors and nine acute phase proteins in healthy human plasma, saliva and urine. J Proteome. 2012;75:4802–19.
18. Reich M, Liefeld T, Gould J, Lerner J, Tamayo P, Mesirov JP. GenePattern 2.0. Nat Genet. 2006;38:500–1.
19. Metsalu T, Vilo J. ClustVis: a web tool for visualizing clustering of multivariate data using principal component analysis and heatmap. Nucleic Acids Res. 2015;43:W566–70.
20. Discovery Assay - Eve Technologies. Eve Technologies Corporation; 2017.
21. Breen EJ, Polaskova V, Khan A. Bead-based multiplex immuno-assays for cytokines, chemokines, growth factors and other analytes: median fluorescence intensities versus their derived absolute concentration values for statistical analysis. Cytokine. 2015;71:188–98.
22. Breen EJ, Tan W, Khan A. The statistical value of raw fluorescence signal in Luminex xMAP based multiplex immunoassays. Sci Rep. 2016;6:26996.
23. SOMAscan Assay: An unprecedented protein biomarker discovery and development tool. SOMALOGIC, INC.; 2017.

18

Kinomic profiling of glioblastoma cells reveals PLCG1 as a target in restricted glucose

Kiera Walker[1], Nathaniel H. Boyd[1], Joshua C. Anderson[2], Christopher D. Willey[2] and Anita B. Hjelmeland[1*]

Abstract

Background: For glioblastoma (GBM) treatments to be effective in vivo, understanding the effects of the tumor microenvironment is imperative. In traditional cell culture conditions, glucose concentrations do not model physiologic levels, nor the diminished concentrations found in tumor niches. We therefore sought to profile the differences in kinase activity in GBM cells cultured in restricted glucose to identify pathways that could be targeted with small molecule inhibitors.

Methods: Using the PamStation12 platform, we examined the ability of GBM lysates from cells cultured in standard or low glucose conditions to phosphorylate 144 tyrosine and 144 serine/threonine peptides that correspond to known protein phosphorylation sites. Potential kinase targets were identified and validated using small molecule kinase inhibitors in GBM spheroid cultures.

Results: Using results from two GBM patient-derived xenografts, we determined common changes to peptides derived from Phospholipase C, Gamma 1 (PLCG1) and Raf-1. Using PLC and Raf inhibitors, we found a significantly stronger growth inhibitory effect of the PLC inhibitor U73122 under restricted glucose conditions. In contrast, Raf inhibitors were significantly growth inhibitory regardless of the nutrient level tested.

Conclusions: Together, our data demonstrate that kinase activity is altered in low glucose conditions and that kinomic profiling can assist with the identification of effective strategies to target GBM growth. Our data further suggest the importance of accurately modeling the tumor microenvironment to reproduce cancer cell signaling and develop drug screens for anti-cancer agents.

Keywords: Glioblastoma, Tumor initiating cell, Cancer stem cell, PLCG1, Tumor microenvironment, Restricted glucose, Kinomics

Background

Glioblastoma (GBM) is a highly aggressive brain tumor and the most commonly occurring primary malignant glioma in adults, accounting for approximately 50% of all primary malignant brain tumor diagnoses [1–3]. Standard of care consists of surgical resection, concurrent radiation and chemotherapy, followed by adjuvant chemotherapy. While this treatment has extended the average survival to 14.6 months and increased 2 year survival to 17%, the overall prognosis still remains poor [4, 5]. GBM has proven difficult to treat due to tumor heterogeneity and the presence of tumor microenvironments such as low pH, oxygen, and nutrients [6–14]. Initially described as the Warburg Effect, tumor cells can activate alternative metabolic pathways for production of ATP and biomolecules to circumvent microenvironmental obstacles and fuel tumor growth [15]. Nutrient restriction is a modulator of the cellular metabolic state and can alter the kinase signaling pathways in the cell, with glucose playing a key role as a precursor for protein, nucleic acid, and lipid synthesis [9, 16–20].

Tyrosine kinase inhibition is a common modality in cancer treatment, as a myriad of components of the protein tyrosine kinase family have been recognized as

* Correspondence: hjelmea@uab.edu
[1]Department of Cell, Developmental and Integrative Biology, University of Alabama at Birmingham, Birmingham, AL 35294, USA

proto-oncogenes [21]. Previous drugs developed to impede tyrosine kinase activity for cancer treatment have had limited success, as one of the major challenges is the presence or development of resistance to treatment with long-term use, such as acquired resistance to epidermal growth factor receptor (EGFR) inhibitors [21]. High-throughput profiling of kinase activity (kinomics) allows direct measurement of targetable activity, without the limitations of using genomic or other molecular surrogates. Paired with an unbiased prediction tool, kinomics has been utilized to help determine responders from non-responders, with the goal to improve drug efficacy by applying this technique to patient stratification [21]. The critical aspect of this technology is its ability to precisely measure the pertinent mechanism of action of a kinase inhibitor [21].

One important group of enzymes that may be altered by kinase activity during cancer progression are phospholipase C (PLC) family members, which serve as modulators of intracellular lipids and are involved in many cancer signaling cascades. Phospholipase C, gamma 1 (PLCG1) is most notably characterized in cancer by activation of cellular proliferation in response to growth factors such as epidermal growth factor receptor (EGFR) and platelet derived growth factor receptor (PDGFR), both common pathways altered in GBM. Elucidating how these kinase pathways change in response to local microenvironments during GBM progression will allow more directed approaches in treatment.

In this study, we sought to determine how kinase activity may be modulated by the tumor microenvironment in GBM, with the goal of identifying important pathways that could be targeted for cancer treatment. Utilizing kinase arrays, we were able to determine differences in peptide phosphorylation that are nutrient dependent and predict pathways important for GBM growth. Our experiments demonstrate the importance of accurately modeling the tumor microenvironment for drug screening.

Methods

Cell culture

Cells from dissociated GBM patient-derived xenografts (PDX) GBM14 and GBM456 were cultured at 37 °C in Dulbecco's Modified Eagle's Medium (DMEM)/F-12 50/50 with no phenol red, containing Gem21 NeuroPlex supplement w/o vitamin A, 1% Penicillin/Streptomycin, 1% Sodium Pyruvate, and 20 ng/mL each of recombinant human EGF and FGF basic 145aa. For kinomic assays, cells were plated from each cell line in high glucose media [Neurobasal-A Medium, 25 mM D-Glucose, 1% Penicillin/Streptomycin, 1% Sodium Pyruvate, 1% L-glutamine, 20 ng/mL hEGF and hFGF, B27] or low glucose media [high glucose media diluted 1:10 with Neurobasal-A supplemented medium without D-Glucose – final concentration of glucose is 450 mg/L or 2.5 mM] and incubated at 37° for a minimum of 3 days prior to harvest. Normal Human Astrocytes (NHA) were purchased from Lonza and cultured and treated in DMEM high glucose supplemented with 10% Fetal Bovine Serum, 1% N2 NeuroPlex, 3μg hEGF, and 1% Penicillin/Streptomycin. NHA cells were split and treated alongside the GBM PDX cells with the indicated inhibitors.

Multiplex in vitro kinase assay

Kinomic profiling was performed in the UAB Kinome Core using standard methods [22–25]. Briefly, the protein lysates were extracted from the cells as described previously and quantified using a standard BCA assay with duplicates of each sample loaded at 15μg/well for tyrosine (PTK) assay or 2μg/well for serine/threonine (STK) assay onto the PamChips (PamGene International, 's-Hertogenbosch, The Netherlands). The in vitro kinase assay images were captured using the PamGene Evolve Software on the PamStation®12 platform and then images were imported to BioNavigator for raw primary analysis. Phosphorylation as measured by FITC intensity was captured multiple times during the course of the assay as the lysate is pumped across the array in cycles for the kinetic portion of the assay. During the kinetic portion, 50 ms exposures were used for image capture at the indicated cycle number. At the end of the reaction, the lysate and kinase assay reagents were rinsed off and multiple camera exposures (10, 20, 50, 100 ms) were integrated into a post wash slope, multiplied by 100 and Log2 transformed to compare and visualize signal in both low and high intensity peptides [21].

Unsupervised clustering analysis

Unsupervised hierarchical clustering of both sample(column) and peptide(row) using Euclidian distance means-based hierarchal clustering method with complete linkage was performed within BioNavigator on all peptides to generate a clustered heatmap, with a heatmap colored by Signal change (from peptide mean across all replicates) and dendrogram trees to show similarity clustering. Additionally, to measure the strength of these relationships, a pvclust algorithm using R (v3.1.1) and Rstudio was used to generate approximately unbiased (au) and bootstrap probability (bp) values for each branch for high signal (> 7.0) peptides.

Inhibitor treatment

Inhibitors were obtained from Selleck Chemicals and resuspended in DMSO to 10 mM stocks that were used via serial dilution to generate 1000× stocks for use at 1 μL/mL to generate the indicated final concentrations. After incubating in high and low glucose media for at least 3 days, GBM14 and GBM456 cells were split without using a dissociation reagent or Accutase was used to split NHA, into 96 well plates in triplicate at a density of 1000 cells/well in their corresponding high or low glucose media. Cells were allowed to recover for 24 h prior to drug or vehicle treatment. Cells were treated with the PLC inhibitor U73122 to a final concentration of 0.5, 2, and 4 μM or the Raf inhibitor AZ628 at a final concentration of 0.5 or 2 μM. Using Cell Titer Glo 2.0 reagent (Promega), growth of cells was measured using a luminometer after treatment with inhibitor at the indicated timepoints. This experiment was replicated a minimum of three times.

Statistical analysis

For inhibitor treatments, a student's t-test was used to compare the effects of treatment under restricted and standard glucose at the indicated time points with the indicated concentration of drug.

Results

Evaluation of the GBM Kinome in physiologic glucose

To better understand the GBM kinome in physiologically relevant tumor microenvironments, we cultured GBM cells in standard (25 mM) or low (2.5 mM) glucose (Fig. 1). GBM cells were obtained from dissociated PDX and subsequently cultured in the absence of serum but in the presence of EGF, FGF, and B27. These conditions have been shown to best recapitulate parental tumors [26]. We then performed kinomics on both serine/threonine and tyrosine kinase arrays to monitor phosphorylation of substrate peptides with known phosphorylatable target sequences. Following quality control examination of the phosphorylation curves, we performed an unsupervised hierarchical clustering analysis to determine how the kinomic signatures of high signal peptides clustered across all samples/conditions. Notably, the most obvious clustering was by xenograft origin (Fig. 2a). These data, and the scoring of the clustering strengths, suggest that any differences in the kinome due to changes in glucose levels do not override the intrinsic differences in the kinome of xenografts derived from different patients (Fig. 2a-b).

We next sought to determine if there were common peptides that were differentially phosphorylated with low glucose culture between the two xenografts. We identified peptides that were uniquely regulated in either GBM456 or GBM14 cells with a Log2 change in restricted glucose greater than 0.3 (Fig. 3a) or less than − 0.3 (Fig. 3b). The phosphorylatable sites in the proteins that correspond to those in the individual peptides are indicated. Of note, the protein modification targets that were identified with culture in low glucose are predominately tyrosine phosphorylation sites.

A subset of peptides also displayed similar changes in phosphorylation in both GBM456 and GBM14. To identify peptides with common increases in phosphorylation, which are shown in both the labels to the right of the clustered heatmap (Fig. 2a) and in the overlapping regions of the Venn diagrams (Fig. 3a), the change was required to be in the same direction with a Log2 of at least 0.3 in both cell types or 0.5 in one cell type and 0.2 in the other. Using these criteria, five peptides were shown to have common increases in phosphorylation with restricted glucose exposure. These were peptides derived from regions of muscarinic acetylcholine receptor M5 (ACM5_498_510), cluster of differentiation CD79A (CD79A_181_193), Forkhead box protein O3 (FOXO3_25_37), phospholipase C, gamma 1 (PLCG1_764_776), and Raf-1 (RAF1_332_344). Among these, only the PLCG1 peptide demonstrated Log2 increases greater than 0.5 for both GBM456 and GBM14. These data suggested common increases in PLCG1 phosphorylation at tyrosine 771 and 775 in the presence of restricted glucose.

We also used a similar approach to identify peptides with common decreases in phosphorylation upon exposure to restricted glucose. Using the criteria of a Log2 change of at most − 0.3 in both cell types or − 0.5 in one cell type and − 0.2 in the other, six peptides were

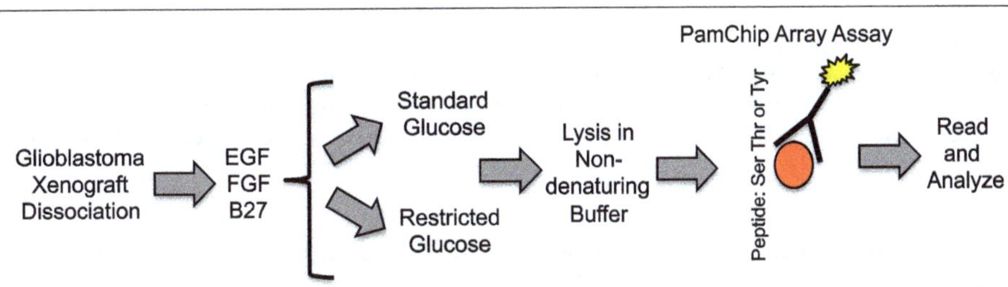

Fig. 1 Overview of the kinomics experimental approach. The PamChip Array Assay permits analysis of peptides with Serine, Threonine, or Tyrosine phosphorylatable sites. We utilized the assay to measure kinase activity in lysates isolated from GBM cells cultured in low or standard glucose as outlined

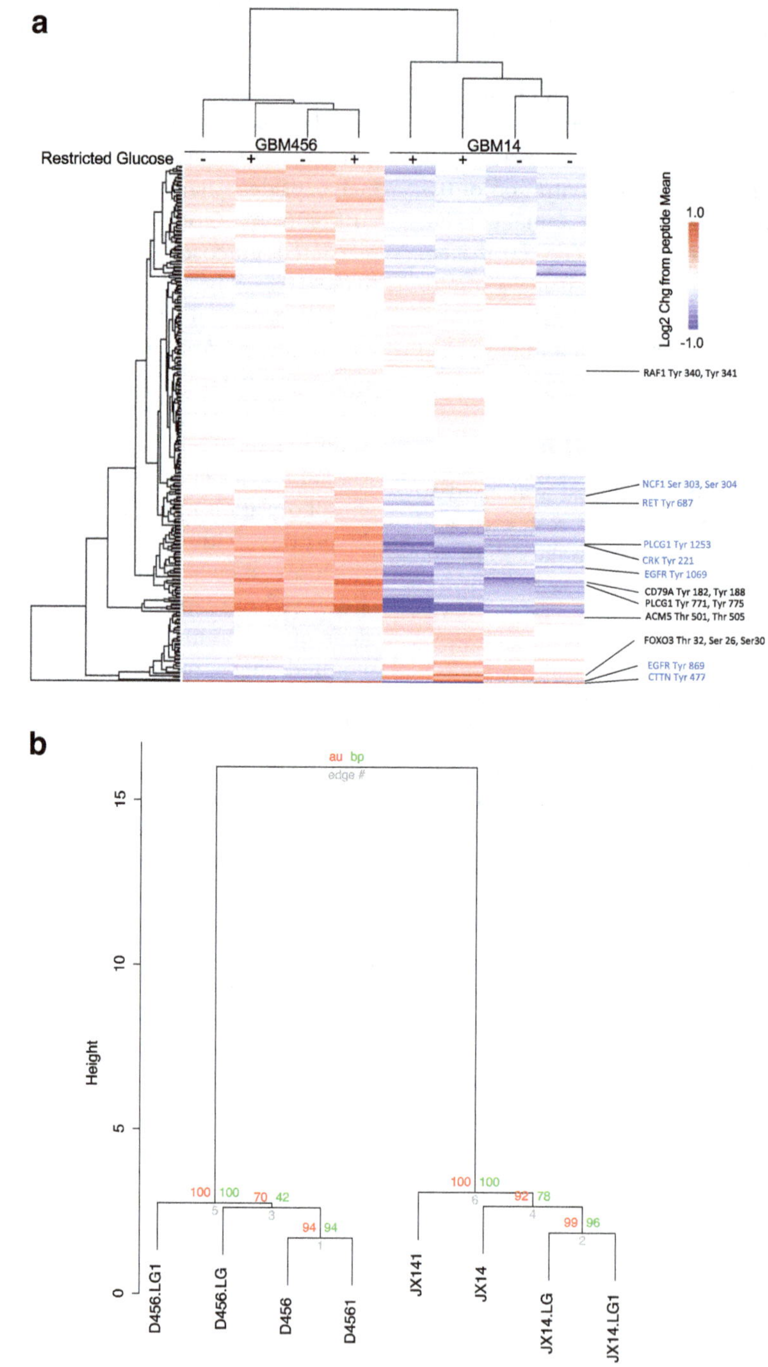

Fig. 2 Heatmap of kinomic profiling with xenograft derived cells cultured in standard or restricted glucose. **a** Unsupervised clustering of kinomic data from cells isolated from two different GBM PDX of distinct subtype indicates grouping by xenograft followed by the treatment condition (standard or restricted glucose) (**b**). Scoring of dendrogram branching using Pvclust with unsupervised clustering (Euclidean/ward) of kinomic data having >7.0 average Log2 values with approximately unbiased (au) and bootstrap probabilities (bp) values superimposed. Nboot iterations = 1000

shown to have common decreases in phosphorylation (Fig. 3b). These peptides corresponded to regions of CRK (CRK_214_226), cortactin (SRC8_CHICK_470_482), epidermal growth factor receptor (EGFR_1062_107), neutrophil cytosol factor 1 (NCF1_296_308), PLCG1 (PLCG1_1246_1258), and RET (RET_680_692). Of these peptides, only the EGFR derived peptide demonstrated Log2 change of of at most -0.5 for both GBM456 and GBM14, but changes in PLCG1 and CRK had a Log2 of -0.4 or less in both cell types.

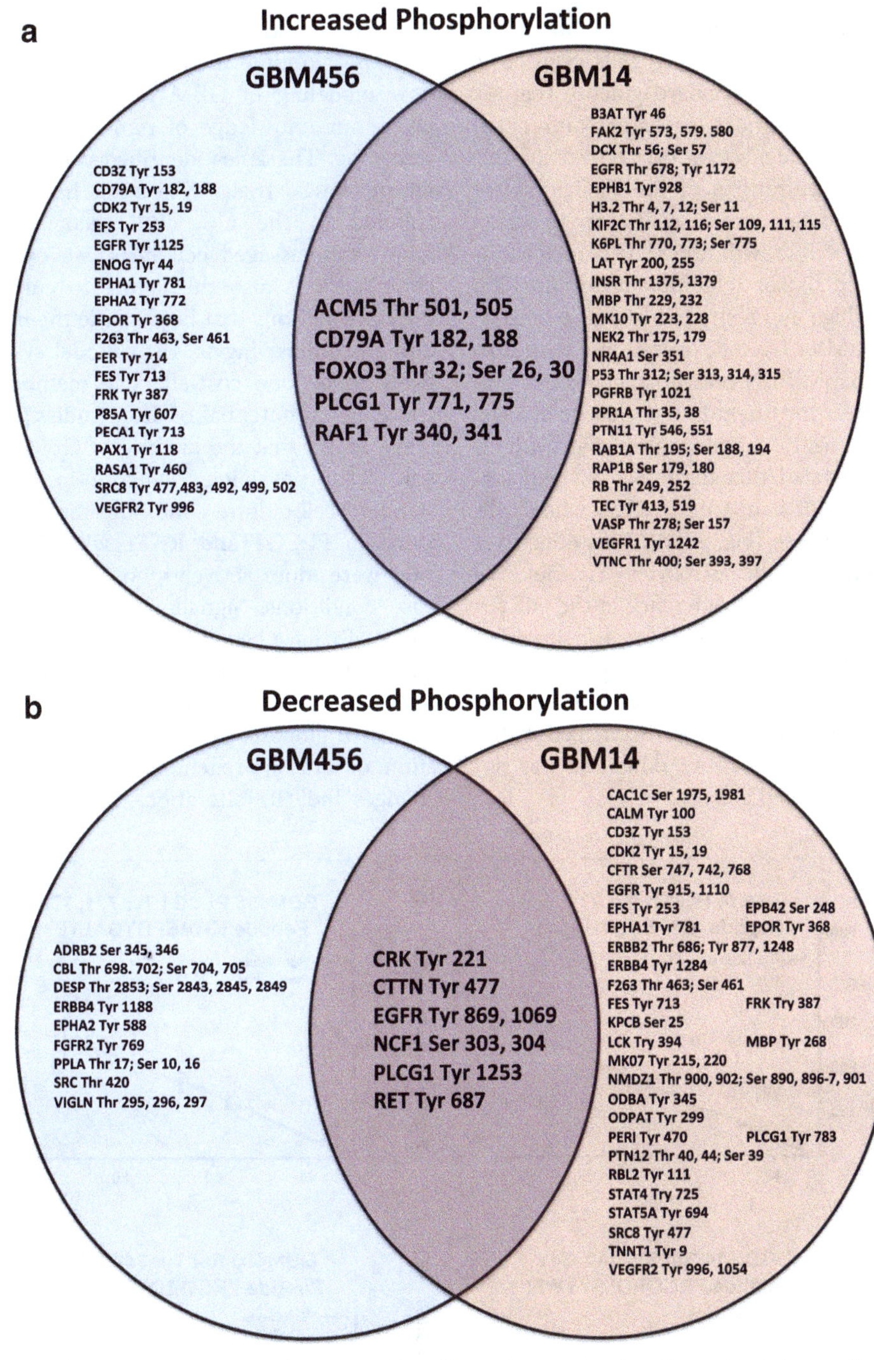

Fig. 3 Proteins and phosphorylation sites corresponding to peptides differentially phosphorylated in restricted glucose. All peptides with a Log2 change > 0.3 (**a**) or < − 0.3 (**b**) when GBM456 (blue) or GBM14 (red) cells were cultured in low glucose in comparison to standard conditions are indicated. The Venn Diagram shows overlapping peptides in the center that have Log2 changes indicated above in both cell types. Peptides for which there was at least a > 0.5 Log2 change in one cell type and > 0.2 Log2 change in the other are also shown in the overlapping region in **a**. Peptides for which there was at least a < − 0.5 in one cell type and < − 0.2 Log2 change in the other are also shown in the overlapping region in **b**. The predominant common changes occur at tyrosine phosphorylation sites

Targeting restricted glucose mediated changes in phosphorylation

As the data suggested increased phosphorylation at a subset of common targets among GBMs, we next considered whether inhibition of these targets could have distinct effects in low glucose. PLC and RAF small molecule inhibitors were commercially available, and we confirmed that the kinetic curves (captured over pumping cycles) for peptides PLCG1_764_776 and RAF1_332_344 demonstrated increased phosphorylation upon incubation with lysates from GBM cells exposed to low glucose in comparison to standard glucose (Fig. 4). The kinetic curves had the most consistent differential slope for the PLCG1 peptide, so we first tested the impact of increasing concentrations of the PLC inhibitor U73122. Using an ATP-based luminescent assay to screen for general changes in cell growth, the highest concentration of U73122 caused similar inhibition of proliferation under both standard/high and restricted/low glucose conditions. However, 2 uM of U73122 caused less than 50% growth inhibition in GBM PDX cells in standard cell culture conditions, whereas treatment in low glucose blocked GBM cell growth (Fig. 5a, b). A time course of growth effects similarly demonstrated that there was a significant increase in the efficacy of 2 uM of U73122 when cells were exposed to low glucose (Fig. 5c, d). This effect was not observed in non-neoplastic astrocytes (Fig. 5e). We also did not observe a significant difference in the efficacy of the RAF inhibitor AZ628 against GBM cells cultured in standard or restricted glucose (Fig. 5f). Together, these data indicate that small molecule inhibitor efficacy may differ depending on the level of glucose in the cell with a specific finding that PLC but not RAF inhibition was significantly different in restricted glucose.

Discussion

We have investigated the impact of restricted glucose on the GBM kinome to develop a better understanding of how modeling of GBM microenvironments could improve our knowledge of tumor cell signaling and drug screening. Therapies identified via in vitro screens often fail in clinical trials. While this has been previously attributed to the now well recognized limitations of long-term passaged cell lines, we expect that a major contributor is also the failure to culture cells in vitro under conditions that best mimic the in vivo microenvironment. Improving in vitro model systems is therefore likely to be one cost-effective method to improve the translational potential of drug studies.

We found that the kinome of GBM cells is altered by culture in physiologic glucose in comparison to the standard cell culture conditions. Specific peptides for regions in PLCG1 and RAF1 with Tyr phosphorylation sites were more actively phosphorylated under low glucose conditions. Signaling pathways related to PLCG1 and RAF1 have been previously identified to be activated and/or mutated upon restricted glucose culture: AKT phosphorylation [27] and RAS mutation [28] increase in restricted glucose. While these data provide some validation of our approach, other peptide phosphorylation changes indicate alterations to pathways that have not

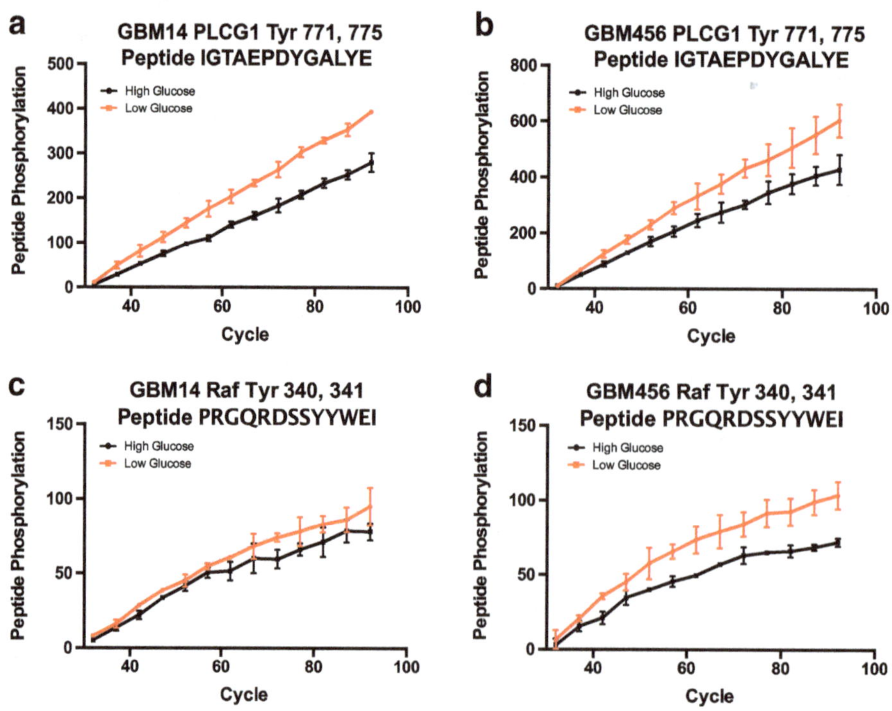

Fig. 4 Kinetic curves for peptides corresponding to regions of PLCG1 and RAF1. Kinomic profiling demonstrated changes in the peptides that contain tyrosine phosphorylation sites corresponding to regions of PLCG1 (**a**, **b**) and Raf-1 (**c**, **d**). Representative curves for results from lysates isolated from GBM14 (**a**, **c**) or GBM456 (**b**, **d**) cells cultured in standard or restricted glucose with measurements over pumping cycles (time) are shown. Phosphorylation as measured by FITC intensity was captured at the indicated cycle number as the lysate was pumped across the array in cycles

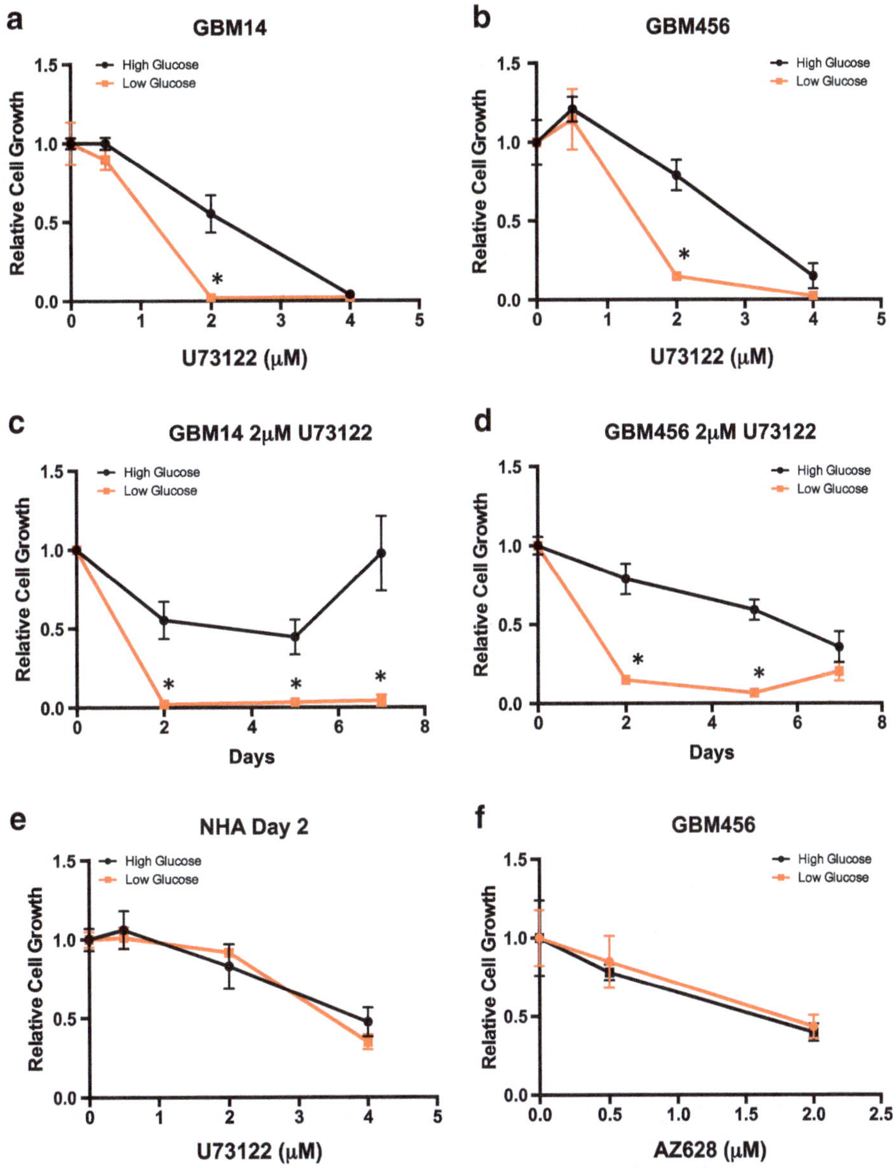

Fig. 5 The efficacy of a PLC, but not Raf, inhibitor was increased when GBM cells were grown in restricted glucose. GBM cells isolated the indicated xenografts (**a-d**) or non-transformed human astrocytes (**e**) were cultured in standard or low glucose with or without U73122 or DMSO as a vehicle control. Data were normalized to the DMSO control of the appropriate glucose condition at the same time point. *, $p < 0.05$ with t-test comparison. **f** No significant difference in efficacy of the Raf inhibitor AZ628 was observed with changes in glucose levels in the media

been thoroughly investigated in GBMs. A peptide corresponding to ACM5 (CHRM5) was differentially phosphorylated in restricted glucose, but there are limited reports on the potential role of this muscarinic receptor in glioma. Data do suggest that acetylcholine can act through muscarinic receptors to induce proliferation of astrocytes and glioma cells [29, 30], potentially via the M3 receptors [31]. In contrast, activation of M2 receptors has been associated with decreased glioma growth [32, 33] and increased cell death [34], including in the tumor initiating cell subset [35]. Changes in phosphorylation to the peptide corresponding to regions of CD79A, the immunoglobulin-associated alpha chain of the B-cell antigen receptor complex, further suggest the importance of studying the impact of tumor microenvironments on immune system function. Thus, our findings suggest additional avenues of investigation to further explore the mechanisms through which restricted glucose impacts cancer growth.

PLCG1 is part of the gamma subclass of PLCs which exclusively contain SH2 and 3 domains, and the enzyme has been reported to be an important effector of activated RTKs such as EGFR and PDGF [36, 37]. The targeting and recruitment of this enzyme to activated RTKs requires the SH2 domain [38]. Therefore, the observed effects in the current study of increased phosphorylation of Tyr771 and Tyr775 in the context of low glucose could reasonably be attributed to increased RTK signaling, as these phosphorylation sites lie within the SH2 homology domain. Indeed, EGFR is predicted to be activated in low glucose when analyzing our results with Kinexus Kinase Predictor (data not shown). While EGFR inhibitors have thus far not led to significant improvements in GBM patient survival, these findings and literature do suggest that other low glucose activated or elevated upstream kinases could be targeted based on the kinomic array results.

Short term exposure to restricted nutrient conditions alters kinase activity in GBM but intrinsic differences in kinomes between patient samples remain: clustering of kinomic data was most strongly dependent on the xenograft rather than the glucose level. These data suggest that the different genetic alterations between tumors are likely to be the dominant force driving a kinomic signature. However, we did not compare the kinome of the GBM cells in distinct cell culture conditions to that in a portion of the non-dissociated tumor directly. The possibility remains that, even when glucose is at physiological levels, cell culture itself promotes kinomic shifts. By comparing parental tumor profiles to those in distinct cell culture conditions, we may identify the optimal in vitro conditions to mimic in vivo cell signals. Such optimization would better improve the translational potential of any molecular, biological, or drug studies.

Conclusions

Our data provide strong evidence that the kinome of GBM does change when physiologically relevant glucose levels are utilized in comparison to the high glucose levels present in standard medias. As a proof of concept, we determined that PLCG1 peptide phosphorylation and efficacy of a PLC inhibitor were significantly altered in low glucose conditions. When considered in the broader context of drug screening, these data demonstrate the utility of high-throughput platforms that incorporate physiologically relevant microenvironments.

Abbreviations

ACM5: Muscarinic acetylcholine receptor M5; GBM: Glioblastoma; NHA: Normal human astrocytes; PDX: patient derived xenografts; PLCG1: Phospholipase C, gamma 1

Funding

This work was supported by National Institutes of Health grant R21NS096531 (ABH), R01NS104339 (ABH), F31CA200085 (NHB), the UAB Brain Tumor SPORE Career Development Award, and startup funds from the University of Alabama at Birmingham, which includes funds from the Department of Cell, Developmental and Integrative Biology, the Comprehensive Cancer Center, the Civitan International Research Center for Glial Biology in Medicine, and the Center for Free Radical Biology.

Authors' contributions

KW, NB, JA, CW, and AB designed the experimental approach, interpreted results, and wrote the manuscript. KW, NB, and JA performed the experiments and analyzed the data. KW, NB, JA, CW, and AB read and approved the final manuscript.

Competing interests

The authors declare that they have no competing interests.

Author details

[1]Department of Cell, Developmental and Integrative Biology, University of Alabama at Birmingham, Birmingham, AL 35294, USA. [2]Department of Radiation Oncology, University of Alabama at Birmingham, Birmingham, AL, USA.

References

1. Ohgaki H, Kleihues P. Epidemiology and etiology of gliomas. Acta Neuropathol. 2005;109(1):93–108.
2. Hottinger AF, Stupp R, Homicsko K. Standards of care and novel approaches in the management of glioblastoma multiforme. Chinese journal of cancer. 2014;33(1):32–9.
3. Stupp R, Hegi ME, Mason WP, van den Bent MJ, Taphoorn MJ, Janzer RC, Ludwin SK, Allgeier A, Fisher B, Belanger K, et al. Effects of radiotherapy with concomitant and adjuvant temozolomide versus radiotherapy alone on survival in glioblastoma in a randomised phase III study: 5-year analysis of the EORTC-NCIC trial. The Lancet Oncology. 2009;10(5):459–66.
4. Balca-Silva J, Matias D, do Carmo A, Girao H, Moura-Neto V, Sarmento-Ribeiro AB, Lopes MC. Tamoxifen in combination with temozolomide induce a synergistic inhibition of PKC-pan in GBM cell lines. Biochim Biophys Acta. 2015;1850(4):722–32.
5. Stupp R, Mason WP, van den Bent MJ, Weller M, Fisher B, Taphoorn MJ, Belanger K, Brandes AA, Marosi C, Bogdahn U, et al. Radiotherapy plus concomitant and adjuvant temozolomide for glioblastoma. N Engl J Med. 2005;352(10):987–96.
6. Vartanian A, Singh SK, Agnihotri S, Jalali S, Burrell K, Aldape KD, Zadeh G. GBM's multifaceted landscape: highlighting regional and microenvironmental heterogeneity. Neuro-Oncology. 2014;16(9):1167–75.
7. Vaupel P. Metabolic microenvironment of tumor cells: a key factor in malignant progression. Exp Oncol. 2010;32(3):125–7.
8. Vaupel P. Blood flow and metabolic microenvironment of brain tumors. J Neuro-Oncol. 1994;22(3):261–7.
9. Vaupel P, Kallinowski F, Okunieff P. Blood flow, oxygen and nutrient supply, and metabolic microenvironment of human tumors: a review. Cancer Res. 1989;49(23):6449–65.
10. Flavahan WA, Wu Q, Hitomi M, Rahim N, Kim Y, Sloan AE, Weil RJ, Nakano I, Sarkaria JN, Stringer BW, et al. Brain tumor initiating cells adapt to restricted nutrition through preferential glucose uptake. Nat Neurosci. 2013;16(10): 1373–82.
11. Heddleston JM, Hitomi M, Venere M, Flavahan WA, Yang K, Kim Y, Minhas S, Rich JN, Hjelmeland AB. Glioma stem cell maintenance: the role of the microenvironment. Curr Pharm Des. 2011;17(23):2386–401.
12. Heddleston JM, Li Z, McLendon RE, Hjelmeland AB, Rich JN. The hypoxic microenvironment maintains glioblastoma stem cells and promotes reprogramming towards a cancer stem cell phenotype. Cell Cycle. 2009; 8(20):3274–84.
13. Hjelmeland AB, Wu Q, Heddleston JM, Choudhary GS, MacSwords J, Lathia JD, McLendon R, Lindner D, Sloan A, Rich JN. Acidic stress promotes a glioma stem cell phenotype. Cell Death Differ. 2011;18(5):829–40.
14. Li Z, Bao S, Wu Q, Wang H, Eyler C, Sathornsumetee S, Shi Q, Cao Y, Lathia J, McLendon RE, et al. Hypoxia-inducible factors regulate tumorigenic capacity of glioma stem cells. Cancer Cell. 2009;15(6):501–13.

15. Warburg O, Wind F, Negelein E. The metabolism of tumors in the body. J Gen Physiol. 1927;8(6):519–30.
16. Abbadi S, Rodarte JJ, Abutaleb A, Lavell E, Smith CL, Ruff W, Schiller J, Olivi A, Levchenko A, Guerrero-Cazares H, et al. Glucose-6-phosphatase is a key metabolic regulator of glioblastoma invasion. Mol Cancer Res. 2014;12(11):1547–59.
17. Lewis CA, Brault C, Peck B, Bensaad K, Griffiths B, Mitter R, Chakravarty P, East P, Dankworth B, Alibhai D, et al. SREBP maintains lipid biosynthesis and viability of cancer cells under lipid- and oxygen-deprived conditions and defines a gene signature associated with poor survival in glioblastoma multiforme. Oncogene. 2015;34(40):5128–40.
18. Savaskan NE, Eyupoglu IY. xCT modulation in gliomas: relevance to energy metabolism and tumor microenvironment normalization. Ann Anat. 2010; 192(5):309–13.
19. Schlappack OK, Zimmermann A, Hill RP. Glucose starvation and acidosis: effect on experimental metastatic potential, DNA content and MTX resistance of murine tumour cells. Br J Cancer. 1991;64(4):663–70.
20. Eckert A, Bock BC, Tagscherer KE, Haas TL, Grund K, Sykora J, Herold-Mende C, Ehemann V, Hollstein M, Chneiweiss H, et al. The PEA-15/PED protein protects glioblastoma cells from glucose deprivation-induced apoptosis via the ERK/MAP kinase pathway. Oncogene. 2008;27(8):1155–66.
21. Versele M, Talloen W, Rockx C, Geerts T, Janssen B, Lavrijssen T, King P, Gohlmann HW, Page M, Perera T. Response prediction to a multitargeted kinase inhibitor in cancer cell lines and xenograft tumors using high-content tyrosine peptide arrays with a kinetic readout. Mol Cancer Ther. 2009;8(7):1846–55.
22. Yang ES, Willey CD, Mehta A, Crowley MR, Crossman DK, Chen D, Anderson JC, Naik G, Della Manna DL, Cooper TS, et al. Kinase analysis of penile squamous cell carcinoma on multiple platforms to identify potential therapeutic targets. Oncotarget. 2017;8(13):21710–8.
23. Ghosh AP, Willey CD, Anderson JC, Welaya K, Chen D, Mehta A, Ghatalia P, Madan A, Naik G, Sudarshan S, et al. Kinomic profiling identifies focal adhesion kinase 1 as a therapeutic target in advanced clear cell renal cell carcinoma. Oncotarget. 2017;8(17):29220–32.
24. Anderson JC, Willey CD, Mehta A, Welaya K, Chen D, Duarte CW, Ghatalia P, Arafat W, Madan A, Sudarshan S, et al. High throughput Kinomic profiling of human clear cell renal cell carcinoma identifies kinase activity dependent molecular subtypes. PLoS One. 2015;10(9):e0139267.
25. Gilbert AN, Shevin RS, Anderson JC, Langford CP, Eustace N, Gillespie GY, Singh R, Willey CD. Generation of microtumors using 3D human biogel culture system and patient-derived Glioblastoma cells for Kinomic profiling and drug response testing. J Vis Exp. 2016;(112).
26. Lee J, Kotliarova S, Kotliarov Y, Li A, Su Q, Donin NM, Pastorino S, Purow BW, Christopher N, Zhang W, et al. Tumor stem cells derived from glioblastomas cultured in bFGF and EGF more closely mirror the phenotype and genotype of primary tumors than do serum-cultured cell lines. Cancer Cell. 2006;9(5):391–403.
27. Zhuang Y, Chan DK, Haugrud AB, Miskimins WK. Mechanisms by which low glucose enhances the cytotoxicity of metformin to cancer cells both in vitro and in vivo. PLoS One. 2014;9(9):e108444.
28. Yun J, Rago C, Cheong I, Pagliarini R, Angenendt P, Rajagopalan H, Schmidt K, Willson JK, Markowitz S, Zhou S, et al. Glucose deprivation contributes to the development of KRAS pathway mutations in tumor cells. Science. 2009; 325(5947):1555–9.
29. Guizzetti M, Costa LG. Possible role of protein kinase C zeta in muscarinic receptor-induced proliferation of astrocytoma cells. Biochem Pharmacol. 2000;60(10):1457–66.
30. Guizzetti M, Wei M, Costa LG. The role of protein kinase C alpha and epsilon isozymes in DNA synthesis induced by muscarinic receptors in a glial cell line. Eur J Pharmacol. 1998;359(2–3):223–33.
31. Guizzetti M, Costa LG. Activation of phosphatidylinositol 3 kinase by muscarinic receptors in astrocytoma cells. Neuroreport. 2001;12(8):1639–42.
32. Ferretti M, Fabbiano C, Di Bari M, Ponti D, Calogero A, Tata AM. M2 muscarinic receptors inhibit cell proliferation in human glioblastoma cell lines. Life Sci. 2012;91(21–22):1134–7.
33. Ferretti M, Fabbiano C, Di Bari M, Conte C, Castigli E, Sciaccaluga M, Ponti D, Ruggieri P, Raco A, Ricordy R, et al. M2 receptor activation inhibits cell cycle progression and survival in human glioblastoma cells. J Cell Mol Med. 2013; 17(4):552–66.
34. Di Bari M, Tombolillo V, Conte C, Castigli E, Sciaccaluga M, Iorio E, Carpinelli G, Ricordy R, Fiore M, Degrassi F, et al. Cytotoxic and genotoxic effects mediated by M2 muscarinic receptor activation in human glioblastoma cells. Neurochem Int. 2015;90:261 70.
35. Alessandrini F, Cristofaro I, Di Bari M, Zasso J, Conti L, Tata AM. The activation of M2 muscarinic receptor inhibits cell growth and survival in human glioblastoma cancer stem cells. Int Immunopharmacol. 2015;29(1):105–9.
36. Rebecchi MJ, Pentyala SN. Structure, function, and control of phosphoinositide-specific phospholipase C. Physiol Rev. 2000;80(4):1291–335.
37. Rhee SG, Bae YS. Regulation of phosphoinositide-specific phospholipase C isozymes. J Biol Chem. 1997;272(24):15045–8.
38. Fukami K. Structure, regulation, and function of phospholipase C isozymes. J Biochem. 2002;131(3):293–9.

19

Epigenetic regulation of cancer progression by EZH2: from biological insights to therapeutic potential

Lu Gan[1,2,3†], Yanan Yang[1,2†], Qian Li[2,3], Yi Feng[2,3], Tianshu Liu[2,3] and Weijian Guo[1,2*]

Abstract

Enhancer of zeste homolog 2 (EZH2), a histone methyltransferase and a catalytic component of PRC2, catalyzes tri-methylation of histone H3 at Lys 27 (H3K27me3) to regulate gene expression through epigenetic machinery. EZH2 also functions both as a transcriptional suppressor and a transcriptional co-activator, depending on H3K27me3 or not and on the different cellular contexts. Unsurprisingly, numerous studies have highlighted the role of EZH2 in cancer development and progression. Through modulating critical gene expression, EZH2 promotes cell survival, proliferation, epithelial to mesenchymal, invasion, and drug resistance of cancer cells. The tumor suppressive effects of EZH2 are also identified. What is more, EZH2 has decisive roles in immune cells (for example, T cells, NK cells, dendritic cells and macrophages), which are essential components in tumor microenvironment. In this review, we aim to discuss the molecular functions of EZH2, highlight recent findings regarding the physiological functions and related regulation of EZH2 in cancer pathogenesis. Furthermore, we summarized and updated the emerging roles of EZH2 in tumor immunity, and current pre-clinical and clinical trials of EZH2 inhibitors in cancer therapy.

Keywords: EZH2, Epigenetic, Histone H3 Lys27 trimethylation, Cancer, Polycomb repressive complex

Background

Epigenetic modification could regulate chromatin state and gene expression through DNA methylation and de-methylation, histone modification, chromatin remodeling etc., without altering DNA sequences [1, 2]. Polycomb group proteins (PcGs), a group of important epigenetic regulators, play an important part in cell proliferation and are critical factors of pluripotency and differentiation of stem cells as well as aberrant gene expression during the malignant transformation [2, 3]. PcG proteins contain two core complexes, respectively are the maintenance complex polycomb repressive complex 1 (PRC1) and the initiation complex polycomb repressive complex 2(PRC2). PRC1 has been known to mono-ubiquitinate the histone H2A at Lys 119 through RING1A and RING1B ubiquitin ligases. PRC2 has been considered to catalyze the mono-, di-, and tri-methylation of histone H3 at Lys 27 to regulate gene transcription [3].

Enhancer of zeste homolog 2 (EZH2) is an evolutionary conserved gene identified in many species, sharing similar structural motifs and domains. As a histone methyltransferase, EZH2 has been identified as a catalytic subunit of PRC2 for tri-methylation of histone H3 at Lys 27 (H3K27me3) by SET domain in its C-terminus, which silences targeted genes and is involved in various biological functions (e.g. cell cycle, cell proliferation, cell differentiation, etc.). The role of EZH2 in cancer progression was also considered and unraveled. EZH2 is aberrantly overexpressed in various malignant tumors, such as prostate cancer, breast cancer, and ovarian cancer.EZH2 mediates H3K27me3 and functions as a critical factor in promoting tumor growth and metastasis in many malignant tumor models [3–5]. In addition, EZH2 gain or loss of function mutations have also been discovered in various cancer [4–6]. Accumulating studies indicate that inhibition of EZH2 by small molecular inhibitors or gene knockdown results in reduced cancer cell growth and tumor formation [4, 7]. Beyond playing its role in a PCR2-dependent manner as a histone modifier, EZH2 also acts in

* Correspondence: guoweijian1@outlook.com
†Equal contributors
[1]Department of Medical Oncology, Fudan University Shanghai Cancer Center, No.270, Dongan Road, Shanghai 200032, China
[2]Department of Oncology, Shanghai Medical college, Fudan University, No.130, Dongan Road, Shanghai 200032, China

a PCR2 and histone independent manner in cancer. For example, EZH2 can methylate non-histone protein STAT3 in glioblastoma, and participate in androgen receptor-associated complexes in castration-resistant prostate cancer (CRPC) as a co-activator [5, 8, 9].The diverse functions of EZH2in cancer derive from its genetic, transcriptional, post-transcriptional and post-translational regulation in different circumstances and different types of cancer [7, 10].

In this review, we aim to discuss the molecular functions of EZH2, highlight recent findings regarding the physiological functions and related regulation of EZH2 in cancer pathogenesis. Additionally, we summarized and updated the emerging roles of EZH2 in tumor immunity, and EZH2 inhibitors in current pre-clinical and clinical trials in cancer therapy.

Action modes of EZH2

As important epigenetic regulators, there are two families of PcG complexes identified in mammals, PRC1 and PRC2. The PRC1 complex catalyzes the monoubiquitylation of histone H2A and is composed of several subunits, such as PCGF, HPH, CBX, and RING1 paralog groups, whereas the PRC2 complex contributes to the methylation of H3K27 and mainly consists of EED, SUZ12, RbAp46/48, and either EZH1 or EZH2 [2, 3]. As a histone methyltransferase, EZH2 is responsible for the H3K27 methylation. Human EZH2 gene is located on the long arm of chromosome 7 at 7q35 and encodes a 746 amino acids protein. EZH2 organizes into several domains: the conserved SET domain at the C-terminus functions for maintaining histone methyl transferase (HMT) activity, CXC domain and ncRBD domain are required for interactions with other PRC2 components and regulatory proteins [2, 3]. Accumulating studies have demonstrated that EZH2 participates in many diverse biological processes and displays different modes of actions. Here, we will firstly briefly summarize the known archetypes of molecular functions of EZH2: a dual-faced molecule acting both as a transcriptional suppressor and a transcriptional co-activator, depending on its interaction with other PRC2 components or not and in different cellular contexts (Fig. 1).

PRC2-dependent H3K27 methylation for gene silencing

EZH2 is essential for epigenetic gene silencing. EZH2 catalyzes H3K27 trimethylation (H3K27me3) in the nucleus and then PRC1 binds to monoubiquitinated histone H2A at lysine 119 (H2AK-119ub1) and H3K27me3. This complex then mediates chromatin compaction followed by transcriptional repression of downstream genes [11].

PRC2-dependent non-histone protein methylation for gene silencing

EZH2 also functions in the cytosol to methylate non-histone proteins in a PRC2 complex dependent way. EZH2 can directly methylate cardiac transcription factor GATA4 at Lys299, thereby attenuating p300-mediated GATA4 acetylation and promoting GATA4 transcriptional repression and gene silencing [12]. EZH2 was also shown to bind to and methylate RAR-related orphan receptor alpha (RORα) at Lys38 to promote DDB1/DCAF1/CUL4 ubiquitin ligase complex-mediated RORα ubiquitination and lead to RORα target gene silencing [13]. Gunawan et al. showed that EZH2 directly methylates talin, a key regulatory molecule in cell migration, to disrupt the binding of talin to F-

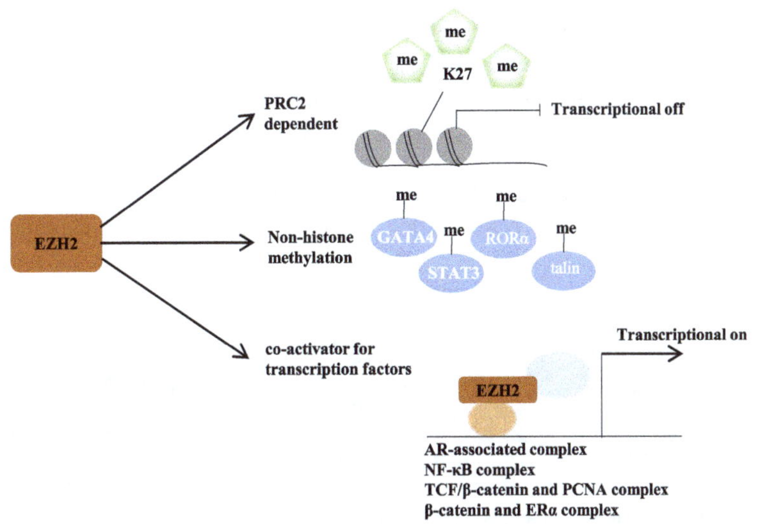

Fig. 1 The action modes of EZH2. (1) EZH2 catalyzes H3K27me3 dependent on PCR2, which contributes to transcriptional silencing. (2) EZH2 is also capable of methylating several non-histone protein substrates (e.g. STAT3, GATA4, talin, and RORα), which contributes to both transcriptional silencing and transcriptional activation. 3) EZH2 also has a PRC2-independent role in transcriptional activation, acting as co-activator for transcription factors, such as AR-associated complex, NF-κB signaling, TCF/β-catenin and PCNA, and β-catenin and ERα

actin and thereby promotes the turnover of adhesion structures [14].

PRC2-independent gene transactivation

In addition to transcriptional repression, emerging researches have shown that EZH2 methylates non-histone targets or directly interacts with other proteins to activate downstream genes in a PRC2-independent manner. Kim et al. found that AKT phosphorylates EZH2 at Ser21. The phosphorylated EZH2 directly binds to and methylates STAT3, leading to enhanced STAT3 activity by increasing phosphorylation of STAT3 at Y705 and thereby promotes the tumorigenicity of glioblastoma and glioblastoma stem-like cells (GSCs) [8].

The phosphorylated EZH2 also acts as a co-activator of critical transcription factors. Xu and colleagues demonstrated that EZH2 acts as a coactivator of androgen receptor-associated complexes to support castration-resistant prostate cancer (CRPC) growth, suggesting novel combination therapies for the treatment of metastatic, hormone-refractory prostate cancer [9]. Lee ST and colleagues identified that EZH2 binds to the NF-κB components to form a ternary complex leading to transcriptional activation of its downstream target genes in ER-negative basal-like breast cancer cells [15]. Similarly, EZH2 is also found to act as a co-activator of other critical transcription factors, such as TCF/β-catenin and the DNA repair protein PCNA-associated factor in colorectal cancer (CRC), β-catenin and ERα in breast cancer, to promote the transcription of their target genes, respectively [16, 17].

Another study by Yan et al. shows that ectopic expression of an EZH2 mutant lacking HMTase activity in NKTL cell lines rescued the tumor growth inhibition resulting from depletion of endogenous EZH2, indicating that the growth promoting function of EZH2 is independent of its HMTase activity [18]. However, further studies are still needed to uncover the detailed mechanism.

Dysregulation of EZH2 in cancers

As various functions of EZH2 were discovered, it has become understandable that EZH2 plays critical roles in the development and progression of various cancers. The significance of EZH2 in cancer was firstly realized in 2002 when Varambally and colleagues elucidated the association betweenEZH2 and prostate cancer prognosis. It was found that the upregulation of EZH2is associated with advanced stage and poor prognosis in prostate cancer [19]. Subsequent studies showed that EZH2 is upregulated in various solid malignancies including lung, hepatocellular, colorectal, breast and pancreatic cancer etc., and is shown to have prognostic significance in a variety of solid cancers [3, 4]. Unsurprisingly, the biological functions of EZH2 in different kinds of tumor cells are under intense investigation. However, both overexpression and loss-of-function mutations of EZH2 gene being detected in myelodysplastic syndrome (MDS) and acute myeloid leukemia (AML) suggests that EZH2 can function as tumor suppressor gene or as an oncogene in myeloid malignancies. In addition to the expression and function of EZH2 in cancer cells, recent studies also revealed that EZH2 might have critical roles in tumor immunity. Here, we will systematically discuss the functions of dysregulated EZH2 in cancers as below (Fig. 2).

Cell cycle, proliferation and apoptosis

EZH2 is involved in regulation of cell cycle progression and dysregulation of EZH2 accelerates cell proliferation and promotes survival, resulting in cancer development, such as CRC, melanoma and breast cancer [20–22]. For example, EZH2 inhibition by its inhibitor, DZNep or gene knockdown, can induce autophagy and apoptosis in CRC cells in vitro [20]. EZH2 inhibition in cholangiocarcinoma cells enhances cell apoptosis and arrests cells in the G1 phase, characteristized by elevated levels of p16 and p21 [23].

Epithelial to mesenchymal transition (EMT) and invasion

Strong evidence demonstrated that EZH2 could promote EMT by interacting with SNAIL1 and down-regulating the expression of E-cadherin [24, 25]. EZH2 can also induce the gene silencing of Disabled Homolog2-Interacting Protein (DAB2IP) to regulate EMT and metastasis in CRC [26]. In addition, EZH2 is demonstrated to promote tumor

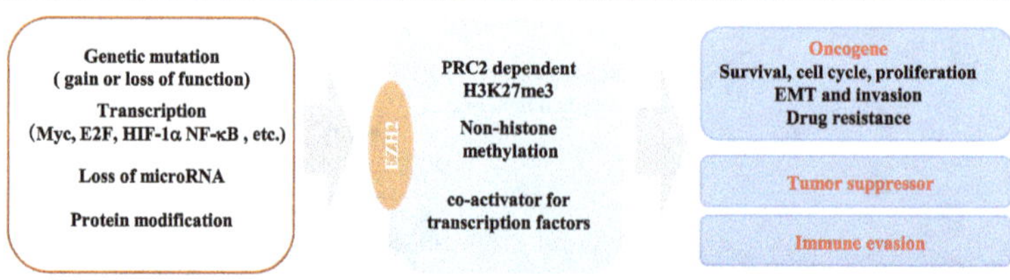

Fig. 2 The physiological functions and related regulation of EZH2 in cancer pathogenesis. The EZH2 expression and activity in cancer cells is regulated at genetic, transcriptional, post-transcriptional and post-translational levels, which leads to diverse functions of EZH2. EZH2, mediating gene transcriptional silencing and activation, promotes cell survival, proliferation, epithelial to mesenchymal, invasionand drug resistance of cancer cells. The tumor suppressive effects of EZH2 are also identified in several cancers, especially T-ALL, pancreatic cancer and clear cell renal carcinoma. What's more, EZH2 has decisive roles in T and NK cells mediated immune evasion

cell invasion. Yi et al. found that EZH2 inhibitsTIMP2 expression via H3K27me3 and DNA methylation, by which mean it relieves MMP repression and facilitates migration and invasion of ovarian cancer cells [27]. Under hypoxia, activation ofHIF-1α results in inactivation of PRC2 and the release of EZH2. Released EZH2 participates in the EZH2/ Forkhead box M1 (FoxM1) complex and induces MMP expression and invasion in triple-negative breast cancer (TNBC) [22]. As mediating the activation of EMT and invasion, EZH2 could increase metastasis in many cancers, such as CRC, melanoma, and breast cancer [22, 26, 28].

EZH2-mediated drug resistance

Despite of the development of cancer therapy, the drug resistance of cancer remains a serious problem. The critical roles of EZH2 in drug resistance of cancer cells were also identified. Several studies showed that EZH2 overexpression enhances chemoresistance in small cell lung cancer, head and neck squamous cell carcinoma (HNSCC) and glioblastoma [29–31]. In small cell lung cancer, EZH2 mediated H3K27me3 suppressed the expression of SLFN11, a factor implicated in DNA-damage repair deficiency, leading to chemoresistance [29]. In glioblastoma, EZH2 promotes the expression of ABC transporter MDR, MRP and BCRP to strengthen chemoresistance [31]. An EZH2 inhibitor combined with standard cytotoxic therapies suppressed emergence of acquired resistance and augmented chemotherapeutic efficacy in both chemosensitive and chemoresistant models.

Acquired and intrinsic resistance to receptor tyrosine kinase inhibitors (RTKi) represents a major hurdle in improving the management of clear cell renal cell carcinoma (ccRCC). Adelaiye et al. highlighted EZH2 as a rational target for therapeutic intervention in sunitinib-resistant ccRCC. Modulating EZH2 expression or activity suppressed phosphorylation of certain RTK, restoring the anti-tumor effects of sunitnib [32]. Inhibitors against poly (ADP-ribose) polymerase (PARP) are promising targeted therapy agents currently used to treat BRCA-mutant ovarian cancer and are in clinical trials for other cancer types, including BRCA-mutant breast cancer. Yamaguchi et al. demonstrated that EZH2 regulates the sensitivity of cancer cells to PARP inhibitors (PARPi). Upon DNA damage, PARP1 interacts and PARylates EZH2, inducing PRC2 complex dissociation and EZH2 downregulation. When PARPi is used, alkylating DNA damage-induced EZH2 downregulation would be disturbed, and EZH2-mediated gene silencing and cancer stem cell property are enhanced, leading to decreased sensitivity of PARPi [33]. However, in acute myeloid leukemia (AML), loss of the histone methyltransferase EZH2 and subsequent reduction of histone H3K27 trimethylation is identified as a novel pathway of acquired resistance to tyrosine kinase inhibitors (TKIs) and cytotoxic drugs in AML. Suppression of EZH2 protein expression reduces chemoresistance of AML cell lines and primary cells in vitro and in vivo. Low EZH2 level results in derepression of HOX genes, and knockdown of HOXB7 and HOXA9 in chemoresistant cells is sufficient to improve cell sensitivity to TKIs and cytotoxic drugs [34].

Tumor suppressive roles of EZH2

Although the oncogenic roles of EZH2 in many cancer types have been reported, the tumor suppressive roles of EZH2 were also identified. Suppression of EZH2 promotes cancer progression in some cancer types. T cell acute lymphoblastic leukemia (T-ALL) is an immature hematopoietic malignancy driven mainly by oncogenic activation of NOTCH1 signaling. Ntziachristos et al. demonstrated loss-of-function mutations and deletions of the EZH2 and SUZ12 genes in 25% of T-ALLs. Activation of NOTCH1 specifically induces loss of the repressive mark H3K27me3 by antagonizing the activity of PRC2, promoting cancer progression of T-ALL [35]. Mallen-St et al. found that loss of EZH2 resulted in impaired pancreatic regeneration and accelerated KRAS (G12D)-driven neoplasia, implicating that EZH2 restricted cancer progression via homeostatic control of pancreatic regeneration [36]. In clear cell renal carcinoma, loss of PRC2-dependent H3K27me3 in cancer cells activates HIF-driven chemokine (C-X-C motif) receptor 4 (CXCR4) expression in support of chemotactic cell invasion, leading to cancer metastasis [37].

Emerging roles of EZH2 in tumor immunity

Aberrant EZH2 expression in cancer cells can help them to modulate immune response and immunotherapy. Peng et al. showed that ovarian tumor EZH2 and DNA methyltransferase 1 (DNMT1) are negatively associated with tumor-infiltrating $CD8^{+}$T cells and patient outcome. EZH2-mediated H3K27me3 and DNMT1-mediated DNA methylation repress the tumor production of T helper 1 (Th1)-type chemokines CXCL9 and CXCL10, and subsequently determine effector T-cell trafficking to the tumor microenvironment. Treatment with epigenetic modulators increases tumor infiltration of effector T cell, slows down tumor progression, and improves the therapeutic efficacy of PD-L1 checkpoint blockade and adoptive T-cell transfusion in tumor-bearing mice [38]. A similar effect of EZH2 was also observed in colorectal cancer. Inhibition EZH2 in colorectal cancer cells augmented CXCL9 and CXCL10 expression to affect the infiltration of effector T cells in tumor [39]. Besides, Zingg et al. showed that during anti-CTLA-4 or IL-2 immunotherapy in mice, intratumoral tumor necrosis factor-αproduction and T cell accumulation results in increased Ezh2 expression in melanoma cells, which in turn silences their own immunogenicity and antigen presentation. Ezh2 inactivation reversed this resistance and synergized with anti-CTLA-4 and IL-2 immunotherapy to lead to intratumorally accumulation of IFN-γ-producing

PD-1^{low} $CD8^+$ T cells and PD-L1 downregulation to suppress melanoma growth [40].

Aberrant EZH2 expression and activity in immune cells in the tumor microenvironment affects tumor progression and therapy. Accumulating evidences have shown that EZH2 has direct roles on T cell response. EZH2 expression in naïve T cells promotes survival, proliferation and function of effector $CD4^+$ and $CD8^+$ T cells but inhibits Th1 and Th2 differentiation [6]. Therefore, EZH2 inhibition in T cells may suppress survival, expansion and effect of tumor-specific effectors T cell to inhibit anti-tumor immunity. Indeed, Zhao et al. demonstrated that EZH2 has a key role for the function of tumor-specific effector T cells, that cancer cells evaded tumor surveillance by targeting T-cell specific expression of EZH2 in the tumor microenvironment. The percentage of $EZH2^+$ $CD8^+$ T cells in ovarian cancer tissues is a stronger predictor of overall and progression-free survival as compared to the percentage of $CD8^+$ T cells. Ovarian cancer cells could induce expression of specific micro-RNAs in $CD4^+$ and $CD8^+$ T cells of the tumor microenvironment, which suppressesEZH2 expression and decreases their survival and immune function. Inhibition of EZH2 in tumor-specific T cells increases the tumor burden and the metastatic potential in mice models of ovarian cancer [41]. Long et al. identified that miR-26a expression is elevated in CTLs responding to tumor microenvironment secretome stimulation, miR-26a inhibits EZH2 to impair CTL function, indicating miR-26a-EZH2 axis as a novel target to improve the efficacy of CTL-based cancer immunotherapy [42].

Besides, EZH2 is considered critical for the recruitment and immunosuppression function of activated regulatory T cells (Tregs) at the sites of inflammation, and EZH2-deficient Tregs fail to protect mice from the development of autoimmunity in a model of naïve T cell-mediated colitis [43, 44]. It has been documented that Tregs can be induced in tumor microenvironment and display negative impact on anti-tumor immunity. Therefore, it is of particular interest to investigate for the regulation of EZH2 expression in Tregs in tumor microenvironment.

A recent study by Yin et al. has provided insight to an epigenetic-based mechanism regulating natural killer (NK) cell development and NK-based cancer immunotherapies. Inhibition of EZH2 expression or activity in hematopoietic stem and progenitor cells (HSPCs) gives rise to increased NK precursors and mature progeny, which displays enhanced cytotoxicity against tumor cells with up-regulation of IL-15R (CD122) and the NKG2D-activating receptor [45]. Gunawan et al. demonstrated that EZH2regulated the integrin signaling and adhesion dynamics of dendritic cells (DCs) to promote the development of experimental autoimmune encephalomyelitis [14], while Donas et al. found that inhibition of H3K27 demethylation induced tolerogenic DCs to inhibit inflammation and the development of experimental autoimmune encephalomyelitis [46]. These indicate a potential role of EZH2 in DC function, and whether EZH2 regulates DC-based cancer immunotherapies is worth further investigation. Another innate immune cell macrophage in tumor microenvironment, named tumor-associated macrophages (TAMs) can promote tumor growth directly, by favoring tumor cell proliferation and survival, and indirectly, by creating an immunosuppressive microenvironment. Qiao et al. demonstrated that EZH2 mediated H3K27me3 promotes IFN-γ-induced macrophage activation and inflammatory response [47]. However, how the dysregulated EZH2 in TAM participates tumor progression is still unknown.

Regulations of EZH2 in cancer

As shown above, EZH2 has diverse functions in different types of cancer. Accumulating evidences have shown that the expression and activity of EZH2 in cancer cells can be regulated at genetic, transcriptional, post-transcriptional and post-translational levels, which may explain these diverse functions of EZH2 (Fig. 2).

Mutation of EZH2

Recent studies have shown that somatic mutations in *EZH2* gene are observed in specific cancer types. Heterozygous point mutations affecting tyrosine 641 (Y641) within the C-terminal catalytic SET domain of EZH2 have been identified in B-cell lymphomas [diffuse large B-cell lymphoma (DLBCL) 22%; follicular lymphoma 7–12%] [48, 49]. Functional analysis has demonstrated that this mutation mediates gain-of-function of EZH2 enzymatic activity leading to increased levels of H3K27me3 and resulting in suppression of gene expression (e.g. TCF4, FOXP1, TCL1A, BIK, RASSF6P, CDKN1A) in lymphomas [50–52]. Otherwise, Souroullas et al. demonstrated that somatic EZH2 gain-of-function mutation (Y641F) in lymphoma and melanoma induces a vast reorganization of chromatin structure, inducing both repression and activation of polycomb-regulated loci. EZH2 mutation (Y641F) globally increased the abundance of H3K27me3 in lymphoma and melanoma, but also caused a widespread redistribution of this repressive mark, including a loss of H3K27me3 that was associated with increased transcription at many loci [53].

In contrast, EZH2 inactivating deletion, frameshift, nonsense and missense mutations have been identified in myelodysplastic syndromes (MDS), myeloproliferative neoplasms (MPN), MDS-MPN overlap disorders and T-cell acute lymphocytic leukemia [54–56], implicating that EZH2 loss-of-function is associated with development of malignancy and EZH2 may function as a tumor suppressor. Consistently with these findings in patients, mice lacking EZH2 gene have enhanced initiation and progression of Runx1-mutant MDS [57]. These studies suggest that the potential tumor suppressive effects of EZH2 should be considered during therapeutic application of EZH2 inhibitors.

Transcriptional regulation of EZH2

EZH2 has been considered to be overexpressed in many cancer types and to be transcriptionally regulated by oncogenic signaling to promote cancer cell proliferation and disease progression. EZH2 expression is correlated with Myc expression in prostate cancer. Myc binds to EZH2 promoter and directly activates its transcription [58]. E2F, another cell cycle regulator, positively controls EZH2 transcription through its direct binding on EZH2 promoter upon Rb/RB1 phosphorylation in bladder and small cell lung cancer [59]. ANCCA, a co-activator of androgen receptor (AR), can bind E2F and enhance E2F-mediated EZH2 transcription in prostate cancer cells [60, 61]. SOX4, one of the key regulators of stem cells, directly regulates the expression of EZH2 mRNA to promote EMT [28].

Besides, many other transcription factors have also been identified to affect the expression of EZH2 gene, including EWS-FLI1 in Ewing tumors [62], MEK- ERK-ELK1 in pancreatic cancer, triple negative and ERBB2 positive breast cancer [63, 64], KRAS mutations and downstream ERK or Akt in non-small cell lung cancer [65], hypoxia-induced HIF-1α in breast cancer [66], and NF-κB in T-cell leukemia [67]. All these findings provide better understanding of EZH2 regulation at the transcriptional level and allow therapeutic combinations of pathway targeting agents and EZH2 inhibitors to achieve maximum therapeutic benefit in cancers.

Post-transcriptional regulation of EZH2

The expression of EZH2 in cancer is also regulated by post-transcriptional mechanisms through microRNAs. These microRNAs can bind to the EZH2 mRNA 3'UTR and modulate its stability, integrity and translation, thereby affecting the levels of EZH2 protein. In specific cancer types, downregulation of these microRNAs leads to EZH2 overexpression and subsequent H3K27me3 accumulation to promote tumor progression. In particular, miR-26a and miR-101 are the most demonstrated as negative regulators of EZH2. Wong et al. firstly found that miRNA-26a, an up-regulated miRNA during myogenesis, binds to the EZH2 mRNA 3'UTR and inhibits its expression in myoblasts [68]. The following studies identified that miR-26a acts as a tumor suppressor, and directly targets and regulatsEZH2 at a post-transcriptional level in cancer cells to inhibit the development of hepatocellular cancer, Burkitt lymphoma, rhabdomyosarcoma, nasopharyngeal carcinoma, and breast cancer. Similarly, Xiaoping et al. demonstrated that down-regulation of miR-101 in glioblastoma cells promotes tumor angiogenesis, cell proliferation and invasion by increasing EZH2-mediated overexpression of cytoplasmic polyadenylation element-binding protein 1 (CPEB1) [69, 70].

Other microRNAs (e.g. miR-126, miR-138, miR-32, miR-506, miR-137) are also reported to directly target EZH2 in different types of cancer and displayed different functions. For example, miR-126 and miR-138 directly target EZH2 transcript and increase the sensitivity of osteosarcoma cells and gastric cancer cells to chemotherapy [71, 72]. miRNA-32, miR-137 and miR-506 also directly target EZH2 transcript and suppress tumor proliferation, angiogenesis and metastasis in melanoma, colon cancer and glioblastoma [73–75].

Post-translational regulation of EZH2

In addition to transcriptional regulation and miRNA-mediated post-transcriptional regulation, the expression and activity of EZH2 can be regulated at the post-translational level, such as protein phosphorylation, ubiquitinylation, palmitoylation, etc.

AKT1-mediated phosphorylation of EZH2 allows it to act as a coactivator of androgen receptor-associated complexes, promoting the expression of androgen receptor-target genes in the absence of androgen and the development and progression of castration-resistant prostate cancer (CRPC) [9]. The phosphorylated EZH2 also can directly bind to and methylate STAT3, leading to enhanced STAT3 activity by increased tyrosine phosphorylation of STAT3 and thereby promote the tumorigenicity of glioblastoma stem-like cells (GSCs) [8]. Cyclin-dependent kinases 1 and 2 (CDK1/2) phosphorylate EZH2 at T492 disrupts the PRC2 assemblies and decreases EZH2 activity, while phosphorylation of EZH2 at T350 and T492 promotes EZH2 ubiquitinylation and degradation, suggesting its decreased methyltransferase activity [76, 77]. While CDK-mediated EZH2 phosphorylation is critical for cancer-cell invasion and osteogenic differentiation of mesenchymal stem cells, further investigation is needed toreveal the role of this interaction in the fate and function of cancer cells. Another study by Yang et al. showed that cyclin E/CDK2 phosphorylates EZH2 at T416 (pT416-EZH2) and enhances the ability of EZH2 to promote triple negative breast cancer cell migration/invasion, tumor sphere formation and in vivo tumor growth [78].

Wang et al. also identified NIMA-related kinase 2 (NEK2) as a functional binding protein of EZH2 that plays a critical role in the posttranslational regulation of EZH2 protein in GSCs. NEK2 is among the most differentially expressed kinase-encoding genes in GSC-containing cultures, and is required for in vitro clonogenicity, in vivo tumor propagation and radioresistance. Mechanistically, the formation of a protein complex comprising NEK2 and EZH2 in glioma spheres phosphorylates and then protectsEZH2 from ubiquitination-dependent protein degradation in a NEK2 kinase activity-dependent manner [79]. Besides, Yan et al. demonstrated that JAK3, a tyrosine kinase activated downstream of cytokine receptors, phosphorylates

EZH2 on tyrosine residue 244, altering EZH2 activity and promotes the survival and proliferation of NK/T-cell lymphoma cells [80].

EZH2 can also be regulated by protein ubiquitination. Sahasrabuddhe et al. identified EZH2 as a novel inter actor and substrate of the SCF E3 ubiquitin ligase FBXW1. FBXW1ubiquitinatesEZH2, and Jak2-mediated phosphorylation on Y641 directsFBXW1-mediated EZH2 degradation, thereby controlling H3K27me3 activity and lymphoma pathogenesis [81]. Jin et al. identified another E3 ubiquitin ligase, FBW7that targets EZH2 in pancreatic cancer cells. The expression of EZH2 protein is negatively correlated with FBW7 protein levels in a cohort of human pancreatic cancer specimens, and FBW7 suppresses EZH2 activity and inhibits tumor migration and invasion via degradation of EZH2 in pancreatic cancer cells [82].

Protein S-palmitoylation is a reversible posttranslational modification in proteins with fatty acids that is regulated by protein acyltransferases (PAT), characterized by a conserved catalytic domain containing an Asp-His-His-Cys (DHHC) motif [83]. A recent study found that the gene-encoding zinc finger DHHC-type-containing (ZDHHC) 5 directly palmitoylates EZH2 to increase EZH2-mediated H3K27me3 but not EZH2 expression, thereby promoting tumorigenicity of GSCs [84]. Yamaguchi et al. reported that during DNA damage, PARP1 mediates PARylation of EZH2, inducing PRC2 complex dissociation and EZH2 downregulation. Inhibition of PARP by PARPi attenuates alkylating DNA damage-induced EZH2 downregulation, thereby promotes EZH2-mediated gene silencing and cancer stem cell property compared with PARPi-untreated cells [33].

Collectively, all these findings strongly suggest that posttranslational regulation of EZH2 might be of particular importance with regards to its diverse and complex implication in cancer development and growth.

Targeting EZH2 for cancer therapy

EZH2 widely regulates gene expression affecting several physiological functions, especially cancer progression. Thus, EZH2 is a potential target for cancer therapy, and EZH2 inhibitors have been under intense pre-clinical and clinical investigation.

3-deazaadenosine A (DZNep) is a non-specific EZH2 inhibitor which decreases the protein level of EZH2 and the H3K27me3 marks, thereby exhibiting anti-tumor effects in various malignancies. However, DZNep was reported to have efficacy but also toxicity in animal models [85].

Recently, some studies referred that targeting histone methylation might be a promising approach for cancer therapy, for example, lysine-specific demethylase 1 inhibition increased histone H3lysine4 methylation and finally induced apoptosis and differentiation of stem-like leukemia cells [86, 87]. In 2012, potent, highly selective S-adenosylmethionine-competitive small molecule inhibitors of EZH2 methyltransferase activity, GSK126 [88] and EPZ005687 [89], were developed.GSK126 and EPZ005687 can bind to wild-type and Y641 mutant EZH2, leading to decreased H3K27me3 level and upregulation of expression of the silenced gene transcription, thereby effectively inhibiting the proliferation of EZH2 mutant DLBCL both in vitro and in xenograft mice models [88, 89]. GSK926 [90] and GSK-343 [91] are also exhibited to inhibit EZH2 activity to suppress H3K27me3 level in breast and prostate cancer cells. An oral inhibitor of EZH2, EPZ6438 (tazemetostat), reportedly decreases the levels of H3K27me3 to reduce tumor growth in EZH2 mutant non-Hodgkin lymphoma [92]. EPZ6438is currently under evaluation in a phase 1/2 clinical trial in patients with B-cell lymphomas and advanced solid tumors (NCT01897571), provided with encouraging preliminary signs of clinical activity. Besides, this compound is being further evaluated in a phase 1 clinical trial for pediatric patients (NCT02601937) and a phase 2 clinical trial for adults (NCT02601950) with relapsed rhabdoid tumors, synovial sarcomas, renal medullary carcinoma and epithelioid sarcoma [5]. In 2015,the selective and orally available EZH2 inhibitor, EPZ011989, was also reported and shown to have significant effects in the mouse xenograft model of B cell lymphoma [93]. Another more recent study introduced that ZLD1039, a highly selective, potent and orally available agent can decrease H3K27 methylation to upregulate tumor suppressor genes in breast cancer and suppress the tumor growth and metastasis in a mouse breast cancer xenograft model [94].

Recent studies demonstrated that inhibition of the interaction between EZH2 with PRC2 complex may also be a specific approach with efficacy against various neoplastic diseases with decreased toxicity. Kim et al. reported that stabilized alpha-helix of EZH2 (SAH-EZH2) peptides selectively inhibited H3K27me3 by disrupting the EZH2-EED complex and reducing EZH2 protein levels, thereby leading to growth arrest and differentiation of MLL-AF9 leukemic cells [95]. Similarly, the small molecule inhibitor Astemizole can also inhibit EZH2/EED interaction which destabilizes PRC2 complex thereby decreasing the proliferation of lymphoma cells [96]. Another inhibitor CPI-1205, disturbing the interaction of EZH2 with PRC2 complex, is currently evaluated in a phase 1 clinical trial in patients with B-cell lymphomas (NCT02395601) [97].

In addition to the competitive inhibitors of EZH2 expression and activity, a novel strategy to suppress EZH2 by protein degradation has been developed by Wang et al. They reported that a gambogenic acid (GNA) derivative, GNA022, specifically and covalently binds to Cys668 within the EZH2-SET domain, subsequently triggersEZH2 degradation through COOH terminus of Hsp70-interacting protein (CHIP)-mediated ubiquitination of EZH2, enhancingEZH2 degradation and inhibiting tumor growth [98].

Conclusions

In conclusion, EZH2 is a methyltransferase and catalytic component of the PRC2, and mediates H3K27me3. Accumulating evidence from in vitro and in vivo models together with clinical studies collectively suggest that EZH2 is involved in the development and progression of several human malignancies. EZH2 activity is upregulated in cancer due to gain-of-function mutations, and overexpression by transcriptional, post-transcriptional and post-translational regulation. EZH2 downregulates expression of tumor suppressor genes and upregulates oncogenes, promoting cancer cell survival, proliferation, epithelial to mesenchymal and invasion. In particular, EZH2 has been also reported to be associated with drug resistance to chemotherapy and targeted therapy. Therefore, several targeted compounds inhibiting EZH2 expression and activity have been introduced in cancer therapeutics with promising results in preclinical studies combination with traditional chemotherapy with or not, and are currently under evaluation in phase 1 and 2 clinical trials.

However, the tumor suppressive roles of EZH2 were also identified that suppression of EZH2 promotes cancer progression in some cancer types, such as T-ALL, pancreatic cancer and clear cell renal carcinoma. Besides, recent studies also revealed that EZH2had complicated roles in tumor immunity. Inhibition of EZH2 in HSPCs gives rise to increased NK precursors and mature progeny displaying enhanced cytotoxicity against tumor cells. But EZH2 is essential for tumor-specific T cells-mediated tumor surveillance. EZH2 has also been shown to regulate the function of Tregs, dendritic cells and macrophage, all of which are critical parts of tumor microenvironment. Therefore, therapeutic targeting EZH2 is posing new challenges and worth future further investigation.

Abbreviations

AML: acute myeloid leukemia; AR: androgen receptor; CcRCC: clear cell renal cell carcinoma; CDK1/2: Cyclin-dependent kinases 1 and 2; CHIP: COOH terminus of Hsp70-interacting protein; CPEB1: cytoplasmic polyadenylation element-binding protein 1; CRC: colorectal cancer; CRPC: castration-resistant prostate cancer; DAB2IP: Disabled Homolog2-Interacting Protein; DCs: dendritic cells; DHHC: Asp-His-His-Cys; DLBCL: diffuse large B-cell lymphoma; DNMT1: DNA methyltransferase 1; EZH2: Enhancer of zeste homolog 2; FoxM1: Forkhead box M1; GNA: gambogenic acid; GSCs: glioblastoma stem-like cells; H2AK-119ub1: histone H2A at lysine 119; H3K27me3: tri-methylation of histone H3 at Lys 27; HMT: histone methyl transferase; HNSCC: head and neck squamous cell carcinoma; HSPCs: hematopoietic stem and progenitor cells; MDS: myelodysplastic syndrome; MPN: myeloproliferative neoplasms; NEK2: NIMA-related kinase 2; NK: natural killer; PARP: poly (ADP-ribose) polymerase; PARPi: PARP inhibitors; PAT: protein acyltransferases; PcGs: Polycomb group proteins; PRC1: polycomb repressive complex 1; PRC2: polycomb repressive complex 2; pT416-EZH2: phosphorylates EZH2 at T416; RORα: RAR-related orphan receptor alpha; RTKi: receptor tyrosine kinase inhibitors; SAH-EZH2: stabilized alpha-helix of EZH2; T-ALL: T cell acute lymphoblastic leukemia; TAMs: tumor-associated macrophages; Th1: T helper 1; TKIs: tyrosine kinase inhibitors; TNBC: triple-negative breast cancer; Tregs: regulatory T cells; ZDHHC: zinc finger DHHC

Acknowledgements
Not applicable.

Funding
Not applicable.

Authors' contributions

LG prepare the manuscript draft, YY contributed the article writing and revising, QL and YF provided the important suggestions, TL critically reviewed the article, WG designed the study, and revised the manuscript. All authors read and approved the final manuscript draft.

Consent for publication

Not applicable.

Competing interests

The authors declare that they have no competing interests.

Author details
[1]Department of Medical Oncology, Fudan University Shanghai Cancer Center, No.270, Dongan Road, Shanghai 200032, China. [2]Department of Oncology, Shanghai Medical college, Fudan University, No.130, Dongan Road, Shanghai 200032, China. [3]Department of Medical Oncology, Zhongshan Hospital, Fudan University, No.180, Fenglin Road, Shanghai 200032, China.

References

1. Greer EL, Shi Y. Histone methylation: a dynamic mark in health, disease and inheritance. Nat Rev Genet. 2012;13(5):343–57.
2. Margueron R, Reinberg D. The Polycomb complex PRC2 and its mark in life. Nature. 2011;469(7330):343–9.
3. Pasini D, Emerging DCL. Roles for Polycomb proteins in cancer. Curr Opin Genet Dev. 2016;36:50–8.
4. Yamagishi M, Uchimaru K. Targeting EZH2 in cancer therapy. Curr Opin Oncol. 2017;29(5):375–81.
5. Kim KH, Roberts CW. Targeting EZH2 in cancer. Nat Med. 2016;22(2):128–34.
6. Karantanos T, et al. Regulation of T cell differentiation and function by EZH2. Front Immunol. 2016;7:172.
7. Yan KS, et al. EZH2 in cancer progression and potential application in cancer therapy: a friend or foe? Int J Mol Sci. 2017;18(6)
8. Kim E, et al. Phosphorylation of EZH2 activates STAT3 signaling via STAT3 methylation and promotes tumorigenicity of glioblastoma stem-like cells. Cancer Cell. 2013;23(6):839–52.
9. Xu K, et al. EZH2 oncogenic activity in castration-resistant prostate cancer cells is Polycomb-independent. Science. 2012;338(6113):1465–9.
10. Christofides A, et al. Epigenetic regulation of cancer biology and anti-tumor immunity by EZH2. Oncotarget. 2016;7(51):85624–40.
11. Cao R, Zhang Y. The functions of E(Z)/EZH2-mediated methylation of lysine 27 in histone H3. Curr Opin Genet Dev. 2004;14(2):155–64.
12. He A, et al. PRC2 directly methylates GATA4 and represses its transcriptional activity. Genes Dev. 2012;26(1):37–42.
13. Lee JM, et al. EZH2 generates a methyl degron that is recognized by the DCAF1/DDB1/CUL4 E3 ubiquitin ligase complex. Mol Cell. 2012;48(4):572–86.
14. Gunawan M, et al. The methyltransferase Ezh2 controls cell adhesion and migration through direct methylation of the extranuclear regulatory protein talin. Nat Immunol. 2015;16(5):505–16.
15. Lee ST, et al. Context-specific regulation of NF-kappaB target gene expression by EZH2 in breast cancers. Mol Cell. 2011;43(5):798–810.
16. Jung HY, et al. PAF and EZH2 induce Wnt/beta-catenin signaling hyperactivation. Mol Cell. 2013;52(2):193–205.
17. Shi B, et al. Integration of estrogen and Wnt signaling circuits by the polycomb group protein EZH2 in breast cancer cells. Mol Cell Biol. 2007;27(14):5105–19.
18. Yan J, et al. EZH2 overexpression in natural killer/T-cell lymphoma confers growth advantage independently of histone methyltransferase activity. Blood. 2013;121(22):4512–20.
19. Varambally S, et al. The polycomb group protein EZH2 is involved in progression of prostate cancer. Nature. 2002;419(6907):624–9.
20. Yao Y, et al. Downregulation of enhancer of Zeste homolog 2 (EZH2) is essential for the induction of autophagy and apoptosis in colorectal cancer cells. Genes (Basel). 2016;7(10)

21. Zingg D, et al. The epigenetic modifier EZH2 controls melanoma growth and metastasis through silencing of distinct tumour suppressors. Nat Commun. 2015;6:6051.
22. Mahara S, et al. HIFI-alpha activation underlies a functional switch in the paradoxical role of Ezh2/PRC2 in breast cancer. Proc Natl Acad Sci U S A. 2016;113(26):E3735–44.
23. Nakagawa S, et al. Enhancer of zeste homolog 2 (EZH2) promotes progression of cholangiocarcinoma cells by regulating cell cycle and apoptosis. Ann Surg Oncol. 2013;20(Suppl 3):S667–75.
24. Ma DN, et al. MicroRNA-26a suppresses epithelial-mesenchymal transition in human hepatocellular carcinoma by repressing enhancer of zeste homolog 2. J Hematol Oncol. 2016;9(1)
25. Cao Q, et al. Repression of E-cadherin by the polycomb group protein EZH2 in cancer. Oncogene. 2008;27(58):7274–84.
26. Wang J, et al. The positive feedback between snail and DAB2IP regulates EMT, invasion and metastasis in colorectal cancer. Oncotarget. 2015;6(29): 27427–39.
27. Yi X, et al. EZH2-mediated epigenetic silencing of TIMP2 promotes ovarian cancer migration and invasion. Sci Rep. 2017;7(1):3568.
28. Tiwari N, et al. Sox4 is a master regulator of epithelial-mesenchymal transition by controlling Ezh2 expression and epigenetic reprogramming. Cancer Cell. 2013;23(6):768–83.
29. Gardner EE, et al. Chemosensitive relapse in small cell lung cancer proceeds through an EZH2-SLFN11 Axis. Cancer Cell. 2017;31(2):286–99.
30. Chang JW, et al. EZH2 is associated with poor prognosis in head-and-neck squamous cell carcinoma via regulating the epithelial-to-mesenchymal transition and chemosensitivity. Oral Oncol. 2016;52:66–74.
31. Fan TY, et al. Inhibition of EZH2 reverses chemotherapeutic drug TMZ chemosensitivity in glioblastoma. Int J Clin Exp Pathol. 2014;7(10):6662–70.
32. Adelaiye-Ogala R, et al. EZH2 modifies sunitinib resistance in renal cell carcinoma by kinome reprogramming. Cancer Res. 2017;
33. Yamaguchi H, et al. EZH2 contributes to the response to PARP inhibitors through its PARP-mediated poly-ADP ribosylation in breast cancer. Oncogene. 2017;
34. Gollner S, et al. Loss of the histone methyltransferase EZH2 induces resistance to multiple drugs in acute myeloid leukemia. Nat Med. 2017;23(1):69–78.
35. Ntziachristos P, et al. Genetic inactivation of the polycomb repressive complex 2 in T cell acute lymphoblastic leukemia. Nat Med. 2012;18(2):298–301.
36. Mallen-St Clair J, et al. EZH2 couples pancreatic regeneration to neoplastic progression. Genes Dev. 2012;26(5):439–44.
37. Vanharanta S, et al. Epigenetic expansion of VHL-HIF signal output drives multiorgan metastasis in renal cancer. Nat Med. 2013;19(1):50–6.
38. Peng D, et al. Epigenetic silencing of TH1-type chemokines shapes tumour immunity and immunotherapy. Nature. 2015;527(7577):249–53.
39. Nagarsheth N, et al. PRC2 epigenetically silences Th1-type chemokines to suppress effector T-cell trafficking in colon cancer. Cancer Res. 2016;76(2):275–82.
40. Zingg D, et al. The histone methyltransferase Ezh2 controls mechanisms of adaptive resistance to tumor immunotherapy. Cell Rep. 2017;20(4):854–67.
41. Zhao E, et al. Cancer mediates effector T cell dysfunction by targeting microRNAs and EZH2 via glycolysis restriction. Nat Immunol. 2016;17(1):95–103.
42. Long H, et al. The tumor microenvironment disarms CD8+ T lymphocyte function via a miR-26a-EZH2 axis. Oncoimmunology. 2016;5(12):e1245267.
43. DuPage M, et al. The chromatin-modifying enzyme Ezh2 is critical for the maintenance of regulatory T cell identity after activation. Immunity. 2015; 42(2):227–38.
44. Yang XP, et al. EZH2 is crucial for both differentiation of regulatory T cells and T effector cell expansion. Sci Rep. 2015;5:10643.
45. Yin J, et al. Ezh2 regulates differentiation and function of natural killer cells through histone methyltransferase activity. Proc Natl Acad Sci U S A. 2015; 112(52):15988–93.
46. Donas C, et al. The histone demethylase inhibitor GSK-J4 limits inflammation through the induction of a tolerogenic phenotype on DCs. J Autoimmun. 2016;75:105–17.
47. Qiao Y, et al. IFN-gamma induces histone 3 lysine 27 Trimethylation in a small subset of promoters to stably silence gene expression in human macrophages. Cell Rep. 2016;16(12):3121–9.
48. Morin RD, et al. Somatic mutations altering EZH2 (Tyr641) in follicular and diffuse large B-cell lymphomas of germinal-center origin. Nat Genet. 2010; 42(2):181–5.
49. Bodor C, et al. EZH2 Y641 mutations in follicular lymphoma. Leukemia. 2011; 25(4):726–9.
50. Yap DB, et al. Somatic mutations at EZH2 Y641 act dominantly through a mechanism of selectively altered PRC2 catalytic activity, to increase H3K27 trimethylation. Blood. 2011;117(8):2451–9.
51. Guo S, et al. EZH2 mutations in follicular lymphoma from different ethnic groups and associated gene expression alterations. Clin Cancer Res. 2014; 20(12):3078–86.
52. Beguelin W, et al. EZH2 is required for germinal center formation and somatic EZH2 mutations promote lymphoid transformation. Cancer Cell. 2013;23(5):677–92.
53. Souroullas GP, et al. An oncogenic Ezh2 mutation induces tumors through global redistribution of histone 3 lysine 27 trimethylation. Nat Med. 2016; 22(6):632–40.
54. Ernst T, et al. Inactivating mutations of the histone methyltransferase gene EZH2 in myeloid disorders. Nat Genet. 2010;42(8):722–6.
55. Nikoloski G, et al. Somatic mutations of the histone methyltransferase gene EZH2 in myelodysplastic syndromes. Nat Genet. 2010;42(8):665–7.
56. Simon C, et al. A key role for EZH2 and associated genes in mouse and human adult T-cell acute leukemia. Genes Dev. 2012;26(7):651–6.
57. Sashida G, et al. Ezh2 loss promotes development of myelodysplastic syndrome but attenuates its predisposition to leukaemic transformation. Nat Commun. 2014;5:4177.
58. Koh CM, et al. Myc enforces overexpression of EZH2 in early prostatic neoplasia via transcriptional and post-transcriptional mechanisms. Oncotarget. 2011;2(9):669–83.
59. Bracken AP, et al. EZH2 is downstream of the pRB-E2F pathway, essential for proliferation and amplified in cancer. EMBO J. 2003;22(20):5323–35.
60. Kalashnikova EV, et al. ANCCA/ATAD2 overexpression identifies breast cancer patients with poor prognosis, acting to drive proliferation and survival of triple-negative cells through control of B-Myb and EZH2. Cancer Res. 2010;70(22):9402–12.
61. Duan Z, et al. Developmental and androgenic regulation of chromatin regulators EZH2 and ANCCA/ATAD2 in the prostate via MLL histone methylase complex. Prostate. 2013;73(5):455–66.
62. Richter GH, et al. EZH2 is a mediator of EWS/FLI1 driven tumor growth and metastasis blocking endothelial and neuro-ectodermal differentiation. Proc Natl Acad Sci U S A. 2009;106(13):5324–9.
63. Fujii S, et al. RAS oncogenic signal upregulates EZH2 in pancreatic cancer. Biochem Biophys Res Commun. 2012;417(3):1074–9.
64. Fujii S, et al. MEK-ERK pathway regulates EZH2 overexpression in association with aggressive breast cancer subtypes. Oncogene. 2011;30(39):4118–28.
65. Riquelme E, et al. Modulation of EZH2 expression by MEK-ERK or PI3K-AKT signaling in lung cancer is dictated by different KRAS oncogene mutations. Cancer Res. 2016;76(3):675–85.
66. Dong M, et al. Aberrant expression of enhancer of zeste homologue 2, correlated with HIF-1alpha, refines relapse risk and predicts poor outcome for breast cancer. Oncol Rep. 2014;32(3):1101–7.
67. Fujikawa D, et al. Polycomb-dependent epigenetic landscape in adult T-cell leukemia. Blood. 2016;127(14):1790–802.
68. Wong CF, Tellam RL. MicroRNA-26a targets the histone methyltransferase enhancer of Zeste homolog 2 during myogenesis. J Biol Chem. 2008; 283(15):9836–43.
69. Smits M, et al. miR-101 is down-regulated in glioblastoma resulting in EZH2-induced proliferation, migration, and angiogenesis. Oncotarget. 2010;1(8): 710–20.
70. Xiaoping L, et al. CPEB1, a histone-modified hypomethylated gene, is regulated by miR-101 and involved in cell senescence in glioma. Cell Death Dis. 2013;4:e675.
71. Wang P, et al. MicroRNA-126 increases chemosensitivity in drug-resistant gastric cancer cells by targeting EZH2. Biochem Biophys Res Commun. 2016;479(1):91–6.
72. Zhu Z, et al. MiR-138 acts as a tumor suppressor by targeting EZH2 and enhances cisplatin-induced apoptosis in osteosarcoma cells. PLoS One. 2016;11(3):e0150026.
73. Ma YB, et al. MicroRNA-32 functions as a tumor suppressor and directly targets EZH2 in uveal melanoma. Genet Mol Res. 2016;15(2)
74. Zhang Y, et al. MicroRNA-506 suppresses tumor proliferation and metastasis in colon cancer by directly targeting the oncogene EZH2. Oncotarget. 2015; 6(32):32586–601.
75. Sun J, et al. MiR-137 inhibits proliferation and angiogenesis of human glioblastoma cells by targeting EZH2. J Neuro-Oncol. 2015;122(3):481–9.

76. Wei Y, et al. CDK1-dependent phosphorylation of EZH2 suppresses methylation of H3K27 and promotes osteogenic differentiation of human mesenchymal stem cells. Nat Cell Biol. 2011;13(1):87–94.
77. Wu SC, Zhang Y. Cyclin-dependent kinase 1 (CDK1)-mediated phosphorylation of enhancer of zeste 2 (Ezh2) regulates its stability. J Biol Chem. 2011;286(32):28511–9.
78. Yang CC, et al. Phosphorylation of EZH2 at T416 by CDK2 contributes to the malignancy of triple negative breast cancers. Am J Transl Res. 2015;7(6): 1009–20.
79. Wang J, et al. Targeting NEK2 attenuates glioblastoma growth and radioresistance by destabilizing histone methyltransferase EZH2. J Clin Invest. 2017;127(8):3075–89.
80. Yan J, et al. EZH2 phosphorylation by JAK3 mediates a switch to noncanonical function in natural killer/T-cell lymphoma. Blood. 2016;128(7): 948–58.
81. Sahasrabuddhe AA, et al. Oncogenic Y641 mutations in EZH2 prevent Jak2/ beta-TrCP-mediated degradation. Oncogene. 2015;34(4):445–54.
82. Jin X, et al. CDK5/FBW7-dependent ubiquitination and degradation of EZH2 inhibits pancreatic cancer cell migration and invasion. J Biol Chem. 2017; 292(15):6269–80.
83. Linder ME, Jennings BC. Mechanism and Function of DHHC S-acyltransferases. Biochem Soc Trans. 2013;41(1):29–34.
84. Chen X, et al. EZH2 Palmitoylation mediated by ZDHHC5 in p53-mutant glioma drives malignant development and progression. Cancer Res. 2017; 77(18):4998–5010.
85. Mayr C, et al. 3-deazaneplanocin a may directly target putative cancer stem cells in biliary tract cancer. Anticancer Res. 2015;35(9):4697–705.
86. Feng Z, et al. Pharmacological inhibition of LSD1 for the treatment of MLL-rearranged leukemia. J Hematol Oncol. 2016;9:24.
87. Song Y, et al. Targeting histone methylation for cancer therapy: enzymes, inhibitors, biological activity and perspectives. J Hematol Oncol. 2016;9(1):49.
88. McCabe MT, et al. EZH2 inhibition as a therapeutic strategy for lymphoma with EZH2-activating mutations. Nature. 2012;492(7427):108–12.
89. Knutson SK, et al. A selective inhibitor of EZH2 blocks H3K27 methylation and kills mutant lymphoma cells. Nat Chem Biol. 2012;8(11):890–6.
90. Amatangelo MD, et al. Three-dimensional culture sensitizes epithelial ovarian cancer cells to EZH2 methyltransferase inhibition. Cell Cycle. 2013; 12(13):2113–9.
91. Verma SK, et al. Identification of potent, selective, cell-active inhibitors of the histone lysine methyltransferase EZH2. ACS Med Chem Lett. 2012;3(12): 1091–6.
92. Knutson SK, et al. Selective inhibition of EZH2 by EPZ-6438 leads to potent antitumor activity in EZH2-mutant non-Hodgkin lymphoma. Mol Cancer Ther. 2014;13(4):842–54.
93. Campbell JE, et al. EPZ011989, a potent, orally-available EZH2 inhibitor with robust in vivo activity. ACS Med Chem Lett. 2015;6(5):491–5.
94. Song X, et al. Corrigendum: selective inhibition of EZH2 by ZLD1039 blocks H3K27methylation and leads to potent anti-tumor activity in breast cancer. Sci Rep. 2016;6:24893.
95. Kim W, et al. Targeted disruption of the EZH2-EED complex inhibits EZH2-dependent cancer. Nat Chem Biol. 2013;9(10):643–50.
96. Kong X, et al. Astemizole arrests the proliferation of cancer cells by disrupting the EZH2-EED interaction of polycomb repressive complex 2. J Med Chem. 2014;57(22):9512–21.
97. Vaswani RG, et al. Identification of (R)-N-((4-Methoxy-6-methyl-2-oxo-1,2-dihydropyridin-3-yl)methyl)-2-methyl-1-(1-(1 -(2,2,2-trifluoroethyl)piperidin-4-yl)ethyl)-1H-indole-3-carboxamide (CPI-1205), a potent and selective inhibitor of histone methyltransferase EZH2, suitable for phase I clinical trials for B-cell lymphomas. J Med Chem. 2016;59(21):9928–41.
98. Wang X, et al. A covalently bound inhibitor triggers EZH2 degradation through CHIP-mediated ubiquitination. EMBO J. 2017;36(9):1243–60.

20

PI3K, p38 and JAK/STAT signalling in bronchial tissue from patients with asthma following allergen challenge

Thomas Southworth[1,3*], Sarah Mason[1], Alan Bell[1], Isabel Ramis[2], Marta Calbet[2], Anna Domenech[2], Neus Prats[2], Montserrat Miralpeix[2] and Dave Singh[1]

Abstract

Background: Inhaled allergen challenges are often used to evaluate novel asthma treatments in early phase clinical trials. Current novel therapeutic targets in asthma include phosphoinositide 3-kinases (PI3K) delta and gamma, p38 mitogen-activated protein kinase (p38) and Janus kinase/Signal Transducer and Activator of Transcription (JAK/STAT) signalling pathways. The activation of these pathways following allergen exposure in atopic asthma patients it is not known.

Methods: We collected bronchial biopsies from 11 atopic asthma patients at baseline and after allergen challenge to investigate biomarkers of PI3K, p38 MAPK and JAK/STAT activation by immunohistochemistry. Cell counts and levels of eosinophil cationic protein and interleukin-5 were also assessed in sputum and bronchoalvelar lavage.

Results: Biopsies collected post-allergen had an increased percentage of epithelial cells expressing phospho-p38 (17.5 vs 25.6%, $p = 0.04$), and increased numbers of sub-epithelial cells expressing phospho-STAT5 (122.2 vs 540.6 cells/mm^2, $p = 0.01$) and the PI3K marker phospho-ribosomal protein S6 (180.7 vs 777.3 cells/mm^2, $p = 0.005$). Type 2 inflammation was increased in the airways post allergen, with elevated levels of eosinophils, interleukin-5 and eosinophil cationic protein.

Conclusions: Future clinical trials of novel kinase inhibitors could use the allergen challenge model in proof of concept studies, while employing these biomarkers to investigate pharmacological inhibition in the lungs.

Keywords: Allergens, Asthma, Bronchoscopy, Immunohistochemistry, JAK-STAT signalling, Kinase, p38 mitogen-activated protein kinase, Phosphoinositide 3-kinase

Background

Novel asthma treatments in early clinical development are often evaluated using the inhaled allergen challenge model [1], which enables rapid evaluation of the potential to suppress allergic inflammation before later phase studies focusing on clinical endpoints. The primary endpoint of allergen challenge studies is usually the fall in lung function caused by allergen inhalation, but biomarkers of lung inflammation can also be measured.

Intracellular kinase inhibition can potentially exert broad immunosuppressive effects on multiple cell types. Examples of kinases that have been considered as therapeutic targets in asthma are phosphoinositide 3-kinases (PI3K) delta and gamma, p38 mitogen-activated protein kinase (p38) and Janus kinase/Signal Transducer and Activator of Transcription (JAK/STAT) [2–4]. PI3Kδ and PI3Kγ are predominantly expressed in leukocytes and play a role in lymphocyte differentiation, activation, cell migration and reactive oxygen species production. In animal models of asthma, PI3K inhibition reduces inflammation and airway remodelling [5]. Furthermore, PI3Kδ expression is increased in the airways of asthma patients compared to controls [6]. p38

* Correspondence: tsouthworth@meu.org.uk
[1]Division of Infection, Immunity & Respiratory Medicine, The Medicines Evaluation Unit, The University of Manchester, Manchester Academic Health Science Centre, Manchester University NHS Foundation Trust, Manchester, UK
[3]The University of Manchester, 2nd Floor Education and Research Center, Wythenshawe Hospital, Southmoor Road, Manchester M23 9LT, UK

MAPK controls inflammatory gene transcription and translation [2] and is involved in the inflammatory responses of many different cell types to a wide range of stimuli [7–9]. In asthma patients the levels of p38 MAPK activity in the blood have been shown to increase with disease severity [10], while there is also evidence of increased alveolar macrophage and bronchial epithelial p38 MAPK activation in severe asthma [11, 12]. The JAK pathway is activated by pro-inflammatory cytokines leading to phosphorylation of STAT transcription factors [3]. JAK/STAT signalling is essential for lymphocyte differentiation and anti-viral mechanisms [13, 14]. Corticosteroids are currently the most commonly used anti-inflammatory treatment for asthma. However, in vitro studies, using human airway cells, have shown that JAK/STAT-dependent mechanisms are corticosteroid-insensitive [15, 16]. Animal models of allergic asthma show activation of PI3K, p38 MAPK and JAK/STAT pathways in the lungs [17, 18]. However, whether allergen exposure activates these pathways in humans with asthma has not been studied.

This study investigated the activation of PI3K, p38 MAPK and JAK/STAT signalling in lungs of asthma patients after allergen challenge; thus assessing the mechanistic involvement of these pathways during the human allergic response. As allergen challenge studies are often used during early clinical development of novel drugs, we also sought to identify biomarkers of PI3K, p38 MAPK and JAK/STAT activation in the lungs after allergen challenge.

Methods

Patients

Twelve steroid naïve atopic asthma patients were recruited; nine were male, with mean age of 45.5 and FEV_1% predicted of 86.2%. Patient demographics and clinical characteristics can be found in Table 1. All subjects demonstrated a positive skin prick test to either cat or house dust mite extract (Aquagen® SQ, ALK Laboratories, Cophenhagen, Denmark); showed methacholine hyperresponsiveness ($PC_{20} < 16$ pg/ml); and previously had shown both an early (from 0 to 2 h) and late (from 4 to 10 h) asthma response following allergen challenge, defined as a decrease in FEV_1 of > 20% and 15% respectively. Allergen challenges were performed using the Cockcroft method [19]. The study was approved by the local research ethics committee (Greater Manchester Central REC reference: 14/NW/0048) and subjects provided written informed consent.

Table 1 Individual Patient demographics, clinical characteristics and allergen challenge information

Number of patients	11
Age	45.5 (7.2)
Gender	Male 9 Female 2
Baseline FEV_1 (% predicted)	101.5 (12.3)
Baseline FeNO (ppb)	34.5 (20.6)
ACQ score	1.2 (0.6)
Methacholine PC_{20}	2.7 (2.2)
Allergen selected for challenge	HDM 9 CAT 2
Cumulative Allergen Concentration Administered (SQU/mL)	22,366.5 (27,672.3)
Maximum % fall in FEV_1 during EAR	29.2 (3.9)

Results shown as mean (sd)
Abbreviations: FEV_1 forced expiratory volume in 1 s, *FeNO* forced exhaled nitric oxide, *ppb* parts per billion, *ACQ* asthma control questionnaire, *PC_{20}* provocation concentration, *HDM* house dust mite, *EAR* early asthmatic response

Study design

Baseline induced sputum and bronchoscopy samples were collected. Induced sputum samples were processed to obtain supernatant for protein analysis and differential cell count cytospins [20]. Bronchoscopy was performed to collect bronchoalveolar lavage (BAL) fluid for protein analysis and bronchial biopsies for immunohistochemical analysis. Bronchial biopsies were collected from right or left lower lobes. At 6 weeks after the baseline bronchoscopy, an allergen challenge was performed. This time period was to allow for patient recovery following baseline bronchoscopy sample collection. Sputum induction and bronchoscopy were carried out at 4 and 6 h post-allergen challenge respectively; this impeded FEV_1 characterisation of the late asthma response.

Immunohistochemistry was used to assess bronchial biopsy expression of the following proteins in both the epithelium and sub-epithelium; phospho-Protein kinase B (pAKT) and phospho-Ribosomal Protein S6 (pRPS6) involved in PI3K signalling; p-p38 and phospho-Heat Shock Protein 27 (p-HSP27) involved in p38 MAPK signalling; and phospho-STATs 1, 3, 5 and 6.

Levels of IL-5 and eosinophil cationic protein (ECP) were assessed in sputum supernatants and bronchoalveolar lavage by MesoScaleDiscovery assay at SGS Cephac Europe, Saint Benoît Cedex, France. Sputum differential cell counts were assessed by Rapi-Diff stain [20].

Cockcroft allergen challenge

Allergen (Aquagen® SQ, ALK Laboratories, Cophenhagen, Denmark) inhalations using the tidal breathing method were performed with a deVilbiss nebuliser operated by air and at a flow rate to give an output of 0.13 ml/min. The subjects wore a nose-clip and aerosol was inhaled through a mouth-piece during tidal volume breathing (V_T). The starting concentration for the allergen was determined with results of the skin sensitivity test and the methacholine PC_{20} according to the formula published by Cockcroft et al., 1987. The starting concentration was 2 doubling doses less than predicted to cause a 20% fall in FEV_1 during the EAR. FEV_1 was measured twice, one minute apart, 10 min after the allergen was administered. If the FEV_1 fell by < 15%, the next dose of allergen was administered. If the FEV_1 fall was ≥ 15% and < 20%, FEV_1 measurements were performed at 15 mins post allergen to see if a ≥ 20% fall was achieved. When the FEV_1 fell by ≥ 20% or the highest dose of allergen was administered, the allergen challenge was discontinued and serial FEV_1 measurements were performed for 4 h before performing a sputum induction. An early asthmatic response (EAR – FEV_1 fall ≥ 20%) was assessed after 2 h.

Methacholine challenge

Methacholine challenges, using Methacholine chloride, Stockport Pharmaceuticals, Stockport, UK, were performed if the FEV_1 was ≥ 65% predicted. Subjects inhaled doubling concentrations of methacholine (0.03125 to 16 mg/ml) for 2 min at V_T with a nose clip, at 5 min intervals using the deVilbiss nebuliser until there was a fall in FEV_1 of ≥ 20%. FEV_1 was measured at 30 and 90 s intervals after each allergen administration and the highest value used for calculating FEV_1 fall. Initially, a diluent control was used. Subjects with a post-diluent decrease ≥ 10% did not continue to the methacholine challenge. The provocation concentration of methacholine required to cause a fall in FEV_1 of 20% (PC_{20}) was calculated from the dose response curve.

Serial skin prick test

The skin sensitivity test was performed to determine the allergen PC_{20} estimation for the tidal breathing challenge. Duplicate skin prick tests were performed with the fold dilutions of the same allergen (Aquagen® SQ, ALK Laboratories, Cophenhagen, Denmark) used for inhalation. The diameter of each wheal diameter was calculated from the average of the two. Cutaneous skin sensitivity was defined as the concentration producing a mean wheal diameter of 2 mm and was obtained from a plot of the log concentrations versus wheal size.

Sputum induction

Sputum samples were obtained at the start of the study (visit 1) and at 4 h post allergen challenge at visit 3. Sputum induction was performed after administration of 200-400 µg of Salbutamol. Increasing saline concentrations (3%, 4%, 5%) was given to the patient as 3 nebulisations (Flaem Nuova EasyNeb II, Milan, Italy) each lasting for 5 min. Spirometry (Micro-loop®, Carefusion, Basingstoke, UK) was performed prior to sputum induction and after each nebulisation cycle as a safety precaution to assess the effect of inhaled saline on FEV_1.

Sputum processing

Selected sputum was weighed, and samples greater than 0.05 g was mixed with eight volumes of phosphate buffered saline (PBS) before centrifugation. Supenatants were collected and stored at -80 °C until required for protein analysis. Remaining cells were mixed with 0.1% DTT for 15 min. Harvested cells were re-suspended in cold PBS so that a cell count could be performed using trypan blue to assess the number of viable cells. Cytopsin slides were prepared for differential count. Cytospin preparations were air dried, fixed with methanol and stained with Rapi-diff (Triangle, Skelmersdale, UK). Each reader scored 400 cells. This was used to determine the percentage of squamous cells as a measure of sputum quality. Samples with < 50% squamous cells were scored as acceptable. The results were expressed as a percentage of the total non-squamous count, and a total cell count/g of sputum.

Bronchoscopy and sample processing

Bronchoscopy was performed after the subjects had been sedated. BAL was collected from the right or left upper lobe. The bronchoscope was wedged in the bronchus and a maximum of 4 × 60 ml aliquots of pre-warmed sterile 0.9% saline solution were instilled. The aspirated fluid was stored on ice before filtration (100 µm filter, Becton Dickenson, Oxford, UK). The filtrate was centrifuged (400 *g*/10 min at 4 °C) and the BAL fluid was stored at -80 °C in 1 ml aliquots for biomarker analysis. The cell pellet resuspended in PBS and viable cell counts were determined by trypan blue exclusion (Neubauer hemocytometer), and the suspension adjusted to 0.5×10^6 BAL cells/ml. Cytospins for differential cell counts were made using 100ul of cell suspension. Bronchial biopsies were collected from the right or left lower lobes.

Immunohistochemistry

Bronchial biopsies were fixed overnight in 10% neutral buffered formalin (CellPath, Powys, UK), and embedded in paraffin wax (Surgipath, Milton Keynes, UK). 3 µm tissue sections were cut and lifted onto a polysine coated glass slides, before dewaxing in xylene and rehydrated with decreasing concentrations of alcohol. Following heat induced epitope retrieval (20 min in microwave at 800 W); tissues were stained overnight with primary antibody, before detection with biotinylated anti-rabbit IgG secondary antibody (Vector Laboratories, Peterborough, UK). Staining was visualised using avidin biotin peroxidase complex (Vector Laboratories). All sections were counterstained with Gill's II haematoxylin (Leica, Milton Keynes, UK). Quantification was performed using the ImagePro Plus 6.0 software. All antibodies were purchased from Cell Signalling Technology, Davers, USA, except for pSTAT6 (Life Technology, Paisley, UK): pAKT product #9271; pRPS6 product #5364; p-p38 product #9211; p-HSP27 product #2401; phospho-STAT 1, 3, 5 and 6 product codes 9167, 9145, 9359 and 700,247, respectively. Sub-epithelial cell counts for neutrophils (neutrophil elastase), eosinophils (Luna stain), $CD4^+$ and $CD8^+$ cells were performed as previously described [21]. Positive staining was confirmed

Cell Type	CD4	CD8	Eosinophil	Neutrophil
Baseline	76.6 (39.0)	117.8 (83.6)	4.1 (8.2)	1.7 (3.3)
Post-Allergen	95.8 (64.7)	130.6 (102.0)	5.1 (4.7)	1.5 (2.2)
p	0.48	0.69	0.75	0.85
Representative image	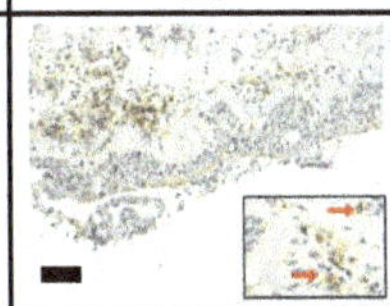	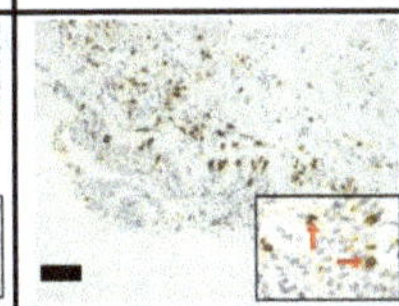	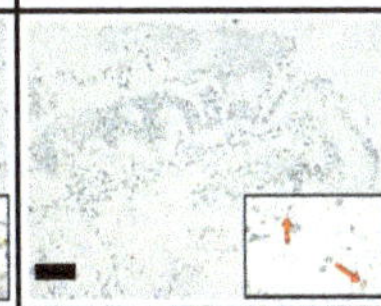	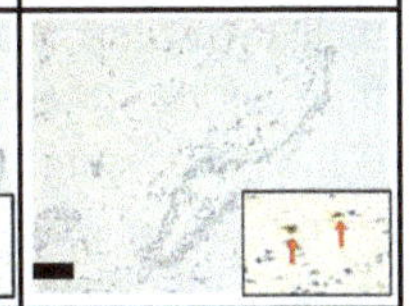
Negative control image	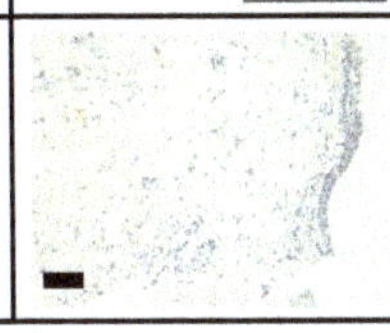	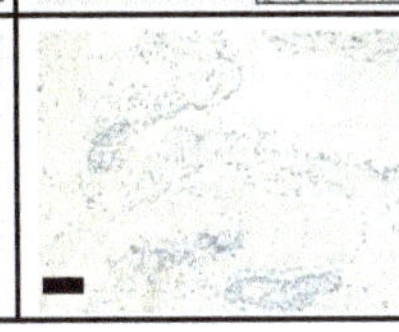	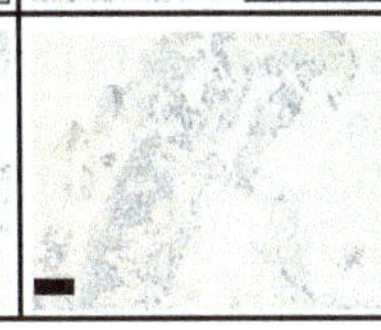	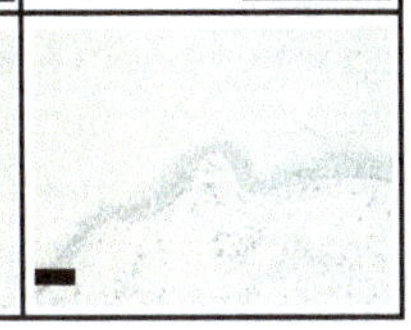

Fig. 1 Inflammatory cell counts in sub-epithelial bronchial tissue at baseline and post-allergen ($n = 11$). Bronchial biopsies were collected from 11 asthma patients at baseline and 6 h post allergen challenge, with CD4, CD8 and neutrophil numbers being assessed by immunohistochemistry and eosinophils with Luna staining. Data presented as mean (sd). Comparisons between Baseline and Post-allergen by paired T-test. Images of staining are at × 200 magnification; Black bars represent 100 μm. Magnified images and red arrows illustrate positive staining. Negative control images represent isotype controls results for CD4, CD8 and neutrophil elastase, and non-Luna staining for eosinophils

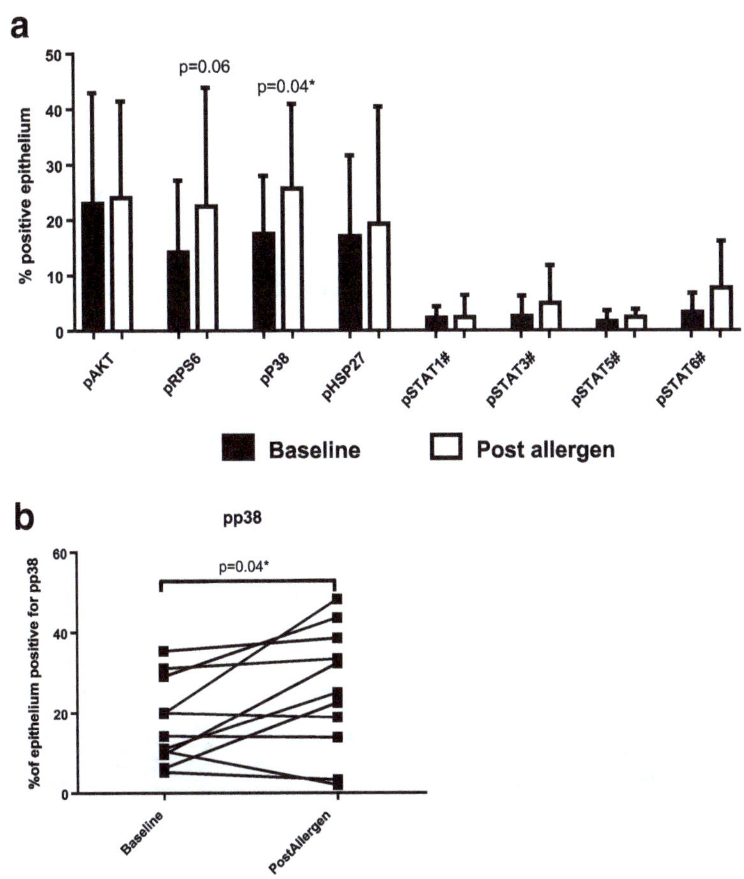

Fig. 2 Levels of PI3K, p38 and JAK/STAT markers in bronchial epithelium at baseline and post allergen ($n = 11$): Bronchial biopsies were collected from 11 asthma patients at baseline and 6 h post allergen challenge, with protein expression analysed in the epithelium (**a**) by immunohistochemistry. Data presented as mean values with standard deviation. Individual patient's data for the statistically significant changes in pp38 are shown in (**b**). Comparisons between baseline and post allergen were by paired T-tests or Wilcoxon tests (#), as appropriate $^*p < 0.05$

by use of two negative controls: (i) exclusion of primary antibody and (ii) use of isotype control antibody.

Differential cell count

Sputum and BAL cell cytospins were fixed in methanol for 10 min and left to air dry, before being stained with Rapi-Diff (GCC Diagnostics) using the following method: (1) stain slide for 2 min in solution A; (2) wash slide in distilled water; (3) stain slide for 2 min in solution B; (4) wash slide under tap water. Slides are then mounted using DPX and cover slipped. 400 non-squamous cells were counted per slide. Neutrophils, macrophages, eosinophils, lymphocytes and bronchial epithelial cells differentiated based on morphology and staining.

Statistical analysis

Data distribution was assessed by Kolmogorov-Smirnov test. Data with non-parametric distribution are highlighted in figures with an asterisk. Changes in cell counts and protein levels pre- and post-allergen challenge were analysed by two-sided paired T-tests or Wilcoxon tests, where appropriate. All analysis was carried out using Prism 7.0. software (Graphpad, La Jolla, California, USA). A *p*-value of less than 0.05 was deemed significant.

Results

One subject was withdrawn after not tolerating the baseline bronchoscopy, with 11 completing the study. All subjects demonstrated an early asthma response with a fall in FEV_1 of > 20% within 20 min of allergen inhalation, with a mean maximum fall of 29.2%.

Paired baseline and post-allergen sputum samples were successfully collected from 10 of the 11 patients. Allergen challenge increased sputum eosinophil percentage (from mean 1.1% to 3.8%; $p = 0.019$) and cell count (from median 0.01 to 0.12×10^6 cells/g sputum;

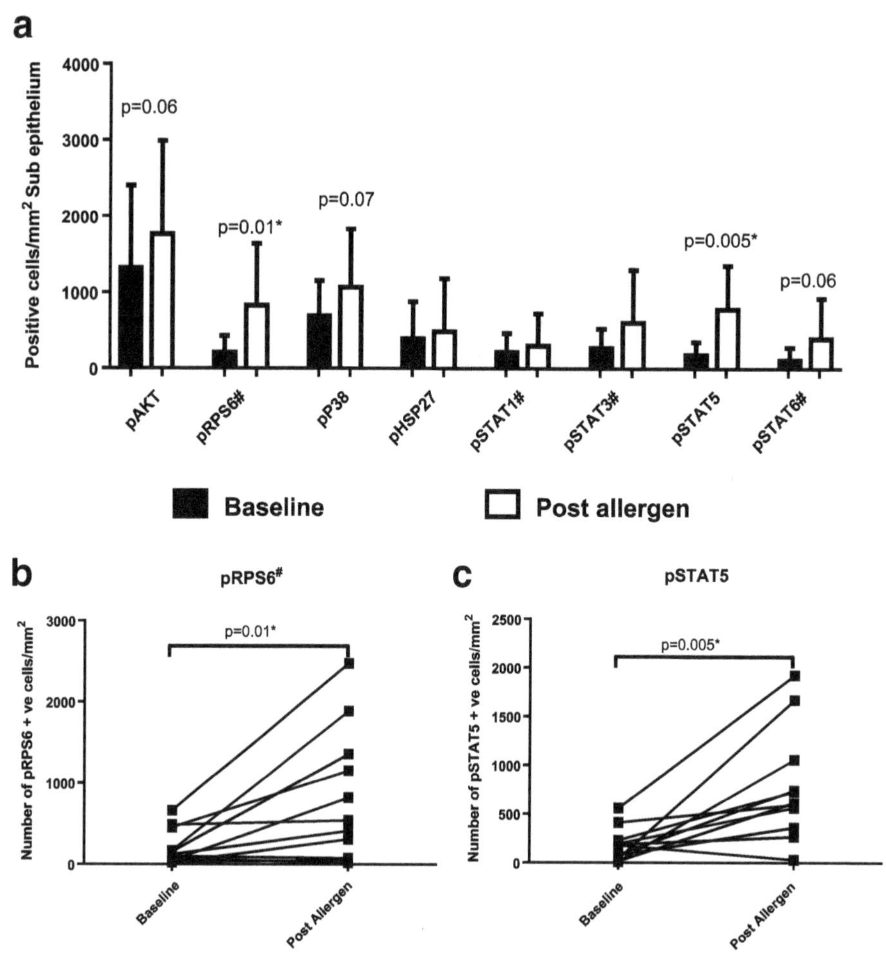

Fig. 3 Levels of PI3K, p38 and JAK/STAT markers in bronchial subepithelium at baseline and post allergen ($n = 11$): Bronchial biopsies were collected from 11 asthma patients at baseline and 6 h post allergen challenge, with protein expression analysed in the epithelium (**a**) by immunohistochemistry. Data presented as mean values with standard deviation. Individual patient's data for the statistically significant changes in pRPS6 and pSTAT5 are shown in (**b**) and (**c**), respectively. Comparisons between baseline and post allergen were by paired T-tests or Wilcoxon tests (#), as appropriate $^*p < 0.05$

$p = 0.008$). Neutrophil percentage and cell counts also increased (from mean 37.9 to 63.4%, $p = 0.004$, and from 0.8 to 2.0×10^6 median neutrophils/g sputum: $p = 0.05$). The macrophage percentage decreased (from mean 49.9 to 28.6%, $p = 0.02$) after allergen challenge. There were no changes in sputum lymphocyte or epithelial cell numbers.

Type 2 inflammation was increased by allergen challenge; sputum supernatant ECP (57 vs 169 ng/ml; $p = 0.049$) and IL-5 (0.9 vs 19.9 pg/ml; $p = 0.016$) levels were higher after allergen challenge. BAL ECP levels were increased by allergen challenge (1.9 vs 3.2 ng/ml; $p = 0.014$). The higher levels measured in sputum supernatant was probably due to the know dilution effect of BAL, but the median fold change in ECP was similar in sputum supernatant and BAL (2.7-fold and 2.0-fold, respectively). Levels of IL-5 in BAL were undetectable, both at baseline and post allergen. Allergen exposure had no effect on neutrophil, macrophage, eosinophil and lymphocyte cell numbers in bronchial tissue (Fig. 1).

In bronchial epithelium there was a significant increase in the percentage of cells expressing p-p38 post-allergen (p = 0.04; Fig. 2). The percentage of pRPS6 positive epithelial cells was also increased, but this did not reach significance ($p = 0.06$). Numbers of sub-epithelial cells expressing pRPS6 and pSTAT5 were increased post-allergen ($p = 0.01$ and $p = 0.005$ respectively, Fig. 3). Numbers of pAKT, p-p38 and pSTAT6 positive sub-epithelial cells were also increased, but these did not reach significance ($p = 0.06$, $p = 0.07$ and $p = 0.06$ respectively). Other proteins analysed in epithelium (pHSP27, pAKT, pSTATs 1, 3, 5 and 6) or sub-epithelium (pHSP27, pSTATs 1 and 3) by immunohistochemistry did not show any change after allergen challenge. Representative images of bronchial tissue staining are shown in Fig. 4.

Discussion

There was an increase in p-p38 MAPK expression in the bronchial epithelia after allergen challenge, while in the sub-epithelium there was evidence of PI3K activation (pRPS6) and JAK/STAT activation (pSTAT5). These observations support involvement of these kinase pathways in the allergic response, but with different roles in the epithelium compared to the sub-epithelium.

Phospho-p38 MAPK expression is increased in the bronchial epithelium of patients with severe asthma [12, 22]. We now show p38 MAPK activation at the same anatomical location after allergen challenge. Overall, these findings suggest that epithelial p38 MAPK activation contributes to the inflammatory cascade in asthma caused by environmental triggers, such as allergen exposure. In vitro studies using human bronchial epithelial cells have shown that the house dust mite antigen, DerP1, induces p38-dependent cell apoptosis and intracellular oxidative stress [5], while in mice p38 is essential for allergen induced epithelial production of IL-25 and thymic stromal lymphopoietin (TSLP), which are both initiators of the Type-2 allergic response in asthma [10].

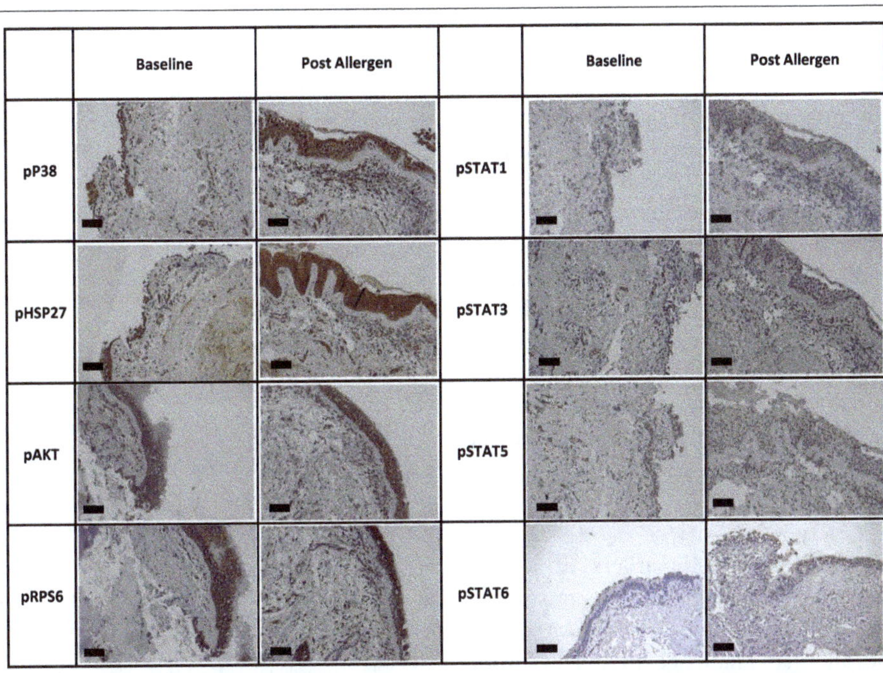

Fig. 4 Representative images of cell signalling markers in bronchial biopsy tissue. Bronchial tissue collect pre and post allergen challenge were stained by immunohistochemistry for phosphorylated cell signalling proteins. All representative images are from the same patient. Black bars represent 100 μm

There is evidence that PI3K activation is increased in severe asthma [23]. PI3Kδ has a central role in T-cell activation [4]. The allergic response involves T-helper 2 cell activation, suggesting that PI3K activation could occur after allergen challenge. RPS6 is a terminal signalling protein of the PI3K/AKT/mTOR pathway, involved in protein synthesis and cell cycle progression [24]. Increased pRPS6 levels in the sub-epithelium suggest PI3K activation by allergen challenge, perhaps due to increased T-cell activity [25], although we did not specifically evaluate this.

Increased pSTAT5 expression suggests JAK/STAT pathway involvement in sub-epithelial leukocyte activation after allergen challenge. In murine lungs, STAT5 in dendritic cells is essential for TSLP-induced Th2 responses following allergen exposure [26], while STAT5 is also involved in mast cell functions, such as expression of the high affinity IgE receptor [27]. Other STAT proteins did not display changes that reached statistical significance.

The increased sub-epithelial expression of pSTAT5 and pRPS6 after allergen challenge was not due to an increase in cell numbers, as there were no increases in sub-epithelial leukocyte numbers. There are inconsistent reports of changes in leukocyte numbers in the bronchial mucosa after allergen challenge, probably due in part to differences in the time-point of sampling [28, 29]. This contrasts with the increase in luminal eosinophilic inflammation after allergen challenge, which we and others have observed [30]. Although we used a limited sample size, it was sufficiently large to observe the expected upregulation of airway luminal eosinophilic inflammation, evidenced by increased eosinophil numbers as well as IL-5 and ECP levels [31].

The expression of protein phosphorylation can be very transient e.g. pAKT expression can be short-lived in contrast to pRPS6 expression [32]. This may explain why we did not observe positive results for all the biomarkers within a kinase pathway e.g. pRPS6 expression, but not pAKT, in the sub-epithelium. We were limited in the quantity of tissue available to perform validation experiments using a different technique, such as Western blotting. Nevertheless, our results demonstrate biomarkers within these kinase pathways that show the most promise for application during the study of allergic responses in human lungs.

Conclusions

This study presents candidate biomarkers of kinase activation during the asthmatic allergic response. Future clinical trials of novel kinase inhibitors could consider using the allergen challenge model in proof of concept studies, while employing these biomarkers to understand the pharmacological effects of kinase inhibition in the lungs.

Abbreviations

ACQ: Asthma control questionnaire; BAL: Bronchoalveolar lavage; DTT: Dithiothreitol; EAR: Early asthma response; ECP: Eosinophil cationic protein; FEV_1: forced expiratory volume in one second; Ig: Immunoglobulin; IL: Interleukin; JAK: Janus Kinase pAKTphosphorylated AKT; PBS: Phosphate buffered saline; PC_{20}: provocation concentration producing a 20% fall in FEV_1; pHSP27: phosphorylated heat shock protein 27; PI3K: Phosphoinositide 3-kinase.; p-p38 MAPK: phosphorylated p38 mitogen-activated protein kinase; pRPS6: phosphorylated ribosomal protein S6; pSTAT: phosphorylated Signal Transducer and Activator of Transcription; TSLP: Thymic stromal lymphopoietin; V_T: Tidal volume breathing

Acknowledgements

This report is independent research supported by National Institute for Health Research South Manchester Respiratory and Allergy Clinical Research Facility at Manchester University NHS Foundation Trust. The views expressed in this publication are those of the author(s) and not necessarily those of the NHS, the National Institute for Health Research or the Department of Health. In addition we would like to thank all study participants for their contribution.

Funding

The authors would like to acknowledge the North West Lung Centre Charity, Manchester, UK and Almirall, S.A, Barcelona, Spain, for financially supporting this project.

Authors' contributions

TS, AB, IR, MC, MM and DS all made substantial contributions to the conception and design of the study. TS, SM, AB, AD and NP were involved in the acquisition of data. All authors were involved in the analysis and interpretation of the results. TS drafted the article, with all other authors revising it critically for important intellectual content. All authors approved the final version of the manuscript prior to submission.

Competing interests

DS has received sponsorship to attend international meetings, honoraria for lecturing or attending advisory boards and research grants from various pharmaceutical companies including Almirall, AstraZeneca, Boehringer Ingelheim, Chiesi, Genentech, GlaxoSmithKline, Glenmark, Johnson and Johnson, Merck, NAPP, Novartis, Pfizer, Skypharma, Takeda, Teva, Therevance and Verona. IR, MC, AD, NP and MM are employees of Almirall S. A. TS, SM and AB declare that they have no competing interests.

Author details

[1]Division of Infection, Immunity & Respiratory Medicine, The Medicines Evaluation Unit, The University of Manchester, Manchester Academic Health Science Centre, Manchester University NHS Foundation Trust, Manchester, UK. [2]Almirall R&D Center, Sant Feliu de Llobregat, Barcelona, Spain. [3]The University of Manchester, 2nd Floor Education and Research Center, Wythenshawe Hospital, Southmoor Road, Manchester M23 9LT, UK.

References

1. Singh D, Leaker B, Boyce M, Nandeuil MA, Collarini S, Mariotti F, Santoro D, Barnes PJ. A novel inhaled phosphodiesterase 4 inhibitor (CHF6001) reduces the allergen challenge response in asthmatic patients. Pulm Pharmacol Ther. 2016;40:1–6.
2. Khorasanizadeh M, Eskian M, Gelfand EW, Rezaei N. Mitogen-activated protein kinases as therapeutic targets for asthma. Pharmacol Ther. 2017;174: 112–26.
3. Vale K. Targeting the JAK-STAT pathway in the treatment of 'Th2-high' severe asthma. Future Med Chem. 2016;8(4):405–19.
4. Yoo EJ, Ojiaku CA, Sunder K, Panettieri RA Jr. Phosphoinositide 3-kinase in asthma: novel roles and therapeutic approaches. Am J Respir Cell Mol Biol. 2016;56(6):700-7.

5. Lin CH, Hong YC, Kao SH. Aeroallergen Der p 2 induces apoptosis of bronchial epithelial BEAS-2B cells via activation of both intrinsic and extrinsic pathway. Cell & bioscience. 2015;5:71.
6. Southworth T, Plumb J, Gupta V, Pearson J, Ramis I, Lehner MD, Miralpeix M, Singh D. Anti-inflammatory potential of PI3Kdelta and JAK inhibitors in asthma patients. Respir Res. 2016;17(1):124.
7. Brusselle GG, Maes T, Bracke KR. Eosinophils in the spotlight: eosinophilic airway inflammation in nonallergic asthma. Nat Med. 2013;19(8):977–9.
8. Cosmi L, Liotta F, Annunziato F. Th17 regulating lower airway disease. Curr Opin Allergy Clin Immunol. 2016;16(1):1–6.
9. Aalbers R, Vogelmeier C, Kuna P. Achieving asthma control with ICS/LABA: a review of strategies for asthma management and prevention. Respir Med. 2016;111:1–7.
10. Yu HS, Angkasekwinai P, Chang SH, Chung Y, Dong C. Protease allergens induce the expression of IL-25 via Erk and p38 MAPK pathway. J Korean Med Sci. 2010;25(6):829–34.
11. Bhavsar P, Hew M, Khorasani N, Torrego A, Barnes PJ, Adcock I, Chung KF. Relative corticosteroid insensitivity of alveolar macrophages in severe asthma compared with non-severe asthma. Thorax. 2008;63(9):784–90.
12. Liu W, Liang Q, Balzar S, Wenzel S, Gorska M, Alam R. Cell-specific activation profile of extracellular signal-regulated kinase 1/2, Jun N-terminal kinase, and p38 mitogen-activated protein kinases in asthmatic airways. J Allergy Clin Immunol. 2008;121(4):893–902. e892
13. Ross JA, Nagy ZS, Cheng H, Stepkowski SM, Kirken RA. Regulation of T cell homeostasis by JAKs and STATs. Arch Immunol Ther Exp. 2007;55(4):231–45.
14. Medrek SK, Parulekar AD, Hanania NA. Predictive biomarkers for asthma therapy. Curr Allergy Asthma Rep. 2017;17(10):69.
15. Southworth T, Metryka A, Lea S, Farrow S, Plumb J, Singh D. IFN-gamma synergistically enhances LPS signalling in alveolar macrophages from COPD patients and controls by corticosteroid-resistant STAT1 activation. Br J Pharmacol. 2012;166(7):2070–83.
16. Peters SP. Asthma phenotypes: nonallergic (intrinsic) asthma. J Allergy Clin Immunol Pract. 2014;2(6):650–2.
17. Dhawale VS, Amara VR, Karpe PA, Malek V, Patel D, Tikoo K. Activation of angiotensin-converting enzyme 2 (ACE2) attenuates allergic airway inflammation in rat asthma model. Toxicol Appl Pharmacol. 2016;306:17–26.
18. Ashino S, Takeda K, Li H, Taylor V, Joetham A, Pine PR, Gelfand EW. Janus kinase 1/3 signaling pathways are key initiators of TH2 differentiation and lung allergic responses. J Allergy Clin Immunol. 2014;133(4):1162–74.
19. Cockcroft DW, Davis BE, Boulet LP, Deschesnes F, Gauvreau GM, O'Byrne PM, Watson RM. The links between allergen skin test sensitivity, airway responsiveness and airway response to allergen. Allergy. 2005;60(1):56–9.
20. Lee WY, Southworth T, Singh D. Different inhaled allergen challenge models give reproducible results. Pulm Pharmacol Ther. 2015;33:57–8.
21. Kolsum U, Ravi A, Hitchen P, Maddi S, Southworth T, Singh D. Clinical characteristics of eosinophilic COPD versus COPD patients with a history of asthma. Respir Res. 2017;18(1):73.
22. Hackett TL, Singhera GK, Shaheen F, Hayden P, Jackson GR, Hegele RG, Van Eeden S, Bai TR, Dorscheid DR, Knight DA. Intrinsic phenotypic differences of asthmatic epithelium and its inflammatory responses to respiratory syncytial virus and air pollution. Am J Respir Cell Mol Biol. 2011;45(5):1090–100.
23. Alliouachene S, Bilanges B, Chicanne G, Anderson KE, Pearce W, Ali K, Valet C, Posor Y, Low PC, Chaussade C, et al. Inactivation of the class II PI3K-C2beta potentiates insulin signaling and sensitivity. Cell Rep. 2015;13(9):1881–94.
24. Meyuhas O. Ribosomal protein S6 phosphorylation: four decades of research. Int Rev Cell Mol Biol. 2015;320:41–73.
25. Khan A, Southworth T, Worsley S, Sriskantharajah S, Amour A, Hessel EM, Singh D. An investigation of the anti-inflammatory effects and a potential biomarker of PI3Kdelta inhibition in COPD T cells. Clin Exp Pharmacol Physiol. 2017;44(9):932–40.
26. Bell BD, Kitajima M, Larson RP, Stoklasek TA, Dang K, Sakamoto K, Wagner KU, Kaplan DH, Reizis B, Hennighausen L, et al. The transcription factor STAT5 is critical in dendritic cells for the development of TH2 but not TH1 responses. Nat Immunol. 2013;14(4):364–71.
27. Li Y, Qi X, Liu B, Huang H. The STAT5-GATA2 pathway is critical in basophil and mast cell differentiation and maintenance. J Immunol. 2015;194(9): 4328–38.
28. Ricciardolo FL, Di Stefano A, Silvestri M, Van Schadewijk AM, Malerba M, Hiemstra PS, Sterk PJ. Exhaled nitric oxide is related to bronchial eosinophilia and airway hyperresponsiveness to bradykinin in allergen-induced asthma exacerbation. Int J Immunopathol Pharmacol. 2012;25(1):175–82.
29. Ravensberg AJ, Ricciardolo FL, van Schadewijk A, Rabe KF, Sterk PJ, Hiemstra PS, Mauad T. Eotaxin-2 and eotaxin-3 expression is associated with persistent eosinophilic bronchial inflammation in patients with asthma after allergen challenge. J Allergy Clin Immunol. 2005;115(4):779–85.
30. Boomer JS, Parulekar AD, Patterson BM, Yin-Declue H, Deppong CM, Crockford S, Jarjour NN, Castro M, Green JM. A detailed phenotypic analysis of immune cell populations in the bronchoalveolar lavage fluid of atopic asthmatics after segmental allergen challenge. Allergy, asthma, clin immunol : offi j Cana Soc Allergy Clin Immunol. 2013;9(1):37.
31. Zissler UM, Esser-von Bieren J, Jakwerth CA, Chaker AM, Schmidt-Weber CB. Current and future biomarkers in allergic asthma. Allergy. 2016;71(4):475–94.
32. Kubota H, Noguchi R, Toyoshima Y, Ozaki Y, Uda S, Watanabe K, Ogawa W, Kuroda S. Temporal coding of insulin action through multiplexing of the AKT pathway. Mol Cell. 2012;46(6):820–32.

21

microRNA based prognostic biomarkers in pancreatic Cancer

Shixiang Guo[1,2], Andrew Fesler[1], Huaizhi Wang[2] and Jingfang Ju[1*]

Abstract: Despite tremendous research efforts focused on diagnosis and treatment, pancreatic ductal adenocarcinoma remains the third leading cause of cancer-related death in the United States, with a 5-year overall survival rate of less than 5%. Although resistance is rather complex, emerging evidence has demonstrated that epigenetic alterations (e.g. miRNA) have important roles in PDAC progression as well as resistance to therapy. Certain miRNAs have been identified as potential prognostic biomarkers in PDAC. In this review, we summarize the recent developments in miRNA research related to PDAC therapeutic resistance mechanisms and the potential of miRNAs as prognostic biomarkers for future clinical management of PDAC.

Keywords: Pancreatic ductal adenocarcinoma, miRNA, Biomarkers, Resistance, Prognosis, Chemotherapy, Gemcitabine

Background

Pancreatic ductal adenocarcinoma (PDAC) is the third deadliest cancer in the United States [1]. It is characterized by late clinical presentation, early metastasis and poor prognosis [2]. A large proportion of patients are diagnosed with locally advanced or metastatic disease at the time of presentation [3]. Current therapy for PDAC mainly involves surgical resection, adjuvant chemotherapy and radiotherapy [4]. Despite the advancement in clinical management (e.g. Abraxane), patient outcomes remain unsatisfactory [5, 6].

In addition to patients presenting with advanced disease, many patients also experience early appearance of post-operative recurrence [7]. Therefore, adjuvant treatments (chemotherapy, radiotherapy etc.) are necessary and critical for management of patients with advanced disease. However, few effective chemotherapeutic options exist for advanced PDAC patients in the clinic. Since 1997, gemcitabine has been approved as the standard first-line chemotherapeutic, several novel therapeutic regimens based on gemcitabine have also been investigated for PDAC treatment [8]. Multiple agents have been assessed in combination with gemcitabine including 5-fluorouracil, oxaliplatin, cisplatin and capecitabine [9–12]. However, the impact on patient survival is rather limited. Such failure is caused, at least in part, by chemoresistance. Chemoresistance is mainly classified into intrinsic and acquired resistance. Compared with intrinsic resistance where therapy is ineffective from the start of treatment, acquired resistance with continuous chemotherapy ultimately causes relapse and metastasis [13]. Over the past decade extensive research efforts have been dedicated to investigate the underlying mechanisms of chemoresistance. Resistance involves PDAC stem cells which have unique characteristics including enhanced epithelial–mesenchymal transition (EMT), autophagy, and altered metabolism that contributes to their plastic nature and chemoresistant phenotype. Altered expression of many different genes (e.g. KRAS, TP53, CCND1, BCL-2, BIRC5) and changes in key signaling pathways (e.g. Notch, PI3K/AKT, NF-κB, Hedgehog, cell cycle, apoptosis) also contribute to resistance [13–16]. Clearly there is an urgent need to develop early detection and/or novel prognostic biomarkers to help better manage PDAC treatment to maximize survival benefits and to avoid toxicity.

Epigenetic regulations mediated by miRNAs in PDAC resistance mechanism

Based on a large body of growing evidence, we know PDAC resistance is regulated, at least in part, by epigenetic alterations including miRNA. miRNAs are small non-coding RNAs 18–22 nucleotides in length that have

* Correspondence: jingfang.ju@stonybrookmedicine.edu
[1]Stony Brook University, Stony Brook, New York 11794, USA
Full list of author information is available at the end of the article

been identified to be associated with tumorigenesis, cell cycle control, apoptosis, proliferation, chemoresistance, invasion and metastasis [17]. In PDAC, miRNAs have been demonstrated to modulate key targets and pathways such as KRAS, TP53, PI3K/AKT, NF-κB and Hedgehog signaling, and their aberrant expression is associated with chemoresistance (14). It has been shown that miR-17-92 cluster counteracts quiescence and chemoresistance in a distinct subpopulation of pancreatic cancer stem cells by acting through the NODAL/ACTIVIN/TGF-β1 signaling cascade [18]. A number of important miRNAs in PDAC are listed in Table 1.

In terms of resistance of PDAC to chemotherapeutic treatment, miR-21 is one of the most investigated oncogenic miRNAs related to gemcitabine resistance. Elevated expression of miR-21 inhibits the anti-tumor activity of gemcitabine, and is significantly associated with shorter survival time [19]. Giovannetti et al. suggests that miR-21 contributes to gemcitabine chemoresistance by inhibiting tumor suppressor gene phosphatase and tensin homologue (PTEN), thereby activating the PI3K/AKT pathway [20]. Park et al. illustrated that silencing miR-21 leads to cell cycle arrest (G1 phase) and induction of apoptosis by up-regulating PTEN [21]. Hwang et al. showed that down-regulation of miR-21 expression correlates with prolong overall survival and benefit from chemotherapeutic treatment [22]. In addition to miR-21, several other miRNAs (miR-34, miR-217, miR-96, miR-145) have been shown to be deregulated and impact the PI3K/AKT pathway in PDAC [14]. EMT/ mesenchymal-epithelial transition (MET) has been shown to be critical in chemoresistance of PDAC and is mediated by key miRNAs. Emerging evidence confirms that the miR-200 family plays a key role in chemoresistance via reversing EMT. Ali et al. reported that down-regulation of miR-21 and restoration of miR-200b and miR-200c inactivates pAKT by reactivation of PTEN and reverses EMT, resulted in enhanced gemcitabine sensitivity [19]. Furthermore, Li et al. show that miR-200b, miR-200c, let-7 family (let-7b, let-7c, let-7d, let-7e) are down-regulated in gemcitabine-resistant PDAC cells. Restoration of miR-200 and let-7 results in a reversal of PDAC from EMT to MET and sensitivity to gemcitabine treatment [23].

Previous studies have demonstrated that the miR-34 family (miR-34a, b and c) is associated with p53 and p38-MAPK pathways in response to DNA damage [24]. Down-regulation of miR-34 is responsible for progression of various malignancies including PDAC, lung, breast, prostate and liver cancer [25]. miR-34 has an anti-cancer role via modulating targets implicated in apoptosis, cell cycle, and DNA repair, such as NOTCH, BCL2, VEGFA, CCND1 and CDK6 [26]. In regards to PDAC resistance, Ji et al. reported that miR-34 is regulated by p53, and inhibits target genes NOTCH and BCL-2. Loss of miR-34 leads to the enrichment of cancer stem cells or tumor-initiating cells and restoration of miR-34 inhibits PDAC cell growth and enhanced chemotherapeutic sensitivity to gemcitabine [27].

Table 1 Critical miRNAs as potential diagnostic, therapeutic, prognostic targets in PDAC

miRNAs	Function	Expression in tumor	Targets	Pathway	Ref.
miR-21	Oncogenic	Up-regulated	PTEN, PDCD4, CDK6, CDKN1A, IL-6R, FAS, TPM1, APAF1, SOCS5	PI3K/AKT	[20–22]
miR-34	Tumor suppressor	Down-regulated	NOTCH, BCL2, VEGFA, CCND1, CDK6	p53/p38-MAPK/NOTCH PI3K/AKT	[14, 24, 26]
miR-200 family	Tumor suppressor	Down-regulated	E-cadherin, ZEB, Vimentin	NOTCH, EMT	[14, 20, 23]
Let-7 family	Tumor suppressor	Down-regulated	KRAS, HRAS, LIN28, HMGA2, NF2, TRIM71	EMT, KRAS	[16]
miR-15a	Tumor suppressor	Down-regulated	WANT3A, FGF7, BMI-1	ERK/AKT, EMT	[28, 29]
miR-506	Tumor suppressor	Down-regulated	SPHK1, PI3M	SPHK1/AKT/NF-κB	[31, 32]
miR-221	Oncogenic	Up-regulated	KIT, CDKN1C, CDKN1B	EMT, PKC/NF-κB, PTEN/PI3K/AKT	[14, 21]
miR-96	Tumor suppressor	Down-regulated	KRAS, AKT	KRAS, PI3K/AKT	[14, 15]
miR-17-92	Tumor suppressor	Down-regulated	p21, p57, TBX3	NODAL/ACTIVIN/TGF-1	[18]
miR-145	Tumor suppressor	Down-regulated	KRAS, RREB1	KRAS, PI3K/AKT	[14]
miR-155	Oncogenic	Up-Regulated	TP53INP	Apoptosis, Exosome Synthesis	[30]

Zhang et al. suggested that miR-214 enhances chemoresistance to gemcitabine by down-regulating the tumor suppressor gene ING4, while miR-15a can suppress the growth of chemoresistant PDAC cells via targeting WNT3A and FGF7, contributing to progression and proliferation through the phosphorylation of the kinases ERK and AKT [28]. Moreover, Guo et al. indicated that miR-15a inhibits cell proliferation and EMT by down-regulating BMI-1 in PDAC [29].

miR-155 expression has been shown to induce gemcitabine resistance. Prolonged exposure to gemcitabine leads to increased miR-155 expression, which inhibits apoptosis and increases exosome production, resulting in gemcitabine resistance [30]. Li et al. reported that miR-506 can inhibit cell proliferation, induce cell cycle arrest, promote apoptosis and enhance chemosensitivity to gemcitabine in PDAC by regulating the SPHK1/AKT/NF-κB signaling pathway [31]. Meanwhile, Du et al. revealed that miR-506 represses PDAC cell proliferation by targeting PIM3, a member of oncogenic PIM family [32]. Based on these studies, it appears that miR-506 plays a tumor suppressor role in PDAC. The functions of several miRNAs in PDAC are shown in Fig. 1.

miRNAs as prognostic biomarkers

Based on the poor prognosis of PDAC, the development of early detection methods, more effective treatment options and better prognostic biomarkers are of critical significance. Besides the significance of miRNAs for early detection and diagnosis, accumulating evidence suggests that miRNAs have great potential as prognostic biomarkers [33, 34]. Dillhoff et al. showed that 79% of PDAC patients with miR-21 high expression have poor outcomes [35]. Bloomston et al. found that six miRNAs (miR-30a-3p, miR-105, miR-127, miR-187, miR-452, and miR-518a-2) are predictive of better prognosis (survival time beyond 2 years) in PDAC patients [36]. One recent study found that over-expression of miR-212 and miR-675 and down-regulation of miR-148a, miR-187, and let-7 g were independent predictors of worse prognosis in PDAC patients [37]. miR-142-5p and miR-204 are found to be down-regulated in chemoresistant PDAC cells, and high expression of these miRNAS in PDAC patients associates with better overall survival [38]. One study has concluded that miR-155, miR-203, miR-210, miR-222, miR-200c and miR-302 are associated with PDAC patients' outcome [39]. In our previous studies, we found that low expression of miR-506 was an independent predictor of poor prognosis in PDAC, while miR-15a is significantly related with prognosis of PDAC patients [29, 31]. Collectively, these studies support the potential role of miRNAs as prognostic biomarkers for PDAC.

Other class of noncoding RNAs in PDAC resistance and prognosis

Beyond miRNA, other types of noncoding RNAs (e.g. lncRNA, circRNA) have also been implicated in cancer resistance and prognosis [40–42]. It has been reported that elevated HOTAIR expression is significantly associated with poor prognosis of PDAC patients. HOTAIR

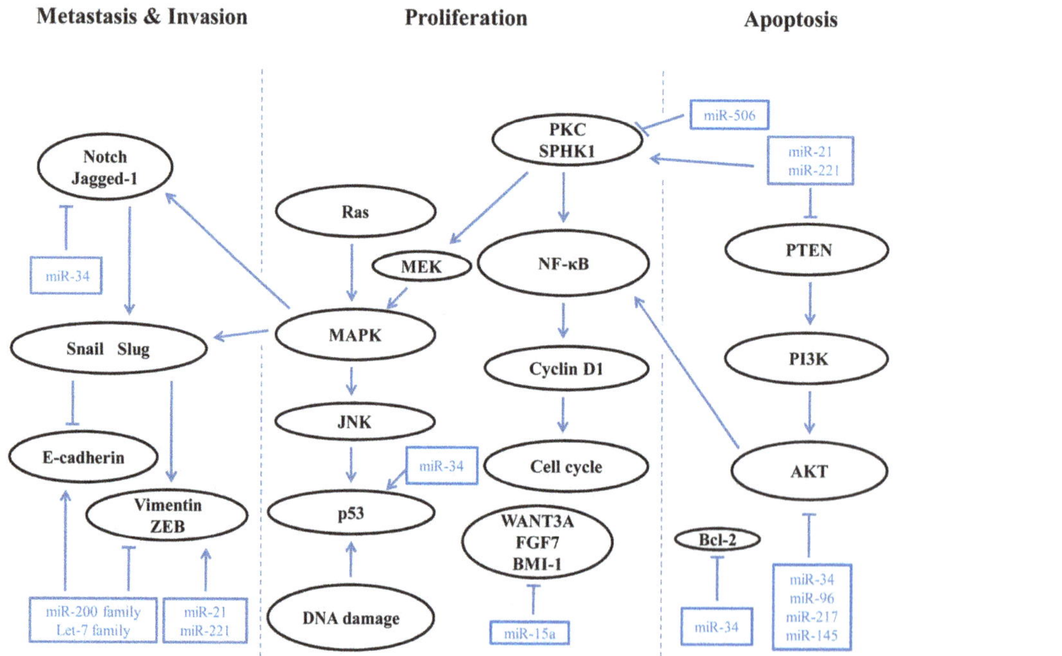

Fig. 1 Schematic illustration of miRNAs that are important in PDAC through regulation key targets and signaling pathways

has oncogenic activity by suppressing a number of interferon-related genes and genes related to cell cycle control [43]. Huang et al. recently reported that circular RNA, hsa_circ_0000977, is upregulated in PDAC. Inhibition of hsa_circ_0000977 suppresses PDAC cell proliferation and induces cell cycle arrest. Hsa_circ_0000977 interferes with hsa-miR-874-3p and increases Polo like kinase 1 (PLK1) expression [44]. It is conceivable that we are still at the early stage of exploring other types of noncoding RNAs in PDAC and there will be more exciting discoveries in the future.

Conclusions

It is clear that PDAC utilizes a variety of mechanisms to maintain a highly resistant phenotype. The highly plastic nature of PDAC resistance is mediated by genetic and epigenetic alterations. The epigenetic controls such as miRNAs allow cells to quickly adapt to the genotoxic stress environment caused by chemotherapy. miRNAs can quickly modulate mRNA translation in PDAC cells in response to chemotherapeutic treatment. As a result, a number of miRNAs have shown great potential as prognostic biomarkers in PDAC. Hopefully these biomarker miRNAs will form a solid foundation to better manage clinical treatment strategies to enhance survival benefits and avoid toxicity. Beyond miRNAs as prognostic biomarkers, as miRNAs are multi-targeted entities that suppress a number of key targets and pathways, some of these miRNAs will be good candidates to develop as novel therapeutics for overcoming PDAC resistance.

Abbreviations

circRNA: circular RNA; EMT: Epithelial–mesenchymal transition; lncRNA: long noncoding RNA; MET: Mesenchymal–epithelial transition; PDAC: Pancreatic ductal adenocarcinoma

Acknowledgements

The authors apologize to those whose work has not been included in this review due to scope and space limitations.

Funding

This study was supported by the National Institute of Health/National Cancer Institute R01CA15501904 (J Ju), R01CA19709801 (J Ju) and the National Natural Science Foundation of China No. 81502550 (SX Guo).

Authors' contributions

SX: Gathered references and drafted the manuscript and made the figure. AF edited the manuscript and figure, and gathered references. HW edited the manuscript and provided additional references. JJ drafted the manuscript, designed the figure and provided funding. All authors read and approved the final manuscript.

Competing interests

The authors declare that they have no competing interests.

Author details

[1]Stony Brook University, Stony Brook, New York 11794, USA. [2]Third Military Medical University, Chongqing 400038, People's Republic of China.

References

1. Siegel RL, Miller KD, Jemal A. Cancer statistics, 2018. CA Cancer J Clin. 2018;68:7–30.
2. Li D, Xie K, Wolff R, Abbruzzese JL. Pancreatic cancer. Lancet. 2004;363:1049–57.
3. Siegel RL, Miller KD, Jemal A. Cancer statistics, 2017. CA Cancer J Clin. 2017;67:7–30.
4. Wagner M, Redaelli C, Lietz M, Seiler CA, Friess H, Buchler MW. Curative resection is the single most important factor determining outcome in patients with pancreatic adenocarcinoma. Br J Surg. 2004;91:586–94.
5. Hartwig W, Werner J, Jager D, Debus J, Buchler MW. Improvement of surgical results for pancreatic cancer. Lancet Oncol. 2013;14:e476–85.
6. Garrido-Laguna I, Hidalgo M. Pancreatic cancer: from state-of-the-art treatments to promising novel therapies. Nat Rev Clin Oncol. 2015;12:319–34.
7. Matsuno S, Egawa S, Fukuyama S, Motoi F, Sunamura M, Isaji S, Imaizumi T, Okada S, Kato H, Suda K, et al. Pancreatic Cancer registry in Japan: 20 years of experience. Pancreas. 2004;28:219–30.
8. Burris HA 3rd, Moore MJ, Andersen J, Green MR, Rothenberg ML, Modiano MR, Cripps MC, Portenoy RK, Storniolo AM, Tarassoff P, et al. Improvements in survival and clinical benefit with gemcitabine as first-line therapy for patients with advanced pancreas cancer: a randomized trial. J Clin Oncol. 1997;15:2403–13.
9. Berlin JD, Catalano P, Thomas JP, Kugler JW, Haller DG, Benson AB 3rd. Phase III study of gemcitabine in combination with fluorouracil versus gemcitabine alone in patients with advanced pancreatic carcinoma: eastern cooperative oncology group trial E2297. J Clin Oncol. 2002;20:3270–5.
10. Heinemann V, Quietzsch D, Gieseler F, Gonnermann M, Schonekas H, Rost A, Neuhaus H, Haag C, Clemens M, Heinrich B, et al. Randomized phase III trial of gemcitabine plus cisplatin compared with gemcitabine alone in advanced pancreatic cancer. J Clin Oncol. 2006;24:3946–52.
11. Louvet C, Labianca R, Hammel P, Lledo G, Zampino MG, Andre T, Zaniboni A, Ducreux M, Aitini E, Taieb J, et al. Gemcitabine in combination with oxaliplatin compared with gemcitabine alone in locally advanced or metastatic pancreatic cancer: results of a GERCOR and GISCAD phase III trial. J Clin Oncol. 2005;23:3509–16.
12. Herrmann R, Bodoky G, Ruhstaller T, Glimelius B, Bajetta E, Schuller J, Saletti P, Bauer J, Figer A, Pestalozzi B, et al. Gemcitabine plus capecitabine compared with gemcitabine alone in advanced pancreatic cancer: a randomized, multicenter, phase III trial of the Swiss Group for Clinical Cancer Research and the central European cooperative oncology group. J Clin Oncol. 2007;25:2212–7.
13. Wang Z, Li Y, Ahmad A, Banerjee S, Azmi AS, Kong D, Sarkar FH. Pancreatic cancer: understanding and overcoming chemoresistance. Nat Rev Gastroenterol Hepatol. 2011;8:27–33.
14. Drakaki A, Iliopoulos D. MicroRNA-gene signaling pathways in pancreatic cancer. Biom J. 2013;36:200–8.
15. Yu S, Lu Z, Liu C, Meng Y, Ma Y, Zhao W, Liu J, Yu J, Chen J. miRNA-96 suppresses KRAS and functions as a tumor suppressor gene in pancreatic cancer. Cancer Res. 2010;70:6015–25.
16. Pai P, Rachagani S, Are C, Batra SK. Prospects of miRNA-based therapy for pancreatic cancer. Curr Drug Targets. 2013;14:1101–9.
17. Bartel DP. MicroRNAs: genomics, biogenesis, mechanism, and function. Cell. 2004;116:281–97.
18. Cioffi M, Trabulo SM, Sanchez-Ripoll Y, Miranda-Lorenzo I, Lonardo E, Dorado J, Reis Vieira C, Ramirez JC, Hidalgo M, Aicher A, et al. The miR-17-92 cluster counteracts quiescence and chemoresistance in a distinct subpopulation of pancreatic cancer stem cells. Gut. 2015;64:1936–48.
19. Ali S, Ahmad A, Banerjee S, Padhye S, Dominiak K, Schaffert JM, Wang Z, Philip PA, Sarkar FH. Gemcitabine sensitivity can be induced in pancreatic cancer cells through modulation of miR-200 and miR-21 expression by curcumin or its analogue CDF. Cancer Res. 2010;70:3606–17.
20. Giovannetti E, Funel N, Peters GJ, Del Chiaro M, Erozenci LA, Vasile E, Leon LG, Pollina LE, Groen A, Falcone A, et al. MicroRNA-21 in pancreatic cancer: correlation with clinical outcome and pharmacologic aspects underlying its role in the modulation of gemcitabine activity. Cancer Res. 2010;70:4528–38.
21. Park JK, Lee EJ, Esau C, Schmittgen TD. Antisense inhibition of microRNA-21 or −221 arrests cell cycle, induces apoptosis, and sensitizes the effects of gemcitabine in pancreatic adenocarcinoma. Pancreas. 2009;38:e190–9.

22. Hwang JH, Voortman J, Giovannetti E, Steinberg SM, Leon LG, Kim YT, Funel N, Park JK, Kim MA, Kang GH, et al. Identification of microRNA-21 as a biomarker for chemoresistance and clinical outcome following adjuvant therapy in resectable pancreatic cancer. PLoS One. 2010;5:e10630.
23. Li Y, VandenBoom TG 2nd, Kong D, Wang Z, Ali S, Philip PA, Sarkar FH. Up-regulation of miR-200 and let-7 by natural agents leads to the reversal of epithelial-to-mesenchymal transition in gemcitabine-resistant pancreatic cancer cells. Cancer Res. 2009;69:6704–12.
24. Kong YW, Ferland-McCollough D, Jackson TJ, Bushell M. microRNAs in cancer management. Lancet Oncol. 2012;13:e249–58.
25. Petrocca F, Lieberman J. Micromanipulating cancer: microRNA-based therapeutics? RNA Biol. 2009;6:335–40.
26. Rokhlin OW, Scheinker VS, Taghiyev AF, Bumcrot D, Glover RA, Cohen MB. MicroRNA-34 mediates AR-dependent p53-induced apoptosis in prostate cancer. Cancer Biol Ther. 2008;7:1288–96.
27. Ji Q, Hao X, Zhang M, Tang W, Yang M, Li L, Xiang D, Desano JT, Bommer GT, Fan D, et al. MicroRNA miR-34 inhibits human pancreatic cancer tumor-initiating cells. PLoS One. 2009;4:e6816.
28. Zhang XJ, Ye H, Zeng CW, He B, Zhang H, Chen YQ. Dysregulation of miR-15a and miR-214 in human pancreatic cancer. J Hematol Oncol. 2010;3:46.
29. Guo S, Xu X, Tang Y, Zhang C, Li J, Ouyang Y, Ju J, Bie P, Wang H. miR-15a inhibits cell proliferation and epithelial to mesenchymal transition in pancreatic ductal adenocarcinoma by down-regulating Bmi-1 expression. Cancer Lett. 2014;344:40–6.
30. Mikamori M, Yamada D, Eguchi H, Hasegawa S, Kishimoto T, Tomimaru Y, Asaoka T, Noda T, Wada H, Kawamoto K, et al. MicroRNA-155 controls exosome synthesis and promotes gemcitabine resistance in pancreatic ductal adenocarcinoma. Sci Rep. 2017;7:42339.
31. Li J, Wu H, Li W, Yin L, Guo S, Xu X, Ouyang Y, Zhao Z, Liu S, Tian Y, et al. Downregulated miR-506 expression facilitates pancreatic cancer progression and chemoresistance via SPHK1/Akt/NF-kappaB signaling. Oncogene. 2016;35:5501–14.
32. Du J, Zheng X, Cai S, Zhu Z, Tan J, Hu B, Huang Z, Jiao H. MicroRNA506 participates in pancreatic cancer pathogenesis by targeting PIM3. Mol Med Rep. 2015;12:5121–6.
33. Huang J, Liu J, Chen-Xiao K, Zhang X, Lee WN, Go VL, Xiao GG. Advance in microRNA as a potential biomarker for early detection of pancreatic cancer. Biomark Res. 2016;4:20.
34. Liang L, Wei DM, Li JJ, Luo DZ, Chen G, Dang YW, Cai XY. Prognostic microRNAs and their potential molecular mechanism in pancreatic cancer: a study based on the Cancer genome atlas and bioinformatics investigation. Mol Med Rep. 2018;17:939–51.
35. Dillhoff M, Liu J, Frankel W, Croce C, Bloomston M. MicroRNA-21 is overexpressed in pancreatic cancer and a potential predictor of survival. J Gastrointest Surg. 2008;12:2171–6.
36. Bloomston M, Frankel WL, Petrocca F, Volinia S, Alder H, Hagan JP, Liu CG, Bhatt D, Taccioli C, Croce CM. MicroRNA expression patterns to differentiate pancreatic adenocarcinoma from normal pancreas and chronic pancreatitis. JAMA. 2007;297:1901–8.
37. Schultz NA, Andersen KK, Roslind A, Willenbrock H, Wojdemann M, Johansen JS. Prognostic microRNAs in cancer tissue from patients operated for pancreatic cancer–five microRNAs in a prognostic index. World J Surg. 2012;36:2699–707.
38. Ohuchida K, Mizumoto K, Kayashima T, Fujita H, Moriyama T, Ohtsuka T, Ueda J, Nagai E, Hashizume M, Tanaka M. MicroRNA expression as a predictive marker for gemcitabine response after surgical resection of pancreatic cancer. Ann Surg Oncol. 2011;18:2381–7.
39. Greither T, Grochola LF, Udelnow A, Lautenschlager C, Wurl P, Taubert H. Elevated expression of microRNAs 155, 203, 210 and 222 in pancreatic tumors is associated with poorer survival. Int J Cancer. 2010;126:73–80.
40. Huang X, Xiao R, Pan S, Yang X, Yuan W, Tu Z, Xu M, Zhu Y, Yin Q, Wu Y, et al. Uncovering the roles of long non-coding RNAs in cancer stem cells. J Hematol Oncol. 2017;10:62.
41. Dong Y, He D, Peng Z, Peng W, Shi W, Wang J, Li B, Zhang C, Duan C. Circular RNAs in cancer: an emerging key player. J Hematol Oncol. 2017;10:2.
42. Ma P, Pan Y, Li W, Sun C, Liu J, Xu T, Shu Y. Extracellular vesicles-mediated noncoding RNAs transfer in cancer. J Hematol Oncol. 2017;10:57.
43. Kim K, Jutooru I, Chadalapaka G, Johnson G, Frank J, Burghardt R, Kim S, Safe S. HOTAIR is a negative prognostic factor and exhibits pro-oncogenic activity in pancreatic cancer. Oncogene. 2013;32:1616–25.
44. Huang WJ, Wang Y, Liu S, Yang J, Guo SX, Wang L, Wang H, Fan YF. Silencing circular RNA hsa_circ_0000977 suppresses pancreatic ductal adenocarcinoma progression by stimulating miR-874-3p and inhibiting PLK1 expression. Cancer Lett. 2018;422:70–80.

Platelet protein biomarker panel for ovarian cancer diagnosis

Marta Lomnytska[1,2,3*], Rui Pinto[4], Susanne Becker[3], Ulla Engström[5], Sonja Gustafsson[6], Christina Björklund[6], Markus Templin[7], Jan Bergstrand[8], Lei Xu[8], Jerker Widengren[8], Elisabeth Epstein[2,9], Bo Franzén[3,6] and Gert Auer[3,6]

Abstract

Background: Platelets support cancer growth and spread making platelet proteins candidates in the search for biomarkers.

Methods: Two-dimensional (2D) gel electrophoresis, Partial Least Squares Discriminant Analysis (PLS-DA), Western blot, DigiWest.

Results: PLS-DA of platelet protein expression in 2D gels suggested differences between the International Federation of Gynaecology and Obstetrics (FIGO) stages III-IV of ovarian cancer, compared to benign adnexal lesions with a sensitivity of 96% and a specificity of 88%. A PLS-DA-based model correctly predicted 7 out of 8 cases of FIGO stages I-II of ovarian cancer after verification by western blot. Receiver-operator curve (ROC) analysis indicated a sensitivity of 83% and specificity of 76% at cut-off >0.5 (area under the curve (AUC) = 0.831, $p < 0.0001$) for detecting these cases. Validation on an independent set of samples by DigiWest with PLS-DA differentiated benign adnexal lesions and ovarian cancer, FIGO stages III-IV, with a sensitivity of 70% and a specificity of 83%.

Conclusion: We identified a group of platelet protein biomarker candidates that can quantify the differential expression between ovarian cancer cases as compared to benign adnexal lesions.

Keywords: Ovarian cancer, Platelet proteome, Biomarker, Liquid biopsy

Background

Epithelial ovarian cancer is characterised by an asymptomatic growth in the abdominal cavity. In 75% of all cases, it is only detected at an advanced stage. The 5-year survival rate in FIGO stages I-II is over 90%, compared to around 30% in stages III-IV [1, 2]. The sensitivity of the CA-125 tumor marker for the detection of non-advanced epithelial ovarian cancer ranges from 50% to 70%, and this parameter alone is not recommended for differentiating between a benign and a malignant adnexal mass [3]. An expertly conducted transvaginal sonography (TVS) is a primary method for evaluation of ovarian and pelvic tumors, as it is able to discriminate between benign and malignant conditions with 90% sensitivity and 94% specificity using the International Ovarian Tumor Analysis (IOTA) pattern recognition [4, 5]. Despite high performance of TVS, the assessment will be inconclusive in around 8% of cases, also in the hands of an expert examiner [4]. Commonly used tumor markers, such as CA-125, HE4 and the Risk of Malignancy Index (RMI), did not improve, but rather deteriorated assessment in these difficult to classify tumors [6].

A several-fold increase in a patient's platelet count is a common observation in cancer. A high preoperative platelet count is associated with early relapse in non-advanced epithelial ovarian cancer [7] and colorectal cancer [8]. Platelets influence angiogenic and immunological processes in cancer [9, 10], as well as directly protect tumor cells [7]. Proteomic analysis of platelets has identified several potential cancer markers [11]. Among them are angiogenic factors that have been shown to be sequestered by platelets [12] and delivered to the site of activated endothelium within an early

* Correspondence: marta.lomnytska@gmail.com
[1]Department of Obstetrics and Gynaecology, Academical Uppsala University Hospital, Uppsala University, SE-751 85 Uppsala, Sweden
[2]Institute of Women's and Children's Health, Karolinska Institute, SE-171 76 Stockholm, Sweden

tumor [11]. Detection of platelet-derived growth factor, platelet factor 4 (PF-4) and platelet-derived endothelial cell growth factor was suggested for diagnosis of several cancers [13]. Upon platelet activation, PF-4, vascular endothelial growth factor (VEGF) and fibrinogen undergo significant spatial rearrangements, detectable only by super resolution stimulated emission depletion (STED) microscopy [14].

The proteome of platelets in ovarian cancer has not been previously studied. The hypothesis of the current study is that knowledge of quantitative alterations of proteins in platelets can become the basis for non-invasive diagnosis of ovarian cancer and evaluation of the malignant potential of adnexal lesions.

Methods

The study comprised three phases:

1. Platelet pellets were prospectively collected from patients with benign adnexal lesions and ovarian cancer. This clinical material was subjected to two-dimensional (2D) gel electrophoresis, statistical analysis of protein expression, and subsequently, mass spectrometry-aided identification of protein biomarker candidates.
2. Antibody identification and confirmation of protein identification by western blot.
3. Verification of our biomarker candidate protein panel using western blot and DigiWest, and evaluation of sensitivity and specificity for detecting ovarian cancer.

Clinical material

Blood samples were obtained from volunteering women with adnexal lesions and suspected ovarian cancer. Approval for the study was given by the local ethical committee of Stockholm County Council, Dnr 2010/504–31. Cases were coded as "TR" followed by a number, and the coding was saved separately from the personal information of patients. Clinical material from 114 patients was prospectively collected between 2011 and 2014 at the Department of Obstetrics and Gynaecology, Karolinska University Hospital-Solna, Stockholm, Sweden (Table 1, Additional file 1: Table S1). Peripheral venous blood was drawn from the antecubital vein of each subject. The requirement for inclusion in the study was collection of a blood sample prior to any invasive diagnostic or treatment procedures. Patients with another known active cancer were excluded from the study. Patient records included age at diagnosis, comorbidities, medication with coagulation and platelet aggregation blockers, optionally - TVS according to IOTA criteria, and post-operative histopathological

Table 1 Description of the clinical material

Diagnosis and International classification of disease (ICD) coding					
Benign lesions		Epithelial ovarian cancer, C56.9			
	n	stages I-II	n	stages III-IV	n
Serous ovarian cyst, N82.3	19	serous	2	serous	47
Ovarian fibrom, N82.3	10	mucinous	1	endometrioid	1
Dermoid ovarian cyst, N82.3	5	endometrioid	2	clear-cell	1
Endometriosis cyst, N80.1	8	clear-cell	3		
Mucinous ovarian cyst, N83.2	10				
Non-cancer ascites, R18.9	1				
Paratubar cyst, Q50.5	2				
Uterine myom, D25.9	2				
Total	57		8		49

Transvaginal sonography, IOTA classification			
Ultrasound assessment	Certainty in the assessment	Histopathology	n
Benign	certainly benign	benign	7
Benign	probably benign	benign	16
Benign	uncertain	benign	6
Borderline tumor	uncertain	benign	4
Malignant	probably malignant	benign	2
Malignant	certainly malignant	malignant	1[a]
Malignant	certainly malignant	malignant	13[b]
no IOTA-based examination		benign	22
no IOTA-based examination		malignant	7[a]
no IOTA-based examination		malignant	36[b]
Total			114

Comorbidities	n	Medication: coagulation/aggregation blockers	n
None	99	none	111
One or few following diseases:	15	Warfarin	1
Breast cancer remission	4	Dabigatran	1
Cardiovascular	14	Aspirin	1
Rheumatic	2	Total	114
Endocrine	4	Experimental setup, n	

Table 1 Description of the clinical material *(Continued)*

Diagnosis and International classification of disease (ICD) coding					
Benign lesions		Epithelial ovarian cancer, C56.9			
	n	stages I-II	n	stages III-IV	n
Astma	2	Method/ Statistics	Benign	Ovarian cancer, stage	
Hepatitis C	1		lesions	I-II	III-IV
Total	114	2D/PCA	28	8	32
		2D/PLS-DA	25	8	30
		Western blot/PLS-DA	20	8	20
		DigiWest/ PLS-DA	29	0	30

[a]stages I-II
[b]stages III-IV

conclusion. Randomization of the material was performed prior to experimental procedures.

Isolation of platelets from peripheral blood

Peripheral venous blood was drawn into 4.5 ml vacutainer plastic whole blood collection tubes with spray-coated K_2EDTA (Vacutainer, BD, Franklin Lakes, NJ, USA) and processed within 30 min. Isolation of platelets was performed by three centrifugation steps. Exclusion of erythrocytes and leucocytes was achieved by centrifugation of whole blood at 1500 relative centrifugal force (RCF) for 10 min at +4 °C, and the platelet-rich plasma obtained was subjected to a second centrifugation at 3000 RCF for 10 min at +4 °C [15]. The resulting platelet pellet was re-suspended in 500 μL 0.9% NaCl and centrifuged at 3000 RCF for 10 min at +6 °C. The quality and purity of the platelet isolation was confirmed by light microscopy after immunostaining with an antibody against CD61 (119,992, Abcam, Cambridge, UK). In addition, fluorescence-activated cell sorting (FACS) of selected cases using the antibody against p-selectin, or CD62 (348,107, BD Biosciences-Europe) was also used to assess quality and purity. Platelet pellets were aliquoted to avoid excess freeze-thaw cycles and stored at −70 °C.

Two-dimensional gel electrophoresis

The platelet fractions for 2D gel electrophoresis were lyophilized and resuspended in lysis buffer; the protein concentration was determined using the Bradford protein analysis protocol [16] and the Versa Max Microplate reader (Molecular Devices, Sunnyvale CA, USA). Samples of 75.0 μg protein were subjected to 2D gel electrophoresis as previously described [17]. One 2D gel per clinical case was included into analysis after evaluation of the gel quality, i.e., absence of protein degradation protein spot smearing or overstraining. The expression level of protein spots in 2D gels was analysed using Progenesis SameSpot software (Nonlinear Dynamics, London, UK). The cut-off for selection of protein spots was a relative expression difference of 1.5-fold, $p < 0.05$, power > 0.8, $q < 0.05$, as evaluated by analysis of variance (ANOVA) by the SameSpot software.

Search parameters and acceptance criteria for MS/MS and peptide mass fingerprint (PMF)

Protein spots selected for identification were excised from the gels, treated for in-gel digestion, and subjected to MALDI TOF mass spectrometry carried out on the Ultraflex III TOF/TOF (Bruker Daltonics, Bremen, Germany). Peptide spectra were internally calibrated using trypsin autolytic peptides. A peak list generating software, Data Analysis 3.2 (Bruker Daltonics, Bremen, Germany), was used. In selected cases, MS/MS was performed with acceptance score exceeding 30. Mass tolerance for fragment ions was 0.5 Da. Based on the obtained peptide spectra, identification of the proteins was performed using the MASCOT (Matrix Science, London, England) and the "NCBInr" database. The deviation of mass did not exceed 0.05 Da. Probability of identification was evaluated according to score value, sequence coverage, and matched peptides. All other steps were performed as previously described [17].

Western blot analysis

A semi-quantitative dual label fluorescent detection western blot analysis was performed using the same patient cases that were subjected to 2D gel electrophoresis (Table 1). Samples were diluted in 4× lithium dodecyl sulfate (LDS) buffer and 10× reducing agent to a concentration of 1 μg/μl, and then incubated for 10 min at 70 °C. Four NuPAGE 4–12% Bis-Tris Gel, 1.0 mm × 15 wells were run in parallel; a total of 10 μg protein per case was loaded. Gel running conditions were as follows: 200 V for 60 min in XCell SureLock Mini-Cell EI0001 (Life Technologies, Stockholm, Sweden), followed by incubation of gels in transfer buffer containing 10% methanol and blotting to a nitrocellulose membrane for 1 h at 30 V (BioRad Power Pac 100 and Hoefer EPS 2A200). Membranes were incubated with Odyssey blocking buffer (Li-Cor Biosciences, East Chesterton Ward, UK) with addition of 0.1% Tween 20 for one hour, and then with the combination of commercially available primary antibodies, GAPDH and anti-14-3-3-gamma for loading controls [18] (Additional file 1: Table S2) with rotation at +4 °C overnight. After washing with PBS, each membrane was incubated with secondary antibodies (IRDye 2nd Ab Goat anti-Rabbit 680, 1:10,000 and IRDye 2nd Ab Goat anti-Mouse 800, 1:15,000, Li-Cor Biosciences, East Chesterton Ward, UK) at room temperature for 1 h. After washing with PBS, each membrane was scanned using the Odyssey SA Infrared Imaging System (Li-Cor Biosciences, East Chesterton Ward, UK).

DigiWest analysis

For each platelet lysate, two technical repeats (20 μg protein per lane) were subjected to SDS-PAGE using 4–12% Bis-Tris gradient gels. After blotting with primary antibodies (Additional file 1: Table S2) and biotinylation of the proteins, individual sample lanes were cut into 96 molecular weight fractions (0.5 mm each) and proteins were eluted. Eluted proteins from each molecular weight fraction were loaded onto color-coded neutravidin-coated Luminex bead sets (MagPlex, Luminex, Austin TX, USA), and the antibody specific signals were analysed (DigiWest analysis, version 3.8.5.2, Excel-based) [19].

Multivariate methods (PCA, PLS-DA, OPLS-DA)

Principal components analysis (PCA) [20] is the most widely used (non-supervised) multivariate method, and the root to most others. By finding covariance between multiple (correlated) variables in a single dataset **X**, it sequentially defines (uncorrelated, or orthogonal) principal components, with decreasing amount of variance explained, built from weighted initial variables. A number of interesting components can be selected, as variation in the dataset is reframed as structured (e.g. biological information) or residual (noise). Each component defines a percentage of variation of the original dataset, and is described by two vectors: scores, representing the score of each sample in the newly created principal component; loadings, representing the weight of each initial variable in the principal component. PCA performs dimensionality reduction, thus allowing one to condense most of the information in a large dataset into a small number of components. Its scores and loadings can be plotted and used as an exploratory technique, to find relations between variables, detect groups and trends in the samples, as well as outliers.

Projection to latent structures (PLS) is a well established (supervised) method for the analysis of complex multivariate datasets, as found in the –omics fields, including proteomics [21, 22]. In originates from partial least squares regression, a multivariate analysis method which relates two matrices (**X** with the actual data or independent variables, and **Y**/**y** as responses or dependent variables) by maximizing the covariance of their latent variables. The 2-class PLS-DA is simply a particular type of PLS in which the dependent variable is a "dummy" binary (0/1) class **y**-vector. PLS-DA targets complementary objectives: as a discriminant method, it allows discrimination/prediction of class for test samples; as a multivariate method it shows the relationship among variables in the dataset through the creation of latent variables, built using weighted original variables; as a linear method, it allows one to visualize and understand which variables in the data are more relevant for the class discrimination.

Orthogonal PLS (OPLS) [23] is a modification of the PLS method, and while both models have the same model statistics and prediction capability, OPLS allows for easier interpretation of the relevant variables than PLS. The reason is because apart from dividing variation into systematic and residual (as PLS), OPLS also divides the systematic variation into predictive (related to the phenomenon in study) and orthogonal (structured variation related to other factors, such as age and gender). This property is advantageous when interpretation of the results, rather than prediction, is the main objective of the analysis. In the context of OPLS-DA the statistically significant predictive loadings show which initial variables are important in the discrimination of class, and in which class these variables have higher values.

(O)PLS-DA number of latent variables and validation [24]

(O)PLS-DA models can separate data variability into systematic and random, and use the systematic one for building the actual model while discarding the random variation, or noise. In order to attain that objective, it is critical to select an appropriate number of latent variables for the model, which is achieved in general through the use sampling methods such as cross-validation (CV). In this strategy, one calculates multiple (O)PLS-DA models using subsets of the **X** data, while predicting the class (**y**) of the samples left out in each round. By doing this for models with different number of latent variables, one can evaluate how well predicted by the model are the samples that were left out in each of those models, and select the best one. It yields the following cross-validation's statistics: R2X- fraction of the variance in **X** explained by each latent variable; R2- fraction of variance of **y** (class) explained by each latent variable; and most importantly Q2- the fraction of variance of **y** predicted by the model. A model with good modelling and predictive power is desired, and while R2X may be low (due to low number of variables in **X** explaining class discrimination), R2Y and Q2 should be the closest possible to each other, as well as close to a maximum of 1.

After a model is built, containing the appropriate number of latent variables, it undergoes appropriate validation procedures, notably cross-validation analysis of variance (CV-ANOVA), permutation test, and evaluation of cross-validation scores. CV-ANOVA compares the y predicted residuals of the model of interest with the variation around the global average using an F-test, resulting in a significance *p*-value for decisional purposes. Permutation test evaluates the statistical significance of estimated predictive power, by comparing R2 and Q2 of multiple models (where **y** was randomized) with R2 and Q2 of the actual model of interest. If the model is significant, its values are expected to be higher than for the y-randomized models. Cross-validation scores are scores that are calculated for each sample during cross validation, and can be visually or systematically evaluated to indicate over-fitting in case they differ from the regular scores.

Prediction of test samples and variable relevance for class discrimination

After proper choice of number of latent variables and method validation, the model can be used for prediction of test samples, and to find out which variables are relevant for class discrimination.

As class membership is defined by the 0/1 dependent variable **y** vector in the training set, class membership of "new" samples in a test set is dependent on their predicted **y** value. Samples similar to class "1" are expected to yield values of **y** similar to 1, thus above a certain threshold, e.g. 0.5, while samples similar to the ones in class "0" will be predicted below that threshold.

To find out which variables are relevant for class discrimination, two methods are commonly used: the variable importance on the projection (VIP) method, which is an (unsigned) compact parameter to summarize the importance of each of the variables in PLS-type models with more than one latent variable; the other method can be used with OPLS-type models and checks if the confidence interval for the mean of the CV-calculated loadings crosses zero or not (in which case it is consistently positive or negative for each of the cross validation models).

PCA, PLS-DA and OPLS-DA were performed using SIMCA P v13.0 software (Umetrics AB).

Experimental design and statistical rationale

Normalized expression values exported from SameSpot software of all protein spots (approximately 2000 spots in one 2D gel) were subjected to PCA analysis and PLS-DA.

PCA analysis was performed using the material from patients with benign adnexal lesions (28 cases), ovarian cancer, International Federation of Gynaecology and Obstetrics (FIGO) stages I-II (8 cases), and ovarian cancer, FIGO stages III-IV (32 cases) (Table 1). The PLS-DA model was based on the expression of all platelet protein spots in 2D gels in benign ovarian lesions (16 cases) and ovarian cancer, FIGO stages III-IV (20 cases). The predictive ability of the model was tested using 8 cases of the ovarian cancer, FIGO stages I-II, 9 cases of benign adnexal lesions and 10 cases of the ovarian cancer, FIGO stages III-IV. Protein spots selected by PLS-DA were ranked as variables of importance in the projection (VIP) by the strength of their input into the model. An analysis of the influence of co-morbidities and the intake of coagulation and platelet aggregation blockers was performed.

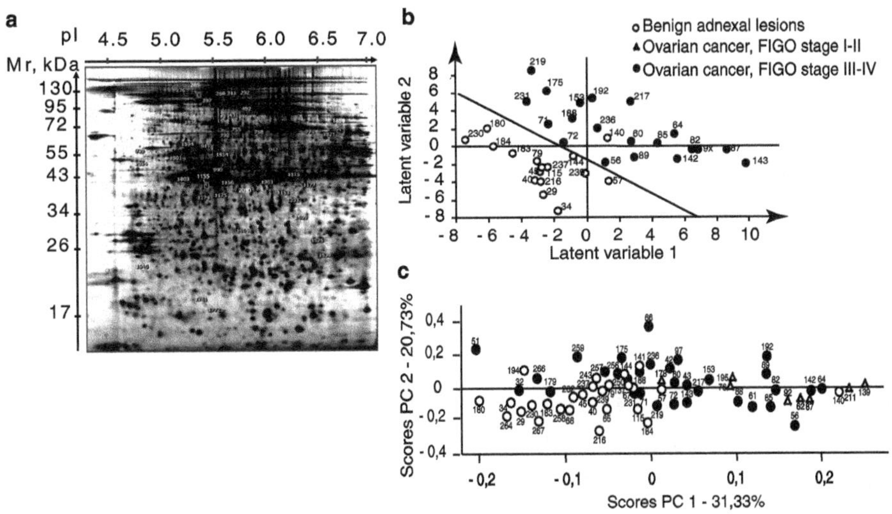

Fig. 1 Proteomics-based analysis of platelet proteins was based on the separation of proteins according to mass (Mr, kDa) and charge (pI) by 2D gel electrophoresis with further analysis of the expression of protein spots for marker identification. **a** 2D gel electrophoresis diagram of platelet proteins. Circles and numbers indicate the identified biomarkers. **b** The PLS-DA-based cross-validated model based on the partial least squares discriminate analysis of 2D gels for benign adnexal lesions (white circle) and ovarian cancer, FIGO stage III-IV (black circle) in accordance to the expression of all protein spots in the gel. **c** Principal component analysis (PCA) showing separation of the generated 2D gels for benign adnexal lesions (white circle), ovarian cancer, FIGO stage I-II (triangle) and FIGO stage III-IV (black circle) in accordance to the expression of selected biomarkers; percentage of variance X explained by the two PCA components shown

Western blot analysis for antibody identification and confirmation of protein identification was performed using 20 cases of benign adnexal lesions, 20 cases of ovarian cancer, FIGO stages III-IV and 8 cases of stages I-II (Table 1). The same cases were used for 2D electrophoresis (Additional file 1: Table S1). For protein panel verification, all analysed samples were randomized and distributed to four sets of gel separation batches. Each batch produced four equal gels, each of which, after transferring, was incubated with four different mixtures of primary antibodies against 16 proteins (Additional file 1: Table S2) for a total of 16 gels per data set. This experiment was repeated three times (sets 1–3). Protein expression levels were subjected to OPLS-DA, logistic regression and receiver-operator curve (ROC) analysis (MedCalc Software, Ostend, Belgium).

Verification using DigiWest analysis [19] was performed on an independent set of prospectively collected randomized platelet samples from patients with ovarian cancer, FIGO stages III-IV ($n = 30$), and benign adnexal control lesions ($n = 29$) (Table 1, Additional file 1: Table S1). Statistical analysis was OPLS-DA based.

Results

Cancer-related expression of platelet proteins in 2D gels

Each 2D gel contained approximately 2000 protein spots (Fig. 1a). Initial PCA (Fig. 1c) of expression levels of significantly differentially expressed protein spots in 2D gels indicated a degree of separation between the three analysed patient groups: benign adnexal lesions, ovarian cancer, FIGO stages I-II and FIGO stages III-IV. PCA scores showing these groups are presented in Fig. 1c.

The PLS-DA cross-validated model based on the expression of all protein spots in 2D gels of benign adnexal lesions and ovarian cancer (FIGO stages III-IV) presented 96% sensitivity and 88% specificity for discrimination between these groups (Table 2a, Fig. 1b). The predictive ability of the built PLS-DA model was tested. We observed that all 8 cases ovarian cancer, FIGO stages I-II were recognised as cancer (1.00 sensitivity), and also 8 of 10 cases of ovarian cancer, FIGO stages III-IV (80%). Four out of 9 cases of benign adnexal lesions were recognised as benign (0.44 specificity) (Table 2a). Forty-three protein variables with VIP > 2 were selected for protein identification.

Table 2 Statistics for PLS-DA, OPLS-DA model, details for predictive and orthogonal parts; ROC analysis

A) PLS-DA-based analysis of protein spots expression in 2D

Component	Latent variables	R2X (cum)	Q2 (cum)	CV-ANOVA, p-value	permutation test, p-value		Sensitivity	Specificity
Model	3	0.318	0.72	8,5 * 10–9	<0.001	calibration set	0.96	0.88
						validation set	1.00	0.44

B) OPLS-DA-based analysis of protein expression in western blot.

Component	Latent variables	R2X (cum)	R2 (cum)	Q2 (cum)	CV-ANOVA, p-value	permutation test, *p*-value		Sensitivity	Specificity
Model	1 + 1	0.203	0.632	0.477	4.41E-14	<0.001	calibration set	0.83	0.89
Predictive	1	0.0717	0.632	0.477			validation set	0.88	not tested
Orthogonal	1	0.131	0						

C) ROC analysis of protein expression in western blot.

Compared groups	AUC	standart deviation	95% confidence interval	z statistics	p-value		Sensitivity	Specificity
ROC 1	0.777	0.0418	0,695 to 0,859	6.639	<0,0001	ROC1	60	83.33
ROC 2	0.831	0.0501	0,733 to 0,930	6.615	<0,0001	ROC2	83.33	76.19

D) OPLS-DA-based analysis of protein expression in Digi west.

Component	Latent variables	R2X (cum)	R2 (cum)	Q2 (cum)	CV-ANOVA, p-value	permutation test, p-value		Sensitivity	Specificity
Model	1 + 2	0.24	0.785	0.345	4.50E-03	<0.001	test set	0.7	0.83
Predictive	1	0.037	0.785	0.345					
Orthogonal	2	0.203							

R2X cumulative percentage of X variance explained, *R2* cumulative percentage of Y variance explained, *Q2* cumulative percentage of variance of Y predicted, *CV-ANOVA p-value* p-value of cross-validation ANOVA, *permutaion test p-value p*-value of (1000 iterations) permutation test

Table 3 Protein identification

Protein spot number on 2D	Gene ontology name	Protein name	theoretical		experimental		NCBI accession number	Sequence coverage, %	Matched peptides	Total peptide count	score	msms
			pI	Mr, kDa	pI	Mr, kDa						
1	2	3	4	5	6	7	8	9	10	11	12	13
285	ACTN1	Alpha-actinin-1 isoform b	5.2	104	5.5	100	NP_001093	25	19	75	98	–
1836	ACTN4	Alpha actinin 4, partial	5.2	74	5.3	72	AAH15620	14	9	30	68	–
1153	ACTB	beta actin variant, partial	5.4	42	6.2	40	BAD96752.1	31	9	48	71	–
1803	ACTB	actin beta	5.2	39	5.3	42	BAG62914.1	30	10	54	81	–
1772	AP4A	Bis(5′-nucleosyl)- tetraphosphatase	5.1	17	5.4	17	NP_001152	27	5	36	52	1
1274	CAPZA1	capping actin protein of muscle Z-line alpha subunit 1	6	32	5.4	40	XP_005542394.1	54	11	60	106	–
911	CD41	Integrin alpha-IIb precursor variant	5.7	60	5.4	60	BAD92789.1	–	–	–	46	1
276	CD41	Integrin, alpha 2b (platelet glycoprotein IIb of IIb/IIIa complex, antigen CD41), isoform CRA_a	5.4	104	5.3	110	EAW51594.1	24	17	49	122	–
1761	CD42A	glycoprotein IX platelet	5.4	18	5.4	20	AAH30229	27	5	43	53	2
792	CD61	Platelet glycoprotein IIIa, partial	5	87	5.6	70	AAA52600	–	–	–	15	1
942	CNDP2	Cytosolic non-specific dipeptidase	5.6	53	6	55	BAG53426	22	8	48	51	3
1539	CRKL	Crk-lke protein	6.3	34	6.5	26	NP_005198	29	9	56	64	1
1525	ERP29	Erp28, endoplasmic reticulum resident protein 29 isoform 1 precursor	6.8	29	6.5	27	NP_006808	28	6	68	44	2
1854	FBG	Fibrinogen gamma chain	5.5	48	5.6	50	EAX04921	40	13	53	113	–
397	GELS	Gelsolin isoform a precursor (782 aa)	5.9	86	5.4	95	NP_000168	–	–	–	61	1
401	GELS	Gelsolin isoform b (731 aa)	5.6	81	5.7	90	NP_937895	12	9	50	45	2
311	HSPA9	Stress-70 potein, mitochondrial precursor	5.8	74	5.7	120	NP_001126860	27	17	66	100	3
1155	HP	Haptoglobin	6.3	38	5.4	42	AAI07588.1	25	10	61	71	–
482	HSPA8	Heat shock 70 kDa protein 1A/1B	5.4	70	5.7	80	P08107	13	6	56	29	–
1115	ILEU	Leukocyte elastase inhibitor	5.9	43	6.3	43	NP_109591	21	7	43	72	–
1177	MPST	3-mercaptopyruvate sulfurtransferase	6.8	35	6.4	37	BAD92061.1	33	8	39	75	–
1231	NSFL1C	NSFL1 cofactor p47 isoform X8	5	31	6.2	38	XP_011527607.1	25	5	46	38	1
1850	PGM1	phosphoglucomutase-1 isoform 1	6.3	62	6.8	70	NP_002624.2	11	5	32	33	–
1464	PHB	Prohibitin	5.5	28	5.7	30	XP_003912755.3	49	12	46	136	–
1054	RNH1	ribonuclease/angiogenin inhibitor 1	4.8	50	4.8	50	AAH11186.1	11	5	25	45	–
999	PRKAR1A	protein kinase cAMP-dependent type I regulatory subunit alpha	5.2	43	5.5	53	XP_004041145.1	35	13	72	102	
939	PRKAR2B	protein kinase cAMP-dependent type II regulatory subunit beta	5	45	4.8	55	BAG54705.1	19	6	27	41	2
1175	SRB6	Serpin B6	4.2	39	5.6	40	XP_011512978.1	34	10	45	76	–
1821	SRC	Protooncogene tyrosine-protein kinase Src	7.1	60	6.6	60	NP_005408.1	13	8	54	39	–
1801	TUBA4A	Tubulin alpha-4A chain	4.9	49	5.1	55	NP_001265481.1	23	10	56	73	–
1801	TUBA1C	tubulin alpha 1c	4.9	59	5.1	55	BAH11541.1	23	10	56	68	
758	TLN1	Talin 1	5.8	272	5.9	70	AAF27330	7	13	43	42	1
755	TLN1	Talin 1	5.8	272	5.8	70	AAF27330	9	15	46	54	–
292	TLN1	Talin 1	5.8	272	5.8	110	AAF27330	14	33	84	106	–

Table 3 Protein identification *(Continued)*

Protein spot number on 2D	Gene ontology name	Protein name	theoretical		experimental		NCBI accession number	Sequence coverage, %	Matched peptides	Total peptide count	score	msms
			pI	Mr, kDa	pI	Mr, kDa						
1	2	3	4	5	6	7	8	9	10	11	12	13
774	TLN1	Talin 1	5.8	272	6.4	70	AAF27330	–	–	–	25	1
1409	TLN1	Talin 1	5.8	272	6.4	34	AAF23322.1	6	15	39	47	–
1640	TPM1	Tropomyosin 1, alpha	5	20	4.7	20	XP_005254707	23	6	64	30	–
1894	TUBA6	Tubulin alpha-6 chain, partial	5	47	5.3	56	EHH66249.1	34	10	56	80	–
1894	TUBA8	tubulin alpha-8	5	43	5.3	56	XP_007469555.1	33	10	56	82	
1894	TUBA1C	tubulin alpha-1C chain	5	47	5.3	56	XP_004646666.1	35	10	56	81	
999	TUBB1	tubulin beta-1 chain isoform X7	5.1	43	5.5	53	XP_018872841.1	42	12	72	93	–
1850	WDR1	WD repeat-containing protein 1 iso 1	6.4	59	6.8	70	AAD05045	35	18	60	135	–

1 - number of a protein spot on 2-D gel,
2 - gene ontology name,
3 - protein name,
4 - isoelectric point of a protein spots according to the position on 2D gel,
5 - protein mass of a protein according to the position of a spot on 2D gel,
6 - isoelectric point of a protein spot as provided by Mascot search database,
7 - protein mass as provided by Mascot search database,
8 - protein accession number according to NCBI,
9 - matching of the experimental peptide sequence to a peptide sequence provided by NCBI,
10 - number of identified peptides that matched to the peptides of a peptide sequence provided by NCBI,
11 - total amount of peptides in a peptide sequence provided by NCBI,
12 - score provided by Mascot search engine,
13 - performed msms for the certainty of protein identification.

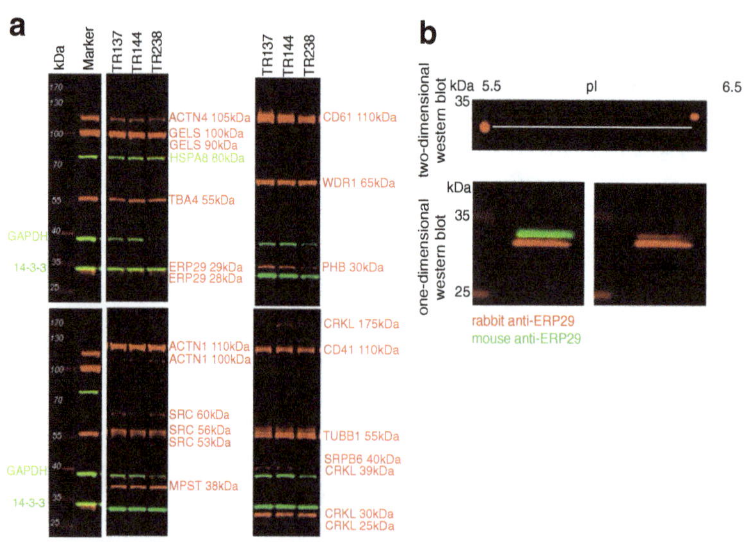

Fig. 2 Western blot analysis. **a** Confirmation of protein identification by western blot using antibodies against 15 selected proteins, and normalisation against14–3-3-gamma (loading control). **b** Western blot detection of ERP29. This example compares Mr/pI from 2D gel and Western blot where the mouse anti-ERP29 detects protein spot #1525, while the rabbit anti-ERP29 detects an additional protein spot, possibly an isoform of ERP29

Co-morbidities and use of of coagulation and platelet aggregation blockers did not influence the predictive ability of the model. The PLS-DA model suggested a list of protein spots for protein identification as potential biomarkers, which could be evaluated from the VIP plot.

Identification of platelet protein biomarkers and confirmation of identification

A total of 35 proteins were identified in 37 protein spots excised from 2D gels (Table 3).

A number of proteins were excluded due to low quality and/or low expression level that made identification by mass spectrometry unfeasible. Visual representation of the location of the identified spots may be found in Fig. 1a.

Confirmation of the protein identification was performed by western blot analysis of the samples used for 2D electrophoresis. Antibodies against 16 proteins were analysed. Protein identities with the highest VIP < 20 were prioritised for analysis. Antibodies were selected based on the qualitative and quantitative recognition of protein bands, and protein detection was confirmed using positive control cell lines (Additional file 1: Table S2). Initially, we analysed several antibodies against each protein and identified useful antibodies for detection of biomarkers from the 2D gels (Fig. 2).

Several isoforms of the identified proteins were detected by western blot. ERP29 was detected in both 2D and western blot at around 29 kDa as a double band, however only the upper band corresponded to protein spot #1525 from the 2D analysis. The identified isoform, with NCBI accession number NP-006808, had both experimental and theoretical pI of around 6.5. The particular band could be singled out by a mouse monoclonal antibody (83,073, Abcam, Cambridge, UK) and was confirmed by 2D Western blot (Fig. 2b). CRKL was located at 25 kDa on 2D and in western blot the correct isoform was identified among four detected bands. Finally, both the 60 kDa and 53 kDa isoforms of SRC were recognised as part of the biomarker panel.

Verification of platelet biomarkers by western blot and DigiWest data

Expression of proteins in western blot was normalized against the levels of 14–3-3-gamma, which is a more stable and relevant loading control for platelet proteins compared to GAPDH [18]. PCA was performed individually in each set of blotted membranes in order to look for major trends and grouping of the samples by observing the scores plots. These represented three repetitions of the experiment, with four groups per experiment. The PCA scores plots showed consistent separation between benign adnexal lesions from the cases of ovarian cancer, FIGO stages III-IV, as it was observed in 10 of the 12 PCA's scores plots.

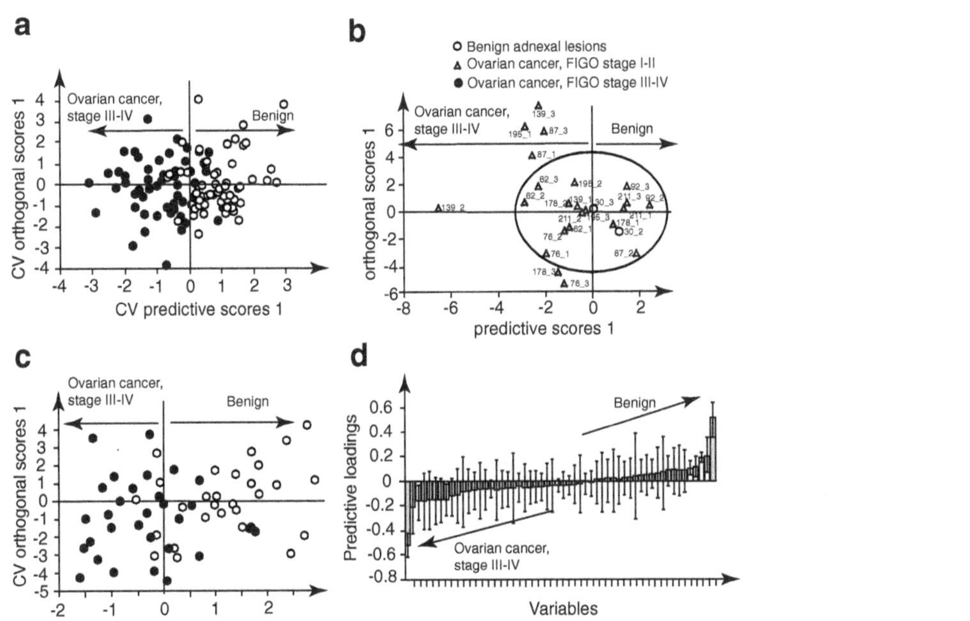

Fig. 3 Statistical analysis of the protein expression levels. **a** Cross-validated model built upon protein expression in benign and ovarian cancer, FIGO stage III-IV – western blot data, **b** Test model detecting the cases of ovarian cancer, FIGO stage I-II – western blot data, **c** Cross-validated model built upon protein expression in benign and of ovarian cancer, FIGO stage III-IV – DigiWest data, **d** Relative contribution of variables within the model on the separation between benign adnexal lesions and ovarian cancer, FIGO stage III-IV – DigiWest data

There was nonetheless some intrinsic batch variability, which could potentially be explained primarily by differences in the gels prepared for each batch, uneven protein transfer from gel to membrane, and suboptimal quantification of the protein bands expressed. Due to such variability, data were centred per batch previous to OPLS-DA modeling. After proper validation of the OPLS-DA model as described in the statistical section, results of the verification by western blot revealed a sensitivity of 83% (50/60) and a specificity of 89% (53/60) for separation between benign adnexal lesions and ovarian cancer, FIGO stages III-IV (Fig. 3a, Table 2b).

Next, model was tested for its predictive capacity. The correct prediction of two out of three samples per case was set as an acceptance criterion. Seven out of eight cases of ovarian cancer, FIGO stages I-II were predicted correctly (88% sensitivity). Sample 30 was reclassified by histology as benign and the prediction model confirmed this reclassification (Fig. 3b). Nine protein variables were suggested as a biomarker panel. In ovarian cancer, FIGO stages III-IV, seven protein variables were up-regulated and two variables were down-regulated. The ROC analysis of the detected nine-variable panel suggested discrimination between benign adnexal lesions and ovarian cancer, FIGO stages III-IV with a sensitivity of 60% and a specificity of 83% (Table 2c – ROC1) and between benign adnexal lesions and ovarian cancer, FIGO stages I-II with a sensitivity of 83% and a specificity of 76% (Table 2c – ROC2).

Next, the panel was verified by DigiWest with inclusion of a new, larger set of samples that were not previously used for 2D gel electrophoresis and western blot analysis. The expression profiles were analysed by OPLS-DA and the DigiWest based prediction model suggested a sensitivity of 70% (21/30) and a specificity of 83% (24/29) for the separation between benign adnexal lesions and ovarian cancer, FIGO stages III-IV (Fig. 3c, Table 2d). The verification of biomarker candidates by DigiWest suggested seven protein variables as seen in the loadings plot in Fig. 3d; three protein variables were increased in ovarian cancer, FIGO stages III-IV and four were decreased. We observed a correspondence between western blot and DigiWest analysis regarding the potential value of six identified proteins as biomarkers, of which three were increased in ovarian cancer, FIGO stages III-IV and three were decreased in both western blot and DigiWest.

Discussion

In this study, we analysed the proteome of platelets isolated from peripheral blood of patients with ovarian cancer, FIGO stages I-II and III-IV, and benign adnexal lesions. By PLS-DA modelling of protein expression in 2D gels we observed the possibility to correctly differentiate between cases of benign adnexal lesions and ovarian cancer, FIGO stages III-IV, and correctly predict cases of FIGO stages I-II. These findings were verified by western blot and DigiWest.

Table 4 Function of proteins biomarkers in relation to ovarian cancer and platelets

Protein name	Associated pathologic conditions	
	ovarian cancer	platelet disorders
ACTN1	not studied	macrotrombocytopenia [37, 38]
ACTN4	↑ in ovarian cancer [39]	myelodysplastic syndrome [38, 40]
CD41/CD61	platelets contribute to ovarian cancer growth [35]	deficient in Glanzmann thrombasthenia type II [41]
CRKL	↑ in ovarian cancer [42]	ST - elevated myocadial infarction [43]
ERP29	not studied	mediator of thrombus formation [44]
GELS	↑ in serum in ovarian cancer [45]	↑ in megakaryoblastic leukemia [46], ↑ in thrombin-activated platelets [47]
HSPA8	↑ in ovarian cancer, a potential therapy target [48]	mediator of thromboembolism [49]
MPST	not studied	not clarified
PHB	↑ in paclitaxel-resistant ovarian cancer [30] ↓ in platinum-resistant ovarian cancer [32]	mediator of platelet aggregation [50]
SRC	therapy-target for thyrosine-kinase inhibitor in ovarian cancer [51], resistance to cis-platin [33]	ST - elevated myocadial infarction [43]
SERPINB6	not studied	inhibitor of thrombin [25]
TLN1	↑ in ovarian cancer [52], resistance to cis-platin [33]	myelodysplastic syndrome [40]
TUBB1, TUBA4	↑ in ovarian cancer, mediator of paclitaxel resistance [31]	↑ in thrombin-activated platelets [47], gene mutation in autosomal dominant macrothrombocytopenia [25]
WDR1	↑ in ovarian cancer [53], resistance to cis-platin [34]	mediator of TLN1-induced activation of CD41/CD61 [54]

↑ corresponds up-regulation, ↓ corresponds down-regulation

In the prospectively collected clinical material, there were 57 cases of benign adnexal lesions, 49 cases of ovarian cancer, FIGO stages III-IV, and 8 cases of ovarian cancer, FIGO stages I-II. Overrepresentation of advanced ovarian cancer patients (80% of all cases) in our study reflects the worldwide situation regarding the detection rate of the disease at its advanced stages [1]. The initial PCA provided an indication of degree of correspondence between protein profiles of the compared groups. PLS-DA allowed us to build a multivariate regression model. Through PLS-DA it became possible to 1) "filter" the high level of biological background noise by using only the latent variables related to the biological variation of interest, 2) build a training model and use it to predict the class of earlier cancer test samples, and 3) identify the most discriminant variables within the multiplex profile by observing their variable importance in projection (VIP), i.e. ranking in the model [22–24].

Our proteome analysis was based on 2D gel electrophoresis, which made it possible to identify full-length proteins and also their isoforms with regards to their relevance for the protein marker panel. The verification of identified platelet proteins suggested the possibility for separating benign adnexal lesions, ovarian cancer, FIGO stages I-II and III-IV. However, verification by western blot has inherently several disadvantages, such as gel batch variability, protein transfer limitations, and semi-quantitive output. DigiWest, a recently developed system that represents a high-throughput multiplex version of the classical western blot method, uses a bead-based microarray platform for signal generation [19]. The sensitivity, signal linearity, and reproducibility of DigiWest are comparable to or exceed the best available western blot systems. Compared to the western blot method, DigiWest provides higher reproducibility with simultaneous analysis of up to 100 samples and quantification of individual cases.

The function of the 16 identified and immunovalidated platelet proteins was described using the Platelet Web database [25] (Additional file 1: Table S3).

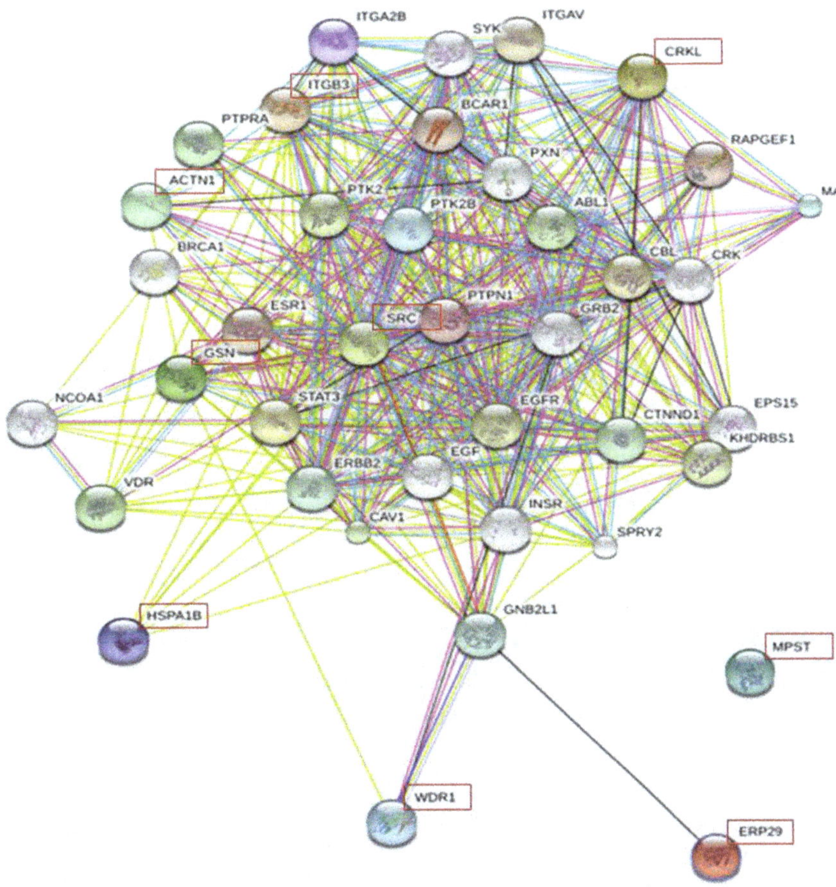

Fig. 4 Functional interaction profile of identified platelet proteins [36]. Lines represent interaction, where thick lines suggest a substantial number of references, thin lines correspond to single studies, arrows point the direction of activation influence, and block signs describe inhibitory actions

Most of these proteins are reported to have a functional relevance to ovarian cancer, normal platelet biology and platelet-associated pathological conditions (Table 4). Published proteomics and molecular biology studies suggest up-regulation of ACTN4, CRKL, GELS, HSPA8, talin-1, tubulins and WDR1 in ovarian cancer. Expression changes and possible functional impact of ACTN1 [26], MPST [27], ERP29 [28] and SERPINB6 [29] are reported for several cancers, but not for ovarian cancer. PHB, SRC, talin-1, tubulins and WDR1 are related to development of ovarian cancer resistance to paclitaxel [30, 31] and cis-platin [32–34]. An interesting observation is an increased expression level of CD41/CD61 in platelets associated with tumor xenografts as well as enhanced tumor growth in the presence of platelets [35].

Using the STRING database [36], we analyzed potential interactions and functional impact of the identified platelet proteins on other known protein targets (Additional file 1: Table S4, Fig. 4). Most described protein interactions are related to CRKL, SRC, CD61, GELS (GSN), and ACTN1, while information is limited regarding the interaction profile of MPST, ERP29, HSPA8, and WDR1.

Limitations of the current study include dependency of sensitivity and specificity on the quantitative properties of the verification method and analysis of relatively small groups of clinical material. Multivariate PLS-DA-based statistics partially allowed us to overcome the problem of small clinical groups, however, further validation using clinical material from patients with early-stage ovarian cancer and borderline ovarian tumors is expected to strengthen the diagnostic sensitivity and specificity. Combination of the marker panel with the TVS protocol, which evaluates malignant potential of adnexal masses, towards a biochemical-instrumental test is the final goal. The objective diagnosis of adnexal lesions will help clinicians to correctly refer patients to a gynaecological cancer specialist, thus minimizing the cost of additional examinations and delays for patients needing advanced treatment. The panel detected is currently being developed as a new non-invasive in vitro diagnostic multivariate index-based analytical method for differentiation of adnexal lesions.

Conclusion

The identified platelet protein panel allows for differentiation between benign adnexal lesions and ovarian cancers of FIGO stages III-IV. Correct prediction of seven out of eight cases of ovarian cancer, FIGO stages I-II was possible through multivariate prediction modeling based on platelet protein expression profiles.

Abbreviations

2D: Two-dimensional; ANOVA: Analysis of variance; AUC: Area under the curve; CV: Cross validation; DA: Discriminant analysis; FIGO: International Federation of Gynaecology and Obstetrics; IOTA: International Ovarian Tumor Association.; LDS: Lithium dodecyl sulfate.; PCA: Principal components analysis.; PF-4: Platelet factor 4.; PLS: Projection to latent structures (or partial least squares).; PMF: Peptide mass fingerprint.; RCF: Relative centrifugal force.; ROC: Receiver-operator curve.; RMI: Risk of malignancy index.; STED: Stimulated emission depletion.; TVS: Transvaginal ultrasound.; VEGF: Vascular endothelial growth factor.; VIP: Variable importance in projection.; X: Data matrix (number of rows equal to number of samples, number of columns equal to number of variables).; Y: Column vector (with one element per sample).

Acknowledgements

We acknowledge Teddy Primack and Michael Vanlandewijck for language assistance.

Funding

This work was supported by grants from the Cancer Research Foundations of Radiumhemmet, Stockholm Count County: HMT 20130704 and HMT 20140754, KI Fonder 2013fobi37433, Dagmar Ferbs Minnesfond 2012–2016, Vinnova 2014–03458 to NeoProteomics AB.

Authors' contributions

LM, FB, AG, WJ, EE planned the project, selected patients, interpreted results, LM and EE recruited patients for the study, BS, BC, GS performed preparation of the platelet fraction, 2D gel electrophoresis, western blot, EU performed mass-spectrometry, TM performed Digi west analysis, XL, BJ performed analysis of platelets using high-resolution microscopy, PR performed statistical analysis, LM performed ROC curve analysis, LM, FB, PR and AG were the major contributors in writing the manuscript. All authors read and approved the final manuscript.

Competing interests

Authors Gustafsson Sonja, Björklund Christina, Franzén Bo and Auer Gert are affiliated to NeoProteomics AB. Other authors declare no competing interests.

Author details

[1]Department of Obstetrics and Gynaecology, Academical Uppsala University Hospital, Uppsala University, SE-751 85 Uppsala, Sweden. [2]Institute of Women's and Children's Health, Karolinska Institute, SE-171 76 Stockholm, Sweden. [3]Department of Oncology and Pathology, Cancer Centre Karolinska, Karolinska Institute, SE-171 76 Stockholm, Sweden. [4]Department of Epidemiology and Biostatistics, MRC-PHE Centre for Environment and Health, School of Public Health, Imperial College London, St. Mary's Campus, Norfolk Place, W2 1PG, London, England, UK. [5]Ludwig Institute for Cancer Research Ltd, Box 595, SE-751 24 Uppsala, Sweden. [6]NeoProteomics AB, Cancer Centre Karolinska, SE-17176 Stockholm, Sweden. [7]NMI Natural and Medical Sciences Institute at the University of Tübingen, 72770 Reutlingen, Germany. [8]Experimental Biomolecular Physics, Department of Applied Physics, Royal Institute of Technology, AlbaNova University Center, SE-106 91 Stockholm, Sweden. [9]Department of Obstetrics and Gynaecology, Department of Clinical Science and Education, Södersjukhuset, SE-118 83 Stockholm, Sweden.

References

1. De Angelis R, Sant M, Coleman MP, Francisci S, Baili P, Pierannunzio D, et al. Cancer survival in Europe 1999-2007 by country and age: results of EUROCARE-5-a population-based study. Lancet Oncol. 2014;15(1):23–34.
2. Jacobs IA, Menon U, Ryan A, Gentry-Maharaj A, Burnell M, Kalsi JK, et al. Ovarian cancer screening and mortality in the UK collaborative trial of ovarian cancer screening (UKCTOCS): a randomised controlled trial. Lancet. 2016;387(10022):945–56.

3. Biggs WS, Marks ST. Diagnosis and Management of Adnexal Masses. Am Fam Physician. 2016;93(8):676–81.
4. Valentin L, Ameye L, Savelli L, Fruscio R, Leone FP, Czekierdowski A, et al. Adnexal masses difficult to classify as benign or malignant using subjective assessment of gray-scale and Doppler ultrasound findings: logistic regression models do not help. Ultrasound in Obstet Gynecol. 2011;38(4):456–65.
5. Timmerman D, Valentin L, Bourne TH, Collins WP, Verrelst H, Vergote I. Terms, definitions and measurements to describe the sonographic features of adnexal tumors: a consensus opinion from the international ovarian tumor analysis (IOTA) group. Ultrasound in Obstet Gynecol. 2000;16(5):500–5.
6. Kaijser J, Van Belle V, Van Gorp T, Sayasneh A, Vergote I, Bourne T, Van Calster B, Timmerman D. Prognostic value of serum HE4 levels and risk of ovarian malignancy algorithm scores at the time of ovarian cancer diagnosis. Int J Gynecol Cancer. 2014;24(7):1173–80.
7. Allensworth SK, Langstraat CL, Martin JR, Lemens MA, McGree ME, Weaver AL, et al. Evaluating the prognostic significance of preoperative thrombocytosis in epithelial ovarian cancer. Gynecol Oncol. 2013;130(3): 499–504.
8. Wan S, Lai Y, Myers RE, Li B, Hyslop T, London J, et al. Preoperative platelet count associates with survival and distant metastasis in surgically resected colorectal cancer patients. J Gastrointest Cancer. 2013;44(3):293–304.
9. Gay LJ, Felding-Habermann B. Contribution of platelets to tumor metastasis. Nat Rev Cancer. 2012;11:123–34.
10. Buergy D, Wenz F, Groden C, Brockmann MA. Tumor-platelet interaction in solid tumors. Int J Cancer. 2012;130:2747–60.
11. Senzel L, Gnatenko DV, Bahou WF. The platelet proteome. Curr Opin Hematol. 2009;16(5):329–33.
12. Klement GL, Yip TT, Cassiola F, Kikuchi L, Cervi D, Podust V, et al. Platelets actively sequester angiogenesis regulators. Blood. 2009;133:2835–42.
13. Folkman J, Klement G. Platelet biomarkers for the detection of disease. Patent US20060204951A1, 2006.
14. Rönnlund D, Yang Y, Blom H, Auer G, Widengren J. Fluorescence nanoscopy of platelets resolves platelet-specific storage, release and uptake of proteins, opening for future diagnostic applications. Adv. Healthcare Mater. 2012;1(6):707–13.
15. Reicheltová Z, Májek P, Riedel T, Suttnar J, Dyr JE. Simplified platelet sample preparation for SDS-PAGE-based proteomic studies. Proteomics Clin Appl. 2012;6(7–8):374–81.
16. Bradford MM. Rapid and sensitive method for the quantitation of microgram quantities of protein utilizing the principle of protein-dye binding. Anal Biochem. 1976;72:248–54.
17. Lomnytska M, Becker S, Gemoll T, Lundgren C, Habermann J, Olsson A, et al. Impact of genomic stability on protein expression in endometrioid endometrial cancer. Br J Cancer. 2012;106(7):1297–305.
18. Baumgartner R, Umlauf E, Veitinger M, Guterres S, Rappold E, Babeluk R, et al. Identification and validation of platelet low biological variation proteins, superior to GAPDH, actin and tubulin, as tools in clinical proteomics. J Proteome. 2013;94:540–51.
19. Treindl F, Ruprecht B, Beiter Y, Schultz S, Döttinger A, Staebler A, et al. A bead-based western for high-throughput cellular signal transduction analyses. Nat Commun. 2016;7:12852.
20. Jolliffe IT. Principal Component Analysis, Series:Springer Series in Statistics. 2nd ed. Springer: NY; 2002.
21. Wold S, Sjöström M, Eriksson L. PLS-regression: a basic tool of chemometrics. Chemom Intell Lab Syst. 2011;58:109–30.
22. Ottervald J, Franzén B, Nilsson K, Andersson LI, Khademi M, Eriksson B, et al. Multiple sclerosis: identification and clinical evaluation of novel CSF biomarkers. J Proteome. 2010;73(6):1117–32.
23. Bylesjo M, Rantalainen M, Cloarec O, Nicholson JK, Holmes E, Trygg JOPLS. Discriminant analysis: combining the strengths of PLS-DA and SIMCA classification. J Chemometrics. 2006;20(9–10):341–51.
24. Pinto R.C. Chemometrics methods and strategies in metabolomics. In: Sussulini a. (eds) metabolomics: from fundamentals to clinical applications. Advances in experimental medicine and biology, vol 965. Springer, Champions, 2017.
25. Boyanova D, Nilla S, Birschmann I, Dandekar T, Dittrich M. PlateletWeb: a systems biologic analysis of signaling networks in human platelets. Blood. 2012;119(3):e22–34.
26. Kanamori H, Kawakami T, Effendi K, Yamazaki K, Mori T, Ebinuma H, et al. Identification by differential tissue proteome analysis of talin-1 as a novel molecular marker of progression of hepatocellular carcinoma. Oncology. 2011;80(5–6):406–15.
27. Bronowicka-Adamska P, Bentke A, Wróbel M. Hydrogen sulfide generation from l-cysteine in the human glioblastoma-astrocytoma U-87 MG and neuroblastoma SHSY5Y cell lines. Acta Biochim Pol. 2017;64(1):171–6.
28. Fan NJ, Gao JL, Liu Y, Song W, Zhang ZY, Gao CF. Label-free quantitative mass spectrometry reveals a panel of differentially expressed proteins in colorectal cancer. Biomed Res Int. 2015:365068.
29. Ha ES, Choi S, In KH, Lee SH, Lee EJ, Lee SY, et al. Identification of proteins expressed differently among surgically resected stage I lung adenocarcinomas. Clin Biochem. 2013;46(4–5):369–77.
30. Cao L, Li X, Zhang Y, Peng F, Yi H, Xu Y, et al. Proteomic analysis of human ovarian cancer paclitaxel-resistant cell lines. Zhong Nan Da Xue Xue Bao Yi Xue Ban. 2010;35(4):286–94.
31. Vergara D, Tinelli A, Iannone A, Maffia M. The impact of proteomics in the understanding of the molecular basis of paclitaxel-resistance in ovarian tumors. Curr Cancer Drug Targets. 2012;12(8):987–97.
32. Dai Z, Yin J, He H, Li W, Hou C, Qian X, et al. Mitochondrial comparative proteomics of human ovarian cancer cells and their platinum-resistant sublines. Proteomics. 2010;10(21):3789–99.
33. Sansing HA, Sarkeshik A, Yates JR, Patel V, Gutkind JS, Yamada KM, Berrier AL. Integrin αβ1, αvβ, α6β effectors p130Cas, Src and talin regulate carcinoma invasion and chemoresistance. Biochem Biophys Res Commun. 2011;406(2):171–6.
34. Kim SW, Kim S, Nam EJ, Jeong YW, Lee SH, Paek JH, et al. Comparative proteomic analysis of advanced serous epithelial ovarian carcinoma: possible predictors of chemoresistant disease. OMICS. 2011;15(5):281–92.
35. Yuan L, Liu X. Platelets are associated with xenograft tumor growth and the clinical malignancy of ovarian cancer through an angiogenesis-dependent mechanism. Mol Med Rep. 2015;11(4):2449–58.
36. Franceschini A, Szklarczyk D, Frankild S, Kuhn M, Simonovic M, Roth A, et al. STRING v9.1: protein-protein interaction networks, with increased coverage and integration. Nucleic Acids Res. 2013;41(Database issue):D808–15.
37. Westbury SK, Shoemark DK, Mumford AD. ACTN1 variants associated with thrombocytopenia. Platelets. 2017;28(6):625–7.
38. Finamore F, Pieroni L, Ronci M, Marzano V, Mortera SL, Romano M, et al. Proteomics investigation of human platelets by shotgun nUPLC-MSE and 2DE experimental strategies: a comparative study. Blood Transfus. 2010; 8(Suppl 3):s140–8.
39. Honda K. The biological role of actinin-4 (ACTN4) in malignant phenotypes of cancer. Cell Biosci. 2015;5:41.
40. Fröbel J, Cadeddu RP, Hartwig S, Bruns I, Wilk CM, Kündgen A, et al. Platelet proteome analysis reveals integrin-dependent aggregation defects in patients with myelodysplastic syndromes. Mol Cell Proteomics. 2013;12(5):1272–80.
41. Mutreja D, Sharma RK, Purohit A, Aggarwal M, Saxena R. Evaluation of platelet surface glycoproteins in patients with Glanzmann thrombasthenia: association with bleeding symptoms. Indian J Med Res. 2017;145(5):629–34.
42. Luo LY, Hahn WC. Oncogenic signaling adaptor proteins. J Genet Genomics. 2015;42(10):521–9.
43. Parguiña AF, Grigorian-Shamagian L, Agra RM, López-Otero D, Rosa I, Alonso J, et al. Variations in platelet proteins associated with ST-elevation myocardial infarction: novel clues on pathways underlying platelet activation in acute coronary syndromes. Arterioscler Thromb Vasc Biol. 2011; 31(12):2957–64.
44. Schulman S, Bendapudi P, Sharda A, Chen V, Bellido-Martin L, Jasuja R, et al. Extracellular thiol isomerases and their role in thrombus formation. Antioxid Redox Signal. 2016;24(1):1–15.
45. Pierredon S, Ribaux P, Tille JC, Petignat P, Cohen M. Comparative secretome of ovarian serous carcinoma: gelsolin in the spotlight. Oncol Lett. 2017; 13(6):4965–73.
46. Zunino R, Li Q, Rosé SD, Romero-Benítez MM, Lejen T, Brandan NC, Trifaró JM. Expression of scinderin in megakaryoblastic leukemia cells induces differentiation, maturation, and apoptosis with release of plateletlike particles and inhibits proliferation and tumorigenesis. Blood. 2001;98(7):2210–9.
47. Peña E, Padro T, Molins B, Vilahur G, Badimon L. Proteomic signature of thrombin-activated platelets after in vivo nitric oxide-donor treatment: coordinated inhibition of signaling (phosphatidylinositol 3-kinase-γ, 14-3-3ζ, and growth factor receptor-bound protein 2) and cytoskeleton protein translocation. Arterioscler Thromb Vasc Biol. 2011;31(11):2560–9.
48. Saini J, Sharma PK. Clinical, prognostic and therapeutic significance of heat shock proteins in cancer. Curr Drug Targets. 2017; https://doi.org/10.2174/1389450118666170823121248.

49. Karmakar S, Banerjee D, Chakrabarti A. Platelet proteomics in thalassemia: factors responsible for hypercoagulation. Proteomics Clin Appl. 2016; 10(3):239–47.
50. Wang YJ, Guo XL, Li SA, Zhao YQ, Liu ZC, et al. Prohibitin is involved in the activated internalization and degradation of protease-activated receptor 1. Biochim Biophys Acta. 2014;1843(7):1393–401.
51. Awasthi N, Schwarz RE. Profile of nintedanib in the treatment of solid tumors: the evidence to date. Onco Targets Ther. 2015;8:3691–701.
52. Tang H, Yao L, Tao X, Yu Y, Chen M, Zhang R, Xu C. miR-9 functions as a tumor suppressor in ovarian serous carcinoma by targeting TLN1. Int J Mol Med. 2013;32(2):381–8.
53. Haslene-Hox H, Oveland E, Woie K, Salvesen HB, Wiig H, Tenstad O. Increased WD-repeat containing protein 1 in interstitial fluid from ovarian carcinomas shown by comparative proteomic analysis of malignant and healthy gynecological tissue. Biochim Biophys Acta. 2013;1834(11):2347–59.
54. Dasgupta SK, Le A, Da Q, Cruz M, Rumbaut RE, Thiagarajan P. Wdr1-dependent actin reorganization in platelet activation. PLoS One. 2016; 11(9):e0162897.

23

SRSF2 mutations in myelodysplasia/ myeloproliferative neoplasms

Amandeep Aujla[1], Katherine Linder[2†], Chaitanya Iragavarapu[3†], Michael Karass[1] and Delong Liu[1,4*]

Abstract

Recurrent gene mutations have been described with varying frequencies in myelodysplasia (MDS) /myeloproliferative neoplasm (MPN) overlap syndromes (MMOS). Recent work has placed significant focus on understanding the role of gene lesions involving the spliceosomal machinery in leukemogeneis. SRSF2 is a gene encoding critical spliceosomal proteins. SRSF2 mutations appear to play an important role in pathogenesis of MMOS, particularly in chronic myelomonocytic leukemia. Inhibition of splicing may be a new therapeutic approach. E7107, a spliceosome inhibitor, has been shown to differentially inhibit splicing more in SRSF2-mutant cells leading to decreased leukemia burden in mice. H3B-8800 is a small molecule modulator of spliceosome complex and has been shown to lower leukemia burden in SRSF2-P95H mutant mice. This review focuses on the incidence of mutant SRSF2 across various MMOS as well as recent clinical development of spliceosome inhibitors.

Background

Myelodysplastic and myeloproliferative overlap syndromes (MMOS) were initially recognized as a unique entity in the third edition of WHO classification of myeloid neoplasms [1]. This group initially had three disorders - chronic myelomonocytic leukemia (CMML), atypical chronic myeloid leukemia, BCR-ABL1$^-$ (aCML), and juvenile myelomonocytic leukemia (JMML). The fourth entity, MDS/MPN with ringed sideroblasts and thrombocytosis (MDS/MPN-RS-T, previously known as RARS-T), was added in the 2016 revision of WHO classification [2]. Currently, MMOS also includes a fifth group, MDS/MPN unclassifiable, which is inclusive of all other MDS/MPN -like syndromes that do not meet diagnostic criteria for the above.

With the increasing use of next-gene sequencing and molecular studies in clinical practice, new patterns of gene mutations are being reported in myeloid neoplasms [3–8]. These mutations are being used as biomarkers for classification and druggable targets [9–12]. A variety of small molecules including ruxolitinib, enasidenib, midostaurin, and AG-120 are in clinical applications and/or late-stage clinical development [13–21].

MDS/MPN overlap syndromes can present with overlapping clinical and morphological features of both MDS (peripheral cytopenia and/or dysplastic bone marrow) and clonal proliferation (leukocytosis, thrombocytosis or organomegaly) during the initial diagnosis [22]. Genomic aberrations have been reported at a frequency as high as 75% along with multiple somatic mutations [23]. Most common mutations reported are TET2, ASXL1 and/or SRSF2 in CMML, NRAS/KRAS in JMML, SETBP1 in aCML and JAK-STAT and/or SF3B1 in MDS/MPN-RS-T [24–27]. This review focuses on SRSF2 mutations across various entities of MMOS.

SRSF2

SRSF2 (Serine and arginine Rich Splicing Factor 2), also called SC35 and SRp30b, belongs to the SR (Serine and Arginine rich) protein family [28, 29]. It was recognized first in 1990 by Fu and Maniatis using a monocloncal antibody developed against mammalian spliceosomes [30]. It was reported to play a role in splicing during spliceosome assembly [31, 32]. SRSF2 has a RNA recognition motif and thus promotes spliceosome assembly at adjacent splice sites to allow appropriate exon inclusion [28, 33, 34]. In addition, SRSF2 was reported to play an active role in transcription elongation and in coupling transcription and splicing processes [35, 36].

* Correspondence: delong_liu@nymc.edu
†Katherine Linder and Chaitanya Iragavarapu contributed equally to this work.
[1]Department of Medicine, New York Medical College and Westchester Medical Center, Valhalla, NY, USA
[4]The affiliated Cancer Hospital of Zhengzhou University and Henan Cancer Hospital, 127 Dongming Road, Zhengzhou 450008, China

SRSF2 in oncogenesis

The oncogenic potential of SRSF2 was first demonstrated in SRSF2 knock-out mouse embryo fibroblasts (MEFs). SRSF2 mutation increased double-strand DNA breaks, p53 hyperphosphorylation and hyperacetylation with cell cycle arrest [37]. Similar findings were also duplicated in mouse hematopoietic cells, with growth arrest, early senescence and apoptosis in SRSF2 deleted cells [38]. In another study based on similar intervention, SRSF2 homozygous knock-out mice showed 70–90% loss of thymocytes with significantly increased CD4-/CD8- T cells and decreased CD4+/CD8+ T cells. Thus, loss of SRSF2 seemed to affect T cell maturation in thymus, possibly secondary to altered splicing of CD45 as reported in the study [39].

While loss of SRSF2 led to decreased survival, mutant SRSF2 (SRSF2-mut) expression was associated with oncogenesis. Direct association of SRSF2 in development of myelodysplasia was demonstrated in SRSF2-P95H mutant mice [40]. P95H is the most common mutation site in the SRSF2 gene [41–45] and its proximity to RRM site of SRSF2 might play a role in altering RNA binding abilities [38] [46]. Heterozygous P95H mutant and homozygous SRSF2 deleted bone marrow mononuclear cells led to development of significant leukopenia and anemia in lethally irradiated recipient mice. However, only P95H mutated mice developed macrocytic RBCs and had normal bone marrow cellularity in contrast to bone marrow aplasia seen with homozygous SRSF2 deletion. Peripheral erythroid and myeloid dysplasia was also seen only with P95H mutant mice [40]. These findings correlate with MDS findings in humans.

SRSF2 mutant cells have been shown to require wild-type (WT) SRSF2 allele for the cell survival, explaining the phenotypic differences between heterozygous and homozygous genotypes [47]. Hemizygous SRSF2P95H/−mice had shorter survival with severe bone marrow aplasia in contrast to SRSF2P95H/+ mice ($p = 0.004$). Hemizygous cells also showed two-fold higher mis-splicing events compared to heterozygous cells [48]. Similar oncogenic associations secondary to mis-splicing have also been reported with other splicing factor mutations such as U2AF1 and SF3B1 [49] [50, 51]. SRSF2 mutation frequently occurs in close association with these and other mutations [26, 42, 44]. During disease progression of MDS, additional mutations are acquired [52].

SRSF2 in MDS/MPN overlap syndromes

CMML

In 2011, Yoshida et al. identified frequently recurring splicing factor mutations in a cohort of adult patients with myeloid neoplasms through performing whole-exome sequencing. SF3B1 (36%) was the most common mutation followed by SRSF2 (25.6%), U2AF35 (16.9%) and ZRSR2 (10.5%) [8]. These mutations were more frequent and comparatively more specific to the diseases with myelodysplastic features (MDS, CMML, t-AML and AML-MRC) [43]. SRSF2 mutation was reported with a high frequency of 28–47% [41–43, 53] in other cohorts of CMML patients and was reported to be significantly associated with higher age, higher hemoglobin, normal karyotype and TET2 mutation [26, 45, 54]. Interestingly, it occurred mutually exclusively with EZH2 mutation [42, 44]. No significant association had been reported with leukocytosis, blast percentage, WHO histologic categories (CMML-1 and CMML-2) or cytogenetic risk categories. No specific morphological or immunohistochemical features in the bone marrow (e.g. dysplasia, CD14 and CD34 positive cells) were significantly associated with SRSF2 mutations in a study done on MDS/MPN entities. SRSF2 testing on bone marrow specimens was shown to be 44.4% sensitive and 88.1% specific in diagnosing CMML over MDS or MPN; with modest positive likelihood ratio of 3.73 [45].

SRSF2 has been associated with worse survival outcomes in low-risk MDS patients and PMF [43, 44, 55] but evidence has not been very clear among MDS/MPN overlap syndromes. Earlier studies investigating SRSF2 mutations in MDS/MPN overlap syndromes reported no influence of SRSF2-mut on overall survival (OS) either in CMML or other MDS/MPN overlap syndromes [26, 42, 56]. The only impact SRSF2-mut had on survival was noted by Meggendorfer et al. analyzing a series of CMML patients. Patients co-harboring RUNX1 and SRSF2 mutations appeared to have improved OS compared to those who possessed wild-type (WT) variants.

An international cohort study showed poor OS outcomes associated with the SRSF2 mutations in CMML patients aged ≤65 years but with non-significant difference among leukemic transformation rates [57]. Similar outcomes with decreased OS along with decreased progression free survival (PFS) or leukemia free survival (LFS) were also reported in two studies that enrolled 56 and 312 CMML patients, respectively [27, 58]. Additional factors that negatively influenced OS as per multivariate analyses were older age (> 65 years, $p = 0.04$), WBC $> 15 \times 10^9$/L ($p < 0.0001$), presence of anemia (hemoglobin < 10 g/dL in women and < 11 g/dL in men; $p = 0.0002$), thrombocytopenia ($< 100 \times 10^9$/L; $p < 0.0001$) and an absolute lymphocyte count (ALC) $> 4 \times 10^9$/L ($p = 0.03$) [27, 56]. Genotypically, ASXL1 was the only mutation which predicted inferior OS and LFS in multivariate analyses.

Multiple prognostic models based on phenotypic and cytogenetic characteristics have been developed for CMML. These include the MD Anderson Prognostic Score (MDAPS) [59], the Spanish Cytogenetic Risk Stratification [60] and the CMML Prognostic Scoring System (CPSS) [61]. The MDAPS and the CPSS were dependent on clinical factors and/or basic laboratory findings. The CPSS also incorporated the Genetic Risk

Score as determined by the Spanish risk stratification. More recently, attempts have been made to incorporate ASXL1 mutation status into these models based on previous data regarding impact on survival. Recently, two more prognostic models were proposed; the Groupe Francophone des Myelodysplasies (GFM) model [27] and the Mayo molecular model [62]. Of note, the GFM model was validated in a separate cohort of 165 patients with a median follow up of 27.3 months [27].

The CPSS was also updated to incorporate the impact of multiple mutations including ASXL1, NRAS, RUNX1 and SETBP1. The updated system, named CPSS-Mol, assigned variable scores to different mutations as well as the cytogenetic abnormalities [63]. A composite score was then determined using phenotypic variables as defined by CPSS and the "Genetic Risk Group". Four risk categories were delineated and the scoring system was validated in a separate cohort of 286 patients. Lastly, prognostic implications of different types of missense mutations occurring at the P95 site of SRSF2 gene have also been reported; the P95H variant being reported to have better outcomes compared to P95L or P95A [42]. Table 1 summarizes the various studies evaluating SRSF2 mutation frequency and reported impact on overall and progression free survival in CMML.

JMML

Among a cohort of 371 children, SRSF2 mutation was only seen in 2 patients and both with normal karyotype along with co-existing RAS mutations [64]. Both patients received HSCT in the study. One relapsed with loss of SRSF2 mutation at relapse; while RAS mutation persisted. In two other studies, only 1/76 patients with JMML carried a SRSF2 mutation [26, 65]. This mutation had not been described previously and was reported as in-frame deletion in contrast to mis-sense mutations seen in adults. Although morphologically similar, genotypic characteristics of JMML are distinct from those of CMML with RAS, PTPN11, NFI and CBL. Rarity of splicing factor mutations in JMML and their loss at progression of disease likely precludes their independent role in its pathogenesis. The frequency of SRSF2 mutations in JMML was summarized in Table 2.

Atypical CML, *BCR-ABL1*$^-$

Atypical CML (aCML) is a rare entity among MDS/MPN overlap syndromes characterized by the absence of the BCR-ABL1 fusion gene as well as rearrangements of the PDGFRA, PDGFRB or FGFR1 genes [24]. ASXL1 (20–70%), SETBP1 (25–30%) and TET2 (43%) mutations are the most common mutations detected in aCML [66, 67]. SETBP1 mutations correlate with worse survival outcomes [68]. A high frequency of SRSF2 mutations (40%) was reported among a cohort of 60 aCML [54] while its frequency has been reported variably in other studies [67, 69, 70]. SRSF2 mutation appears more frequently with ASXL1-mut ($p = 0.01$) and SETBP1-mut ($p = 0.004$) compared to WT.

MDS/MPN-RS-t (RARS-t)

This entity was previously known as refractory anemia with ringed sideroblasts and thrombocytosis (RARS-T)

Table 1 SRSF2 mutations in chronic myelomonocytic leukemia

Reference	Disease	Frequency of SRSF2 mutation	Effect on Survival	Effect on disease progression
[8]	CMML	28.4%	NR	NR
[42]	CMML	47% (129/275)	No	No
[53]	CMML	46% (173/409)	NR	NR
[41]	CMML	40% (90/226)	No	No
[43]	CMML	28%	NR	NR
[64]	CMML	20% (1/5)	NR	NR
[26]	CMML	32% (28/87)	No	NR
[77]	CMML (Chinese population)	20% (10/50)	No	No
[45]	CMML	44% (16/36)	No	NR
[57]	CMML (aged < 65 years)	45% (72/161)	Yes	No
[58]	CMML	25% (14/56)	Yes	Yes
[27]	CMML	46% (143/312)	Yes	Yes
[56]	CMML	40% (90/226)	No	No
[52]	CMML	45% (116/274	NR	No
[54]	CMML	51% (74/146)	NR	NR
[67]	CMML	53% (31/58)	NR	NR

CMML Chronic Myelomonocytic Leukemia, *NR* not reported

Table 2 Frequency of SRSF2 mutations in myelodysplasia/myeloproliferative neoplasms*

Studies	Disease	Frequency of SRSF2
[64]	JMML	1.7% (2/116)
[26]	JMML	0%
[65]	JMML	3.7% (1/27)
[69]	aCML	0% (0/3)
[70]	aCML	12% (3/25)
[78]	aCML	40% (24/60)
[67]	aCML	34% (12/35)
	MDS/MPN-RS-T	9% (4/45)
[71]	RARS-T	6.7% (5/75)
[72]	RARS-T	2% (1/48)
[67]	MDS/MPN-U	15% (6/39)

Abbreviations: *MDS* myelodysplasia, *MPN* myeloproliferative neoplasm, *CMML* Chronic Myelomonocytic Leukemia, *JMML* Juvenile Myelomonocytic Leukemia, *aCML* atypical Chronic Myeloid Leukemia, *MPN/MDS-U* unclassifiable MDS/MPN. * SRSF2 mutations in CMML are listed in a separate table

and defined under the MDS/MPN-U umbrella diagnosis. This disease has now been accepted as a separate entity in 2016 revision of WHO classification [2]. Splicing factor mutations are common in this group, with SF3B1 being the most frequently occurring mutation (85–91%) [67, 71, 72]. SF3B1 mutation status is strongly associated with increased number of ringed sideroblasts ($p = 0.006$). JAK2 (33–59%), TET2 (10–31%) and ASXL1 (20–29%) are the other frequently occurring mutations in this entity. SRSF2 is comparatively less common (2–9%) and is mostly present in association with other mutations in genotypes carrying high mutation burden [71]. In a cohort of 75 patients, SRSF2 was present in 5 cases and all of them carried ≥4 mutations [60], suggesting that it is less likely to play a driver mutation role in this entity (Table 2).

MDS/MPN – Unclassifiable

MDS/MPN-U is another rare entity with heterogenous dysplastic and proliferative features except some distinct associations such as isolated trisomy 8 seen in about 15% of cases compared to MDS (5%) and MPN (4%) [73]. JAK2 mutation is one of the most common (23–66%) mutations reported in this group [67] but has not been reported to have prognostic importance. Other mutations occur in comparable frequencies, ASXL1 and TET2 (36%), U2AF1 (18%), SRSF2 (15%) and SF3B1 (13%). Overall, MDS/MPN-U presents a mixed picture as opposed to other MMOS. Thrombocytosis has been associated with improved survival in this group [73] but role of SRSF2 in pathogenesis or as prognostic indicator has not been well defined yet (Table 2).

Therapeutic implications of SRSF2

Aberrant spliceosome function secondary to mutated SRSF2 has been associated with mis-splicing of multiple genes (e.g. EZH2, RUNX1, BCOR, IKAROS and CASP8, etc.) that are implicated in pathogenesis of myeloid neoplasms [40, 43]. Inhibition of splicing has been analyzed as possible therapeutic target. E7107, a spliceosome inhibitor, has shown to differentially inhibit splicing more in SRSF2-mut cells leading to decreased leukemia burden in mice [47]. A phase 1 clinical trial investigating E7107 in metastatic or locally advanced solid tumors was discontinued prematurely due to vision loss reported as adverse event in 2 cases [74]. A parallel phase I trial conducted in Europe also reported one instance of grade 4 visual disturbance secondary to optic neuritis which improved after treatment with steroids. Nevertheless, the study was discontinued for safety concerns [75].

Another compound, H3B-8800, acts as a modulator of the SF3b complex. It has demonstrated a preferential cytotoxic effect on SF3B1-mutant cells secondary to GC-rich intronic retention [76]. Decreased leukemic burden was reported in SRSF2-P95H mutant mice compared to SRSF2-WT variants. A phase I clinical trial (NCT02841540) is underway to evaluate safety of this compound in patients with MDS, AML and CMML.

Conclusion

SRSF2 is a frequent mutation seen in MDS/MPN overlap syndromes, especially CMML. It has been shown to play a multi-faceted role during the oncogenesis of these disorders influencing transcription, splicing, translation and genomic stability. There is insufficient evidence to establish it as a primary driver mutation. Conflicting data on its prognostic role especially in CMML demand further evaluation to differentiate worse prognostic outcomes due to presence of SRSF2 mutation as opposed to other factors (e.g. presence of increased mutation burden). Targeting mis-splicing events secondary to splicing factor mutations with novel spliceosome inhibitors is an exciting approach with multiple possible therapeutic implications.

Abbreviations

aCML: atypical Chronic Myeloid Leukemia; CMML: Chronic Myelomonocytic Leukemia; JMML: Juvenile Myelomonocytic Leukemia; MDS: myelodysplasia; MPN: myeloproliferative neoplasm; MPN/MDS-U: unclassifiable MDS/MPN

Funding

The study was partly supported by the Affiliated Cancer Hospital of Zhengzhou University, Zhengzhou, China.

Authors' contributions

DL designed the study. All authors drafted and approved the final manuscript.

Competing interests
The authors declare that they have no competing interests.

Author details
[1]Department of Medicine, New York Medical College and Westchester Medical Center, Valhalla, NY, USA. [2]Section of Hematology-Oncology, Department of Medicine, Baylor College of Medicine, Houston, TX, USA. [3]Division of Blood and Marrow Transplantation, Department of Medicine, Stanford University, Stanford, CA, USA. [4]The affiliated Cancer Hospital of Zhengzhou University and Henan Cancer Hospital, 127 Dongming Road, Zhengzhou 450008, China.

References

1. Vardiman JW, Harris NL, Brunning RD. The World Health Organization (WHO) classification of the myeloid neoplasms. Blood. 2002;100(7):2292–302.
2. Arber DA, Orazi A, Hasserjian R, Thiele J, Borowitz MJ, Le Beau MM, Bloomfield CD, Cazzola M, Vardiman JW. The 2016 revision to the World Health Organization classification of myeloid neoplasms and acute leukemia. Blood. 2016;127(20):2391–405.
3. Döhner H, Weisdorf DJ, Bloomfield CD. Acute Myeloid Leukemia. N Engl J Med. 2015;373(12):1136–52.
4. Hwang SM, Kim SY, Kim JA, Park H-S, Park SN, Im K, Kim K, Kim S-M, Lee DS. Short telomere length and its correlation with gene mutations in myelodysplastic syndrome. J Hematol Oncol. 2016;9(1):62.
5. Nangalia J, Massie CE, Baxter EJ, Nice FL, Gundem G, Wedge DC, Avezov E, Li J, Kollmann K, Kent DG, Aziz A, Godfrey AL, Hinton J, Martincorena I, Van Loo P, Jones AV, Guglielmelli P, Tarpey P, Harding HP, Fitzpatrick JD, Goudie CT, Ortmann CA, Loughran SJ, Raine K, Jones DR, Butler AP, Teague JW, O'Meara S, McLaren S, Bianchi M, et al. Somatic CALR mutations in myeloproliferative neoplasms with nonmutated JAK2. N Engl J Med. 2013; 369(25):2391–405.
6. Papaemmanuil E, Gerstung M, Malcovati L, Tauro S, Gundem G, Van Loo P, Yoon CJ, Ellis P, Wedge DC, Pellagatti A, Shlien A, Groves MJ, Forbes SA, Raine K, Hinton J, Mudie LJ, McLaren S, Hardy C, Latimer C, Della Porta MG, O'Meara S, Ambaglio I, Galli A, Butler AP, Walldin G, Teague JW, Quek L, Sternberg A, Gambacorti-Passerini C, Cross NC, et al. Clinical and biological implications of driver mutations in myelodysplastic syndromes. Blood. 2013; 122(22):3616–27.
7. Tirado CA, Siangchin K, Shabsovich DS, Sharifian M, Schiller G. A novel three-way rearrangement involving ETV6 (12p13) and ABL1 (9q34) with an unknown partner on 3p25 resulting in a possible ETV6-ABL1 fusion in a patient with acute myeloid leukemia: a case report and a review of the literature. Biomarker Research. 2016;4(1):16.
8. Yoshida K, Sanada M, Shiraishi Y, Nowak D, Nagata Y, Yamamoto R, Sato Y, Sato-Otsubo A, Kon A, Nagasaki M, Chalkidis G, Suzuki Y, Shiosaka M, Kawahata R, Yamaguchi T, Otsu M, Obara N, Sakata-Yanagimoto M, Ishiyama K, Mori H, Nolte F, Hofmann WK, Miyawaki S, Sugano S, Haferlach C, Koeffler HP, Shih LY, Haferlach T, Chiba S, Nakauchi H, et al. Frequent pathway mutations of splicing machinery in myelodysplasia. Nature. 2011;478(7367): 64–9.
9. Geyer HL, Mesa RA. Therapy for myeloproliferative neoplasms: when, which agent, and how? Hematology Am Soc Hematol Educ Program. 2014;2014(1): 277–86.
10. Papaemmanuil E, Gerstung M, Bullinger L, Gaidzik VI, Paschka P, Roberts ND, Potter NE, Heuser M, Thol F, Bolli N, Gundem G, Van Loo P, Martincorena I, Ganly P, Mudie L, McLaren S, O'Meara S, Raine K, Jones DR, Teague JW, Butler AP, Greaves MF, Ganser A, Döhner K, Schlenk RF, Döhner H, Campbell PJ. Genomic classification and prognosis in acute myeloid leukemia. N Engl J Med. 2016;374(23):2209–21.
11. Schlenk RF, Döhner K, Krauter J, Fröhling S, Corbacioglu A, Bullinger L, Habdank M, Späth D, Morgan M, Benner A, Schlegelberger B, Heil G, Ganser A, Döhner H. Mutations and treatment outcome in cytogenetically normal acute myeloid leukemia. N Engl J Med. 2008;358(18):1909–18.
12. Welch JS, Petti AA, Miller CA, Fronick CC, O'Laughlin M, Fulton RS, Wilson RK, Baty JD, Duncavage EJ, Tandon B, Lee Y-S, Wartman LD, Uy GL, Ghobadi A, Tomasson MH, Pusic I, Romee R, Fehniger TA, Stockerl-Goldstein KE, Vij R, Oh ST, Abboud CN, Cashen AF, Schroeder MA, Jacoby MA, Heath SE, Luber K, Janke MR, Hantel A, Khan N, et al. TP53 and Decitabine in acute myeloid leukemia and myelodysplastic syndromes. N Engl J Med. 2016;375(21):2023–36.
13. Amatangelo MD, Quek L, Shih A, Stein EM, Roshal M, David MD, Marteyn B, Farnoud NR, de Botton S, Bernard OA, Wu B, Yen KE, Tallman MS, Papaemmanuil E, Penard-Lacronique V, Thakurta A, Vyas P, Levine RL. Enasidenib induces acute myeloid leukemia cell differentiation to promote clinical response. Blood. 2017;130(6):732–41.
14. Maffini E, Giaccone L, Festuccia M, Brunello L, Buondonno I, Ferrero D, Boccadoro M, Dellacasa C, Busca A, Novero D, Bruno B. Ruxolitinib in steroid refractory graft-vs.-host disease: a case report. J Hematol Oncol. 2016;9(1):67.
15. Stein EM, DiNardo CD, Pollyea DA, Fathi AT, Roboz GJ, Altman JK, Stone RM, DeAngelo DJ, Levine RL, Flinn IW, Kantarjian HM, Collins R, Patel MR, Frankel AE, Stein A, Sekeres MA, Swords RT, Medeiros BC, Willekens C, Vyas P, Tosolini A, Xu Q, Knight RD, Yen KE, Agresta S, de Botton S, Tallman MS. Enasidenib in mutant IDH2 relapsed or refractory acute myeloid leukemia. Blood. 2017;130(6):722–31.
16. Stone RM, Mandrekar SJ, Sanford BL, Laumann K, Geyer S, Bloomfield CD, Thiede C, Prior TW, Dohner K, Marcucci G, Lo-Coco F, Klisovic RB, Wei A, Sierra J, Sanz MA, Brandwein JM, de Witte T, Niederwieser D, Appelbaum FR, Medeiros BC, Tallman MS, Krauter J, Schlenk RF, Ganser A, Serve H, Ehninger G, Amadori S, Larson RA, Dohner H. Midostaurin plus chemotherapy for acute myeloid leukemia with a FLT3 mutation. N Engl J Med. 2017;377(5):454–64.
17. Verstovsek S, Odenike O, Singer JW, Granston T, Al-Fayoumi S, Deeg HJ. Phase 1/2 study of pacritinib, a next generation JAK2/FLT3 inhibitor, in myelofibrosis or other myeloid malignancies. J Hematol Oncol. 2016;9(1):137.
18. Yacoub A, Prochaska L. Ruxolitinib improves symptoms and quality of life in a patient with systemic mastocytosis. Biomarker Research. 2016;4(1):2.
19. Saygin C, Carraway HE. Emerging therapies for acute myeloid leukemia. J Hematol Oncol. 2017;10(1):93.
20. Verstovsek S, Gotlib J, Mesa RA, Vannucchi AM, Kiladjian J-J, Cervantes F, Harrison CN, Paquette R, Sun W, Naim A, Langmuir P, Dong T, Gopalakrishna P, Gupta V. Long-term survival in patients treated with ruxolitinib for myelofibrosis: COMFORT-I and -II pooled analyses. J Hematol Oncol. 2017;10(1):156.
21. Verstovsek S, Mesa RA, Gotlib J, Gupta V, DiPersio JF, Catalano JV, Deininger MWN, Miller CB, Silver RT, Talpaz M, Winton EF, Harvey JH, Arcasoy MO, Hexner EO, Lyons RM, Paquette R, Raza A, Jones M, Kornacki D, Sun K, Kantarjian H. Long-term treatment with ruxolitinib for patients with myelofibrosis: 5-year update from the randomized, double-blind, placebo-controlled, phase 3 COMFORT-I trial. J Hematol Oncol. 2017;10(1):55.
22. Orazi A, Germing U. The myelodysplastic/myeloproliferative neoplasms: myeloproliferative diseases with dysplastic features. Leukemia. 2008;22(7):1308–19.
23. Tiu RV, Gondek LP, O'Keefe CL, Elson P, Huh J, Mohamedali A, Kulasekararaj A, Advani AS, Paquette R, List AF, Sekeres MA, McDevitt MA, Mufti GJ, Maciejewski JP. Prognostic impact of SNP array karyotyping in myelodysplastic syndromes and related myeloid malignancies. Blood. 2011;117(17):4552–60.
24. Mughal TI, Cross NC, Padron E, Tiu RV, Savona M, Malcovati L, Tibes R, Komrokji RS, Kiladjian JJ, Garcia-Manero G, Orazi A, Mesa R, Maciejewski JP, Fenaux P, Itzykson R, Mufti G, Solary E, List AF. An international MDS/MPN working Group's perspective and recommendations on molecular pathogenesis, diagnosis and clinical characterization of myelodysplastic/ myeloproliferative neoplasms. Haematologica. 2015;100(9):1117–30.
25. Reiter A, Invernizzi R, Cross NC, Cazzola M. Molecular basis of myelodysplastic/ myeloproliferative neoplasms. Haematologica. 2009;94(12):1634–8.
26. Kar SA, Jankowska A, Makishima H, Visconte V, Jerez A, Sugimoto Y, Muramatsu H, Traina F, Afable M, Guinta K, Tiu RV, Przychodzen B, Sakaguchi H, Kojima S, Sekeres MA, List AF, McDevitt MA, Maciejewski JP. Spliceosomal gene mutations are frequent events in the diverse mutational spectrum of chronic myelomonocytic leukemia but largely absent in juvenile myelomonocytic leukemia. Haematologica. 2013;98(1):107–13.
27. Itzykson R, Kosmider O, Renneville A, Gelsi-Boyer V, Meggendorfer M, Morabito M, Berthon C, Ades L, Fenaux P, Beyne-Rauzy O, Vey N, Braun T, Haferlach T, Dreyfus F, Cross NC, Preudhomme C, Bernard OA, Fontenay M, Vainchenker W, Schnittger S, Birnbaum D, Droin N, Solary E. Prognostic score including gene mutations in chronic myelomonocytic leukemia. J Clin Oncol. 2013;31(19):2428–36.
28. Kielkopf CL. Insights from structures of cancer-relevant pre-mRNA splicing factors. Curr Opin Genet Dev. 2018;48:57–66.
29. Fu XD, Maniatis T. Isolation of a complementary DNA that encodes the mammalian splicing factor SC35. Science. 1992;256(5056):535–8.
30. Fu XD, Maniatis T. Factor required for mammalian spliceosome assembly is localized to discrete regions in the nucleus. Nature. 1990;343(6257):437–41.
31. Fu XD, Maniatis T. The 35-kDa mammalian splicing factor SC35 mediates specific interactions between U1 and U2 small nuclear ribonucleoprotein

particles at the 3′ splice site. Proc Natl Acad Sci U S A. 1992;89(5):1725–9.
32. Wahl MC, Will CL, Luhrmann R. The spliceosome: design principles of a dynamic RNP machine. Cell. 2009;136(4):701–18.
33. Liu HX, Chew SL, Cartegni L, Zhang MQ, Krainer AR. Exonic splicing enhancer motif recognized by human SC35 under splicing conditions. Mol Cell Biol. 2000;20(3):1063–71.
34. Howard JM, Sanford JR. The RNAissance family: SR proteins as multifaceted regulators of gene expression. Wiley Interdiscip Rev RNA. 2015;6(1):93–110.
35. Lin S, Coutinho-Mansfield G, Wang D, Pandit S, Fu XD. The splicing factor SC35 has an active role in transcriptional elongation. Nat Struct Mol Biol. 2008;15(8):819–26.
36. Das R, Yu J, Zhang Z, Gygi MP, Krainer AR, Gygi SP, Reed R. SR proteins function in coupling RNAP II transcription to pre-mRNA splicing. Mol Cell. 2007;26(6):867–81.
37. Xiao R, Sun Y, Ding JH, Lin S, Rose DW, Rosenfeld MG, Fu XD, Li X. Splicing regulator SC35 is essential for genomic stability and cell proliferation during mammalian organogenesis. Mol Cell Biol. 2007;27(15):5393–402.
38. Komeno Y, Huang YJ, Qiu J, Lin L, Xu Y, Zhou Y, Chen L, Monterroza DD, Li H, DeKelver RC, Yan M, Fu XD, Zhang DE. SRSF2 is essential for hematopoiesis, and its myelodysplastic syndrome-related mutations dysregulate alternative pre-mRNA splicing. Mol Cell Biol. 2015;35(17):3071–82.
39. Wang HY, Xu X, Ding JH, Bermingham JR Jr, Fu XD. SC35 plays a role in T cell development and alternative splicing of CD45. Mol Cell. 2001;7(2):331–42.
40. Kim E, Ilagan JO, Liang Y, Daubner GM, Lee SC, Ramakrishnan A, Li Y, Chung YR, Micol JB, Murphy ME, Cho H, Kim MK, Zebari AS, Aumann S, Park CY, Buonamici S, Smith PG, Deeg HJ, Lobry C, Aifantis I, Modis Y, Allain FH, Halene S, Bradley RK, Abdel-Wahab O. SRSF2 mutations contribute to myelodysplasia by mutant-specific effects on exon recognition. Cancer Cell. 2015;27(5):617–30.
41. Patnaik MM, Lasho TL, Finke CM, Hanson CA, Hodnefield JM, Knudson RA, Ketterling RP, Pardanani A, Tefferi A. Spliceosome mutations involving SRSF2, SF3B1, and U2AF35 in chronic myelomonocytic leukemia: prevalence, clinical correlates, and prognostic relevance. Am J Hematol. 2013;88(3):201–6.
42. Meggendorfer M, Roller A, Haferlach T, Eder C, Dicker F, Grossmann V, Kohlmann A, Alpermann T, Yoshida K, Ogawa S, Koeffler HP, Kern W, Haferlach C, Schnittger S. SRSF2 mutations in 275 cases with chronic myelomonocytic leukemia (CMML). Blood. 2012;120(15):3080–8.
43. Makishima H, Visconte V, Sakaguchi H, Jankowska AM, Abu Kar S, Jerez A, Przychodzen B, Bupathi M, Guinta K, Afable MG, Sekeres MA, Padgett RA, Tiu RV, Maciejewski JP. Mutations in the spliceosome machinery, a novel and ubiquitous pathway in leukemogenesis. Blood. 2012;119(14):3203–10.
44. Wu SJ, Kuo YY, Hou HA, Li LY, Tseng MH, Huang CF, Lee FY, Liu MC, Liu CW, Lin CT, Chen CY, Chou WC, Yao M, Huang SY, Ko BS, Tang JL, Tsay W, Tien HF. The clinical implication of SRSF2 mutation in patients with myelodysplastic syndrome and its stability during disease evolution. Blood. 2012;120(15):3106–11.
45. Federmann B, Abele M, Rosero Cuesta DS, Vogel W, Boiocchi L, Kanz L, Quintanilla-Martinez L, Orazi A, Bonzheim I, Fend F. The detection of SRSF2 mutations in routinely processed bone marrow biopsies is useful in the diagnosis of chronic myelomonocytic leukemia. Hum Pathol. 2014;45(12): 2471–9.
46. Daubner GM, Clery A, Jayne S, Stevenin J, Allain FH. A syn-anti conformational difference allows SRSF2 to recognize guanines and cytosines equally well. EMBO J. 2012;31(1):162–74.
47. Lee SC, Dvinge H, Kim E, Cho H, Micol JB, Chung YR, Durham BH, Yoshimi A, Kim YJ, Thomas M, Lobry C, Chen CW, Pastore A, Taylor J, Wang X, Krivtsov A, Armstrong SA, Palacino J, Buonamici S, Smith PG, Bradley RK, Abdel-Wahab O. Modulation of splicing catalysis for therapeutic targeting of leukemia with mutations in genes encoding spliceosomal proteins. Nat Med. 2016;22(6):672–8.
48. Hou HA, Kuo YY, Tang JL, Chou WC, Yao M, Lai YJ, Lin CC, Chen CY, Liu CY, Tseng MH, Huang CF, Chiang YC, Lee FY, Liu MC, Liu CW, Huang SY, Ko BS, Wu SJ, Tsay W, Chen YC, Tien HF. Clinical implications of the SETBP1 mutation in patients with primary myelodysplastic syndrome and its stability during disease progression. Am J Hematol. 2014;89(2):181–6.
49. Yip BH, Steeples V, Repapi E, Armstrong RN, Llorian M, Roy S, Shaw J, Dolatshad H, Taylor S, Verma A, Bartenstein M, Vyas P, Cross NC, Malcovati L, Cazzola M, Hellstrom-Lindberg E, Ogawa S, Smith CW, Pellagatti A, Boultwood J. The U2AF1S34F mutation induces lineage-specific splicing alterations in myelodysplastic syndromes. J Clin Invest. 2017;127(6):2206–21.
50. Dolatshad H, Pellagatti A, Fernandez-Mercado M, Yip BH, Malcovati L, Attwood M, Przychodzen B, Sahgal N, Kanapin AA, Lockstone H, Scifo L, Vandenberghe P, Papaemmanuil E, Smith CW, Campbell PJ, Ogawa S, Maciejewski JP, Cazzola M, Savage KI, Boultwood J. Disruption of SF3B1 results in deregulated expression and splicing of key genes and pathways in myelodysplastic syndrome hematopoietic stem and progenitor cells. Leukemia. 2015;29(8):1798.
51. Mortera-Blanco T, Dimitriou M, Woll PS, Karimi M, Elvarsdottir E, Conte S, Tobiasson M, Jansson M, Douagi I, Moarii M, Saft L, Papaemmanuil E, Jacobsen SEW, Hellstrom-Lindberg E. SF3B1-initiating mutations in MDS-RSs target lymphomyeloid hematopoietic stem cells. Blood. 2017;130(7):881–90.
52. Patnaik MM, Wassie EA, Lasho TL, Hanson CA, Ketterling R, Tefferi A. Blast transformation in chronic myelomonocytic leukemia: risk factors, genetic features, survival, and treatment outcome. Am J Hematol. 2015;90(5):411–6.
53. Wassie EA, Itzykson R, Lasho TL, Kosmider O, Finke CM, Hanson CA, Ketterling RP, Solary E, Tefferi A, Patnaik MM. Molecular and prognostic correlates of cytogenetic abnormalities in chronic myelomonocytic leukemia: a Mayo Clinic-French consortium study. Am J Hematol. 2014;89(12):1111–5.
54. Meggendorfer M, Haferlach T, Alpermann T, Jeromin S, Haferlach C, Kern W, Schnittger S. Specific molecular mutation patterns delineate chronic neutrophilic leukemia, atypical chronic myeloid leukemia, and chronic myelomonocytic leukemia. Haematologica. 2014;99(12):e244–6.
55. Lasho TL, Jimma T, Finke CM, Patnaik M, Hanson CA, Ketterling RP, Pardanani A, Tefferi A. SRSF2 mutations in primary myelofibrosis: significant clustering with IDH mutations and independent association with inferior overall and leukemia-free survival. Blood. 2012;120(20):4168–71.
56. Patnaik MM, Padron E, LaBorde RR, Lasho TL, Finke CM, Hanson CA, Hodnefield JM, Knudson RA, Ketterling RP, Al-kali A, Pardanani A, Ali NA, Komrokji RS, Tefferi A. Mayo prognostic model for WHO-defined chronic myelomonocytic leukemia: ASXL1 and spliceosome component mutations and outcomes. Leukemia. 2013;27(7):1504–10.
57. Patnaik MM, Wassie EA, Padron E, Onida F, Itzykson R, Lasho TL, Kosmider O, Finke CM, Hanson CA, Ketterling RP, Komrokji R, Tefferi A, Solary E. Chronic myelomonocytic leukemia in younger patients: molecular and cytogenetic predictors of survival and treatment outcome. Blood Cancer J. 2015;5:e270.
58. Ouyang Y, Qiao C, Chen Y, Zhang SJ. Clinical significance of CSF3R, SRSF2 and SETBP1 mutations in chronic neutrophilic leukemia and chronic myelomonocytic leukemia. Oncotarget. 2017;8(13):20834–41.
59. Onida F, Kantarjian HM, Smith TL, Ball G, Keating MJ, Estey EH, Glassman AB, Albitar M, Kwari MI, Beran M. Prognostic factors and scoring systems in chronic myelomonocytic leukemia: a retrospective analysis of 213 patients. Blood. 2002;99(3):840–9.
60. Such E, Cervera J, Costa D, Sole F, Vallespi T, Luno E, Collado R, Calasanz MJ, Hernandez-Rivas JM, Cigudosa JC, Nomdedeu B, Mallo M, Carbonell F, Bueno J, Ardanaz MT, Ramos F, Tormo M, Sancho-Tello R, del Canizo C, Gomez V, Marco V, Xicoy B, Bonanad S, Pedro C, Bernal T, Sanz GF. Cytogenetic risk stratification in chronic myelomonocytic leukemia. Haematologica. 2011;96(3):375–83.
61. Such E, Germing U, Malcovati L, Cervera J, Kuendgen A, Della Porta MG, Nomdedeu B, Arenillas L, Luno E, Xicoy B, Amigo ML, Valcarcel D, Nachtkamp K, Ambaglio I, Hildebrandt B, Lorenzo I, Cazzola M, Sanz G. Development and validation of a prognostic scoring system for patients with chronic myelomonocytic leukemia. Blood. 2013;121(15):3005–15.
62. Patnaik MM, Itzykson R, Lasho TL, Kosmider O, Finke CM, Hanson CA, Knudson RA, Ketterling RP, Tefferi A, Solary E. ASXL1 and SETBP1 mutations and their prognostic contribution in chronic myelomonocytic leukemia: a two-center study of 466 patients. Leukemia. 2014;28(11):2206–12.
63. Elena C, Galli A, Such E, Meggendorfer M, Germing U, Rizzo E, Cervera J, Molteni E, Fasan A, Schuler E, Ambaglio I, Lopez-Pavia M, Zibellini S, Kuendgen A, Travaglino E, Sancho-Tello R, Catricala S, Vicente AI, Haferlach T, Haferlach C, Sanz GF, Malcovati L, Cazzola M. Integrating clinical features and genetic lesions in the risk assessment of patients with chronic myelomonocytic leukemia. Blood. 2016;128(10):1408–17.
64. Hirabayashi S, Flotho C, Moetter J, Heuser M, Hasle H, Gruhn B, Klingebiel T, Thol F, Schlegelberger B, Baumann I, Strahm B, Stary J, Locatelli F, Zecca M,

Bergstraesser E, Dworzak M, Van den Heuvel-Eibrink MM, De Moerloose B, Ogawa S, Niemeyer CM, Wlodarski MW, European working group of MDSiC. Spliceosomal gene aberrations are rare, coexist with oncogenic mutations, and are unlikely to exert a driver effect in childhood MDS and JMML. Blood. 2012;119(11):e96–9.
65. Takita J, Yoshida K, Sanada M, Nishimura R, Okubo J, Motomura A, Hiwatari M, Oki K, Igarashi T, Hayashi Y, Ogawa S. Novel splicing-factor mutations in juvenile myelomonocytic leukemia. Leukemia. 2012;26(8):1879–81.
66. Li B, Gale RP, Xiao Z. Molecular genetics of chronic neutrophilic leukemia, chronic myelomonocytic leukemia and atypical chronic myeloid leukemia. J Hematol Oncol. 2014;7:93.
67. Meggendorfer M, Jeromin S, Haferlach C, Kern W, Haferlach T. The mutational landscape of 18 investigated genes clearly separates four subtypes of myelodysplastic/myeloproliferative neoplasms. Haematologica. 2018;103(5):e192–5.
68. Linder K, Iragavarapu C, Liu D. SETBP1 mutations as a biomarker for myelodysplasia/myeloproliferative neoplasm overlap syndrome. Biomark Res. 2017;5:33.
69. Senin A, Arenillas L, Martinez-Aviles L, Fernandez-Rodriguez C, Bellosillo B, Florensa L, Besses C, Alvarez-Larran A. Molecular characterization of atypical chronic myeloid leukemia and chronic neutrophilic leukemia. Med Clin (Barc). 2015;144(11):487–90.
70. Patnaik MM, Barraco D, Lasho TL, Finke CM, Reichard K, Hoversten KP, Ketterling RP, Gangat N, Tefferi A. Targeted next generation sequencing and identification of risk factors in World Health Organization defined atypical chronic myeloid leukemia. Am J Hematol. 2017;92(6):542–8.
71. Jeromin S, Haferlach T, Weissmann S, Meggendorfer M, Eder C, Nadarajah N, Alpermann T, Kohlmann A, Kern W, Haferlach C, Schnittger S. Refractory anemia with ring sideroblasts and marked thrombocytosis cases harbor mutations in SF3B1 or other spliceosome genes accompanied by JAK2V617F and ASXL1 mutations. Haematologica. 2015;100(4):e125–7.
72. Patnaik MM, Lasho TL, Finke CM, Hanson CA, King RL, Ketterling RP, Gangat N, Tefferi A. Predictors of survival in refractory anemia with ring sideroblasts and thrombocytosis (RARS-T) and the role of next-generation sequencing. Am J Hematol. 2016;91(5):492–8.
73. DiNardo CD, Daver N, Jain N, Pemmaraju N, Bueso-Ramos C, Yin CC, Pierce S, Jabbour E, Cortes JE, Kantarjian HM, Garcia-Manero G, Verstovsek S. Myelodysplastic/myeloproliferative neoplasms, unclassifiable (MDS/MPN, U): natural history and clinical outcome by treatment strategy. Leukemia. 2014; 28(4):958–61.
74. Hong DS, Kurzrock R, Naing A, Wheler JJ, Falchook GS, Schiffman JS, Faulkner N, Pilat MJ, O'Brien J, LoRusso P. A phase I, open-label, single-arm, dose-escalation study of E7107, a precursor messenger ribonucleic acid (pre-mRNA) splicesome inhibitor administered intravenously on days 1 and 8 every 21 days to patients with solid tumors. Investig New Drugs. 2014; 32(3):436–44.
75. Eskens FA, Ramos FJ, Burger H, O'Brien JP, Piera A, de Jonge MJ, Mizui Y, Wiemer EA, Carreras MJ, Baselga J, Tabernero J. Phase I pharmacokinetic and pharmacodynamic study of the first-in-class spliceosome inhibitor E7107 in patients with advanced solid tumors. Clin Cancer Res. 2013;19(22): 6296–304.
76. Seiler M, Yoshimi A, Darman R, Chan B, Keaney G, Thomas M, Agrawal AA, Caleb B, Csibi A, Sean E, Fekkes P, Karr C, Klimek V, Lai G, Lee L, Kumar P, Lee SC, Liu X, Mackenzie C, Meeske C, Mizui Y, Padron E, Park E, Pazolli E, Peng S, Prajapati S, Taylor J, Teng T, Wang J, Warmuth M, et al. H3B-8800, an orally available small-molecule splicing modulator, induces lethality in spliceosome-mutant cancers. Nat Med. 2018;24(4):497–504.
77. Sun C, Zhang S, Qiao C, Yang X, Li J. Clinical manifestation of the SRSF2 gene mutation in Chinese patients with chronic myelomonocytic leukemia. Chin Med J. 2014;127(24):4215–9.
78. Alpermann T, Haferlach T, Schrauder C, Konietschke R, Haferlach C, Kern W, Schnittger S. Mutational screening of CSF3R, ASXL1, SETBP1, and SRSF2 in chronic neutrophilic leukemia (CNL), atypical CML and CMML cases. Blood. 2013;122(21):105–5.

NKX2.2, PDX-1 and CDX-2 as potential biomarkers to differentiate well-differentiated neuroendocrine tumors

Michelle X. Yang[1*], Ryan F. Coates[1], Abiy Ambaye[1], Valerie Cortright[1], Jeannette M. Mitchell[1], Alexa M. Buskey[1], Richard Zubarik[2], James G. Liu[3], Steven Ades[4] and Maura M. Barry[4]

Abstract

Background: Well-differentiated neuroendocrine tumors (NET) most frequently arise from the gastrointestinal tract (GI), pancreas, and lung. Patients often present as metastasis with an unknown primary, and the clinical management and outcome depend on multiple factors, including the accurate diagnosis with the tumor primary site. Determining the site of the NET with unknown primary remains challenging. Many biomarkers have been investigated in primary NETs and metastatic NETs, with heterogeneous sensitivity and specificity observed.

Methods: We used high-throughput tissue microarray (TMA) and immunohistochemistry (IHC) with antibodies against a panel of transcriptional factors including NKX2.2, PDX-1, PTF1A, and CDX-2 on archived formalin-fixed paraffin-embedded NETs, and investigated the protein expression pattern of these transcription factors in 109 primary GI ($N = 81$), pancreatic ($N = 17$), and lung ($N = 11$) NETs.

Results: Differential expression pattern of these markers was observed. In the GI and pancreatic NETs ($N = 98$), NKX2.2, PDX-1, and CDX-2 were immunoreactive in 82 (84%), 14 (14%), and 52 (52%) cases, respectively. PDX-1 was expressed mainly in the small intestinal and appendiceal NETs, occasionally in the pancreatic NETs, and not in the colorectal NETs. All three biomarkers including NKX2.2, PDX-1, and CDX-2 were completely negative in lung NETs. PTF1A was expressed in all normal and neuroendocrine tumor cells.

Conclusions: Our findings suggest that NKX2.2 was a sensitive and specific biomarker for the GI and pancreatic neuroendocrine tumors. We proposed that a panel of immunostains including NKX2.2, PDX-1, and CDX-2 may show diagnostic utility for the most common NETs.

Keywords: Well-differentiated neuroendocrine tumor, Biomarker, NKX2.2, PDX-1, CDX-2, Gastrointestinal, Pancreas, Lung

Background

Gastrointestinal tract (GI), pancreas, and lung are among the most common sites to develop well-differentiated neuroendocrine tumors (NET). The incidence of GI NET is increasing, based on recent Surveillance, Epidemiology and End Results (SEER) data [1]. Patients with NET may initially present as liver metastasis in up to 19% of cases [2, 3], and the clinical management and outcome depend on multiple factors, including the primary tumor site [1, 4]. Although primary NET often shows a predominate architectural growth pattern at a particular site, tumor heterogeneity with mixed growth patterns do occur [5]. Using morphological features to diagnose the NET with an unknown primary can be challenging based on the hematoxylin and eosin staining alone, and a panel of immunohistochemistry (IHC) is often required to determine the site of primary tumor. General neuroendocrine markers including chromogranin and synaptophysin are very useful markers to determine the neuroendocrine differentiation. However, they lack specificity for the lineage or site of the tumor. Caudal type homeobox 2 (CDX-2) has been investigated previously by multiple groups and showed high sensitivity and specificity for small intestinal NET, but variable sensitivity for colorectal and pancreatic

* Correspondence: xfyang60@yahoo.com
[1]Department of Pathology and Laboratory Medicine, University of Vermont Medical Center, 111 Colchester Avenue, Burlington, VT 05401, USA

NETs. [6–9] PAX-8 and Islet-1 (ISL-1) have been investigated for their role to identify primary and metastatic pancreatic neuroendocrine tumors and variable sensitivity and specificity has been reported [10–13]. An extended panel of biomarkers including CDX-2, pancreatic and duodenal homeobox 1 (PDX-1), TTF-1, and NESP-55 has been reported in NETs from the pancreas, GI and lung, and these results also showed relatively low sensitivity for the tumors from the rectum and pancreas [14]. More recently, the expression pattern of CDX-2, PAX-6, ISL-1, ER, and PR in the GI and pancreatic NET was investigated and showed small differences between the primary and metastatic NETs [15, 16]. However, these markers showed relatively low sensitivity for pancreatic NETs. Investigation of more biomarkers to distinguish common NETs of different site remains necessary.

For this purpose, we focused on a panel of transcription factors (TFs) including CDX-2, NK2 homeobox 2 (NKX2.2), PDX-1, and pancreas specific transcription factor 1a (PTF1A) [17, 18], and simultaneously investigated their protein expression pattern in the NETs of the most common sites, including GI, pancreas and lung. PDX-1 is a transcription factor essential for both pancreatic ductal and islet cell development during early embryogenesis [18]. After development, PDX-1 is predominantly expressed in the islet cells of pancreas, but not in the ductal epithelium or acinar cells [19]. Interestingly, NKX2.2 is critical for the differentiation of beta cells in the islet cells of the pancreas [20–26], and important for the differentiation of enteroendocrine cells of the intestine [27, 28], as well as oligodendrocytes of the central nervous system [29, 30]. During early pancreatic development, NKX2.2 protein expression is initiated with PDX-1 and PTF1A in the dorsal and ventral pancreatic buds [31]. In the intestine, NKX2.2 is expressed in the endocrine cells located in the villi and deep crypts, and a rare subset of NKX2.2-positive cells is coexpressed with intestinal stem cell markers [32, 33]. We compared the results with the well-known transcriptional factor of intestinal differentiation, CDX-2.

Methods

Study population

A total of 109 primary NETs were retrospectively retrieved from archived blocks at our institution from January 2010 to December 2015, including 92 resections and 17 biopsies. The tumor grade for all cases was extracted from original pathological report for all NETs, based on current World Health Organization (WHO) criteria for each tumor site on the H&E stain. Particularly, 11 lung NETs included 7 typical carcinoids and 4 atypical carcinoids based on 2015 WHO criteria for lung NETs. All the slides were reviewed by two pathologists and representative blocks were selected for this study. This study was approved by our Institutional Review Board (IRB #CHRMS 17–0009).

Tissue microarray (TMA) and immunohistochemistry (IHC)

Using duplicated 2-mm core punch (Beecher Instruments Inc., Sun Prairie, WI), TMA was constructed from formalin-fixed and paraffin-embedded tumor or normal blocks for resection cases, and 2–3 levels of whole tissue section were mounted on the slides for all biopsies. PDX-1 (clone 2A12, 1:100 dilution, Abcam, Cambridge, MA), PTF1A (clone 1A2, 1:200 dilution, Abcam), and NKX2.2 (clone NX2/294, 1:100 dilution, Abcam) immunohistochemistry was initially validated in normal pancreatic tissues. CDX-2 (clone EP25, Leica Biosystems, Buffalo Grove, IL) has been validated according to the College of American Pathologists (CAP) guidelines in the histology lab for routine clinical use. Antigen retrieval was obtained as follows: CDX-2 in H2 buffer (Leica Biosystems) for 10 min, NKX2.2 and PTF1A in H1 buffer (Leica Biosystems) for 30 min, and PDX-1 in H1 for 10 min. All IHCs were performed on BOND-III automated IHC stainer (Leica Biosystems).

Results

Demographics and tumor site

Among the 109 patients, 51 were males and 58 were females with a median age of 57 years (ranging from 12 to 90 years). In this study population, the tubular GI tract was the most common site for NET, followed by the pancreas and lung (Table 1). For 11 lung NETS, 7 cases were typical carcinoid and 4 cases were atypical carcinoid tumors.

Expression of NKX2.2, PDX-1 and PTF1A in normal GI and pancreaticobiliary endocrine cells

In normal GI tract, scattered NKX2.2 immunoreactive nuclei were observed in the endocrine cells predominantly located in the deep crypts of the entire tubular GI tract, including stomach, duodenum, jejunum, ileum,

Table 1 List of well-differentiated neuroendocrine tumors used in this study

Site	Grade 1	Grade 2	Total No.
Rectum	15	1	16
Colon	4	1	5
Appendix	20	2	22
Ileum	11	1	12
Jejunum	4	6	10
Duodenum	3	1	4
Stomach	11	1	12
Pancreas	12	5	17
Total Number	80	18	98

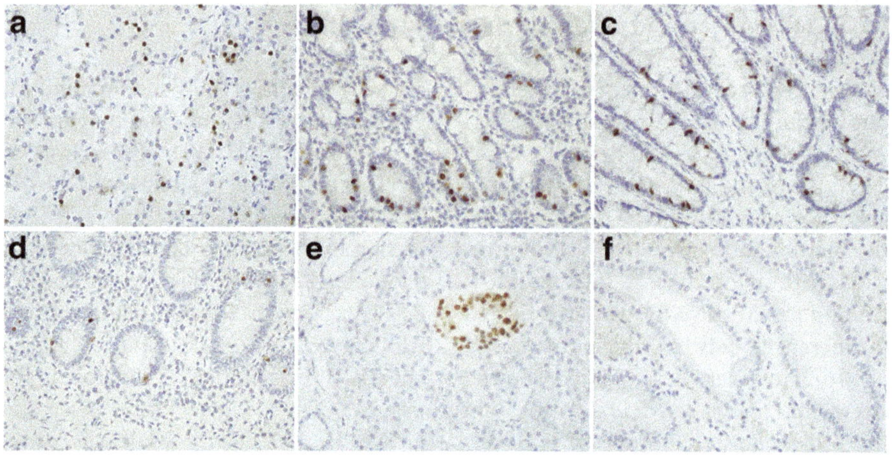

Fig. 1 NKX2.2 immunoreactivity in endocrine cells of normal stomach (**a**), duodenum (**b**), colon (**c**), appendix (**d**), and pancreas (**e**). No NKX2.2 positive cells identified in the gallbladder (**f**). Original magnification, 400×

appendix, colon, and rectum (Fig. 1a, d). No nuclear staining for PDX-1 was seen in the tubular GI tract. PTF1A was immunoreactive in all normal GI tract mucosa.

In normal pancreas, both NKX2.2 (Fig. 1e) and PDX-1 (data not shown) were expressed in the nucleus of islet cells, and were completely negative in normal ductal epithelium and acinar cells. In normal gallbladder, no NKX2.2 or PDX-1 immunoreactive cells were detected (Fig. 1f). PTF1A expression was seen in all types of parenchymal cells in the pancreas (data not shown).

NKX2.2, PDX-1 and CDX-2 expression in NETs of the GI tract

Although IHC interpretation was defined as positive if > 5% of tumor cells had nuclear staining for NKX2.2, CDX-2, PDX-1 and PTF1A, the majority of positive cases demonstrated diffuse nuclear immunoreactivity in both TMA and biopsy cases, and focal or patchy staining in rare cases were seen only in the gastric and pancreatic NETs. We performed IHC on whole sections of 8 of 92 resection cases (8.7%) of the NETs from the GI tract and pancreas, and all positive and negative results were consistent with those on TMA with either diffuse positivity or completely negativity.

In 98 GI and pancreatic NETs, the sensitivity and 95% confidence interval (95% CI) for NKX2.2, PDX-1, and CDX-2 were 84% (95% CI, 75% - 90%), 14% (95% CI, 8% - 23%), and 53% (95% CI, 43% - 63%), respectively. There was no significant difference in all 3 biomarkers between G1 and G2 tumors. Along the GI tract, NKX2.2 immunoreactivity was strong and diffuse in the tumor nuclei of the majority of NETs along the GI tract (Table 2; Fig. 2). Although NKX2.2-positive endocrine cells were seen in normal gastric pits as shown in Fig. 1a, the majority of gastric NETs showed negative and only rare cases with patchy immunoreactivity for NKX2.2 (Fig. 2g). For PDX-1, immunoreactivity was seen in 75% duodenum, 32% appendix, 20% jejunum, 8% ileum, and 6% pancreas NETs (Table 2; Fig. 2). None of the gastric, colonic, and rectal NETs was immunoreactive to PDX-1 (Table 2 and Fig. 2). NKX2.2 IHCs were repeated on all gastric NETs and results remained the same. For 17 pancreatic NETs, NKX2.2 was diffusely immunoreactive in 71% cases (Table 2 and Fig. 3a, b). However, PDX-1 was immunoreactive in only 1 of 17 pancreatic NETs.

As expected, CDX-2 was diffusely positive in all 22 appendiceal, 96% small intestinal, and 60% of colonic NETs. Consistent with the literature, no immunoreactivity for CDX-2 was seen in all 16 rectal NETs, and only 2 of 17 pancreatic NETs showed patchy immunoreactivity for CDX-2 (Table 2 and Fig. 3c). In other words, both CDX-2 and NKX2.2 showed similarly high immunoreactivity rate in the appendiceal, ileal and jejunum NETs. For pancreatic, duodenal, colonic and rectal NETs, NKX2.2 showed much higher immunoreactivity than

Table 2 Immunoreactivity of NKX2.2, PDX-1 and CDX-2 in 109 well-differentiated neuroendocrine tumors

Site	Total = 109	NKX2.2 +	PDX-1 +	CDX-2 +
Rectum	16	16 (100%)	0	0
Colon	5	5 (100%)	0	3 (60%)
Appendix	22	22 (100%)	7 (32%)	22 (100%)
Ileum	12	11 (92%)	1 (8%)	12 (100%)
Jejunum	10	10 (100%)	2 (20%)	10 (100%)
Duodenum	4	4 (100%)	3 (75%)	3 (75%)
Stomach	12	2 (17%)	0	0
Pancreas	17	12 (71%)	1 (6%)	2 (11%)
Lung	11	0	0	0
Total GI-pancreas	98	82 (84%)	14 (14%)	52 (53%)

Abbreviation: GI, gastrointestinal

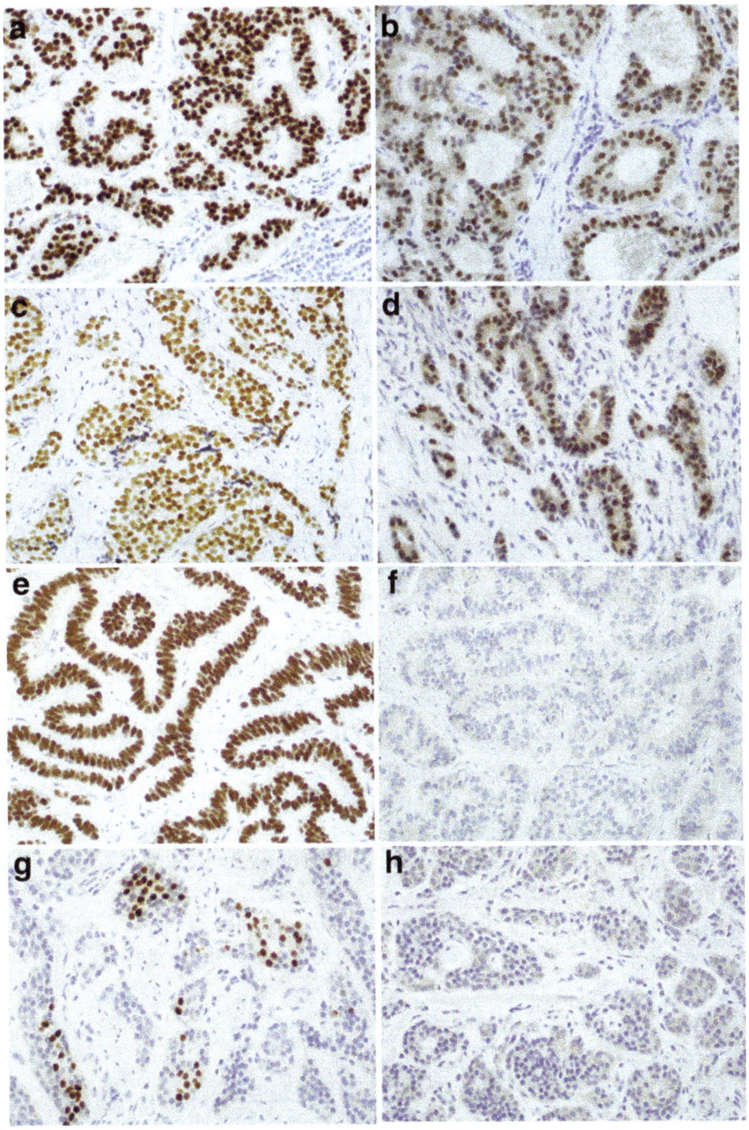

Fig. 2 Representative immunostain of NKX2.2 and PDX-1 in well-differentiated neuroendocrine tumor of the duodenum (**a**, **b**), appendix (**c**, **d**), colorectum (**e**, **f**), and stomach (**g**, **h**), respectively. Original magnification, 400×

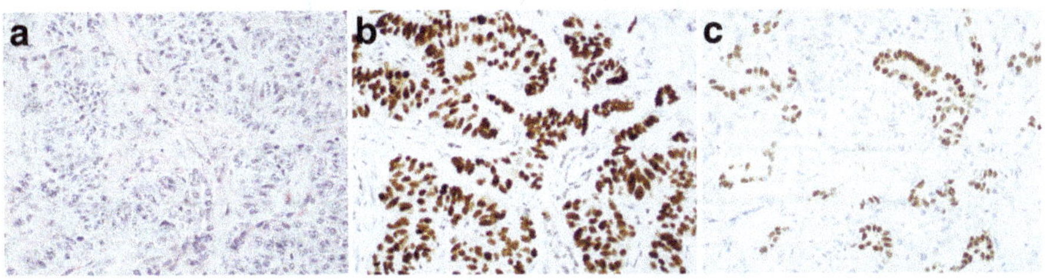

Fig. 3 Diffuse immunoreactivity of NKX2.2 compared to patchy immunoreactivity of CDX-2 in representative pancreatic well-differentiated neuroendocrine tumors. **a** H&E staining. **b** NKX2.2. **c** CDX-2. Original magnification, 400×

CDX-2. All three biomarkers including NKX2.2, PDX-1, and CDX-2 were completely negative in all 11 lung NETs (Table 2).

Non-specific PTF1A expression pattern in all NETs

Unlike the NKX2.2, PDX-1, and CDX-2 that had restricted expression pattern in NETs of different site, PTF1A was expressed in all normal and neuroendocrine tumor cells (data not shown). Therefore, PTF1A appeared to be a non-specific biomarker for all NETs, although a different source of antibody may be tested before a final conclusion can be made.

Discussion

In this study, four transcriptional factors including CDX-2, NKX2.2, PDX-1, and PTF1A were simultaneously investigated for their protein expression in the most common NETs from the GI, pancreatic, and lung by IHC. We found that these transcription factors were differentially expressed in NETs at these anatomic sites. NKX2.2 was a highly sensitive biomarker for neuroendocrine differentiation of pancreatic and intestinal neuroendocrine origin. PDX-1 was expressed in NETs of small intestine and appendix with variable but higher immunoreactivity at these sites, but not in the gastric, colonic or rectal NETs. NKX2.2 was positive in over 2/3 pancreatic NETs. Although PDX-1 immunopositivity was seen in less than 1/3 pancreatic NETs in previous reports, it was positive in 6% of pancreatic NETs in this study probably due to different source of antibodies, since it was positive in all internal controls. Although PTF1A was characterized as one of the pancreatic lineage-specific transcription factors (TFs), its expression was non-specific and was not a useful biomarker for NETs. Consistent with other's results, CDX-2 can be a useful biomarker for NETs arising from the small intestine and appendix. However, it showed only 50% immunoreactivity in colonic NETs and no immunoreactivity in all rectal NETs. CDX-2 was patchy positive in 11% of pancreatic NETs similarly seen in a previous study [14]. Overall, NKX2.2 showed much higher sensitivity for both rectal and pancreatic NETs, compared to PDX-1 and CDX-2 for the tumors at these sites. Most importantly, these biomarkers were completely negative in all lung NETs, pancreatic ductal adenocarcinomas, or other carcinomas (data not shown).

Previous studies showed that NKX2.2 was negative in 13 bronchopulmonary carcinoid tumors, whereas 24 of 26 GI carcinoids (including 1 stomach, 1 duodenum, 2 ampullary, 14/16 pancreas, 5 ileum, and 1 colon), were immunoreactive for NKX2.2 [34]. In this study, we argue that a panel of PDX-1, CDX-2, and NKX2.2 would significantly increase the sensitivity of NETs from the GI tract and pancreas. Although TTF-1 was not tested in this cohort, it has been studied to determine NETs of pulmonary origin by several groups [8, 35–38]. Considering the fact that the majority of neuroendocrine tumors arise from the tubular GI tract, pancreas, and lung, we proposed a diagnostic algorithm using a panel of IHC stains including NKX2.2, PDX-1, CDX-2, and TTF-1 would aid the diagnosis of the primary tumor site in the setting of metastasis (Fig. 4). Although ISL-1, PAX-6, and PAX-8, were not investigated in the primary NETs in our

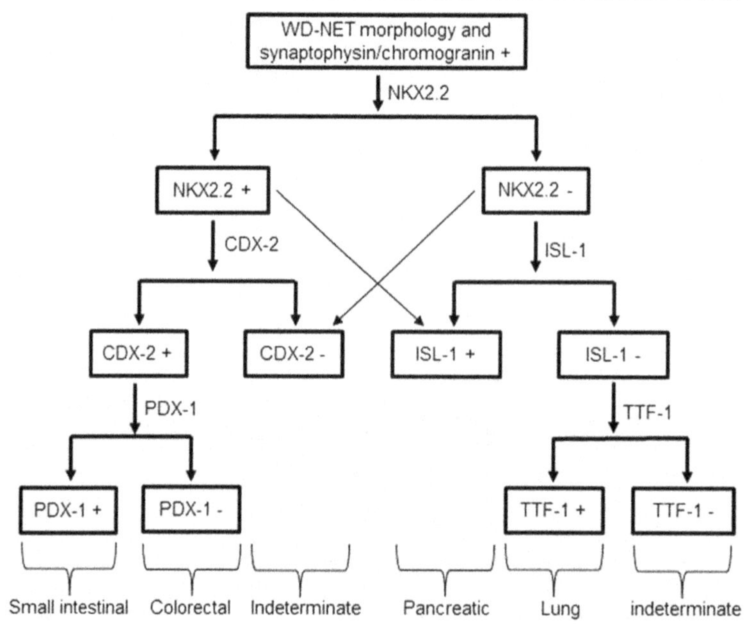

Fig. 4 Proposed diagnostic algorithm for WD-NETs

study, they can be added into the panel when the results are indeterminate for the pancreatic tumor or to increase the confidence of prediction [12], although the specificity of PAX-8 and ISL-1 was variable in different studies [39, 40]. Interestingly, a recent study showed high sensitivity of NKX2.2 in 85 liver metastatic NETs of the digestive system [41].

Conclusions

Using IHC, we found differential immunoreactivity of NKX2.2, CDX-2, and PDX-1 to the NETs from a different anatomic site. NKX2.2 showed higher sensitivity than CDX-2 and PDX-1 in both GI and pancreatic NETs. PDX-1 was expressed mainly in the small intestinal and appendiceal NETs, occasionally in the pancreatic NETs, and not in the colorectal NETs. Importantly, NKX2.2, CDX-2, and PDX-1 were not expressed in 11 lung NETs, and we understand the limitation of small sample size for a final conclusion on the specificity of these markers. These findings suggest that a panel of biomarkers including NKX2.2, PDX-1, and CDX-2 may provide additional insights in clinical diagnosis for the most common NETs especially in the setting of metastasis with an unknown origin.

Abbreviations

CDX-2: Caudal type homeobox 2; ER: Estrogen receptor; GI: Gastrointestinal tract3; IHC: Immunohistochemistry; ISL-1: Islet 1; NET: Well-differentiated neuroendocrine tumors; NKX2.2: NK2 homeobox 2; PAX-6: Paired box gene 6; PAX-8: Paired box gene 8; PDX-1: Pancreatic and duodenal homeobox 1; PR: Progesterone receptor; PTF-1A: Pancreas specific transcription factor 1a; SEER: Surveillance, Epidemiology and End Results; TF: Transcription factor; TMA: Tissue microarray; TTF-1: Transcription termination factor 1; WHO: World Health Organization

Acknowledgements

We would like to thank the Department of Pathology and Laboratory Medicine for funding the initial pilot study.

Funding

This work was supported by funding from University of Vermont Medical Group Research Award to M.X.Y.

Authors' contributions

MXY initiated the design of this study. AA, RZ, JGL, SA, and MMB all participated in the design of this study. RFC and MXY interpreted the protein expression and collected clinical data and wrote the manuscript. VC, JMM, AA, and ABM validated antibodies and constructed TMAs. All authors read, revised and approved the final manuscript.

Competing interests

The authors declare that they have no competing interests.

Author details

[1]Department of Pathology and Laboratory Medicine, University of Vermont Medical Center, 111 Colchester Avenue, Burlington, VT 05401, USA. [2]Gastroenterology, University of Vermont Medical Center, Burlington, VT, USA. [3]Applied Pathology Systems, Worcester, MA, USA. [4]Medical Oncology, University of Vermont Medical Center, Burlington, VT, USA.

References

1. Tsikitis VL, Wertheim BC, Guerrero MA. Trends of incidence and survival of gastrointestinal neuroendocrine tumors in the United States: a seer analysis. J Cancer. 2012;3:292–302.
2. Eriksson J, Stalberg P, Nilsson A, Krause J, Lundberg C, Skogseid B, et al. Surgery and radiofrequency ablation for treatment of liver metastases from midgut and foregut carcinoids and endocrine pancreatic tumors. World J Surg. 2008;32:930–8.
3. Filosso PL, Ruffini E, Oliaro A, Papalia E, Donati G, Rena O. Long-term survival of atypical bronchial carcinoids with liver metastases, treated with octreotide. Eur J Cardiothorac Surg. 2002;21:913–7.
4. Bellizzi AM. Assigning site of origin in metastatic neuroendocrine neoplasms: a clinically significant application of diagnostic immunohistochemistry. Adv Anat Pathol. 2013;20:285–314.
5. Soga J, Tazawa K. Pathologic analysis of carcinoids. Histologic reevaluation of 62 cases. Cancer. 1971;28:990–8.
6. Erickson LA, Papouchado B, Dimashkieh H, Zhang S, Nakamura N, Lloyld RV. Cdx2 as a marker for neuroendocrine tumors of unknown primary sites. Endocr Pathol. 2004;15:247–52.
7. Barbareschi M, Roldo C, Zamboni G, Capelli P, Cavazza A, Macri E, et al. CDX-2 homeobox gene product expression in neuroendocrine tumors: its role as a marker of intestinal neuroendocrine tumors. Am J Surg Pathol. 2004;28:1169–76.
8. Saqi A, Alexis D, Remotti F, Bhagat G. Usefulness of CDX2 and TTF-1 in differentiating gastrointestinal from pulmonary carcinoids. Am J Clin Pathol. 2005;123:394–404.
9. Lin X, Saad RS, Luckasevic TM, Silverman JF, Liu Y. Diagnostic value of CDX-2 and TTF-1 expressions in separating metastatic neuroendocrine neoplasms of unknown origin. Appl Immunohistochem Mol Morphol. 2007;15:407–14.
10. Long KB, Srivastava A, Hirsch MS, Hornick JL. PAX8 expression in well-differentiated pancreatic endocrine tumors: correlation with clinicopathologic features and comparison with gastrointestinal and pulmonary carcinoid tumors. Am J Surg Pathol. 2010;34:723–9.
11. Sangoi AR, Ohgami RS, Pai RK, Beck AH, McKenney JK, Pai RK. PAX8 expression reliably distinguishes pancreatic well-differentiated neuroendocrine tumors from ileal and pulmonary well-differentiated neuroendocrine tumors and pancreatic acinar cell carcinoma. Mod Pathol. 2011;24:412–24.
12. Koo J, Mertens RB, Mirocha JM, Wang HL, Dhall D. Value of islet 1 and PAX8 in identifying metastatic neuroendocrine tumors of pancreatic origin. Mod Pathol. 2012;25:893–901.
13. Schmitt AM, Riniker F, Anlauf M, Schmid S, Soltermann A, Moch H, et al. Islet 1 (Isl1) expression is a reliable marker for pancreatic endocrine tumors and their metastases. Am J Surg Pathol. 2008;32:420–5.
14. Srivastava A, Hornick JL. Immunohistochemical staining for CDX-2, PDX-1, NESP-55, and TTF-1 can help distinguish gastrointestinal carcinoid tumors from pancreatic endocrine and pulmonary carcinoid tumors. Am J Surg Pathol. 2009;33:626–32.
15. Zimmermann N, Lazar-Karsten P, Keck T, Billmann F, Schmid S, Brabant G, et al. Expression pattern of CDX2, estrogen and progesterone receptors in primary Gastroenteropancreatic neuroendocrine tumors and metastases. Anticancer Res. 2016;36:921–4.
16. Maxwell JE, Sherman SK, Stashek KM, O'Dorisio TM, Bellizzi AM, Howe JR. A practical method to determine the site of unknown primary in metastatic neuroendocrine tumors. Surgery. 2014;156:1359–65.
17. Magenheim J, Klein AM, Stanger BZ, Ashery-Padan R, Sosa-Pineda B, Gu G, et al. Ngn3(+) endocrine progenitor cells control the fate and morphogenesis of pancreatic ductal epithelium. Dev Biol. 2011;359:26–36.
18. Berneman-Zeitouni D, Molakandov K, Elgart M, Mor E, Fornoni A, Domingguez MR, et al. The temporal and hierarchical control of transcription factors-induced liver to pancreas transdifferentiation. PLoS One. 2014;9:e87812.
19. Sussel L, Kalamaras J, Hartigan-O'Connor DJ, Meneses JJ, Pedersen RA, Rubenstein JL, et al. mice lacking the homeodomain transcription factor Nkx2.2 have diabetes due to arrested differentiation of pancreatic beta cells. Development. 1998;125:2213–21.

20. Sander M, Sussel L, Conners J, Scheel D, Kalamaras J, Dela Cruz F, et al. Homeobox gene Nkx6.1 lies downstream of Nkx2.2 in the major pathway of beta-cell formation in the pancreas. Development. 2000;127:5533–40.
21. Wang J, Elghazi L, Parker SE, Kizilocak H, Asano M, Sussel L, et al. The concerted activities of Pax4 and Nkx2.2 are essential to initiate pancreatic beta-cell differentiation. Dev Biol. 2004;266:178–89.
22. Doyle MJ, Loomis ZL, Sussel L. Nkx2.2-repressor activity is sufficient to specify alpha-cells and a small number of beta-cells in the pancreatic islet. Development. 2007;134:515–23.
23. Doyle MJ, Sussel L. Nkx2.2 regulates beta-cell function in the mature islet. Diabetes. 2007;56:1999–2007.
24. Kordowich S, Collombat P, Mansouri A, Serup P. Arx and Nkx2.2 compound deficiency redirects pancreatic alpha- and beta-cell differentiation to a somatostatin/ghrelin co-expressing cell lineage. BMC Dev Biol. 2011;11:52.
25. Mastracci TL, Wilcox CL, Arnes L, Panea C, Golden JA, May CL, et al. Nkx2.2 and Arx genetically interact to regulate pancreatic endocrine cell development and endocrine hormone expression. Dev Biol. 2011;359:1–11.
26. Papizan JB, Singer RA, Tschen SI, Dhawan S, Friel JM, Hipkens SB, et al. Nkx2. 2 repressor complex regulates islet beta-cell specification and prevents beta-to-alpha-cell reprogramming. Genes Dev. 2011;25:2291–305.
27. Desai S, Loomis Z, Pugh-Bernard A, Schrunk J, Doyle MJ, Minic A, et al. Nkx2. 2 regulates cell fate choice in the enteroendocrine cell lineages of the intestine. Dev Biol. 2008;313:58–66.
28. Wang YC, Gallego-Arteche E, Iezza G, Yuan X, Matli MR, Choo SP, et al. Homeodomain transcription factor NKX2.2 functions in immature cells to control enteroendocrine differentiation and is expressed in gastrointestinal neuroendocrine tumors. Endocr Relat Cancer. 2009;16:267–79.
29. Briscoe J, Sussel L, Serup P, Hartigan-O'Connor D, Jessell TM, Rubenstein JL, et al. Homeobox gene Nkx2.2 and specification of neuronal identity by graded sonic hedgehog signalling. Nature. 1999;398:622–7.
30. Qi Y, Cai J, Wu Y, Wu R, lee J, Fu H, et al. control of oligodendrocyte differentiation by the Nkx2.2 homeodomain transcription factor. Development. 2001;128:2723–33.
31. Jorgensen MC, Ahnfelt-Ronne J, Hald J, Madsen OD, Serup P, Kecksher-Sorensen J. An illustrated review of early pancreas development in the mouse. Endocr Rev. 2007;28:685–705.
32. Lin W, Xu P, Guo Y, Jia Q, Tao T. Nuclear import of Nkx2-2 is mediated by multiple pathways. Biochem Biophys Res Commun. 2017;482:1511–6.
33. Gross S, Balderes D, Liu J, Asfaha S, Gu G, Wang TC, et al. Nkx2.2 is expressed in a subset of enteroendocrine cells with expanded lineage potential. Am J Physiol Gastrointest Liver Physiol. 2015;309:G975–87.
34. Wang YC, Iezza G, Zuraek MB, Jablons DM, Theodore PR, Bergsland EK, et al. Lack of NKX2.2 expression in bronchopulmonary typical carcinoid tumors: implications for patients with neuroendocrine tumor metastases and unknown primary site. J Surg Res. 2010;163:47–51.
35. Agoff SN, Lamps LW, Philip AT, Amin MB, Schmidt RA, True LD, et al. Thyroid transcription factor-1 is expressed in extrapulmonary small cell carcinomas but not in other extrapulmonary neuroendocrine tumors. Mod Pathol. 2000;13:238–42.
36. Bi Y, Deng Y, Li S, Zhou X, Chen Y, Ma D, et al. Immunophenotypic and prognostic analysis of PAX8 and TTF-1 expressions in neuroendocrine carcinomas of thymic origin: a comparative study with their pulmonary counterparts. J Surg Oncol. 2016;114:697–702.
37. Hirsch MS, Faquin WC, Krane JF. Thyroid transcription factor-1, but not p53, is helpful in distinguishing moderately differentiated neuroendocrine carcinoma of the larynx from medullary carcinoma of the thyroid. Mod Pathol. 2004;17(6):631.
38. Cai YC, Banner B, Glickman J, Odze RD. Cytokeratin 7 and 20 and thyroid transcription factor 1 can help distinguish pulmonary from gastrointestinal carcinoid and pancreatic endocrine tumors. Hum Pathol. 2001;32:1087–93.
39. Lai JP, Mertens RB, Mirocha J, Koo J, Venturina M, Chung F, et al. Comparison of PAX6 and PAX8 as immunohistochemical markers for pancreatic neuroendocrine tumors. Endocr Pathol. 2015;26:54–62.
40. Agaimy A, Erlenbach-Wunsch K, Konukiewitz B, Schmitt AM, Rieker RJ, Vieth M, et al. ISL1 expression is not restricted to pancreatic well-differentiated neuroendocrine neoplasms, but is also commonly found in well and poorly differentiated neuroendocrine neoplasms of extrapancreatic origin. Mod Pathol. 2013;26:995–1003.
41. Yang Z, Klimstra DS, Hruban RH, Tang LH. Immunohistochemical characterization of the origins of metastatic well-differentiated neuroendocrine tumors to the liver. Am J Surg Pathol. 2017;41:915–22.

25

Heterogeneous expression of EPCAM in human circulating tumour cells from patient-derived xenografts

Chiara Agnoletto[1], Linda Minotti[1], Laura Brulle-Soumare[2], Lorenzo Pasquali[3], Marco Galasso[1], Fabio Corrà[1], Federica Baldassari[1], Jean-Gabriel Judde[2], Stefano Cairo[2] and Stefano Volinia[1*]

Abstract

Background: We aim to characterize the heterogeneous circulating tumour cells (CTCs) in peripheral blood, independently of physical or immunological purification, by using patient-derived xenografts (PDXs) models. CTC studies from blood generally rely on enrichment or purification. Conversely, we devised a method for the inclusive study of human cells from blood of PDX models, without pre-selection or enrichment.

Methods: A qRT-PCR assay was developed to detect human and cancer-related transcripts from CTCs in PDXs. We quantified the EPCAM and keratins CTC markers, in a PDX cohort of breast cancer. The murine beta actin gene was used for normalization. Spearman's rho coefficients were calculated for correlation.

Results: We demonstrated, for the first time, that we can quantify the content of CTCs and the expression of human CTC markers in PDX blood using human-specific qRT-PCR. Our method holds strong potential for the study of CTC heterogeneity and for the identification of novel CTC markers.

Conclusions: The identification and the relative quantification of the diverse spectrum of CTCs in patients, irrespective of EPCAM or other currently used markers, will have a great impact on personalized medicine: unrestricted CTCs characterization will allow the early detection of metastases in cancer patients and the assessment of personalized therapies.

Keywords: CTCs, RT-qPCR, PDX

Background

Metastases from primary tumours account for the great majority of cancer-related deaths [1]. This process is thought to involve a series of sequential steps, including the release of circulating tumour cells (CTCs) into blood stream [1, 2]. CTCs have been detected in the peripheral blood of patients with advanced cancers of different origin [3]. Recently, liquid biopsy focusing on the analysis of CTCs has received enormous attention because of its clinical implications [4–6]. The elucidation of CTC's role might represent a turning point in understanding the evolution of tumours during treatment and progression [3]. Clinical applications of CTC detection include early cancer diagnosis, risk prediction for relapse or progression, monitoring the effects of systemic therapies, and stratification of patients [4]. CTC analysis might provide an alternative route for primary diagnosis of tumours, and for restaging/molecular analysis of metastatic lesions. At present, CTCs are used as biomarkers in > 270 clinical trials registered at ClinicalTrials.gov [5]. In on-going interventional studies, the clinical utility of CTC use for therapeutic decisions is being evaluated [7].

To date, however, only incomplete information is available on CTC molecular and biological heterogeneity, and significance. The fact that CTCs are extremely rare, even in patients with advanced metastatic cancers (estimated at one CTC/ billion normal blood cells), and that they may be poised on the verge of apoptosis, has made their analysis contingent upon technological constraints, posing a

* Correspondence: stefano.volinia@unife.it
[1]Department of Morphology, Surgery and Experimental Medicine, LTTA Centre, University of Ferrara, 44121 Ferrara, Italy

serious challenge to any analytical system [8–10]. Thus, although the potential CTC applications appear very promising, there is a critical need for increased detection sensitivity, requiring appropriate, high throughput, and reliable platforms for the isolation or rare tumour cells from blood.

It is thought that only a minor and variable fraction of CTCs represents viable metastatic precursors or tumour-initiating cells [11]. Aberrant activation of epithelial-mesenchymal transition (EMT) in adherent epithelial cells has been implicated in preclinical models as a prerequisite for invasive growth and metastatic spread [12–14]. EMT results in a reduced expression of epithelial markers, increased plasticity and capacity for migration and invasion, thus enabling detachment of tumour cells from a primary site and their passage into the circulation [12]. It also reduces their competence to initiate overt metastasis [15]. Therefore, the most accepted view is currently that tumour cells with a partial EMT have the highest plasticity and represent tumour cells with stem cell-like properties (i.e. metastatic potential) [4, 16, 17]. The detection of CTCs with such an intermediate phenotype seems to be now of the utmost importance, and thus the definition of a wider range of specific markers is required. In general, this plastic phenotype is characterized by partial down-regulation of epithelial markers, and partial up-regulation of mesenchymal markers [5]. Overall, thus far, there is still an incomplete knowledge on the heterogeneity of CTCs [18, 19]; further molecular characterization may give better insights, and help to distinguish clinically relevant CTCs [20]. Most of the current CTC isolation techniques rely on antibody-based capture. Epithelial markers expressed by tumours but not on blood cells have been frequently used to purify cancer cells [6, 21]. The CellSearch system (Menarini Silicon Biosystems), is highly standardized and is currently being evaluated for clinical applications, with CTCs defined as the subset of EpCAM (epithelial cell adhesion molecule)-captured cells, that are confirmed as positive for cytokeratins (KRT8, 18, and 19) and negative for CD45 [22]. However, this technique suffers from relatively low sensitivity: only a fraction of patients with metastatic cancer scores positive for CTCs, with a median yield of approximately one CTC per millilitre and typically low purity [23]. Thus, while progress has been made in the development of microfluidic devices, the discovery and validation of CTC markers is still in its infancy. Indeed, studies on CTCs have been hampered by reliance on a restricted pool of markers [3, 24], often leading to false-negative results [25]. To address these technical challenges, methods for the detection of CTCs from clinical samples should measure both the epithelial and the mesenchymal-like populations, as well as tumour cells with stem cell-like properties [16, 26]. In other words, there is a need for a broad-spectrum enrichment of CTCs based on cell surface epithelial and mesenchymal markers [12, 27], to avoid loss of CTCs with high phenotypic plasticity.

Here, we describe a novel approach that does not rely on the use of epithelial markers such as EPCAM for detection of CTCs in patient-derived xenografts (PDXs). PDXs are generated by transplanting patients' tumour cells or tissues, obtained either by surgical resection or biopsy, into immunodeficient mice [28, 29]. The development of PDXs has significantly enhanced cancer research: these models have been established for different types of cancers, are biologically stable and reflect the patients' tumours in terms of histology, gene profiles, inflammation, and therapeutic response. Thus, PDX models found general application in preclinical screening and evaluation of drugs, identification of therapeutic targets and biomarkers, biological studies, and personalized medicine strategies [29]. At present, CTCs have also been used to generate PDX models, with a great potential for studying tumorigenicity, and for the phenotypic and genetic characterization of CTCs themselves [29]. In this study, we took advantage of PDXs to study human CTCs in a murine genetic background, using human-specific RT-quantitative PCR (RT-qPCR) on RNA from total blood mononuclear cells. By using this highly specific and sensitive approach, without any CTC pre-isolation, we could identify and measure human CTC mRNAs irrespectively of the EPCAM content. In turn this procedure has the potential to identify membrane proteins, that could represent molecular handles for the immune-isolation of viable CTCs. Our approach could represent a major step towards the complete coverage of molecular and cellular heterogeneity in CTCs.

Methods

Patient-derived xenograft models establishment and blood samples collection

All PDXs used in the study were established upon approval of hospitals' ethical committees, and an informed consent was signed for each patient. The major clinical characteristics of the PDX models used in this study are reported in Additional file 1: Table S1. Tumour samples were grafted in the interscapular region of 6- to 8-week-old female athymic nude mice (Athymic Nude-Foxn1nu, ENVIGO-Harlan Laboratories, Gannat, France). Growing tumours were serially transplanted onto recipient mice, underwent comparative examination to confirm preservation of their histological features and were live-frozen to immortalize the model. Blood was collected from mice with tumours reaching the ethical size (tumour volume > 1500 mm^3) and eventually sacrificed in compliance with the indications provided in the protocol, as approved by the animal ethical committee and by the French Ministry of agriculture food and forestry. Briefly, at least 600–800 μl of whole blood were collected from mice by intra-cardiac sampling and under xylazine-ketamine anaesthesia. Blood samples were transferred in Eppendorf tubes containing 0.5 M EDTA, and erythrocytes were lysed at room temperature using the ACK Lysing Buffer (Lonza Walkersville, Inc., Allendale, NJ, USA). PBMC (Peripheral Blood Mononuclear Cells) were frozen in liquid nitrogen and stored at – 80 °C.

RNA isolation and species-specific primers design

For gene expression studies, mouse or PDX PBMC, with or without human CTCs, were lysed by adding 500 µl of Trizol (Invitrogen, Carlsbad, CA, USA). RNA quantity and purity were assessed using a NanoDrop ND-1000 Spectrophotometer (Thermo Fischer Scientific, Wilmington, DE, USA). Total RNA (~ 1 µg) was reverse-transcribed in a final volume of 20 µl using random hexamers and SuperScript II (Life Technologies, Carlsbad, CA, USA). For each gene, human-specific primers were designed using Primer-BLAST at the National Center for Biotechnology Information and verified using the Genome Browser UCSC In-Silico PCR tool; primers with sequence homologies between *Homo sapiens* and *Mus musculus* were excluded. If possible, primers that amplified regions spanning two or more exons or the 5′- or 3′-UTR regions of the transcript were selected, to avoid amplification of genomic sequences and operator or laboratory contamination (Additional file 2: Table S2). To validate species-specificity, all oligonucleotides were tested in RT-PCR on RNA pools from human cell lines (ZR-75-1, MCF-7, MDA-MB-231 breast cancer, and MDA-MB-435 melanoma cells) and Sv/129 mouse blood. One µl of cDNA was amplified using DreamTaq DNA Polymerase (Life Technologies), according to the manufacturer's instructions. Single nested PCR was performed with 1 µl of a 1:10 diluted pre-amplification reaction, by using DreamTaq DNA Polymerase (Life Technologies). PCR products were then analyzed on a 2% low melting point agarose gel.

Quantitative PCR

Gene specific primers and conditions used in qPCR are listed in Additional file 2: Table S2. To ensure detection of very rare human transcripts, one µl of each cDNA was subjected to 14-cycles pre-amplification with DreamTaq DNA Polymerase, and human specific oligonucleotides: for both human reference and target transcripts, pre-amplification was performed with annealing at 58 °C for 5 min. qPCR was then performed using nested specific primers and Dual-Lock™ Taq DNA polymerase on a CFX96 Touch (Bio-Rad Laboratories, Inc., Hercules, CA, USA). qPCR was carried out in 10 µl volume using PowerUp SYBR Green Master Mix (Applied Biosystems™), and 1 µl of a 1:10 diluted pre-amplification reaction. Primers were added to a final concentration of 0.2 µM or 0.3 µM each, depending on the gene, as detailed in Additional file 2: Table S2. After the initial step (2 min at 50 °C for polymerase activation and 2 min of denaturation at 95 °C), 40 cycles were carried out by denaturation at 95 °C for 15 s, and annealing/extension as indicated in Additional file 2: Table S2. The melting curves were evaluated, to confirm the specificity of each reaction. Samples were analyzed in duplicate for mouse Actb reference (mActb), while for each human transcripts qPCR was repeated in four or five independent assays. RNAs from naïve mouse blood (negative control) and human cell lines (positive control) were included in each PCR assay.

The method based on the expectation–maximization (EM) algorithm, as implemented in the R *'nondetects'* package, was applied to estimate missing C_t values [30]. This function returns a qPCRset object with non-detects replaced by their imputed values. Non-detects in qPCR data represent data missing not at random, and the EM algorithm provides a method to obtain maximum likelihood estimates in the presence of missing data by iteratively calculating the conditional expectation. This requires estimating the distribution of gene expression given a non-detect; the process is repeated until convergence. Lastly, estimates of the missing data will be obtained and used to impute the non-detect values. PDX samples with at least one replicate for each human reference, having estimated C_t value larger than 40, were deemed as CTC-negative and excluded from further analyses. Estimated C_t values for target genes higher than 40 were thresholded to 40, and median C_t values used for each gene. The relative quantities of human reference genes normalized on the mouse Actb gene were calculated with the ΔC_t method using the R *'HTqPCR'* package. Conversely, for CTC relative measures, the quantities of human target genes were normalized on the quantities of each human reference gene. All statistical analyses, i.e. Spearman's *rho* correlation coefficient calculation, were performed using SPSS (version 23) and *p* values were two-sided.

Results

Species-specific PCR for detection of human circulating tumour cells in PDX blood

Peripheral blood samples were collected from 28 PDXs and 3 naïve mice (negative controls). Following chemical erythrocytes depletion, RNA was extracted from the whole blood cell pellet, reverse-transcribed and tested for expression of the human EPCAM and KRT19 CTC markers. Human coding region-specific primers were also designed for two reference genes, OAZ1 and ACTB, to avoid detection of mouse homologues and amplification of human genomic DNA (Additional file 2: Table S2). The species-specificity of the protocol was assessed using naïve mouse blood samples and human cell lines as negative and positive controls, respectively. For primer optimization, cDNA from human cell lines and control mice was pre-amplified, and further subjected to single-gene nested PCR (representative assays are reported in Fig. 1). Once verified the species-specificity of the primers, the cDNA from the PDX cohort was tested for the expression of human genes.

Human-specific quantitative RT-PCR on CTCs in blood of PDX mice

RNAs extracted from PDX blood samples were subjected to three independent reverse-transcription reactions and qPCR assays were performed on the pooled cDNAs. The expression levels of the murine reference gene Actb (mActb) and human reference genes OAZ1 and ACTB were measured in each sample. Human cDNAs were pre-amplified, and then subjected to nested-qPCR by using human-specific primers (Additional file 2: Table S2). No detection was obtained in control mice (no PDX) for both human reference genes (no control mice had C_t lower than 40), indicating that in our protocol the human specific quantitative PCR did not lead to false positives. The human references were amplified in five independent qPCRs for each sample (replicated). Undetermined C_t values were estimated by using the expectation–maximization (EM) algorithm, as previously described [30]. The blood from three PDX mice, HB-214-FOI(b), T180R(c), HBCx-28(a), was negative for the human reference genes, therefore had no detectable CTC and the samples were thus excluded from further studies.

Expression of human CTC markers in blood from PDX mice

The expression levels of human EPCAM, KRT19, ACTB and OAZ1 in the blood of PDX models were measured using qPCR (Additional file 3: Table S3 and Additional file 4: Table S4). The normalized expression values for human genes were calculated relative to murine Actb and shown in Fig. 2, sorted by the level of the human OAZ1 reference gene (as approx. indicator of CTC content). As expected for two 'housekeeping' genes, the RNA levels of the two human reference genes (ACTB and OAZ1) were significantly correlated (Spearman's *rho* = 0.462, $p < 0.05$). Ideally ACTB, OAZ1, or any other human 'housekeeping' gene, would act as proxies for the assessment of human CTC content in the PDX blood. We then studied the expression of EPCAM and KRT19 epithelial markers within the human CTC component. The normalized expression values for human target genes were calculated relative to each human reference gene, using the ΔC_t method, obviously with no difference whether the human genes were previously normalized on murine Actb. The expected plots for the different hypotheses that EPCAM levels were not (A), positively (B) or negatively (C) correlated with the total human RNA content are shown in Additional file 5: Figure S1, and describe the predictions of EPCAM profiles relative to human OAZ1. Because the plots report ΔC_t values, the PDX samples with higher

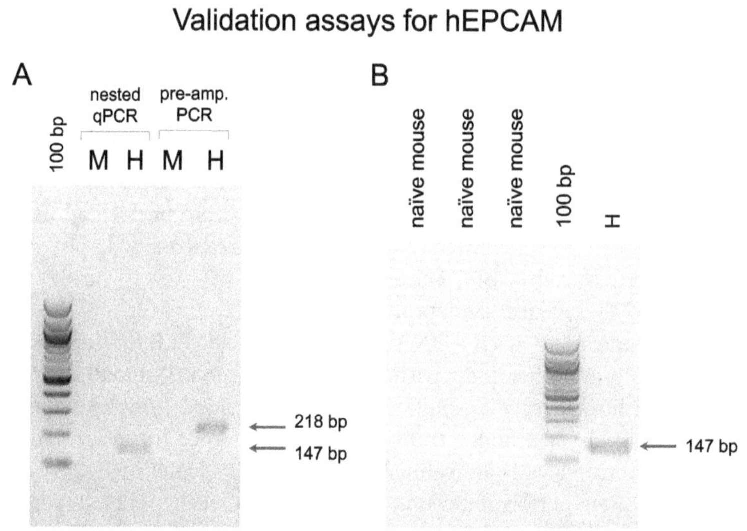

Fig. 1 Representative results from RT- PCR assays for human EPCAM detection in PDX blood. **a** RT-PCR assays confirming PCR specificity on human gene were performed on pooled RNAs from human cell lines: ZR-75-1, MCF-7, MDA-MB-231 breast cancer, and MDA-MB-435 melanoma cells (H), and on RNA from Sv/129 mouse PBMC (M). Each primer set was tested at least in two independent assays. The expected size fragments are indicated. Molecular weight marker: 100 bp DNA Ladder (NE Biolabs). **b** The specificity of the nested-PCR assays was assessed on blood RNA from the naïve mouse used to generate the PDX models (naïve mouse) and on the pooled human cell lines RNA (H), used as negative and positive controls respectively. Each assay was performed at least twice. The expected size fragment is indicated. Molecular weight marker: 100 bp DNA Ladder (NE Biolabs)

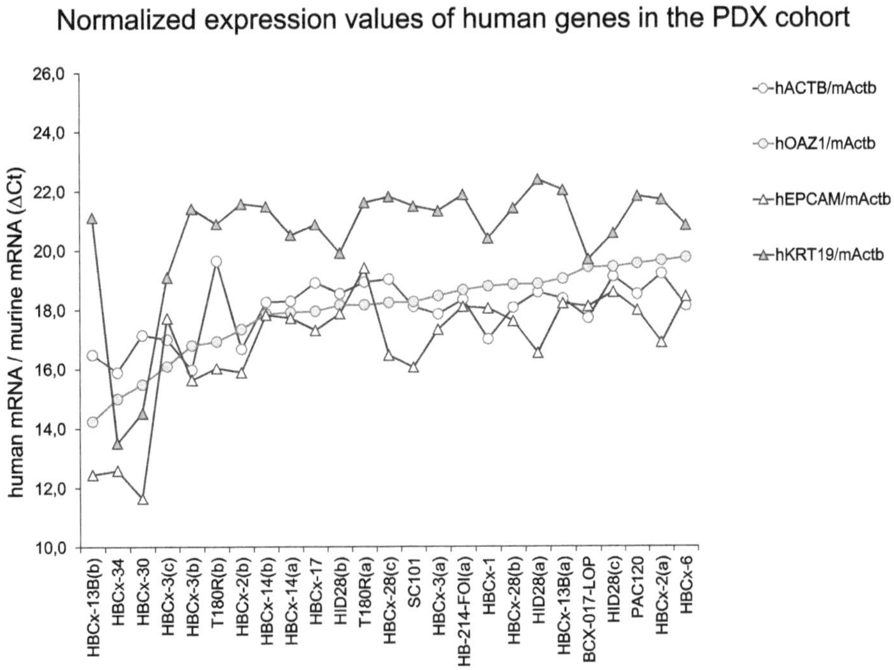

Fig. 2 Normalized expression levels of human genes. The expression levels of human ACTB and OAZ1 reference genes and EPCAM and KRT19 epithelial markers were normalized on murine reference gene Actb, for each PDX sample. Data were expressed as ΔCt values and graphed, sorted on human OAZ1 content. Samples were analyzed in two independent assays for mActb; for human transcripts, qPCR was repeated in four (KRT19) or five (ACTB, OAZ1, EPCAM) independent assays for each gene. In each run, each RNA was measured in duplicate

CTC content (more RNA from OAZ1 housekeeping gene) are towards the left, and those with higher EPCAM in CTC are towards the bottom. The null hypothesis was that EPCAM, if present, was expressed by the CTCs at constant cellular levels (RNA molecules per CTC cell) in different PDXs; thus as human RNA content increases, EPCAM levels should be correspondingly higher (resulting in relatively constant ΔC_t(hEPCAM - hOAZ1) values); this would correspond to the panel A in Additional file 5: Figure S1 (flat line, no correlation). In Fig. 3 we report the

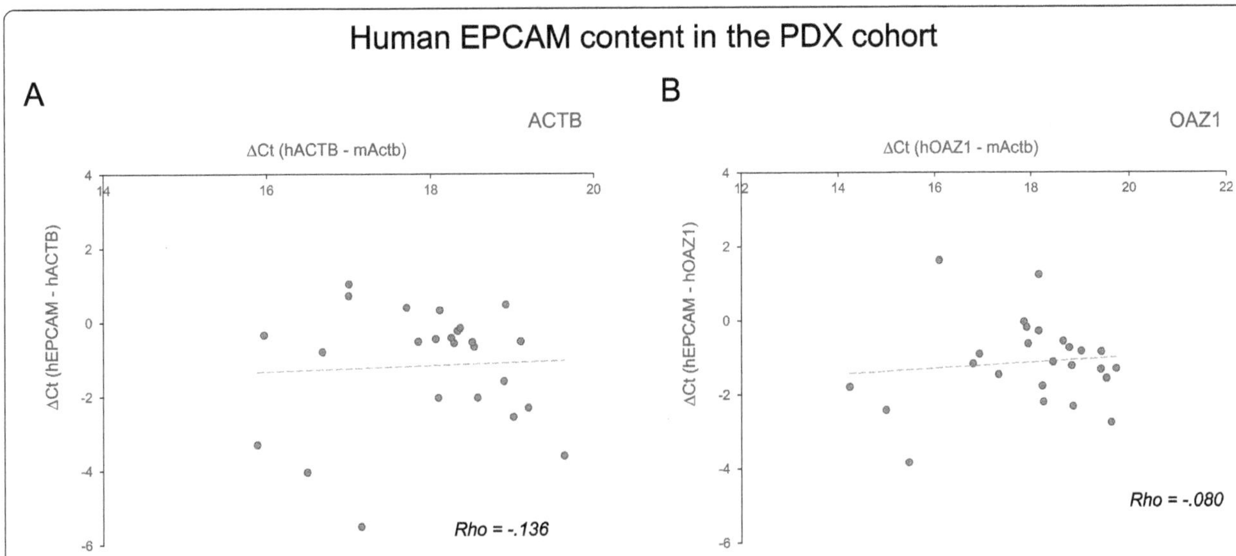

Fig. 3 Correlation of EPCAM expression and human RNA content in PDX cohort. The correlation between EPCAM expression relative to human references ACTB (in **a**) or OAZ1 (in **b**) and the human reference content relative to murine Actb was graphed. Each PDX blood sample gene expression levels were graphed as a scatterplot. Human reference gene Ct values were normalized on the murine Actb gene. Human EPCAM Ct values were normalized on human reference gene. The linear regression fit lines and Spearman's rho correlation coefficients are reported

real data for measured EPCAM levels, relative to two human reference RNAs. In the PDX cohort, the EPCAM levels showed to be relatively constant, as the human content increased, indicative of a pattern similar to A in Additional file 5: Figure S1 (stable reservoir of EPCAM+ cells). The same protocol was applied to KRT19, the most common alternative marker for CTCs detection. As observed for EPCAM, also KRT19 was expressed at similar content in PDXs with diverse amounts of human reference RNAs (Fig. 4). No significant correlation was measured between the two epithelial markers (Spearman's rho = 0.219, relative to ACTB, and rho = 0.152, relative to OAZ1; both $p > 0.05$) [31].

Discussion

Detection of circulating tumour cells in the blood of patients with cancer shows great potential as a 'liquid biopsy', and multiple technologies have been developed for CTC capture [4]. The limitations in current CTC detection are mainly due to reduced specificity and sensitivity and should be carefully considered when interpreting the literature [3]. The quest for technical developments has slowed down the introduction of CTCs into clinical diagnostics. However, new important insights into the biology of CTCs have been reported [32], and tools for combined enrichment, detection, and characterization of CTCs are emerging.

Although the prognostic value of CTC has been demonstrated [33–35], metastatic patients frequently present little or undetectable CTCs when using epithelial markers [12]. Otherwise, higher numbers of CTCs could be detected using alternative methods, suggesting that a mixture of EPCAM+ and EPCAM- tumour cells circulate in the blood [12, 36]. Therefore EpCAM-based CTC isolation might suffer of limitations in the clinical settings since its sensitivity is significantly dependent on EpCAM expression [37]. Also, non-epithelial CTCs might exert a more relevant function in tumorigenesis: indeed, mouse models and in vitro experiments evidenced that EMT, together with stem-like properties in circulating cancer cells, is associated with increased cellular migration and resistance to therapy [16, 38]. Thus, the pre-selection for cells that have retained significant expression of epithelial markers represents an intrinsic challenge in studying CTCs [27]. To overcome these limitations the isolation of CTCs based on size has been described [8], reportedly leading to higher CTC yields. A larger set of tumour-specific markers would be then useful in establishing the identity of the heterogeneous CTCs enriched by filtration strategies, and to rescue those that might escape.

To develop a method for the identification of undifferentiated (or EPCAM-) CTCs, we used human specie-specific qRT-PCR and blood from PDXs. PDX models represent an ideal system for our study, allowing to exclusively profile the human transcriptome in the CTCs, excluding a priori the possible contamination of human mononuclear cells. Species-specific primers were designed and validated in human cell lines and naïve mouse blood. Nested quantitative human-specific qRT-PCR was established as a highly specific and sensitive method to detect and measure the expression of human CTC genes, with no detection of murine genes. Human RNAs for reference genes and epithelial markers were quantified in the blood of patient-derived xenografts from breast cancer. The null

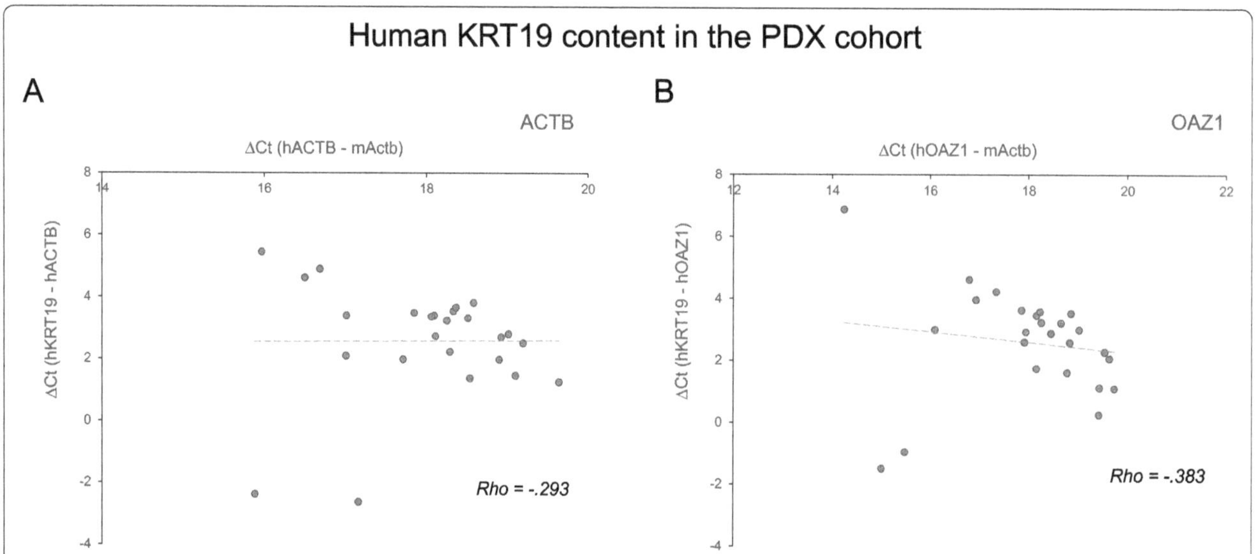

Fig. 4 Correlation of KRT19 expression and human RNA content in PDX cohort. The correlation between KRT19 expression relative to human references ACTB (in **a**) or OAZ1 (in **b**) and the human reference content relative to murine Actb was graphed. Each PDX blood sample gene expression levels were graphed as a scatterplot. Human reference gene Ct values were normalized on the murine Actb gene. Human KRT19 Ct values were normalized on human reference gene. The linear regression fit lines and Spearman's rho correlation coefficients are reported

hypothesis in our study was that EPCAM, when present, would be expressed in CTCs at levels correlated to those of the human housekeeping genes. These results were obtained by using two different reference genes, OAZ1 and ACTB (found to be correlated between them, as expected for housekeeping genes), and also mirrored by another epithelial marker, KRT19. Our findings confirmed that we could reliably measure mRNA from rare CTCs, in the peripheral blood, with the highest degree of sensitivity and specificity. Therefore our assay is able to determine the presence of occult circulating tumour cells in the peripheral blood and has the potential to identify novel CTC markers using PDX mice. For the accurate measure of human CTC content in PDX blood, genomic DNA would be used. Tumour DNA content is more stable than RNA content, thus in principle this measure could result in absolute CTC counts. We decided to focus at first on human mRNA to avoid any environmental contamination, which could greatly affect the results of this extremely sensitive protocol.

The follow-up of this pilot study involves: *i)* identification of novel CTC markers from PDX cohorts; *ii)* test of these novel CTC markers in blood from human cancer patients. Genes detected in the EPCAM-negative subset of samples would lead to isolate CTC subpopulations with intermediate or not well defined phenotype. Eventually a novel set of genes for CTCs capture would be identified, allowing for capture of viable heterogeneous CTCs in murine human cancer xenograft models. Transcripts with no, or very low, expression in PBMC from healthy donors could be used for CTC monitoring in blood of tumour patients for clinical and research applications. At last, human genes expressed in blood of PDX models, originating from circulating tumour cells, will need to be validated in human blood specimens. The application of our approach was originally addressed to the detection and capture of human circulating tumour cells deriving from solid tumours, first in PDX models and then in patients. However, it can be applied in PDX models also for human hematologic malignancies. Recently, a model of human AML has been developed, which efficiently recapitulated the pathological features, including myeloid sarcoma, spleen enlargement, and infiltration of leukemic cells from bone marrow [39]. Since our method is designed to discriminate the transcripts from murine and human species in murine blood samples, circulating leukemic stem cells, which are believed to influence engraftment potential in recipient mice and are responsible for disease resistance or relapse in patients, could be easily examined.

Conclusions

It is in our plans to extend the number of human CTC markers in the assay, the cohort of PDX mice, to incorporate CTC counting by genomic DNA and to perform in parallel single-cell RNA sequencing. Using multiple targets for CTC capture and identification would increase the comprehensiveness of CTC detection. Our work shows the presence of heterogeneous molecular phenotypes in CTCs from a PDX breast cancer cohort and provides the basis for the detection of the diverse spectrum of tumour cells that circulate in blood. Ultimately, alternative methods for detection of CTCs from human samples would be implemented. Extended molecular characterization of CTCs may provide further insight into the biology of these cells and their link to metastasis. Furthermore, molecular profiles of CTCs could lead to novel non-invasive diagnostic tools, and allow real-time monitoring of treatment responses. In this context, we consider our protocol as a proof of concept, with a great potential in opening up a new way towards the identification of novel markers for CTC capture.

Abbreviations

ACTB: Actin beta [*Homo sapiens*]; CTC: Circulating tumour cells; EPCAM: Epithelial cell adhesion molecule [*Homo sapiens*]; KRT19: Keratin 19 [*Homo sapiens*]; mActb: Actin beta [*Mus musculus*]; OAZ1: Ornithine decarboxylase antizyme 1 [*Homo sapiens*]; PDX: Patient-derived xenografts

Funding

S.V. is supported by Associazione Italiana Ricerca sul Cancro AIRC (IG 17063), and Italian PRIN MIUR 2010 (2010W4J4RM).

Authors' contributions

CA and SV designed the research, LBS and SC collected the samples and the clinical data; CA performed in vitro experiments and analyzed the data; CA and SV performed data analysis and biostatistics analysis. CA, SV, JGJ and SC interpreted the results; CA and SV wrote the manuscript. LM, LP, MG, FC and FB participate in paper revision. All authors read and approved the final manuscript.

Competing interests

The authors declare that they have no competing interests.

Author details

[1]Department of Morphology, Surgery and Experimental Medicine, LTTA Centre, University of Ferrara, 44121 Ferrara, Italy. [2]Xentech, Paris, France. [3]Dermatology and Venereology Unit, Department of Medicine, Center for Molecular Medicine, Karolinska University Hospital, SE-17176 Stockholm, Sweden.

References

1. Nguyen DX, Bos PD, Massagué J. Metastasis: from dissemination to organ-specific colonization. Nat Rev Cancer. 2009;9:274–84. https://doi.org/10.1038/nrc2622.
2. Aceto N, Bardia A, Miyamoto DT, Donaldson MC, Wittner BS, Spencer JA, et al. Circulating tumor cell clusters are oligoclonal precursors of breast cancer metastasis. Cell. 2014;158:1110–22. https://doi.org/10.1016/j.cell.2014.07.013.
3. Yu M, Stott S, Toner M, Maheswaran S, Haber DA. Circulating tumor cells: approaches to isolation and characterization. J Cell Biol. 2011;192:373–82. https://doi.org/10.1083/jcb.201010021.
4. Alix-Panabières C, Pantel K. Clinical applications of circulating tumor cells and circulating tumor DNA as liquid biopsy. Cancer Discov. 2016;6:479–91. https://doi.org/10.1158/2159-8290.CD-15-1483.

5. Alix-Panabières C, Pantel K. Challenges in circulating tumour cell research. Nat Rev Cancer. 2014;14:623–31. https://doi.org/10.1038/nrc3820.
6. Pantel K, Alix-Panabières C. Circulating tumour cells in cancer patients: challenges and perspectives. Trends Mol Med. 2010;16:398–406. https://doi.org/10.1016/j.molmed.2010.07.001.
7. Bidard F-C, Fehm T, Ignatiadis M, Smerage JB, Alix-Panabières C, Janni W, et al. Clinical application of circulating tumor cells in breast cancer: overview of the current interventional trials. Cancer Metastasis Rev. 2013;32: 179–88. https://doi.org/10.1007/s10555-012-9398-0.
8. Nagrath S, Sequist LV, Maheswaran S, Bell DW, Irimia D, Ulkus L, et al. Isolation of rare circulating tumour cells in cancer patients by microchip technology. Nature. 2007;450:1235–9. https://doi.org/10.1038/nature06385.
9. Ozkumur E, Shah AM, Ciciliano JC, Emmink BL, Miyamoto DT, Brachtel E, et al. Inertial focusing for tumor antigen-dependent and -independent sorting of rare circulating tumor cells. Sci Transl Med. 2013;5:179ra47. https://doi.org/10.1126/scitranslmed.3005616.
10. Stott SL, Hsu C-H, Tsukrov DI, Yu M, Miyamoto DT, Waltman BA, et al. Isolation of circulating tumor cells using a microvortex-generating herringbone-chip. Proc Natl Acad Sci U S A. 2010;107:18392–7. https://doi.org/10.1073/pnas.1012539107.
11. Hodgkinson CL, Morrow CJ, Li Y, Metcalf RL, Rothwell DG, Trapani F, et al. Tumorigenicity and genetic profiling of circulating tumor cells in small-cell lung cancer. Nat Med. 2014;20:897–903. https://doi.org/10.1038/nm.3600.
12. Yu M, Bardia A, Wittner BS, Stott SL, Smas ME, Ting DT, et al. Circulating breast tumor cells exhibit dynamic changes in epithelial and mesenchymal composition. Science. 2013;339:580–4. https://doi.org/10.1126/science.1228522.
13. Pecot CV, Bischoff FZ, Mayer JA, Wong KL, Pham T, Bottsford-Miller J, et al. A novel platform for detection of CK+ and CK- CTCs. Cancer Discov. 2011;1: 580–6. https://doi.org/10.1158/2159-8290.CD-11-0215.
14. Thiery JP. Epithelial-mesenchymal transitions in tumour progression. Nat Rev Cancer. 2002;2:442–54. https://doi.org/10.1038/nrc822.
15. Kang Y, Pantel K. Tumor cell dissemination: emerging biological insights from animal models and cancer patients. Cancer Cell. 2013;23:573–81. https://doi.org/10.1016/j.ccr.2013.04.017.
16. Mani SA, Guo W, Liao M-J, Eaton EN, Ayyanan A, Zhou AY, et al. The epithelial-mesenchymal transition generates cells with properties of stem cells. Cell. 2008;133:704–15. https://doi.org/10.1016/j.cell.2008.03.027.
17. Tam WL, Weinberg RA. The epigenetics of epithelial-mesenchymal plasticity in cancer. Nat Med. 2013;19:1438–49. https://doi.org/10.1038/nm.3336.
18. Wan L, Pantel K, Kang Y. Tumor metastasis: moving new biological insights into the clinic. Nat Med. 2013;19:1450–64. https://doi.org/10.1038/nm.3391.
19. Lohr JG, Adalsteinsson VA, Cibulskis K, Choudhury AD, Rosenberg M, Cruz-Gordillo P, et al. Whole-exome sequencing of circulating tumor cells provides a window into metastatic prostate cancer. Nat Biotechnol. 2014;32: 479–84. https://doi.org/10.1038/nbt.2892.
20. Wicha MS, Hayes DF. Circulating tumor cells: not all detected cells are bad and not all bad cells are detected. J Clin Oncol. 2011;29:1508–11. https://doi.org/10.1200/JCO.2010.34.0026.
21. Pantel K, Alix-Panabières C. Real-time liquid biopsy in cancer patients: fact or fiction? Cancer Res. 2013;73:6384–8. https://doi.org/10.1158/0008-5472.CAN-13-2030.
22. Riethdorf S, Fritsche H, Müller V, Rau T, Schindlbeck C, Rack B, et al. Detection of circulating tumor cells in peripheral blood of patients with metastatic breast cancer: a validation study of the CellSearch system. Clin Cancer Res. 2007;13:920–8. https://doi.org/10.1158/1078-0432.CCR-06-1695.
23. Attard G, Swennenhuis JF, Olmos D, Reid AHM, Vickers E, A'Hern R, et al. Characterization of ERG, AR and PTEN gene status in circulating tumor cells from patients with castration-resistant prostate cancer. Cancer Res. 2009;69: 2912–8. https://doi.org/10.1158/0008-5472.CAN-08-3667
24. Pantel K, Brakenhoff RH, Brandt B. Detection, clinical relevance and specific biological properties of disseminating tumour cells. Nat Rev Cancer. 2008;8: 329–40. https://doi.org/10.1038/nrc2375.
25. Bednarz-Knoll N, Alix-Panabières C, Pantel K. Clinical relevance and biology of circulating tumor cells. Breast Cancer Res. 2011;13:228. https://doi.org/10.1186/bcr2940.
26. Aktas B, Tewes M, Fehm T, Hauch S, Kimmig R, Kasimir-Bauer S. Stem cell and epithelial-mesenchymal transition markers are frequently overexpressed in circulating tumor cells of metastatic breast cancer patients. Breast Cancer Res. 2009;11:R46. https://doi.org/10.1186/bcr2333.
27. Sieuwerts AM, Kraan J, Bolt J, van der Spoel P, Elstrodt F, Schutte M, et al. Anti-epithelial cell adhesion molecule antibodies and the detection of circulating normal-like breast tumor cells. J Natl Cancer Inst. 2009;101:61–6. https://doi.org/10.1093/jnci/djn419.
28. Hidalgo M, Amant F, Biankin AV, Budinská E, Byrne AT, Caldas C, et al. Patient-derived xenograft models: an emerging platform for translational cancer research. Cancer Discov. 2014;4:998–1013. https://doi.org/10.1158/2159-8290.CD-14-0001.
29. Aparicio S, Hidalgo M, Kung AL. Examining the utility of patient-derived xenograft mouse models. Nat Rev Cancer. 2015;15:311–6. https://doi.org/10.1038/nrc3944.
30. McCall MN, McMurray HR, Land H, Almudevar A. On non-detects in qPCR data. Bioinformatics. 2014;30:2310–6. https://doi.org/10.1093/bioinformatics/btu239.
31. Mikolajczyk SD, Millar LS, Tsinberg P, Coutts SM, Zomorrodi M, Pham T, et al. Detection of EpCAM-negative and cytokeratin-negative circulating tumor cells in peripheral blood. J Oncol. 2011;2011:252361. https://doi.org/10.1155/2011/252361.
32. Pantel K, Speicher MR. The biology of circulating tumor cells. Oncogene. 2016;35:1216–24. https://doi.org/10.1038/onc.2015.192.
33. Cohen SJ, Punt CJA, Iannotti N, Saidman BH, Sabbath KD, Gabrail NY, et al. Prognostic significance of circulating tumor cells in patients with metastatic colorectal cancer. Ann Oncol. 2009;20:1223–9. https://doi.org/10.1093/annonc/mdn786.
34. Cristofanilli M, Budd GT, Ellis MJ, Stopeck A, Matera J, Miller MC, et al. Circulating tumor cells, disease progression, and survival in metastatic breast cancer. N Engl J Med. 2004;351:781–91. https://doi.org/10.1056/NEJMoa040766.
35. de Bono JS, Scher HI, Montgomery RB, Parker C, Miller MC, Tissing H, et al. Circulating tumor cells predict survival benefit from treatment in metastatic castration-resistant prostate cancer. Clin Cancer Res. 2008;14:6302–9. https://doi.org/10.1158/1078-0432.CCR-08-0872.
36. Thurm H, Ebel S, Kentenich C, Hemsen A, Riethdorf S, Coith C, et al. Rare expression of epithelial cell adhesion molecule on residual micrometastatic breast cancer cells after adjuvant chemotherapy. Clin Cancer Res. 2003;9: 2598–604.
37. Gorges TM, Tinhofer I, Drosch M, Röse L, Zollner TM, Krahn T, et al. Circulating tumour cells escape from EpCAM-based detection due to epithelial-to-mesenchymal transition. BMC Cancer. 2012;12:178. https://doi.org/10.1186/1471-2407-12-178.
38. Polyak K, Weinberg RA. Transitions between epithelial and mesenchymal states: acquisition of malignant and stem cell traits. Nat Rev Cancer. 2009;9: 265–73. https://doi.org/10.1038/nrc2620.
39. Her Z, Yong KSM, Paramasivam K, Tan WWS, Chan XY, Tan SY, et al. An improved pre-clinical patient-derived liquid xenograft mouse model for acute myeloid leukemia. J Hematol Oncol. 2017;10:162. https://doi.org/10.1186/s13045-017-0532-x.

Permissions

All chapters in this book were first published in BR, by BioMed Central; hereby published with permission under the Creative Commons Attribution License or equivalent. Every chapter published in this book has been scrutinized by our experts. Their significance has been extensively debated. The topics covered herein carry significant findings which will fuel the growth of the discipline. They may even be implemented as practical applications or may be referred to as a beginning point for another development.

The contributors of this book come from diverse backgrounds, making this book a truly international effort. This book will bring forth new frontiers with its revolutionizing research information and detailed analysis of the nascent developments around the world.

We would like to thank all the contributing authors for lending their expertise to make the book truly unique. They have played a crucial role in the development of this book. Without their invaluable contributions this book wouldn't have been possible. They have made vital efforts to compile up to date information on the varied aspects of this subject to make this book a valuable addition to the collection of many professionals and students.

This book was conceptualized with the vision of imparting up-to-date information and advanced data in this field. To ensure the same, a matchless editorial board was set up. Every individual on the board went through rigorous rounds of assessment to prove their worth. After which they invested a large part of their time researching and compiling the most relevant data for our readers.

The editorial board has been involved in producing this book since its inception. They have spent rigorous hours researching and exploring the diverse topics which have resulted in the successful publishing of this book. They have passed on their knowledge of decades through this book. To expedite this challenging task, the publisher supported the team at every step. A small team of assistant editors was also appointed to further simplify the editing procedure and attain best results for the readers.

Apart from the editorial board, the designing team has also invested a significant amount of their time in understanding the subject and creating the most relevant covers. They scrutinized every image to scout for the most suitable representation of the subject and create an appropriate cover for the book.

The publishing team has been an ardent support to the editorial, designing and production team. Their endless efforts to recruit the best for this project, has resulted in the accomplishment of this book. They are a veteran in the field of academics and their pool of knowledge is as vast as their experience in printing. Their expertise and guidance has proved useful at every step. Their uncompromising quality standards have made this book an exceptional effort. Their encouragement from time to time has been an inspiration for everyone.

The publisher and the editorial board hope that this book will prove to be a valuable piece of knowledge for researchers, students, practitioners and scholars across the globe.

List of Contributors

Gakuro Yoshida, Ichijiro Murata and Nagisa Miyazaki
Department of Nephrology, Gifu University Graduate School of Medicine, Gifu, Japan

Masanori Kawasaki, Yuka Hayakawa, Takuma Aoyama, Yoshihisa Yamada, Kazuhiko Nishigaki and Shinya Minatoguchi
Department of Cardiology, Gifu University Graduate School of Medicine, Yanagido 1-1, Gifu 501-1194, Japan

Yoshie Arai and Fumiaki Suzuki
Faculty of Applied Biological Sciences, Gifu University, Gifu, Japan

Sofie Sølvsten Sørensen and Thomas Christensen
Department of Neurology, Nordsjællands Hospital, University of Copenhagen, Dyrehavevej 29, 3400 Hillerød, Denmark

Ann-Britt Nygaard
Department of Clinical Biochemistry, Nordsjællands Hospital, Hillerød, Denmark

Anting Liu Carlsen and Niels H. H. Heegaard
Department of Autoimmunology and Biomarkers, Statens Serum Institut, Copenhagen, Denmark

Mads Bak
Department of Cellular and Molecular Medicine, Panum Institute, University of Copenhagen, Copenhagen, Denmark

Qinglong Hu
Tucson Pathology Associates, PC Carondelet Saint Joseph Hospital, 351 North Wilmot Road, Tucson, AZ 85711, USA

Yizhuo Zhang
Department of Hematology, Tianjin Medical University Cancer Institute and Hospital, National Clinical Research Center of Cancer, Tianjin Key Laboratory of Cancer Prevention and Therapy, Tianjin 300060, China

Xiaoyan Zhang and Kai Fu
Department of Pathology and Microbiology, University of Nebraska Medical Center, 983135 Nebraska Medical Center, Omaha, NE 68198, USA

John Ha, Aysha Chaudhri, Abhishek Avirineni and Jen-Jung Pan
Department of Internal Medicine, The University of Texas Health Science Center at Houston, 6431 Fanin St, MSB 1.150, Houston, TX 77030, USA

Jen-Jung Pan
Division of Gastroenterology, Hepatology and Nutrition, Department of Internal Medicine, The University of Texas Health Science Center at Houston, 6431 Fanin St, MSB 4.234, Houston, TX 77030, USA

Cheng Zhang, Jun Liu and Xi Zhang
Department of Hematology, Xinqiao Hospital, Third Military Medical University, Chongqing 400037, People's Republic of China

Jiang F. Zhong
Division of Periodontology, Diagnostic Sciences & Dental Hygiene, and Division of Biomedical Sciences, Herman Ostrow School of Dentistry, University of Southern California, Los Angeles, CA, USA

Marcin Krzystanek, Zoltan Szallasi and Aron Charles Eklund
Department of Systems Biology, Center for Biological Sequence Analysis, Technical University of Denmark, Lyngby, Denmark

Judit Moldvay
Department of Tumor Biology, National Koranyi Institute - Semmelweis University, Budapest, Hungary

David Szüts
Institute of Enzymology, Research Centre for Natural Sciences, Hungarian Academy of Sciences, Budapest, Hungary

Zoltan Szallasi
Computational Health Informatics Program (CHIP), Boston Children's Hospital, Boston, USA
Harvard Medical School, Boston, USA

Li Yang and Yi Zhang
Biotherapy Center and Cancer Center, The First Affiliated Hospital of Zhengzhou University, No.1 Jianshe East Road, Zhengzhou, Henan Province 450052, China

Yi Zhang
School of Life Sciences, Zhengzhou University, No.100 Kexue Road, Zhengzhou, Henan Province 450001, China

Tsung-Rong Kuo
Graduate Institute of Nanomedicine and Medical Engineering, College of Biomedical Engineering, Taipei Medical University, Taipei 11031, Taiwan
International Ph.D. Program in Biomedical Engineering, College of Biomedical Engineering, Taipei Medical University, Taipei 11031, Taiwan

Chih-Hwa Chen
Bone and Joint Research Center, Department of Orthopedics and Traumatology, Taipei Medical University Hospital, Taipei 11031, Taiwan
School of Medicine, College of Medicine, Taipei Medical University, Taipei 11031, Taiwan

Christine Y. Yeh
Department of Biomedical Informatics, Stanford University School of Medicine, Stanford, CA 93405, USA

Christine Y. Yeh, Ravali Adusumilli, Majlinda Kullolli, Parag Mallick and Sharon J. Pitteri
Department of Radiology, Canary Center at Stanford for Cancer Early Detection, Stanford University School of Medicine, Palo Alto, CA 94304, USA

Christine Y. Yeh
Department of Genetics, Stanford University School of Medicine, Stanford, CA 93405, USA

Parag Mallick, Esther M. John and Sharon J. Pitteri
Stanford Cancer Institute, Stanford University School of Medicine, Stanford, CA 94305, USA
Cancer Prevention Institute of California, Fremont, CA 94538, USA

Protus Arrey Tarkang
Centre for Research on Medicinal Plants and Traditional Medicine, Institute of Medical Research and Medicinal Plants Studies (IMPM), Yaoundé, Cameroon

Protus Arrey Tarkang, Regina Appiah-Opong and Alexander K. Nyarko
Department of Clinical Pathology, Noguchi Memorial Institute for Medical Research, University of Ghana, Legon, Accra, Ghana

Michael F. Ofori
Department of Immunology, Noguchi Memorial Institute for Medical Research, University of Ghana, Legon, Accra, Ghana

Lawrence S. Ayong
Malaria Research Laboratory, Centre Pasteur Cameroon, BP 1274 Yaoundé, Cameroon

Alexander K. Nyarko
School of Pharmacy, University of Ghana, Legon, Accra, Ghana

Elena Flowers and Bradley E. Aouizerat
Department of Physiological Nursing, School of Nursing, University of California, 2 Koret Way #N605L, CA 94143 San Francisco, USA

Meghana Gadgil and Alka M. Kanaya
Division of General Internal Medicine, University of California, San Francisco, USA

Bradley E. Aouizerat
Institute for Human Genetics, University of California, San Francisco, USA

Alka M. Kanaya
Department of Epidemiology and Biostatistics, University of California, San Francisco, USA

Shih-Chieh Chien
Department of Critical Care Medicine, MacKay Memorial Hospital, No. 92, Sec. 2, Zhongshan N. Rd, Taipei City 10449, Taiwan, Republic of China

Shih-Chieh Chien, Chun-Yen Chen, Chao-Feng Lin and Hung-I Yeh
Cardiovascular Division, Department of Internal Medicine, MacKay Memorial Hospital, Mackay Medical College, No. 92, Sec. 2, Zhongshan N. Rd, Taipei City 10449, Taiwan, Republic of China

Hsiu-Wan Meng
Department of Periodontics, University of Texas School of Dentistry at Houston, Houston, TX, USA

Esther Yun Chien
College of Dentistry, The Ohio State University, Columbus, OH, USA

Hua-Hong Chien
Division of Periodontology, College of Dentistry, The Ohio State University, 305 West 12th Avenue, Columbus, OH 43210, USA

Wiltrud Prinzhorn, Michael Stehle, Helga Kleiner, Sabrina Ruppenthal, Martin C. Müller, Wolf-Karsten Hofmann, Alice Fabarius and Wolfgang Seifarth
Medizinische Klinik (Hämatologie und Onkologie), Wissenschaftliches Labor, Medizinische Fakultät Mannheim der Universität Heidelberg, Pettenkofer Str. 22, 68169 Mannheim, Germany

Chih-Chieh Huang, Tzung-Jiun Tsai and Ping-I Hsu
Division of Gastroenterology, Department of Internal Medicine, Kaohsiung Veterans General Hospital and National Yang-Ming University, Kaohsiung, Taiwan

Kuo-Wang Tsai
Department of Medical Education and Research, Kaohsiung Veterans General Hospital, Kaohsiung, Taiwan

Tzung-Jiun Tsai and Ping-I Hsu
Taiwan Acid-related Disease (TARD) Study Group, Kaohsiung, Taiwan

Ping-I Hsu
Division of Gastroenterology, Department of Internal Medicine, Kaoshiung Veterans General Hospital, 386 Ta Chung 1st Road, Kaohsiung 813, Taiwan, ROC

Ali Esfahani and Mohammad hossein Somi
Gastroenterology, Liver & Gastrointestinal Diseases Research Center, Tabriz University of Medical Sciences, Tabriz, Iran

Hormoz Ayromlou
Neurosciences Research Center, Tabriz University of Medical Sciences, Tabriz, Iran

Alireza Nikanfar
Hematology and Oncology Research Center, Tabriz University of Medical Sciences, Tabriz, Iran

Mohammad Asghari Jafarabadi
Tabriz Health Services Management Research Center and Department of Statistics and Epidemiology, Faculty of Health and Nutrition, Tabriz University of Medical sciences, Tabriz, Iran

Bina Eftekhar Sadat
Physical Medicine & Rehabilitation Research Center, Tabriz University of Medical Sciences, Tabriz, Iran

Zohreh Ghoreishi
Nutrition Research Center, Tabriz University of Medical Sciences, Tabriz, Iran

Su Yin Lim, Jenny H. Lee, Sarah J. Welsh, Seong Beom Ahn and Helen Rizos
Faculty of Medicine and Health Sciences, Macquarie University, Sydney, Australia

Su Yin Lim, Jenny H. Lee, Sarah J. Welsh, Matteo S. Carlino, Alexander M. Menzies, Richard F. Kefford, Richard A. Scolyer, Georgina V. Long and Helen Rizos
Melanoma Institute Australia, Sydney, Australia

Edmond Breen and Alamgir Khan
Australian Proteome Analysis Facility, Macquarie University, Sydney, Australia

Matteo S. Carlino, Alexander M. Menzies, Richard A. Scolyer and Georgina V. Long
Sydney Medical School, University of Sydney, Sydney, Australia

Matteo S. Carlino and Richard F. Kefford
Westmead Hospital, Sydney, Australia

Alexander M. Menzies and Georgina V. Long
Royal North Shore and Mater Hospitals, Sydney, Australia

Helen Rizos
Department of Biomedical Sciences, Faculty of Medicine and Health Sciences, 2 Technology Place, Macquarie University, Sydney, NSW 2109, Australia

Kiera Walker, Nathaniel H. Boyd and Anita B. Hjelmeland
Department of Cell, Developmental and Integrative Biology, University of Alabama at Birmingham, Birmingham, AL 35294, USA

Joshua C. Anderson and Christopher D. Willey
Department of Radiation Oncology, University of Alabama at Birmingham, Birmingham, AL, USA

Lu Gan, Yanan Yang and Weijian Guo
Department of Medical Oncology, Fudan University Shanghai Cancer Center, No.270, Dongan Road, Shanghai 200032, China

Lu Gan, Yanan Yang, Qian Li, Yi Feng, Tianshu Liu and Weijian Guo
Department of Oncology, Shanghai Medical college, Fudan University, No.130, Dongan Road, Shanghai 200032, China

Lu Gan, Qian Li, Yi Feng and Tianshu Liu
Department of Medical Oncology, Zhongshan Hospital, Fudan University, No.180, Fenglin Road, Shanghai 200032, China

Thomas Southworth, Sarah Mason, Alan Bell and Dave Singh
Division of Infection, Immunity & Respiratory Medicine, The Medicines Evaluation Unit, The University of Manchester, Manchester Academic Health Science Centre, Manchester University NHS Foundation Trust, Manchester, UK

Isabel Ramis, Marta Calbet, Anna Domenech, Neus Prats and Montserrat Miralpeix
Almirall R&D Center, Sant Feliu de Llobregat, Barcelona, Spain

Thomas Southworth
The University of Manchester, 2nd Floor Education and Research Center, Wythenshawe Hospital, Southmoor Road, Manchester M23 9LT, UK

Shixiang Guo, Andrew Fesler and Jingfang Ju
Stony Brook University, Stony Brook, New York 11794, USA

Shixiang Guo and Huaizhi Wang
Third Military Medical University, Chongqing 400038, People's Republic of China

Marta Lomnytska
Department of Obstetrics and Gynaecology, Academical Uppsala University Hospital, Uppsala University, SE-751 85 Uppsala, Sweden

Marta Lomnytska and Elisabeth Epstein
Institute of Women's and Children's Health, Karolinska Institute, SE-171 76 Stockholm, Sweden

Marta Lomnytska, Susanne Becker, Bo Franzén and Gert Auer
Department of Oncology and Pathology, Cancer Centre Karolinska, Karolinska Institute, SE-171 76 Stockholm, Sweden

Rui Pinto
Department of Epidemiology and Biostatistics, MRC-PHE Centre for Environment and Health, School of Public Health, Imperial College London, St. Mary's Campus, Norfolk Place, W2 1PG, London, England, UK

Ulla Engström
Ludwig Institute for Cancer Research Ltd, Uppsala, Sweden

Sonja Gustafsson and Christina Björklund
NeoProteomics AB, Cancer Centre Karolinska, SE-17176 Stockholm, Sweden

Markus Templin
NMI Natural and Medical Sciences Institute at the University of Tübingen, 72770 Reutlingen, Germany

Jan Bergstrand, Lei Xu and Jerker Widengren
Experimental Biomolecular Physics, Department of Applied Physics, Royal Institute of Technology, AlbaNova University Center, SE-106 91 Stockholm, Sweden

Elisabeth Epstein
Department of Obstetrics and Gynaecology, Department of Clinical Science and Education, Södersjukhuset, SE-118 83 Stockholm, Sweden

Amandeep Aujla, Michael Karass and Delong Liu
Department of Medicine, New York Medical College and Westchester Medical Center, Valhalla, NY, USA

Katherine Linder
Section of Hematology-Oncology, Department of Medicine, Baylor College of Medicine, Houston, TX, USA

Chaitanya Iragavarapu
Division of Blood and Marrow Transplantation, Department of Medicine, Stanford University, Stanford, CA, USA

Delong Liu
The affiliated Cancer Hospital of Zhengzhou University and Henan Cancer Hospital, 127 Dongming Road, Zhengzhou 450008, China

Michelle X. Yang, Ryan F. Coates, Abiy Ambaye, Valerie Cortright, Jeannette M. Mitchell and Alexa M. Buskey
Department of Pathology and Laboratory Medicine, University of Vermont Medical Center, 111 Colchester Avenue, Burlington, VT 05401, USA

Richard Zubarik
Gastroenterology, University of Vermont Medical Center, Burlington, VT, USA

James G. Liu
Applied Pathology Systems, Worcester, MA, USA

Steven Ades and Maura M. Barry
Medical Oncology, University of Vermont Medical Center, Burlington, VT, USA

Chiara Agnoletto, Linda Minotti, Marco Galasso, Fabio Corrà, Federica Baldassari and Stefano Volinia
Department of Morphology, Surgery and Experimental Medicine, LTTA Centre, University of Ferrara, 44121 Ferrara, Italy

Laura Brulle-Soumare, Jean-Gabriel Judde and Stefano Cairo
Xentech, Paris, France

Lorenzo Pasquali
Dermatology and Venereology Unit, Department of Medicine, Center for Molecular Medicine, Karolinska University Hospital, SE-17176 Stockholm, Sweden

Index

www.ingramcontent.com/pod-product-compliance
Lightning Source LLC
LaVergne TN
LVHW080714210926
848485LV00003B/462